Assisting With Patient Care

Assisting With Patient Care

Sheila A. Sorrentino, RN, PhD
Curriculum Consultant
Normal, Illinois

with 873 illustrations

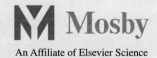

Mosby

An Affiliate of Elsevier Science

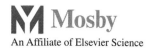
Mosby
An Affiliate of Elsevier Science

Publisher: Sally Schrefer
Senior Editor: Susan R. Epstein
Associate Developmental Editor: Maria Mercurio
Project Manager: John Rogers
Project Specialists: Kathy Teal and Betty Hazelwood
Designers: Pati Pye and David Scott
Cover Design: David Scott
Manufacturing Manager: Linda Ierardi

Printed in the United States of America

Mosby, Inc.
An Affiliate of Elsevier Science
11830 Westline Industrial Drive
St. Louis, Missouri 63146

ISBN 0-8151-2033-8

03 04 / 9 8 7 6 5 4

To my nephews, Christopher Michael and Kyle Anthony
Because I enjoy spoiling them

Aunt Sheila

REVIEWERS

Phyllis J. Nichols, RN
Patient Care Technician Instructor
Tucson, College
Tucson, Arizona

Janet Sesser, BS
Corporate Training Director
High-Tech Institute
Phoenix, Arizona

Carol S. Wells, RN, BSN, MS
Nurse Educator
St. Vincent's Medical Center
Jacksonville, Florida

Denise R. York, RNC, MS, MEd
Assistant Professor
Columbus State Community College
Columbus, Ohio

ACKNOWLEDGMENTS

Textbooks are written and published by the combined efforts of many people. The planning, manuscript development and review, and production processes involve the insights, talents, and contributions of many individuals. I am especially grateful to:

Carol Miller, Employment Specialist at OSF St. Joseph Medical Center in Bloomington, Illinois, for helping me secure job descriptions, employee handbooks, and other information.

Jane DeBlois, Education Coordinator at OSF St. Joseph Medical Center for sharing materials and information, reviewing art, and for helping me problem solve.

Becky Powell, Pam Ward, Rita Schlomer, Kathy Coyle, and Joan Stralow at OSF St. Joseph Medical Center for sharing information and providing clinical expertise.

Pat Nolan, Patient Education Coordinator at Genesis Medical Center in Davenport, Iowa, for sharing information.

Wendy Woith, formerly Director of Clinical Practice at BroMenn Regional Medical Center in Bloomington, Illinois, for sharing competency materials.

Anne Perry and Pat Potter, authors of *Clinical Nursing Skills and Techniques* (fourth edition), for sharing galleys with me. Their sections on "Delegation Considerations" were invaluable in resolving content issues.

Bernie Gorek, co-author of *Mosby's Textbook for Long-Term Care Assistants* (third edition) and Director of Nursing Services and Community Health Services at Bonell Good Samaritan Center in Greeley, Colorado, for her insights and advice.

Julie White, Director of Medical Careers at Wright College—one of the City Colleges of Chicago—for sharing her insights and expertise on content issues.

Jack Tandy of St. Louis for his artwork.

Rick Brady of Riva, Maryland, for his photography.

Phyllis J. Nichols, Janet Sesser, Carol S. Wells, and Denise R. York for reviewing the manuscript and for their candor and suggestions. They have contributed to the thoroughness and accuracy of this book.

Connie Leinicke, freelance editor in St. Louis, for helping with the manuscript review process.

The people at Mosby, especially Suzi Epstein, Maria Mercurio, Betty Hazelwood, and Kathy Teal. Suzi provided me with valuable insights, guidance, and support. Maria Mercurio handled numerous details and clerical needs. Betty Hazelwood was again amazing as a copy editor. Her attention to detail enhanced the quality of this book. Kathy Teal again produced an excellent page layout making the proofreading and production process easy and pleasant.

To all those who contributed to this effort in any way, I am sincerely grateful.

Sheila A. Sorrentino

PREFACE TO THE INSTRUCTOR

The rising cost of health care has forced hospitals and other health care agencies to restructure the delivery of nursing care and other patient care services. Of the many strategies that emerged, the return to a nursing staff mix and patient-focused care affected the traditional nursing assistant role. New titles and new job descriptions developed. Patient care technician, health care assistant, nurse extender, and patient care attendant are some titles that attempt to describe the expanding role of unlicensed assistive personnel. Job descriptions include tasks traditionally delegated to nursing assistants and complex nursing tasks and activities such as wound care, catheterizations, suctioning, and assisting with IV therapy. Phlebotomy and obtaining an ECG are examples of cross-training for purposes of moving hospital services from departments to the bedside.

Assisting With Patient Care is intended to prepare students for the roles that include traditional nursing assistant skills and the expanded role of assistive personnel. It combines the content of *Mosby's Textbook for Nursing Assistants* (fourth edition) and the recently published *Clinical Skills for Assistive Personnel*. Like *Clinical Skills for Assistive Personnel*, *Assisting With Patient Care* was created in response to the teaching and learning needs that result when assistive personnel assume tasks and activities beyond the traditional nursing assistant role. Although much controversy exists about the expanding role of assistive personnel, an ethical and legal imperative exists to provide such individuals with the necessary education and training for safe and effective functioning. Inherent in safe functioning is the need to understand the legal aspects of the role and delegation principles.

Content Issues

Unlike nursing assistant education, which has minimum standards set by the Omnibus Budget Reconciliation Act of 1987, no standardization exists for the expanded role of assistive personnel. Functions vary from hospital to hospital within the same community. Assistive personnel in the same hospital may have different titles and functions in different nursing areas. Some hospitals are more liberal than others in what assistive personnel are allowed to do. State guidelines vary. Some states issued advisory opinions based on their nurse practice acts while others enacted legislation specific to the role. Thus content issues were created.

In deciding content issues, a multitude of resources were studied. The content in this book reflects a critical analysis and synthesis of information collected from:

- State laws, guidelines, and advisory opinions
- State curricula
- Job descriptions
- The current literature
- Research studies
- Training programs developed by health care agencies, educational institutions, and associations
- Focus groups
- Personal interviews

Trends

Several trends emerged in the process of resolving content issues and were accommodated in the organization and development of the book.

- Nursing assistant education and training is often a requisite for the expanded assistive role. Therefore the book focuses on traditional nursing assistant education. Building on that foundation, knowledge and skills common to the expanded role are presented.
- Other than the umbrella title of "unlicensed assistive personnel" or "UAP," no universal title exists to describe the role under discussion. Although it serves a legal purpose, many individuals interviewed consider "unlicensed" to have negative connotations. And New Hampshire, for example, does license nursing assistants. For these reasons, using "unlicensed" was deemed undesirable. Therefore "assistive personnel" is the term used in the title and throughout the book in referring to persons who assist nurses in providing patient care.
- The need for good "work ethics" was a consistent theme among individuals participating in Mosby's market research. Thus an entire chapter (Chapter 3) focuses on behavior in the workplace.
- Effective delegation was a common theme in the literature and is a major focus of the National Council of State Boards of Nursing. RNs must make responsible delegation decisions. However, assistive personnel must decide whether or not to accept or refuse a delegated task or activity. Delegation is discussed in Chapter 2. Throughout the book the student is cautioned to perform a task or activity only if certain conditions are met.

Features and Design

Considerable attention was given to making the text readable and user friendly. By building on Mosby's *Textbook for Nursing Assistants* (fourth edition) several design elements were retained and new ones added (see Preface to the Student, p. xi).

- Key terms with definitions appear at the beginning of each chapter and are in bold print throughout the text. The definition is presented in the text.
- Chapters are organized into units. The units follow the principle that learning proceeds from the simple to the complex. The concepts, principles, and procedures integral to other activities and functions are presented first (Unit I: Assistive Personnel in Health Care, Unit II: Focusing on the Person, and Unit III: Assisting With Protection Needs [Safety, Infection Control, and Body Mechanics]). Content and skills that are easy to learn and basic to the role of assistive personnel are then presented (Unit IV: Assisting With Comfort Needs and Unit V: Assisting With Physical Needs). More complex content follows (Unit VI: Assisting With Assessment, Unit VII: Assisting With the Healing Process, and Unit VIII: Assisting With Clinical Situations). Unit titles reflect the assistive role. *(New!)*
- Icons in section headings alert the reader to an associated procedure. Procedure boxes contain the same icon. *(New!)*
- Procedure boxes are divided into pre-procedure, procedure, and post-procedure steps. Labeling and color gradients differentiate the sections.
- Procedures traditional to the role of assistive personnel are shaded in *blue.* Procedures shaded in *magenta* signal procedures not allowed in all states. This alerts students to the differences between the traditional and advanced roles of assistive personnel. *(New!)*
- Procedure alerts in special procedure boxes caution the student about performing procedures beyond the traditional role of assistive personnel. *(New!)*
- Age-specific differences are highlighted in *Focus on Children* and *Focus on Older Persons* boxes. These segments provide insight into the needs, considerations, and special circumstances of children and older persons. In addition, this feature is useful in meeting age-specific training requirements of the Joint Commission on the Accreditation of Healthcare Organizations (JCAHO). *(New!)*
- Long-term care and home care differences also are highlighted in *Focus on Long-Term Care* and *Focus on Home Care* boxes. This feature is useful for educational programs that prepare students for specific settings and for those that prepare students for a variety of settings. *(New!)*
- Review questions are found at the end of each chapter. They are followed by the page number where the answers are listed.
- Boxes are used to list principles, rules, signs and symptoms, and other information. The boxes present an efficient way for instructors to highlight content and provide useful study guides for students.
- Bullets are used for each item in a list rather than numbering.

Values

The importance of caring and treating the patient as a *person* is an important message throughout this book. The words "person" or "persons" are used whenever possible in reference to the individual to instill the value that the recipient of care is more than a "patient."

Other values and principles include:

- Safe functioning within the legal limits of the assistive role while recognizing that such limits may vary among states.
- Respect for the person and recognition that each person is a physical, social, psychological, social, and spiritual human being with basic needs.
- The importance of personal choice and dignity of person.
- The appreciation of cultural diversity and how culture influences health and illness practices.
- The need for assistive personnel to be aware of and understand their work environment and the individuals in that environment.
- That understanding body structure and function and normal growth and development are helpful for developing desirable attitudes toward individuals and for performing nursing skills safely and competently.
- That the nursing process is the basis for planning and delivering nursing care and that assistive personnel must follow the nursing care plan.

I hope that this book will serve you and your students well. My intent is to provide you and your students with the information needed to teach and learn safe and effective care during this time of dynamic change in health care.

Sheila A. Sorrentino, RN, BSN, MA, MSN, PhD

PREFACE TO THE STUDENT

This book was designed for you. It was designed to help you learn. The book is a useful resource as you gain experience and expand your knowledge.

This preface gives some study guidelines and helps you use the book. When given a reading assignment, do you read from the first page to the last page without stopping? How much do you remember? You will learn more if you use a study system. A useful study system has these steps:

- Survey or preview
- Question
- Read and record
- Recite and review

Preview

Before you start a reading assignment, preview or survey the assignment. This gives you an idea of what the assignment covers. It also helps you recall what you already know about the subject. Carefully look over the assignment. Preview the chapter title, headings, subheadings, and terms or ideas in bold print or italics. Also survey the objectives, key terms, first paragraph, boxes and the summary and review questions at the end of the chapter. Previewing only takes a few minutes. Remember, previewing helps you become familiar with the material.

Question

After previewing, you need to form questions to answer while you read. Questions should relate to what might be asked on a test or how the information applies to giving care. Use the title, headings, and subheadings to form questions. Avoid questions that have one word answers. Questions that begin with what, how, or why are helpful. While reading, you may find that a question does not help you study. If so, just change the question. Remember, questioning sets a purpose for reading. So changing a question only makes this step more useful.

Read and Record

Reading is the next step. Reading is more productive after determining what you already know and what you need to learn. Read to find answers to your questions. The purpose of reading is to:

- Gain new information
- Connect the new information to what you know already

Break the assignment into smaller parts. Then answer your questions as you read each part. Also, mark important information. The information can be marked by underlining, highlighting, or making notes. Underlining and highlighting remind you what you need to learn. You need to go back and review the marked parts later. Making notes results in more immediate learning. When making notes, you write down important information in the margins or in a notebook. Use words and summary statements that will jog your memory about the material.

After reading the assignment, you need to remember the information. To remember the material, you must work with the information. This step involves organizing information into a study guide. Study guides have many forms. Diagrams or charts help show relationships or steps in a process. Much of the information in this text is organized in this manner to help you learn. Note taking in outline format is also very useful. The following is a sample outline.

I. Main heading
   a. Second level
   b. Second level
     1. Third level
     2. Third level
II. Main heading

Recite and Review

Finally, recite and review. Use your notes and the study guides. Answer the questions you formed earlier. Also answer any other questions that came up during the reading and the review questions at the end of the chapter. Answer all questions out loud (recite).

Reviewing is more about *when* to study rather than *what* to study. You already determined what to study during the preview, question, and reading steps. The best times to review the material are right after the first study session, 1 week later, and regularly before a test, midterm, or final exam.

The editors at Mosby and I want you to enjoy learning. We also want you to enjoy your work. You and your work are important. You and the care you give may be bright spots in a person's day.

This book was also designed to help you study. Special design features are described on the next pages.

Objectives tell you what will be presented and what you need to learn.

Key terms are the important words and phrases in the chapter. Definitions are given for each term. The key terms introduce you to the chapter content. They are also useful study guides.

Bolded type is used to highlight the key terms in the text. You again see the key term and read its definition. This helps reinforce your learning.

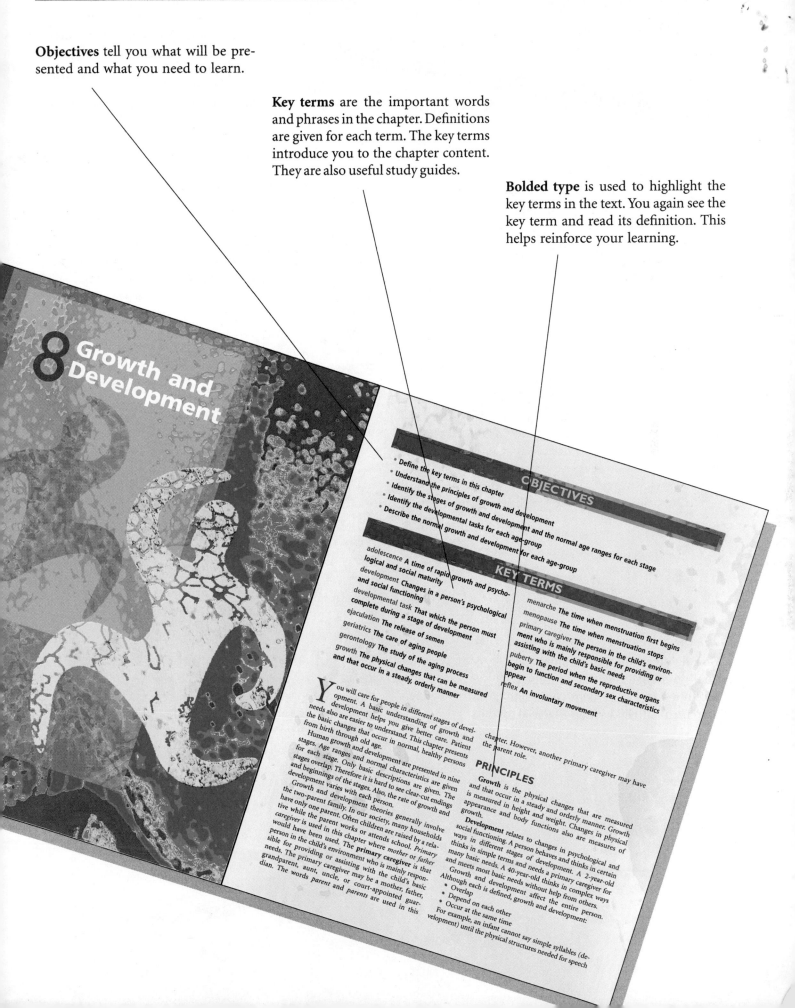

8 Growth and Development

OBJECTIVES

- Define the key terms in this chapter
- Understand the principles of growth and development
- Identify the stages of growth and development and the normal age ranges for each stage
- Identify the developmental tasks for each age-group
- Describe the normal growth and development for each age-group

KEY TERMS

adolescence A time of rapid growth and psychological and social maturity

development Changes in a person's psychological and social functioning

developmental task That which the person must complete during a stage of development

ejaculation The release of semen

geriatrics The care of aging people

gerontology The study of the aging process

growth The physical changes that can be measured and that occur in a steady, orderly manner

menarche The time when menstruation first begins

menopause The time when menstruation stops

primary caregiver The person in the child's environment who is mainly responsible for providing or assisting with the child's basic needs

puberty The period when the reproductive organs begin to function and secondary sex characteristics appear

reflex An involuntary movement

You will care for people in different stages of development. A basic understanding of growth and development helps you give better care. Patient needs also are easier to understand. This chapter presents the basic changes that occur in normal, healthy persons from birth through old age.

Human growth and development are presented in nine stages. Age ranges and normal characteristics are presented for each stage. Only basic descriptions are given. The stages overlap. Therefore it is hard to see clear-cut endings and beginnings of the stages. Also, the rate of growth and development varies with each person.

Growth and development theories generally involve the two-parent family. In our society, many households have only one parent. Often children are raised by a relative while the parent works or attends school. *Primary caregiver* is used in this chapter where *mother* or *father* would have been used. The **primary caregiver** is that person in the child's environment who is mainly responsible for providing or assisting with the child's basic needs. The primary caregiver may be a mother, father, grandparent, aunt, uncle, or court-appointed guardian. The words *parent* and *parents* are used in this

chapter. However, another primary caregiver may have the parent role.

PRINCIPLES

Growth is the physical changes that are measured and that occur in a steady and orderly manner. Growth is measured in height and weight. Changes in physical appearance and body functions also are measures of growth.

Development relates to changes in psychological and social functioning. A person behaves and thinks in certain ways in different stages of development. A person thinks in simple terms and needs a primary caregiver for many basic needs. A 40-year-old thinks in complex ways and meets most basic needs without help from others.

Growth and development affect the entire person. Although each is defined, growth and development:

- Overlap
- Depend on each other
- Occur at the same time

For example, an infant cannot say simple syllables (development) until the physical structures needed for speech

Boxes and tables contain important rules, principles, guidelines, signs and symptoms, and other information in a list format. They identify important information and are useful study guides for reviewing.

Icons in the headings alert the reader to an associated procedure. Procedure boxes contain the same icon.

Color illustrations and photographs visually present a key idea, concept, or procedure step. They help you apply and remember the written material.

238 ASSISTING WITH PROTECTION NEEDS

BOX 12-1

RULES FOR BODY MECHANICS

- Keep your body in good alignment with a wide base of support.
- Use the stronger and larger muscles in your shoulders, upper arms, thighs, and hips.
- Keep objects close to your body when you lift, move, or carry them (see Fig. 12-2). Adjust the overbed table so it is at your waist level.
- Avoid unnecessary bending and reaching. Raise the bed so it is close to your waist.
- Face your work area. This prevents unnecessary twisting.
- Push, slide, or pull heavy objects whenever you can rather than lifting them. Move your front leg forward when pushing. Move your rear leg back when pulling (Fig. 12-3).
- Widen your base of support when pushing or pulling.
- Use both hands and arms to lift, move, or carry heavy objects.
- Turn your whole body when changing the direction of your movement. Move your feet in the direction of the turn.
- Work with smooth and even movements. Avoid sudden or jerky motions.
- Get help from a co-worker if the patient cannot assist with turning or moving.
- Get help from a co-worker to move heavy objects or persons. Avoid lifting or moving patients by yourself.
- Bend your hips and knees to lift heavy objects from the floor (see Fig. 12-2). Straighten your back as the object reaches thigh level. Your leg and thigh muscles work to raise the item off the floor and to waist level.
- Do not lift objects higher than chest level. Do not lift above your shoulders. Use a step stool to reach an object higher than chest level.
- Wear a body support (Fig. 12-4) to help you use good body mechanics.

Fig. 12-3 Move your rear leg back when pulling

316 ASSISTING WITH COMFORT NEEDS

THE BACK MASSAGE

The back massage (back rub) relaxes muscles and stimulates circulation. A massage is normally given after the bath and with HS care. It should last 3 to 5 minutes. Observe the skin before starting the procedure. Look for breaks in the skin, bruises, reddened areas, and other signs of skin breakdown.

Lotion reduces friction when giving the massage. It is warmed before being applied. Warm lotion by placing the bottle in the bath water or holding it under warm water. Or rub some between your hands.

The prone position is best for a massage. The side-lying position is often used. Use firm strokes, and always keep your hands in contact with the person's skin. After the massage, apply some lotion to the elbows, knees, and heels to keep the skin soft. These bony areas are at risk for skin breakdown.

Some persons should not have back massages as described in this procedure. They are dangerous for those with certain heart diseases, back injuries, back surgeries, skin diseases, and some lung disorders. Check with the RN before giving back massages to persons with these conditions.

Fig. 14-18 The person lies in the prone position for a back massage. Stroke upward from the buttocks to the shoulders, down over the upper arms, back up the upper arms, across the shoulders, and down the back to the buttocks.

Fig. 14-19 Kneading is done by picking up tissue between the thumb and fingers.

Procedures are written in a step-by-step format. They are divided into pre-procedure, procedure, and post-procedure sections for easy studying. Procedures traditional to the role of assistive personnel are shaded in blue. Procedures shaded in magenta signal procedures not allowed in all states.

BRUSHING THE PERSON'S TEETH

PRE-PROCEDURE

1 Explain the procedure to the person.
2 Wash your hands.
3 Collect gloves and items listed in *Assisting the Person to Brush the Teeth.*
4 Place the paper towels on the overbed table. Arrange items on top of them.
5 Identify the person. Check the ID bracelet, and call the person by name.
6 Provide for privacy.
7 Raise the bed to the best level for good body mechanics.

PROCEDURE

8 Raise the head of the bed so the person can sit comfortably. Position the person in a side-lying position on the side near you if he or she cannot sit up.
9 Lower the bed rail near you. Make sure the far bed rail is up.
10 Place the towel over the person's chest. This protects the gown and linens from spills.
11 Position the overbed table so you can reach it with ease. Adjust the height as needed.
12 Put on the gloves.
13 Apply toothpaste to the toothbrush.
14 Hold the toothbrush over the kidney basin. Pour some water over the brush.
15 Brush the person's teeth gently as shown in Figure 14-1 on p. 296.
16 Let the person rinse the mouth with water. Hold the kidney basin under the person's chin (Fig. 14-2, p. 296). Repeat this step as necessary.
17 Floss the person's teeth (see *Flossing the Person's Teeth, p. 297*).
18 Let the person use mouthwash. Hold the kidney basin under the chin.
19 Remove the towel when done.
20 Remove and discard the gloves.

POST-PROCEDURE

27 Lower the overbed table to a level appropriate for the person.
28 Unscreen the person.
29 Follow agency policy for dirty linen.
   Wash your hands.
   Report your observations to the RN.

USING A PULSE OXIMETER

PROCEDURE ALERT

• Does your state allow assistive personnel to perform the procedure?
• Is the procedure in your job description?
• Do you have the necessary training and education?
• Is an RN available to answer questions and to supervise you?

PRE-PROCEDURE

1 Review the procedure with the RN.
2 Ask the RN what site to use.
3 Explain the procedure to the person.
4 Collect the following:
   • Oximeter and sensor
   • Nail polish remover
   • Cotton balls
   • SpO₂ flow sheet
   • Tape
   • Towel
5 Identify the person. Check the ID bracelet against your assignment sheet.
6 Provide for privacy.

PROCEDURE

7 Make sure the person is comfortable.
8 Remove nail polish using a cotton ball. (If a toe site is used, remove any nail polish).
9 Dry the site with a towel.
10 Clip or tape the sensor to the site. Make sure the site is dry.
11 Turn on the oximeter.
12 Check the person's pulse (apical or radial) with the pulse on the display. The pulses should be equal. Tell the RN if the pulses are not equal.
13 Read the SpO₂ on the display. Note the value on the flow sheet.
14 Leave the sensor in place for continuous monitoring. Otherwise, turn off the oximeter and remove the sensor.

POST-PROCEDURE

15 Make sure the person is comfortable.
16 Place the call bell within the person's reach.
17 Raise or lower bed rails as instructed by the RN.
18 Unscreen the person.
19 Return the pulse oximeter to its proper place if continuous monitoring is not ordered.
20 Wash your hands.
21 Report the SpO₂ and your other observations to the RN.

Procedure alerts caution the reader about performing procedures beyond the traditional role of assistive personnel.

Focus on boxes highlight special considerations for children, older persons, long-term care, and home care.

HOME CARE

Home health care assistants also must be able to work alone and have self-discipline. You work alone in the home. An RN can be reached by phone. The RN makes some home visits. However, an RN is not immediately available to you at the bedside if problems occur. You must be able to perform procedures skillfully and safely.

Self-discipline also is essential. You must arrive at homes on time. Organize activities so personal care needs and housekeeping tasks are fulfilled. Avoid temptations. This includes watching TV, talking on the telephone, visiting, and stopping for an extra cup of coffee.

Honesty is very important. You may be asked to shop. You must be honest and thrifty with the person's money. Accurately report to the person or family the items purchased, their cost with receipts, total amount spent, and amount of money returned.

Respecting the person's property also is important. Assistive personnel handle valuables and personal property in health care settings. However, access to the person's property is greater in the home. Home furnishings, appliances, linens, and household items are used for personal care and housekeeping. Treat personal and family property with respect. Prevent damage. Read the manufacturer's instructions before using any appliance. Clean the appliance after use.

LONG-TERM CARE

The Omnibus Budget Reconciliation Act of 1987 (OBRA) requires that long-term centers hire nursing assistants who have completed a state-approved training and competency evaluation program. The employer requests proof of training and also checks your record in the state nursing assistant registry.

HOME CARE

Home care agencies receiving Medicare funds must meet OBRA requirements. Assistive personnel must meet the training and competency evaluation requirements outlined in OBRA. Some states have additional training requirements for assistive personnel employed by home care agencies.

Give the employer a copy of your certificate, transcript, or grade report. Never give the original to the employer. Keep the original for future use. The employer may request that a transcript be sent directly from the school college. (See Focus on Long-Term Care and Focus Home Care.)

Job Applications

The agency asks you to complete a job applica 3-3, pp. 40-42). You get the application from nel office or human resources office. You may

complete the application in that office. Some agencies the application home and return it by mail have you are well groomed and behave or in ... ing a job application. It ple ... d impression. m ... hen com-

Safety is a basic need. In a safe environment a person has little risk of illness or injury. The person feels safe and secure physically and mentally. Risk of falling, burns, poisoning, or other injuries is low. The person and the person's property are safe from fire and intruders. The person is not afraid and has few worries and concerns.

ACCIDENT RISK FACTORS

Certain factors increase a person's risk for injury. Age, poor vision, and loss of hearing are some examples. Some people cannot protect themselves. They rely on others for safety.

- *Awareness of surroundings*—People must be aware of their surroundings to protect themselves from injury. Some persons are unconscious or in a **coma**. A person in a coma cannot react or respond to people, places, or things. Other people must protect the person. Confused and disoriented persons may not understand what is happening to and around them. They can be dangerous to themselves and others.
- *Vision*—People who have difficulty seeing are at risk for falls. They also can trip on toys, rugs, furniture, or electrical cords. They also may have problems reading labels on medicines, cleaners, and other containers. Taking the wrong medicine or the wrong dose or poisoning can result.
- *Hearing*—Hearing-impaired persons have problems hearing explanations and instructions. For example, a person does not hear well and takes the wrong medicine or takes it the wrong way. Fire alarms, sirens, weather warnings, car horns, and oncoming cars may not be heard. The person does not know to move to safety.
- *Smell and touch*—Illness and aging affect the senses of smell and touch. The person may have problems smelling smoke or gas. Persons with a reduced sense of touch are easily burned. They have problems sensing heat and cold.
- *Paralysis*—**Paraplegia** is paralysis from the waist down. **Quadriplegia** is paralysis from the neck down. Those with **hemiplegia** are paralyzed on one side of the body. Paralyzed persons may not sense pain, heat, or cold. They may be aware of danger but unable to move to safety.
- *Medications*—Medications have side effects. Loss of balance, dizziness, light-headedness, difficulty concentrating, vision changes, reduced awareness, confusion, disorientation, drowsiness, and loss of coordination are some examples. The person may be fearful or uncooperative or act in unusual ways as a result. (See Focus on Children and Focus on Older Persons.)

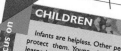

CHILDREN

Infants are helpless. Other people must protect them. Young children have not learned the difference between safety and danger. They normally explore their surroundings, put objects in their mouths, and touch and feel new things. Therefore they are at risk for falls, poisoning, choking, burns, and other accidents. Practice the safety measures listed in Box 10-1 when caring for infants and children. Also practice the safety measures to prevent falls (p. 161), burns (p. 164), poisoning (p. 164), and suffocation (p. 165).

OLDER PERSONS

The physical changes of aging increase the older person's risk for injury. Movements are slower and less steady. Balance may be affected. Decreased sensitivity to heat and cold, poor vision, hearing problems, and a decreased sense of smell are common in older persons. Confusion, poor judgment, memory problems, and disorientation may occur.

SAFETY MEASURES

Common sense and simple safety measures can prevent most accidents. You must protect patients, yourself, and co-workers from accidents and injuries. The safety measures in this section apply to everyday activities. They also apply to hospital, long-term care, and home settings. The nursing care plan lists other safety measures needed by the person.

Preventing Falls

Most falls occur in bedrooms and bathrooms. They are caused by throw rugs, poor lighting, cluttered floors, furniture that is out of place, and pets underfoot. Slippery floors, bathtubs, and showers are other causes. The need to urinate also is a major cause of falls. For example, Mrs. Ford urgently needs to urinate. She falls trying to get out of bed quickly and without help.

Review questions are a useful study guide. They help you to review what you have learned. They can also be used when studying for a test or the competency evaluation. Answers are given at the back of the book beginning on page 850.

REVIEW QUESTIONS

Circle the best answer.

1 Which is *not* a warning sign of cancer?
a Painful, swollen joints
b A sore that does not heal
c Unusual bleeding or discharge from a body opening
d Nagging cough or hoarseness

2 Martha Powers has arthritis. Care does *not* include
a Measures to prevent contractures
b Range-of-motion exercises
c A cast or traction
d Assistance with activities of daily living

3 A cast needs to dry. Which is *false*?
a The cast is covered with blankets or plastic.
b The person is turned as directed so the cast dries evenly.
c The entire length of the cast is supported with pillows.
d The cast is supported by the palms when lifted.

4 A person has a cast. Which are reported immediately?
a Pain, numbness, or inability to move the fingers or toes
b Chills, fever, or nausea and vomiting
c Odor, cyanosis, or temperature changes of the skin
d All of the above

5 A person is in traction. You should do the following *except*
a Perform range-of-motion exercises as directed
b Keep the weights off the floor
c Remove the weights if the person is uncomfortable
d Give skin care at frequent intervals

6 After a hip pinning, the operated leg is
a Abducted at all times
b Adducted at all times
c Externally rotated at all times
d Flexed at all times

7 Martha Powers has osteoporosis. She is at risk for
a Fractures
b An amputation
c Phantom limb pain
d All of the above

8 A person has had a stroke. The RN tells you to do the following. Which should you question?
a Elevate the head of the bed to a semi-Fowler's position.
b Do range-of-motion exercises every 2 hours.
c Turn, reposition, and give skin care every 2 hours.
d Keep the bed in the highest horizontal position.

9 Receptive aphasia means that the person
a Cannot talk
b Cannot write
c Has trouble understanding messages
d All of the above

10 A person has Parkinson's disease. Which is *false*?
a Parkinson's disease affects part of the brain.
b The person's mental function is affected first.
c Signs and symptoms include stiff muscles, slow movements, and a shuffling gait.
d The person is protected from injury.

11 A person has multiple sclerosis. Which is *false*?
a Nerve impulses are sent to and from the brain in a normal manner.
b Symptoms begin in young adulthood.
c There is no cure.
d The person is eventually paralyzed and totally dependent on others for care.

12 Persons with head or spinal cord injuries require
a Rehabilitation
b Speech therapy
c Long-term care
d Psychiatric care

CONTENTS

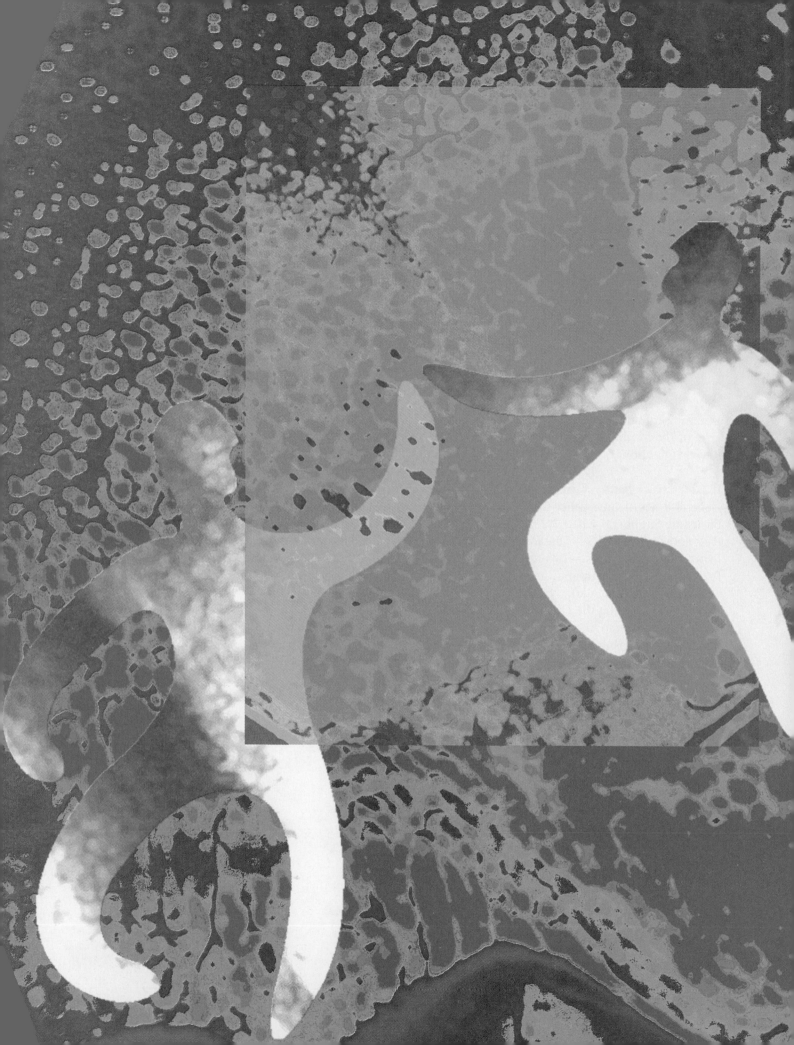

Unit I
Assistive Personnel in Health Care

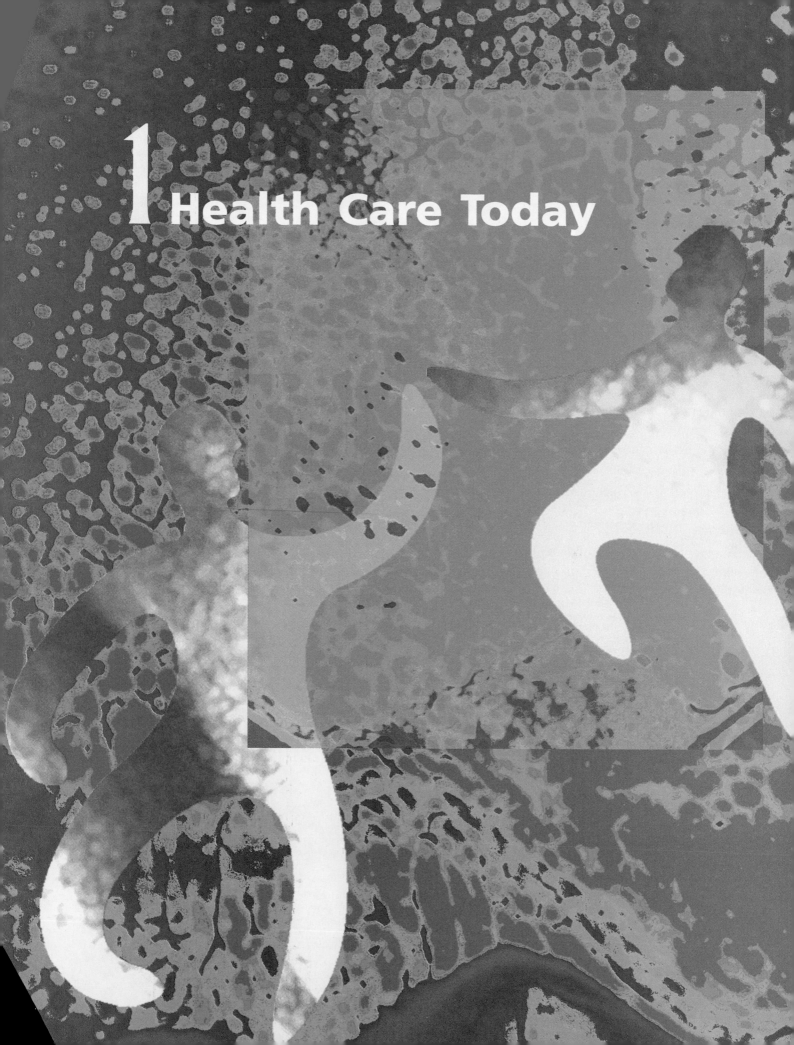

1 Health Care Today

- Define the key terms in this chapter
- Explain the purposes and services of health care agencies
- Identify the members of the health team and the nursing team
- Describe the nursing service department
- Know the differences between RNs, LPNs/LVNs, and assistive personnel
- Explain how assistive personnel are members of the nursing team
- Describe four nursing care patterns
- Describe the programs that pay for health care

acute illness A sudden illness from which a person is expected to recover

assistive personnel Individuals who give basic nursing care under the supervision of RNs; other titles include nursing assistants, nursing attendants, patient care assistants, patient care technicians, and nurse extenders

case management A nursing care pattern; a case manager (an RN) coordinates a person's care from admission through discharge and into the home setting

chronic illness An illness, slow or gradual in onset, for which there is no known cure; the illness can be controlled and complications prevented

functional nursing A nursing care pattern that focuses on tasks and jobs; nursing personnel have specific tasks to do

health team Staff members who work together to provide health care

hospice A health care agency or program for persons who are dying

licensed practical nurse (LPN) An individual who completed a 1-year nursing program and passed a licensing examination; called licensed vocational nurse (LVN) in some states

nursing team Individuals who provide nursing care—RNs, LPNs/LVNs, and assistive personnel

primary nursing A nursing care pattern; an RN is responsible for patients' total care

registered nurse (RN) An individual who studied nursing for 2, 3, or 4 years and passed a licensing examination

team nursing A nursing care pattern; the team leader (an RN) delegates the care of specific persons to RNs and LPNs/LVNs and delegates nursing tasks to assistive personnel

terminal illness An illness or injury for which there is no reasonable expectation of recovery

The many types of health care agencies include hospitals, long-term care centers, and home care agencies. Mental health hospitals, community centers, adult day care centers, hospices, doctors' offices, clinics, homes for mentally retarded persons, and centers for disabled persons are other health care agencies. There are also centers for drug and alcohol treatment and crisis centers for rape, abuse, suicide, and other mental health emergencies.

The people working in these agencies have special talents, knowledge, and skills. All work to meet the patient's needs. The patient—a person—is the focus of care.

HEALTH CARE AGENCIES

Health care agencies offer services to persons who need health care. The many services range from the simple to the complex. Some offer only one type of service.

Purpose

Health care agencies are concerned with health promotion, disease prevention, the detection and treatment of disease, and rehabilitation:

- *Health promotion* includes physical and mental health. The goal is to reduce the risk of illness. Health is promoted by teaching and counseling people about healthy living and about how to manage and cope with existing diseases.
- *Disease prevention* involves identifying the risk factors and early warning signs of disease. Measures are taken to reduce the risk factors and prevent the disease. Simple life-style changes can prevent major health problems.
- *Detection and treatment of disease* are done by diagnostic testing, physical examinations, surgery, emergency care, and medications. Treatment often involves respiratory therapy, physical therapy, and occupational therapy.
- *Rehabilitation* helps persons return to their highest possible level of physical and psychological functioning. Rehabilitation helps persons learn or relearn the skills needed to live, work, and enjoy life. Maintaining function is also an important part of rehabilitation. The person is assisted also with making needed changes to the home setting.

Many agencies provide work-based learning experiences for students. Students study to become nurses, doctors, x-ray and laboratory technicians, dietitians, or assistive personnel. These students also assist in health promotion, disease prevention, disease detection and treatment, and rehabilitation.

Types of Agencies

Assistive personnel work in many settings. Some work in doctors' offices. Most work in the following agencies.

Hospitals

Hospital services include emergency care, surgery, nursing care, x-ray procedures and treatments, and laboratory testing. Services also include respiratory therapy, physical therapy, occupational therapy, and speech therapy. People of all ages need hospital care. They go to hospitals to have babies, for treatment of mental health problems, to have surgery, for treatment of broken bones, for diagnosis and treatment of medical problems, or to die. Persons can have an acute, terminal, or chronic illness:

- **Acute illness** begins suddenly. The person is expected to recover.
- **Terminal illness** eventually results in death (see Chapter 36).
- **Chronic illness** often begins slowly and has no cure. With treatment, the illness can be controlled and complications prevented.

Some hospital stays may be very short, less than 24 hours. Others may last days, weeks, or months depending on the person's condition and illness. Outpatient services are common. The person needs hospital services but does not stay 24 hours. Some surgeries, diagnostic procedures, and therapies do not require 24-hour stays.

Subacute care agencies

Hospital stays are shorter because of changes in insurance coverage. A person may not need hospital care but may still need medical care or rehabilitation. Subacute care units are found in hospitals and long-term care centers. The number of separate agencies for subacute care is growing. Persons needing subacute care may fully recover. Others need long-term care.

Long-term care centers

Long-term care centers (nursing homes or nursing facilities) provide services to persons who cannot care for themselves at home but who do not need hospital care. These agencies provide medical, nursing, dietary, recreational, rehabilitative, and social services.

Persons in long-term care centers are called residents, not patients. They are residents because the center is their temporary or permanent home. Most residents are elderly, with chronic diseases, poor nutrition, or poor health. Long-term care centers are designed to meet the special needs of older persons.

Not all residents are old. Some residents are permanently disabled from birth defects, accidents, or diseases. People are often discharged from hospitals while they are still sick or still recovering from surgery (see Paying for Health Care, p. 11). Home care is an option for some. Others need long-term care. Some residents recover and return home; others need nursing care until death.

Mental health agencies

Mental health centers or hospitals care for and treat persons with mental illnesses. Some persons have difficulty dealing with events in life. Others are dangerous to themselves or others because of how they think and behave. Outpatient treatment is common. Some persons need hospital care for a short time or for life.

Home care agencies

Home care agencies provide care for persons in their homes. Public health departments, private businesses, and hospitals provide home care services. Services range from health teaching and supervision to bedside nursing care. Some elderly persons and persons who are dying often need home care. Besides nursing care, home care agencies may provide physical therapy, rehabilitation, and food services.

Hospices

A **hospice** is a health care agency or program for persons who are dying. The physical, emotional, social, and spiritual needs of the patient and family are provided for in a setting that allows much freedom. The patient and family are given as much control as possible over the patient's quality of life. Children and pets usually can visit at any time. Family and friends can take part in giving care. Hospice care is provided by hospitals, long-term care centers, and home care agencies.

Health care systems

A health care system involves health care agencies joining together as one provider of care. The system usually includes one or more hospitals, long-term care centers, home care agencies, hospice settings, and doctors (Fig. 1-1). Ambulance services and medical supply stores for home care are common. The system may serve a community or a large geographical area.

A health care system intends to serve all health care needs. A person entering the system is referred to other system providers as needed.

Organization

An agency has a governing body called the board of trustees. The board makes policies for the agency to ensure that the agency gives good, safe care at the lowest possible cost. An administrator manages the agency and reports directly to the board. Directors or department heads are responsible for specific areas. Figure 1-2 on p. 6 is a sample organizational chart.

The health team

The **health team** involves staff members whose skills and knowledge are directed to the person's total care (Table 1-1, pp. 8-9). Their goal is to provide quality care. Health team members work together to meet the person's needs. The person is the focus of the health care team (Fig. 1-3, p. 7).

Nursing service

Nursing service is a major department. The director of nursing (DON) is an RN. (Other titles include vice president of nursing and vice president of patient services.) Usually a bachelor's or master's degree is required for the position. The DON is responsible for the entire nursing staff. This includes the activities involved in giving safe nursing care. Nurse managers (also RNs) assist

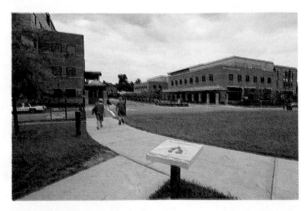

Fig. 1-1 *The hospital and doctors' offices are part of a health care system. (Courtesy Anne Arundel Health System, Inc., Annapolis, Md.)*

the director in managing and carrying out the department's functions.

Nurse managers are responsible for a work shift or nursing area. The nursing areas may be a surgical nursing unit, medical nursing unit, intensive care unit, maternity department, pediatric unit, operating and recovery rooms, an emergency department, or a mental health nursing unit. Nurse managers are responsible for all patient care and the actions of nursing staff in their areas.

Each nursing area has RNs. They provide nursing care and supervise the work of LPNs/LVNs and assistive personnel. Staff RNs report to the head nurse or nurse manager. LPNs/LVNs report to staff RNs or to the head nurses or nurse managers. You report to the RN who supervises your work.

A nursing education department is also part of nursing service. Nursing education staff plan and present educational programs to nursing personnel so that current and safe care is given. This department also educates and trains assistive personnel. New employee orientation also is a responsibility of the nursing education department.

THE NURSING TEAM

The **nursing team** involves RNs, LPNs/LVNs, and assistive personnel. Each has different roles and responsibilities. All are concerned with the physical, social, emotional, and spiritual needs of patients and families.

Registered Nurses

A **registered nurse (RN)** studies for 2 years at a community college, 2 or 3 years in a hospital-based diploma program, or 4 years at a college or university. Nursing and the biological, social, and physical sciences are studied. The graduate nurse takes a licensing examination offered

Text continued on p. 10

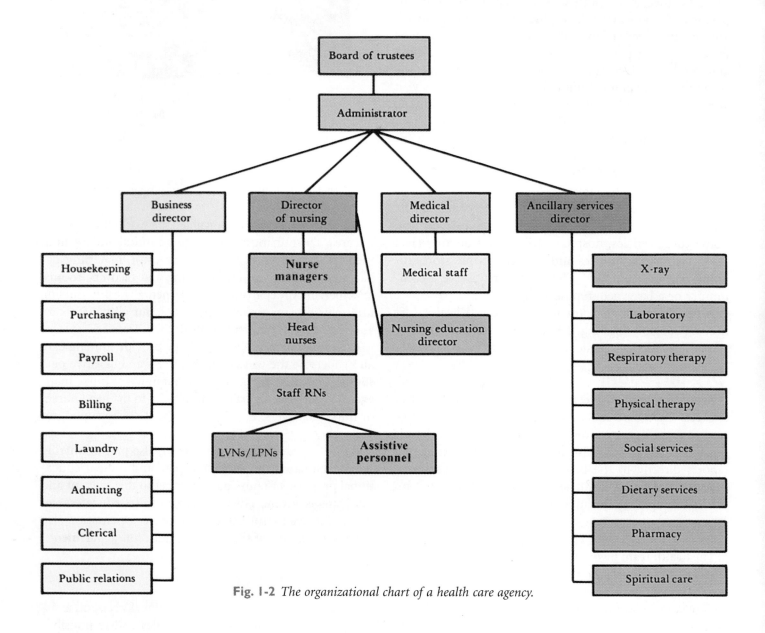

Fig. 1-2 *The organizational chart of a health care agency.*

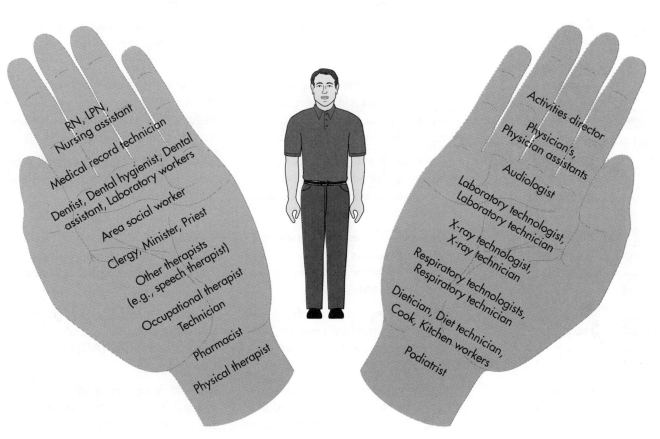

Fig. 1-3 *Members the of the health team with the person as the focus of care.*

TABLE 1-1

HEALTH TEAM MEMBERS

Title	Description	Credentials
Activities Director	Assesses, plans, and implements recreational needs	Required training varies with state and/or employer; ranges from no training to bachelor's degree
Assistive personnel	Assist RNs and LPNs in giving bedside nursing care; must be supervised by an RN	Certified nursing assistant required in some agencies; regulated training forthcoming in some states
Audiologist	Tests hearing; prescribes hearing aids; works with hearing impaired persons	Master's degree in audiology, 1 year of supervised employment, and a national examination
Cleric	Assists persons with their spiritual needs	Priest, minister, rabbi, sister (nun), deacon, or other cleric with pastoral training
Dietitian	Assesses and plans for nutritional needs; teaches individuals and families about good nutrition, food selection, and preparation	Bachelor's degree; registered dietitian (RD) must pass a national registration examination; some states require licensure
Licensed practical/ vocational nurse (LPN/LVN)	Provides direct patient care, including the administration of medications, under the direction of an RN	Graduate of a state-approved program (usually 1 year in length) and state licensure
Medical laboratory technician (MLT)	Collects samples and performs laboratory tests on blood, urine, and other body fluids, secretions, and excretions	Graduate of a 2-year program and national certifying examination; state licensure may be required
Medical records technician	Maintains medical records: transcribes medical reports, files records, completes required reports	Graduate of a 2-year program; takes the national accredited record technician (ART) examination
Medical technologist (MT)	Performs complicated laboratory tests on blood, urine, and other body fluids, secretions, and excretions; organizes, supervises, and performs diagnostic analyses; supervises MLTs	Bachelor's degree in medical technology; national certification examination; licensure required in some states
Occupational therapist (OT)	Assists persons to learn or retain skills needed to perform activities of daily living; designs adaptive equipment for activities of daily living	Bachelor's degree in occupational therapy and national certification; licensure required in some states

TABLE 1-1

HEALTH TEAM MEMBERS—cont'd

Title	Description	Credentials
Occupational therapy assistant	Performs tasks and services supervised by an OT	Graduate of an accredited program (usually 2 years in length) and national certification; licensure required in some states
Pharmacist	Fills medication orders written by a doctor; monitors and evaluates drug interactions; consults with doctors and nurses about drug actions and interactions	Bachelor's degree in pharmacy and state licensure
Physical therapist (PT)	Assists persons with musculo-skeletal problems; focuses on restoring function and preventing disability from illness or injury	Bachelor's degree in physical therapy and state licensure
Physician (doctor)	Diagnoses and treats diseases and injuries	Medical school graduation, residency, and national board examination; state licensure
Podiatrist	Prevents, diagnoses, and treats foot disorders	Doctor of podiatric medicine (DPM); state and/or national certification
Radiographer/ radiologic technologist	Takes x-rays, and processes film for viewing	Graduate of an accredited program and national registry examination
Registered nurse (RN)	Assesses, makes nursing diagnoses, plans, implements, and evaluates nursing care; supervises LPNs/ LVNs and assistive personnel	Graduate of a state-approved pro-gram with an associate degree, diploma, or bachelor's degree; state licensure
Respiratory therapist	Assists in treatment of lung and heart disorders; gives respiratory treatments and therapies	Graduate of a 1- or 2-year program and certification by National Board of Respiratory Therapy
Social worker	Helps patients and families with social, emotional, and environ-mental issues affecting illness and recovery; coordinates community agencies to assist patients and families	Bachelor's or master's degree in social work
Speech-language therapist	Evaluates speech and language and treats persons with speech, voice, hearing, communication, and swallowing disorders	Master's degree in speech/language pathology, 1 year supervised work experience, and national examination

by a state board of nursing. The nurse must pass the examination to become registered and receive a license to practice. RNs must be licensed by the state in which they practice.

RNs assess the patient, make nursing diagnoses, and plan, implement, and evaluate nursing care (see p. 62). An RN identifies a person's nursing problems and develops a care plan. The RN carries out the plan. The RN also delegates nursing care to LPNs/LVNs and assistive personnel. The RN then evaluates the effect of the care plan and nursing care on the person. The person is helped to become independent and is taught ways to stay or become healthy. Family teaching is provided.

The RN is responsible for carrying out the doctor's orders. The RN may carry out the orders or delegate them to LPNs/LVNs or assistive personnel. RNs do not diagnose diseases or illnesses or prescribe treatments or medications. However, RNs can study to become clinical nurse specialists or nurse practitioners. Special certification is required. These RNs are involved in diagnosing and prescribing.

RNs work as staff nurses, nurse managers, directors of nursing, and instructors. Their job opportunities depend on their education, professional abilities, and experience.

Licensed Practical Nurses and Licensed Vocational Nurses

A **licensed practical nurse (LPN)** completes 1 year of study in a hospital-based nursing program, community college, vocational school, or technical school. Some programs are 18 months long. Some public high schools offer 2-year programs. Students study nursing, body structure and function, basic psychology, arithmetic, and communication skills. Graduates take a licensing examination for practical nursing. After passing the test, the nurse receives a license to practice and the title of *licensed practical nurse*. The title *licensed vocational nurse (LVN)* is used in some states. As do RNs, practical or vocational nurses must have a license to practice nursing.

LPNs/LVNs work under the supervision of RNs, licensed doctors, and licensed dentists. Their responsibilities and functions are more limited than are those of RNs. LPNs/LVNs have less education in the biological, physical, and social sciences. They function with little supervision when the person's care is simple and the person's condition is stable. LPNs/LVNs assist RNs in providing care to acutely ill persons and in carrying out complex procedures.

Assistive Personnel

Assistive personnel give basic nursing care under the supervision of RNs. Box 1-1 lists the common titles for

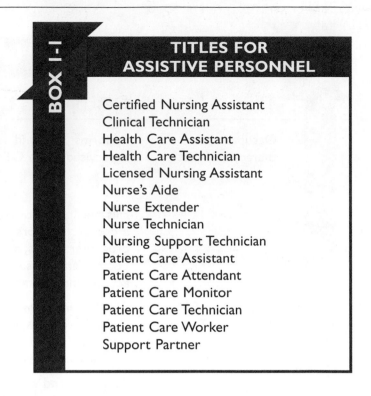

BOX 1-1

TITLES FOR ASSISTIVE PERSONNEL

Certified Nursing Assistant
Clinical Technician
Health Care Assistant
Health Care Technician
Licensed Nursing Assistant
Nurse's Aide
Nurse Extender
Nurse Technician
Nursing Support Technician
Patient Care Assistant
Patient Care Attendant
Patient Care Monitor
Patient Care Technician
Patient Care Worker
Support Partner

assistive personnel. Hospitals, long-term care centers, community colleges, technical schools, and high school vocational programs offer courses for assistive personnel. Assistive personnel are discussed in greater detail in Chapter 2.

NURSING CARE PATTERNS

Safe and effective nursing care is provided in different ways. The nursing care pattern depends on how many patients need care, the available staff, and the cost.

Functional nursing focuses on tasks and jobs. Each nursing team member has specific functions or tasks to do. For example, one RN gives all medications. Another RN changes all dressings and gives all treatments. LPNs/LVNs give baths, take vital signs, and weigh all patients. Assistive personnel make beds, serve meal trays, and feed patients.

Team nursing involves a team of nursing staff led by an RN. The RN determines the amount and kind of care needed by each person. The team leader delegates the care of specific persons to other RNs and to LPNs/LVNs. The team leader delegates nursing tasks, procedures, and activities to assistive personnel. The team leader delegates according to the patients' needs and team members' abilities. Team members report to the team leader about observations made and the care given.

Primary nursing involves total patient care. The primary nurse (an RN) is responsible for the person's total care. Other RNs, LPNs/LVNs, and assistive personnel are involved in the person's care as needed. The RN gives bedside nursing care and teaches and counsels the person and family. The RN also plans the person's discharge.

Case management is like primary nursing. A case manager (an RN) coordinates the person's care from admission through discharge and into the home setting. The case manager communicates with the person's doctor and with community agencies involved in the person's care. Some case managers work with the patients of certain doctors. Others work only with patients having certain health problems.

PAYING FOR HEALTH CARE

Health care is costly. Even after the person leaves the hospital or long-term care center, bills often continue for doctor visits, medicines, medical supplies, and home care. Most people cannot afford large medical bills. Some avoid medical care because they cannot pay. Others pay doctor bills even if it means going without food or medicine. Worry, fear, and emotional upset occur about paying for health care. If the person has health care insurance, part of or all health care costs are covered.

Health care is a major focus in today's society. The goals are to provide health care access to everyone and to reduce the high cost of care. Government leaders have proposed many changes. Efforts to reduce health care costs include managed care and prospective payment systems. More changes are likely. Before managed care and prospective payment are presented, a general discussion of insurance programs is necessary:

- *Private insurance plans* are purchased by individuals and families. Depending on the plan, the insurance company pays for some or all health care costs.
- *Group insurance plans* cover individuals belonging to a group. Many employers provide health insurance for employees under group coverage.
- *Medicaid* is a health insurance program sponsored by federal and state governments. Benefits, regulations, and eligibility requirements vary from state to state. Older, blind, and disabled people are usually eligible. So are those with low incomes. There is no insurance premium to pay.
- *Medicare* is a health insurance plan administered by the Social Security Administration of the federal government. Benefits are for older persons. Younger persons with a disability may be eligible. Medicare has two parts. Part A is for hospital costs. Part B helps pay for doctors' services, ambulance services, laboratory fees, and equipment and supplies. Part B is voluntary. That is, a person can choose to enroll in Part B and pay the required premium.

Managed Care

Managed care deals with the delivery and payment of health care. Insurance companies contract with doctors and hospitals for reduced rates or discounts. The insured person uses those doctors and agencies who provide the lower rates. If other doctors and agencies are used, the cost of care may be covered only in part or not at all. The person pays for costs not covered by insurance.

Types of managed care

Managed care limits the person's choice of where to go for health care and the services covered. It also places limits on which doctors provide the care. Health maintenance organizations (HMOs) and preferred provider organizations (PPOs) (Box 1-2) are common managed care arrangements. Managed care generally involves private and group insurance plans. However, many states require managed care for Medicaid and Medicare participants.

Managed care as preapproval for services

Many insurance companies must approve the need for health care services. If the need is approved, the insurance company pays for the services. If preapproval or precertification is not obtained, the person pays for the health care. This preapproval process and the monitoring of care is also called managed care. The purpose of managed care in this sense is to reduce unneeded medical and surgical services and procedures. The insurance company decides what to pay. With HMO or PPO contracts, the insurance company may decide where the person goes for the services.

Insurance companies have RNs who handle the preapproval process. The process varies depending on the insurance plan.

Prospective Payment Systems

Prospective payment systems limit the amounts paid by insurance companies, Medicare, and Medicaid. Prospective relates to *before* care. The amount paid for services is determined before the person enters the hospital.

Diagnosis-related groups (DRGs) help reduce Medicare and Medicaid costs. Under the DRG system, Medicare and Medicaid payments are determined before the person receives hospital care.

Each DRG has specific diagnoses. Length of stay and treatment costs are determined for each diagnosis. The hospital is paid the predetermined amount for persons covered by Medicare and Medicaid. If the hospital's treatment costs are less than the DRG amount, the hospital keeps the extra money. If costs are greater, the hospital takes the loss.

BOX 1-2

TYPES OF MANAGED CARE

Health Maintenance Organization (HMO)—provides health care services for a prepaid fee. For the fee, persons receive all needed services offered by the organization. Some need only an annual physical examination, but others require hospital care. Whatever services are used, the cost is covered by the prepaid fee. HMOs emphasize preventing disease and maintaining health. Keeping someone healthy costs far less than treating illness.

Preferred Provider Organization (PPO)—is a group of doctors and hospitals that provides health care at reduced rates. Usually the arrangement is made between the PPO and an employer or an insurance company. Employees or those insured are given reduced rates for the services used. The person can choose any doctor or hospital in the PPO.

REVIEW QUESTIONS

Circle the best *answer.*

1 Helping a person return to the best possible physical and psychological functioning is known as
   a Detection and treatment of disease
   b Promotion of health
   c Rehabilitation
   d Disease prevention

2 The governing body of a health care agency is called the
   a Director of nursing
   b Health team
   c Board of trustees
   d Nursing team

3 The nursing team includes the following *except*
   a Registered nurses
   b Doctors
   c Assistive personnel
   d LVNs/LPNs

4 Members of the nursing team perform certain functions and tasks for all persons. This is
   a Functional nursing
   b Primary nursing
   c Team nursing
   d Case management

5 These statements are about insurance programs. Which is *false?*
   a Preferred provider organizations (PPOs) provide health care at reduced rates.
   b Health maintenance organizations (HMOs) provide health care for a prepaid fee.
   c Medicare and Medicaid are government programs for anyone in need.
   d Diagnosis related groups (DRGs) affect Medicare payments.

Circle T *if the statement is true or* F *if the statement is false.*

6 T F The director of nursing is responsible for the entire nursing staff and the activities involved in providing safe nursing care.

7 T F Assistive personnel are members of both the health team and the nursing team.

8 T F An LPN/LVN functions under the supervision of an RN, licensed doctor, or licensed dentist.

9 T F An RN can diagnose health problems and prescribe the appropriate treatment.

10 T F Assistive personnel help RNs provide nursing care.

Answers to these questions are on p. 850.

2 Roles and Functions of Assistive Personnel

- Define the key terms in this chapter
- Explain the history and current trends affecting assistive personnel
- Describe nurse practice acts and how they affect assistive personnel
- Describe the Omnibus Budget Reconciliation Act of 1987
- Explain the functions, roles, responsibilities, and role limits of assistive personnel
- Explain why a job description is important
- Describe the educational requirements for assistive personnel
- Describe the delegation process and the "five rights of delegation"
- Explain how you will use the "five rights of delegation"
- Explain your responsibilities when accepting or not accepting a delegated task
- Explain how to prevent negligent acts
- Give examples of false imprisonment, defamation, assault, battery, and fraud
- Describe how to protect the right to privacy
- Explain the purpose of informed consent
- Describe child, elderly, and domestic abuse

KEY TERMS

accountable Being responsible for one's actions and the actions of others who perform delegated tasks; answering questions about and explaining one's actions and the actions of others

assault Intentionally attempting or threatening to touch a person's body without the person's consent

battery Unauthorized touching of a person's body without the person's consent

civil law Laws concerned with relationships between people; private law

crime An act that violates a criminal law

criminal law Laws concerned with offenses against the public and society in general; public law

defamation Injuring a person's name and reputation by making false statements to a third person

delegate Authorizing another person to perform a task

ethics Knowledge of what is right conduct and wrong conduct

false imprisonment Unlawful restraint or restriction of a person's movement

fraud Saying or doing something to trick, fool, or deceive another person

invasion of privacy Violating a person's right not to have his or her name, photograph, or private affairs exposed or made public without giving consent

law A rule of conduct made by a government body

libel Defamation through written statements

malpractice Negligence by a professional person

negligence An unintentional wrong in which a person fails to act in a reasonable and careful manner and causes harm to a person or to the person's property

preceptor A staff member who guides and teaches

responsibility The duty or obligation to perform some act or function

slander Defamation through oral statements

task A function, procedure, activity, or work that does not require an RN's professional knowledge or judgment

tort A wrong committed against a person or the person's property

Federal and state laws and agency policies combine to define the roles and functions of each health team member. All health care personnel must protect patients from harm. To protect patients from harm, you must understand your roles and responsibilities. You need to know what you can and cannot do, what is right conduct and wrong conduct, and your legal limits. Supervised by RNs, you perform selected nursing tasks. Laws, job descriptions, and the patient's condition influence how you function. So does the amount of supervision you need.

Protecting patients from harm also involves a complex set of rules and standards of conduct. These rules and standards form the legal and ethical aspects of care.

HISTORY AND CURRENT TRENDS

Nursing practice has a long history involving assistive personnel. For decades they assisted nurses in giving patient care. Commonly called nurse's aides or nursing assistants, assistive personnel gave basic bedside nursing care. Bathing and feeding patients were common tasks. So were making beds, repositioning patients, and assisting with elimination. Their work was similar in hospitals and nursing homes throughout the United States. Until the 1980s, no training or experience was required. RNs gave on-the-job training. Some hospitals, nursing homes, and schools offered nursing assistant courses.

Before the 1980s, team nursing was a common nursing care pattern. Team members included RNs, LPNs/LVNs, and nursing assistants. An RN was the team leader. The RN made team member assignments according to each patient's needs and condition. The education and experiences of each staff member also influenced assignments. Team members communicated with the team leader about patient care and observations.

Primary nursing became popular in the 1980s. RNs planned and gave patient care. With this nursing care pattern, hospitals eliminated many LPN/LVN and nursing assistant positions. Often only RNs were hired to give patient care.

Meanwhile, nursing homes relied on nursing assistants for resident care. To improve the quality of life of nursing home residents, the U.S. Congress passed the Omnibus Budget Reconciliation Act of 1987 (OBRA). This law sets minimum training and competency evaluation requirements for nursing assistants who work in nursing homes. This law requires each state to set rules for nursing assistant training and evaluation. A state's requirements must be met before a person can work as a nursing assistant in a nursing home in that state.

Home care also increased during the 1980s. Prospective payment systems greatly affected this trend. Prospective payment systems limit how much insurance companies, Medicare, and Medicaid pay for health care (see p. 11). To reduce care costs, hospitals limit how long patients stay in the hospital. Therefore patients are discharged earlier than in the past. These persons are often still quite ill. Home care is often required.

The rising costs of health care became a major political issue in the early 1990s. The goal was to control and reduce these costs and to provide all persons with access to health care. Insurance companies, Medicare, and Medicaid further reduced payments for treating specific illnesses. Meanwhile, health care costs continued to increase.

Efforts to reduce health care costs included:

- *Hospital closings*—Many hospitals closed for financial reasons. The amount of money coming into the hospital was not enough to meet expenses.
- *Hospital mergers*—Hospitals merged to share resources and to avoid offering the same costly services. For example, instead of two hospitals offering cardiac surgery services, only one does. The other hospital may offer maternity and pediatric services.
- *Health care systems*—Health care agencies join together as one provider of care. For example, a hospital patient needs long-term care. The system's ambulance service is used to transfer the person from the hospital to the system-owned nursing home. When the person is ready for discharge from the nursing home, home care is arranged with the system's home care agency. The person's care is kept within the system. This maximizes the system's resources.
- *Managed care*—Many insurance companies have contracts with doctors, hospitals, and health care systems (see Chapter 1). The contracts provide for reduced rates or discounts. The insured person uses those doctors and agencies offering the lower rates. If others are used, the care is covered only in part or not at all. The patient pays for costs not covered by insurance.
- *Return to a nursing staff mix*—Instead of hiring only RNs, hospitals began hiring assistive personnel. Today more and more hospitals are hiring assistive personnel. Some hospitals train assistive personnel. Others require completion of a state-approved nursing assistant training and competency evaluation program. Additional training is given for those nursing tasks that are not included in the training program but that are part of the person's job description.
- *Patient-focused care and cross-training*—This moves hospital services from departments to the bedside. Staff members are cross-trained to perform basic

skills provided by other health team members. Nurses and assistive personnel are often cross-trained to collect blood specimens (phlebotomy) and take electrocardiograms (ECGs, EKGs). For example, a doctor orders a blood test for Ms. Tyler. The nurse tells the unit secretary, who then calls the laboratory. The laboratory secretary tells a medical laboratory technician. The technician sends a staff member to Ms. Tyler's room to draw the blood sample. Five people are involved so far. With patient-focused care and cross-training, Ms. Tyler's blood is drawn by a nurse or assistive person when the order is given. Ms. Tyler does not wait for laboratory staff to be notified and arrive. She is served faster and with fewer staff members. Staff members are used in efficient and productive ways. The number of people caring for each patient also is reduced, which also reduces care costs.

STATE AND FEDERAL LAWS

The tasks performed by assistive personnel vary from state to state and among agencies. Variation often occurs within agencies. For example, assistive personnel in the emergency room may perform tasks different from those performed by assistive personnel on a surgical nursing unit. The tasks may differ for assistive personnel working in the hospital's home care department.

Unlike long-term care, the work of assistive personnel in hospitals is currently not well defined. Concerns about assistive personnel training and job descriptions are prompting states to study the issue. Many states are regulating the training and practice of assistive personnel working in hospitals. State nurse practice acts and OBRA provide some direction.

Nurse Practice Acts

Each state has a nurse practice act. Intended to protect the public's welfare and safety, the law regulates nursing practice in that state. Definitions are given for RNs and LPNs/LVNs. Their scope of practice and education and licensing requirements are described. The law protects the public from persons practicing nursing without a license. That is, it prevents persons who do not meet the state's education and licensing requirements from performing nursing functions.

Under the law, a nurse's license may be revoked or suspended. The reasons for such action include:
- Being convicted of a crime in any state
- Selling or distributing drugs
- Using the patient's drugs for oneself
- Placing patients in danger from the excessive use of alcohol or drugs

- Demonstrating grossly negligent nursing practice
- Being convicted of abusing or neglecting children or elderly persons
- Violating the act and its rules and regulations
- Demonstrating incompetent behaviors
- Aiding or assisting another person to violate the act and its rules and regulations
- Making medical diagnoses or prescribing medicines and treatments

A state's nurse practice act is used to determine the nursing tasks that assistive personnel can perform. Legal and advisory opinions about assistive personnel are based on the act. So are any state laws that regulate assistive personnel. If you perform a task beyond the legal limits of your role, you could be practicing nursing without a license. This creates serious legal problems for you and the RN supervising your work.

The Omnibus Budget Reconciliation Act of 1987

In 1987 the U.S. Congress passed the Omnibus Budget Reconciliation Act (OBRA). This law applies to all 50 states. The law addresses training for nursing assistants working in long-term care. It requires each state to have a nursing assistant training and competency evaluation program. Assistive personnel working in nursing centers and hospital long-term care units must meet federal and state training and competency requirements.

State requirements vary. However, OBRA requires at least 75 hours of instruction. Sixteen of those hours involves supervised practical training. Such training occurs in a laboratory or clinical setting. The student actually performs nursing care and procedures on another person. An RN supervises this practical training (clinical practicum or clinical experience).

The training program includes the knowledge and skills needed by nursing assistants to give basic nursing care. Areas of study include:
- Communication
- Infection control
- Safety and emergency procedures
- Residents' rights
- Basic nursing skills
- Personal care skills
- Feeding techniques
- Elimination procedures
- Skin care
- Transferring, positioning, and turning techniques
- Dressing
- Ambulating residents
- Range-of-motion exercises

The competency evaluation program includes a written test and a skills test. The number of test questions on the *written test* varies from state to state. The *skills* evaluation involves demonstrating nursing skills learned in the training program.

OBRA requires that each state have a nursing assistant registry. The registry is an official record or listing of persons who have successfully completed a state-approved nursing assistant training and competency evaluation program. Information about a nursing assistant abusing or neglecting a resident is part of the registry information. So are findings about the dishonest use of property. Registry information is available to any agency needing the information. Before a nursing assistant is hired in long-term care, the employer is required to check the registry.

Current knowledge and skills are important. Employers are required to provide regular inservice education and performance reviews. If a nursing assistant has not worked for 2 years (24 months), OBRA requires retraining and a new competency evaluation program. (See Focus on Home Care.)

---

focus on

HOME CARE

Many states have training and competency requirements for home health care assistants (home health aides). If a home care agency receives Medicare funds, assistive personnel must meet OBRA's training and competency evaluation requirements.

BOX 2-1

RULES FOR ASSISTIVE PERSONNEL

- You are an assistant to the nurse.
- An RN determines and supervises your work.
- You do not decide what should or should not be done for a person.
- Clarify directions or instructions with the RN before going to the person.
- Perform no function or task that you have not been prepared to do or that you do not feel comfortable performing without an RN's supervision.
- Perform only those functions and tasks that are allowed by your state and that are in your job description.

ROLES AND RESPONSIBILITIES

Nurse practice acts, OBRA, state laws, and legal and advisory opinions give direction to what assistive personnel can do. To protect patients from harm, you must understand what you can do, what you cannot do, and the legal limits of your role. In some states this is called scope of practice.

Assistive personnel function under the supervision of RNs. You assist RNs and LPNs/LVNs in giving care. You also perform nursing procedures and tasks involved in the person's care. Often you function without an RN in the room. At other times you help nurses give bedside nursing care. In some agencies you assist doctors with diagnostic procedures. The rules listed in Box 2-1 will help you understand your role.

Assistive personnel functions and responsibilities vary among states and agencies. The procedures in this textbook are performed by assistive personnel. Some are more complex and advanced than others. *(Procedures in this book are shaded in two colors. Cyan is used for procedures that are commonly performed by assistive personnel. Magenta signals procedures not allowed in all states.)* Before you perform a procedure make sure that:

- Your state allows assistive personnel to perform the procedure
- The procedure is in your job description
- You have the necessary training and education
- An RN is available to answer questions and to supervise you

Generally, you assist RNs in meeting the hygiene, safety, nutrition, exercise, elimination, and oxygen needs of patients. Related functions include lifting and moving patients, observing them, and helping promote physical comfort. You also assist with patient admissions and discharges and measure temperatures, pulses, respirations, and blood pressures. Assistive personnel often perform sterile procedures such as urinary catheterizations, dressing changes, and collection of blood specimens. Obtaining electrocardiograms is a common task for assistive personnel (Fig. 2-1). (See Focus on Home Care on p. 19.)

Box 2-2 describes the limits of your role. These are the procedures and tasks that assistive personnel never perform. As stated previously, you must understand what you *cannot* do.

You must remember that state laws and legal and advisory opinions differ. Therefore you must know what assistive personnel can do in the state in which you are working. For example, if you live in Utah and move to New Hampshire, you must become familiar with the laws and rules in New Hampshire. Sometimes assistive personnel work in two states. For example, you work part-time at a hospital in Illinois and part-time at a hospital in Iowa. What you are allowed to do in Illinois may be different from what you do in Iowa. You must know the laws and rules of each state.

Some assistive personnel are also emergency medical technicians (EMTs). EMTs are trained to give emergency care outside of health care settings. These settings are called "in the field." EMTs work under the direction of doctors who are in hospital emergency rooms. Each state has laws and rules that apply to EMTs. These laws and rules are different from those for assistive personnel. What

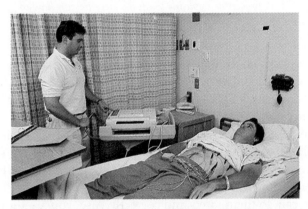

Fig. 2-1 *Assistive personnel often obtain electrocardiograms.*

focus on HOME CARE

Home health care assistants provide personal care and home services. Home services depend on the needs of the person and family. They may include:

- Doing light housekeeping so rooms are clean and neat.
- Doing laundry. Clothing and linens are washed, ironed, and mended as needed. Family laundry may be done also.
- Shopping for groceries and household items as needed and directed.
- Preparing and serving nutritious meals. This includes planning menus, following special diets, and feeding the person if necessary.
- Home health care assistants do not do heavy housekeeping. This includes moving heavy furniture, waxing floors, shampooing carpets, washing windows, cleaning rugs or drapes, and carrying firewood, coal, or ash containers.

BOX 2-2 ROLE LIMITS FOR ASSISTIVE PERSONNEL

- **Never give medications.** This includes medications given orally, rectally, by injection, by application to the skin, or directly into the bloodstream through an intravenous line. Licensed nurses are responsible for giving medications. This responsibility cannot be delegated to assistive personnel. However, some states allow assistive personnel to give medications under certain conditions. One condition is completing a state-required education and training program. Other conditions include having the function in your job description and having the necessary supervision.
- **Never insert tubes or objects into body openings or remove them from the body unless allowed by your state and job description.** For example, some states allow assistive personnel to insert catheters (tubes) into the urinary bladder. Other states do not.
- **Never take oral or telephone orders from doctors.** Politely give your name and title, ask the doctor to wait, and promptly find a nurse to speak with the doctor.
- **Never tell the patient or family the person's diagnosis or medical or surgical treatment plans.** The doctor is responsible for informing the person and family about the diagnosis and treatment. Nurses may further clarify what the doctor said.
- **Never diagnose or prescribe treatments or medications for anyone.** Only doctors can diagnose and prescribe.
- **Never supervise other assistive personnel.** RNs are legally responsible for supervising the work of assistive personnel. You will not be trained or paid to supervise the work of others. Supervising other assistive personnel can have serious legal consequences.
- **Never ignore an order or request to do something that you cannot do or that is beyond your legal limits.** Promptly explain to the nurse why you cannot carry out the order or request. The nurse assumes you are doing what you were told to do unless you explain otherwise. Patient care cannot be neglected.

EMTs do "in the field" is very different from the work of assistive personnel. For example, Joan Woods is an EMT for a fire department. When off duty, she works as a patient care assistant at St. John's Hospital. Her state allows EMTs to start intravenous infusions (IVs) in the field. However, assistive personnel do not start IVs. Despite knowing how to start an IV, Joan cannot start IVs when working at the hospital as a patient care assistant.

The situation is similar for persons who served as medics or corpsmen in military service. Medics or corpsmen may suture wounds. Assistive personnel cannot do so. When employed as assistive personnel, medics and corpsmen must follow the laws and rules that apply to assistive personnel in that state. As with EMTs, the ability to perform a task does not give a person the right to perform that task in all settings.

The functions of assistive personnel are limited by state laws and rules. Job descriptions for assistive personnel reflect those laws and rules.

Job Description

The job description lists the responsibilities and functions the agency expects you to perform (Box 2-3, pp. 21-23). Always request a written job description when you apply for a job. Ask questions about the job description during your job interview. Before accepting a job, tell the employer about any functions you do not know how to do. Also advise the employer of functions you are opposed to doing for moral or religious reasons. Have a clear understanding of what is expected of you before taking a job. Do not take a job that requires you to:

- Act beyond the legal limits of your role
- Function beyond your educational limits
- Perform acts that are against your moral or religious principles

No one can force you to perform a function, task, or procedure that is beyond the legal limits of assistive personnel. Jobs may be threatened for refusing to follow an RN's orders. Often staff obey out of fear. That is why you must understand the roles and responsibilities of assistive personnel. You also need to know the functions you can safely perform, the things you should never do, and your job description. Understanding the ethical and legal aspects of your role is equally important (see pp. 26-31).

Educational Requirements

Each agency has its own educational requirements for assistive personnel. These requirements are based on state laws or recommendations that limit what assistive per-

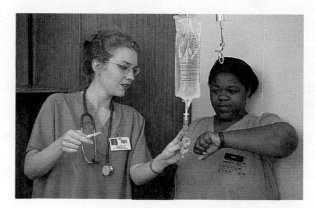

Fig. 2-2 *A preceptor explains to an assistive person how to prime IV tubing.*

sonnel can do. In the future it is likely that states will have laws that regulate the training and practice of assistive personnel. Such laws are for your own and the patient's protection.

When employed, you will complete the agency's orientation program. Agency policies and procedures are explained and your skills checked. That is, the agency has you perform nursing procedures and tasks to make sure you can do them safely and correctly. Also, you are shown how to use the agency's supplies and equipment.

Some agencies have clinical **preceptor** programs. A preceptor is a staff member who guides and teaches. In a clinical preceptor program, staff RNs teach and train assistive personnel in the clinical area (Fig. 2-2). For example, you complete a training program for assistive personnel. You are assigned to an RN preceptor who works with you and supervises your work for a period of time. The RN helps you adjust to your role, shows you how to use the agency's equipment and supplies, answers your questions, and makes sure that you give safe care. Depending on the agency, the preceptor program can last from 6 weeks to 3 months. It is designed to help you succeed in your new role and to ensure quality and safe patient care.

DELEGATION

Nurse practice acts give RNs and LPNs/LVNs certain responsibilities and the authority to perform nursing tasks. A **responsibility** is the duty or obligation to perform some act or function. For example, RNs are responsible for supervising LPNs/LVNs and assistive personnel. Only RNs can carry out this responsibility.

In nursing, a **task** is a function, procedure, activity, or work that does not require an RN's professional knowledge or judgment. **Delegate** means authorizing another person to perform a task. The person must be competent to perform the task in a given situation. For example, you

BOX 2-3

JOB DESCRIPTION FOR ASSISTIVE PERSONNEL

OSF Saint Francis Medical Center
Peoria, Illinois

Job Description

Job Title: **Patient Care Technician**
Department: **Various Services**
Division: **Patient Services**

General Summary:

Reporting to the Patient Care Manager and according to department standards, functions as a member of the Patient Care Team to provide appropriate basic care to patients based on the ages of the patients served on the unit. This includes taking vital signs, assisting patients with activities of daily living, blood draws, dressing changes, Foley catheterizations, EKGs, and observing patients for physical/emotional changes. Records pertinent information in patient charts and communicates with other patient care team members to ensure continuity of care. The following are general characteristics of this job, although duties may vary by assigned shift.

Corporate Philosophy:

It is the obligation of each employee of OSF Saint Francis Medical Center to abide by and promote the Corporate Philosophy, Values, Mission, and Vision of The Sisters of the Third Order of St. Francis.

Principal Duties and Responsibilities:

(The following duties and responsibilities are all essential job functions, as defined by the ADA, except for those that begin with the word "May.")

1. Takes and records patients' vital signs including temperature, pulse, BP, weight, respiration as prescribed by nursing protocol or physician order.
2. Assists patients with activities of daily living including personal hygiene and grooming, bathing, eating, back rubs, etc. Provides patients with bedpans or urinals, empties and cleans, or assists patients to commode or bathroom.
3. Performs various technical nursing procedures according to protocol, including: maintaining oxygen equipment, performing oral and nasopharyngeal suctioning, routine incisional care, performing urinary bladder catheterization, giving tube feedings, changing sterile dressings, providing skin care, sitz baths, enemas, applying and changing nonsterile dressings and pads, applying warm and cold compresses, ointments, etc. Records activities in patient records.
4. Monitors, measures, and records patients' intake and output according to established nursing protocol and physician orders.
5. Observes patients (physical appearance, attitude) and communicates any changes or pertinent information related to the patient's health to appropriate team members.
6. Assists patients with ambulating or exercising. Ensures patient safety by following established safety standards. Repositions patients in chairs and beds.
7. Delivers patient meals and nourishments. In doing so, feeds or assists patients that require assistance in feeding and documents portion of meal completed. Collects meal trays at end of meal and assists with menu marking as needed, including appropriate substitutions and initiates snacks according to patient needs.

Modified from OSF Saint Francis Medical Center, Peoria, Illinois.

Continued

BOX 2-3

JOB DESCRIPTION FOR ASSISTIVE PERSONNEL—cont'd

Principal Duties and Responsibilities—cont'd:

8. Collects patient specimens (e.g., urine, stool, sputum, blood), labels, and sends to laboratory for analysis, and communicates to appropriate team member.

9. Completes EKGs per physician orders. In doing so, attaches electrode leads to various parts of the patients arms and chest. Conducts the EKG and records the heart rhythms. Monitors patients during test to ensure patients are relaxed and remain still in effort to reduce artifacts. Monitors rhythms for abnormal patterns and notifies appropriate patient care team members of critical heart irregularities. Keys information into EKG machine to note position of electrodes and/or manually marks rhythm strips.

10. Obtains blood specimens from patients per physician's order. Applies tourniquet to arm, locates accessible vein, swabs puncture site with antiseptic, and inserts needle into vein to draw blood into collection tube. May prick finger to draw blood, depending on type of specimen test required/requested.

11. As a member of the patient care team, provides support to other patient care team members by assisting in patient care and clerical functions including, but not limited to:
    - Responding to patients' call lights. In doing so, identifies patient needs and provides patient with appropriate response or communicates needs to appropriate team member
    - Passing water, assisting patients when dressing, etc.
    - Providing patients with blankets, pillows, and additional linen when needed
    - Collecting trash, red bagging as needed
    - Assisting in transporting patients to various departments as needed
    - Providing directions to patients/visitors

12. Transfers patients from beds onto gurneys or into wheelchairs (with assistance of other patient care team members when required). Ensures patients' safety by following proper lifting and patient transferring techniques.

13. Keeps patient rooms neat, clean, and orderly. Changes patients' bed linens on a regularly scheduled basis or as needed. Cleans unit's ancillary rooms upon request.

14. Ensures patient and supply rooms are properly stocked with necessities including clean linen, ice water, etc.

15. Attends mandatory department of Medical Center meetings, inservices, and appropriate work-related educational programs.

16. Develops and maintains a positive working relationship with team members, department and Medical Center personnel, and patients/visitors.

17. Supports and is involved in the Medical Center's continuous quality improvement efforts designed to increase patient outcomes, increase patient satisfaction, and improve the utilization of the Medical Center's human, capital, and physical resources.

Knowledge, Skills, and Abilities Required:

1. The job incumbent is required to demonstrate the knowledge and skills necessary to provide patient care appropriate to the age of the patients served on the unit. This requires that the incumbent demonstrate knowledge of the principles of growth and development as well as the physical, emotional and psycho-social needs of the patient population served.

2. Work requires ability to read, write, and communicate effectively at a level generally acquired through completion of a high school education. Must be 17 years old to be considered for position.

BOX 2-3

JOB DESCRIPTION FOR ASSISTIVE PERSONNEL—cont'd

Knowledge, Skills, and Abilities Required—cont'd:

3. Work requires 3 to 4 months of unit-specific orientation and on-the-job training to become familiar with work routines and location of equipment and supplies and to develop proficiencies in patient care tech duties.
4. Work requires the interpersonal skills necessary to comfort patients, family members, and/or significant others; and to communicate effectively with other patient care providers.
5. Work requires analytical ability necessary to prioritize work load.

Physical Requirements:

(The following statements describe the physical abilities required to perform the essential job functions, although exceptions may be made to these requirements based on the principle of reasonable accommodation.)

1. Work requires the ability to lift objects weighing up to 60 pounds on a daily basis.
2. Work requires ability to carry objects weighing up to 20 pounds on a daily basis.
3. Work requires ability to stand for 3 or more hours at a time.
4. Work requires ability to stoop and bend, ability to reach and grab with arms and hands, manual dexterity, ability to communicate with others, and color vision.
5. Work requires ability to push and/or pull wheelchairs, gurneys, beds, or supply carts on a hourly basis.
6. Work requires ability to lift and position patients on a hourly basis.

Reporting Relationships:

1. Reports to the Patient Care Manager.
2. Functions as a member of a self-directed work team. In doing so, provides support to patient care team members by assisting in patient care duties and clerical functions as needed.

Working Conditions:

1. Works on a patient care unit where there is exposure to infectious disease, although potential for personal harm or bodily injury is limited when employee follows all safety procedures and uses appropriate safety equipment.
2. Work requires the performance of various unpleasant patient care tasks on a daily basis.

The above is intended to describe the general content of and requirements for the performance of this job. It is not to be construed as an exhaustive statement of duties, responsibilities, or requirements.

know how to give a complete bed bath. However, Mr. Jones has multiple injuries from an auto accident. He has neck injuries and is at risk for paralysis. His left leg is fractured in three places, and he has a full leg cast. His right lung was punctured, and he has chest tubes. He has two IVs, a retention catheter, a nasogastric tube, and a tracheostomy. In this situation, giving a bed bath to Mr. Jones is complicated. The RN gives the bath and asks you to assist.

Who Can Delegate

Nurse practice acts allow RNs to delegate tasks to LPNs/LVNs and assistive personnel. Some states allow LPNs/LVNs to delegate tasks to assistive personnel. RNs and LPNs/LVNs can delegate tasks only within their scope of practice.

When making delegation decisions, nurses must protect the patient's health and safety. The delegating nurse remains accountable for the delegated task. To be

focus on LONG-TERM CARE

Some states allow LPNs/LVNs to have supervisory roles in long-term care settings. The LPN/LVN delegates tasks to assistive personnel. The LPN/LVN follows the delegation process and the "five rights of delegation."

accountable means to be responsible for one's actions and the actions of others who perform delegated tasks. It also involves answering questions about and explaining one's actions and the actions of others.

The delegating nurse must make sure that the task was completed safely and correctly. If the RN delegates, the RN is responsible for the delegated task. If the LPN/LVN delegates, the LPN/LVN is responsible for the delegated task. Remember, the RN is also responsible for supervising the practice of LPNs/LVNs. Therefore the RN also is accountable for the tasks that LPNs/LVNs delegate to assistive personnel. The RN is accountable for all patient care.

Assistive personnel cannot delegate. You cannot delegate any task to other assistive personnel. You can ask another assistive person to help you. However, you cannot ask or tell another person to do your work. (See Focus on Long-Term Care.)

Delegation Process

Delegated tasks must be within the legal limits of what assistive personnel can do. Before delegating tasks to you, the RN must know:

- What tasks your state allows assistive personnel to perform
- The tasks included in your job description
- What you were taught in your training program
- What skills you learned and how they were evaluated
- About your work experiences

The RN uses this information to make delegation decisions. The RN is likely to discuss this information with you. This is so the RN can get to know you, your abilities, and your concerns. Whenever you work with a new RN, you should meet to discuss your training and work experience. You may be a new employee or new to the nursing unit. Or the RN may be someone new. In any case, it is wise for the RN to get to know you and for you to get to the know the RN.

Agency policies, guidelines, and the job description for assistive personnel state what tasks RNs can delegate to you. These documents must be consistent with state laws, rules, and legal opinions about the roles and functions of assistive personnel. However, even if a task is in your job description, an RN does not have to delegate it to you. The RN must consider the circumstances when delegating.

The RN makes delegation decisions after considering the questions in Box 2-4. The patient's needs, the task, and the person performing the task must fit. The RN can decide to delegate the task to you. Or the RN can decide not to delegate the task. If the patient's needs and the task require the knowledge, judgment, and skill of an RN, the RN completes the task. You may be asked to assist.

You must not be offended or get angry if you are not allowed to perform a task that is part of your job description and that is usually delegated to you. The RN makes a decision that is best for the patient at the time. That decision is also best for you at that time. You do not want to perform a task that requires an RN's judgment and critical thinking skills. For example, you cared for Mrs. Mills while she was in the hospital. You gave personal care, assisted with ambulation, and gave wound care. After discharge, she stayed with her son. A week later she was admitted to the hospital again. She has a hip fracture and bruises on her face and arms. She reported falling down the stairs. The RN suspects abuse. Instead of asking you to bathe Mrs. Mills, the RN does so. The RN wants to assess Mrs. Mills for other signs of abuse and to talk with her. Although you are able to give Mrs. Mills a bath, at this time she needs the RN's knowledge and judgment.

The person's circumstances are central factors in making delegation decisions. Delegation decisions should always result in the best care for the patient. An RN places a patient's health and safety at risk with poor delegation decisions. Also, the RN may face serious legal problems. If you perform a task that places the patient at risk, you also can face serious legal problems.

The five rights of delegation

The National Council of State Boards of Nursing's five rights of delegation summarize the delegation process:

- *The right task*—Can the task be delegated? Does the state's nurse practice act allow the RN or LPN/LVN to delegate the task? Is the task in the job description for assistive personnel?
- *The right circumstances*—What are the patient's physical, mental, emotional, and spiritual needs at this time?
- *The right person*—Do you have the training and experience to safely perform the task for this patient?

BOX 2-4

FACTORS AFFECTING DELEGATION DECISIONS

- What is the patient's condition? Is it stable or likely to change?
- What are the patient's basic needs at this time?
- What is the patient's mental function at this time?
- What are the patient's emotional and spiritual needs at this time?
- Can the patient assist with his or her care? Does the patient depend on others for care?
- Is the task something the nurse can delegate?
- For this patient, does the task require the knowledge, judgment, and skill of an RN or LPN/LVN?
- How often will the RN have to assess the patient?
- Can the task harm the patient? If yes, how?
- What effect will the task have on the patient?
- Is it safe for the patient if the task is delegated to you?
- Do you have the training and experience to perform the task, given the patient's current status? Is your training documented? How were your training and skills evaluated?
- How often have you performed the task?
- What other tasks were delegated to you?
- Do you have the time to perform the task safely?
- Is an RN available to supervise you?
- How much supervision will you need?
- Will you need more directions as you perform the task?
- Is an RN available to help or take over if the patient's condition changes or problems arise?

- *The right directions and communication*—The RN must give clear directions. The RN tells you what to do, when to do it, what observations to make, and when to report back. The RN allows questions and helps you set priorities.
- *The right supervision*—The RN guides, directs, and evaluates the care you give. The RN demonstrates tasks as necessary and is available to answer questions. The less experience you have performing a task, the more supervision you need. Complex tasks require greater supervision than basic tasks. Also, the patient's circumstances affect how much supervision you need. The RN assesses how the task affected the patient and how well you performed the task. To help you learn and give better care, the RN tells you what you did well and what you can do to improve your work.

Your Role in Delegation

You must remember that you perform delegated tasks for or on a *person*. You must perform the task safely to protect the person from harm.

You have two choices when an RN delegates a task to you. You either *agree* or *refuse* to do the task. You should use the "five rights of delegation" to make your choice. Before accepting a delegated task, you need to answer the questions in Box 2-5 on p. 26.

Accepting a task

When you agree to perform a task, you are responsible for your own actions. Remember, what you do or fail to do can bring harm to the patient. *You must complete the task safely.* You must ask for help when you are unsure or have questions about a task. You must communicate with the RN by reporting what you did and your observations.

Refusing a task

You have the right to say "no." Sometimes refusing to follow the RN's directions is your right and duty. You should refuse to perform a task when:
- The task is beyond the legal limits of your role.
- The task is not in your job description.
- You were not prepared to perform the task safely.
- The task could harm the patient.
- The patient's condition has changed.
- You do not know how to use the supplies or equipment.
- The RN's directions are unethical, illegal, or against agency policies.
- The RN's directions are unclear or incomplete.
- An RN is not available for supervision.

Protect patients and yourself by using common sense. Ask yourself if what you are doing is safe for the person.

THE FIVE RIGHTS OF DELEGATION FOR ASSISTIVE PERSONNEL

The Right Task
- Does your state allow assistive personnel to perform the task?
- Were you trained to do the task?
- Do you have experience peforming the task?
- Is the task in your job description?

The Right Circumstances
- Do you have experience performing the task given the patient's condition and needs?
- Do you understand the purpose of the task for the patient?
- Can you perform the task safely under the current circumstances?
- Do you have the equipment and supplies to safely complete the task?
- Do you know how to use the equipment and supplies?

The Right Person
- Are you comfortable performing the task?
- Do you have concerns about performing the task?

The Right Directions and Communication
- Did the RN give clear directions and instructions?
- Did you review the task with the RN?
- Do you understand what the RN expects?

The Right Supervision
- Is an RN available to answer questions?
- Is an RN available if the patient's conditions changes or if problems occur?

(Modified from the National Council of State Boards of Nursing, Inc.)

As explained in Box 2-2, you must never ignore an order or request to do something. You must communicate your concerns to the RN. If the task is within the legal limits of your role and in your job description, the RN can help you feel more comfortable with the tasks. The RN can answer your questions, demonstrate the task, and show you how to use supplies and equipment. The RN can help you as needed, observe you performing the task, and check on you often. The RN also can arrange for needed training.

With good communication, you and the RN should be able to work out the problem. If not, try talking to the RN's supervisor. When work problems continue, talk to someone whom you trust and can confide in. For example, your instructor or another professional can help you sort out work problems.

You must not refuse a delegated task simply because you do not like or want to do the task. You must have sound reasons for your refusal. Otherwise, you could place the patient at risk for harm. You also risk losing your job.

ETHICAL ASPECTS

Ethics is concerned with what is right conduct and wrong conduct. It involves morals and making choices or judgments about what should or should not be done. An ethical person behaves and acts in the right way and does not bring harm to the person.

Ethical behavior also involves not being *prejudiced* or *biased*. A person who is prejudiced or biased makes judgments and has opinions before knowing the facts. Judgments and opinions usually are based on a person's own values and standards. Such values are derived from the person's culture, religion, education, and life experiences. The patient's situation may be very different from your own. For example:
- Children decide that their elderly mother needs nursing home care after leaving the hospital. In your culture, children take care of elderly parents at home.
- A patient has multiple tattoos and body piercings. You do not believe in tattooing or body piercing.

BOX 2-6

RULES OF CONDUCT FOR ASSISTIVE PERSONNEL

- Respect each person as an individual.
- Perform no act that is not within the legal limits of your role.
- Perform no act for which you have not been adequately prepared.
- Take no drug without the prescription and supervision of a doctor.
- Carry out the directions and instructions of the nurse to your best possible ability.
- Complete each task safely.
- Be loyal to your employer and co-workers.
- Act as a responsible citizen at all times.
- Recognize the limits of your role and knowledge.
- Keep patient information confidential.
- Consider the patient's needs to be more important than your own.

- An 80-year-old man has a living will that says he should not be resuscitated. You believe that everything possible should be done to save life.

You must not judge the person by your own values or standards. You must not avoid persons whose standards and values are different from your own.

Ethical dilemmas involve making choices. You must decide what is the right thing to do. For example:

- A co-worker was late for work 3 days this week. You find her in an empty room drinking from a thermos. You also smell alcohol on her breath. She asks you not to tell anyone.
- An older patient has bruises all over her body. She told the RN that they are from a fall. Later she tells you that her son is very mean to her. She asks you not to tell anyone.

Professional groups have codes of ethics. The code involves rules, or standards of conduct, for group members to follow. The American Nurses Association (ANA) has a code of ethics for RNs. The National Federation of Licensed Practical Nurses (NFLPN) has one for LPNs/LVNs. No formal code of ethics exists for assistive personnel. However, the rules of conduct in Box 2-6 can guide your thinking and behavior. See Chapter 3 for ethical behavior in the workplace.

LEGAL ASPECTS

Whereas ethics is concerned with what you *should or should not do,* laws tell you what you *can and cannot do.* A law is a rule of conduct made by a government body such as the U.S. Congress or a state legislature. Laws protect the public welfare and are enforced by the government.

Criminal laws are concerned with offenses against the public and against society in general. A violation of a criminal law is called a **crime.** A person found guilty of a crime is fined or sent to prison. Murder, robbery, rape, and kidnapping are examples of crimes.

Civil laws deal with the relationships between people. Examples of civil laws are those that involve contracts and nursing practice. A person found guilty of breaking a civil law usually has to pay a sum of money to the injured person.

Torts

Tort comes from a French word meaning *wrong.* Torts are part of civil law. A tort is committed by an individual against another person or the person's property. Torts may be intentional or unintentional.

Unintentional torts

Negligence is an unintentional wrong. The person did not mean or intend to cause harm. The negligent person failed to act in a reasonable and careful manner and thereby caused harm to the person or property of another. The person at fault failed to do what a reasonable and careful person would have done. Or the individual did what a reasonable and careful person would not have done. The negligent individual may have to pay damages (a sum of money) to the injured person.

Malpractice is negligence by professionals. A person has professional status because of training, education, and the service provided. Nurses, doctors, dentists, lawyers, and pharmacists are examples of professional people.

You are legally responsible *(liable)* for your own actions. What you do or do not do can lead to a lawsuit if harm results to the person or property of another. An RN may

BOX 2-7

PROTECTING THE PATIENT'S RIGHT TO PRIVACY

- Keep all patient information confidential.
- Make sure the patient is covered when being moved in corridors.
- Screen the patient as in Figure 2-3, and close the door when giving care. Also close drapes and window shades.
- Expose only the body part involved in a treatment or procedure.
- Do not discuss the patient or the patient's treatment with anyone except the nurse supervising your work. "Shop talk" is a common cause of invasion of privacy.
- Ask visitors to leave the room when care is given.
- Do not open the patient's mail.
- Allow the patient to visit with others and to use the telephone in private.

direct you to do something beyond the legal limits of your role. Or you may be asked to do something beyond your education. Giving medications is an example. You may be told not to worry, that the RN will be responsible if anything happens. The RN is liable as your supervisor. However, you are not relieved of personal liability. *You are responsible for your own actions.* Remember, sometimes refusing to follow the RN's directions is your right and duty (see p. 25).

Intentional torts

Intentional torts are acts meant to be harmful. Defamation (libel and slander), assault and battery, false imprisonment, invasion of privacy, and fraud are intentional torts.

Defamation is injuring the name and reputation of a person by making false statements to a third person. **Libel** is making false statements in print, writing, or through pictures or drawings. **Slander** is making false statements orally. Protect yourself from defamation by never making false statements about a patient, a co-worker, or any other person. Examples of defamation include:

- Implying or suggesting that a person has a sexually transmitted disease
- Saying that a person is insane or mentally ill
- Implying or suggesting that a person is corrupt or dishonest

Assault and battery may result in both civil and criminal charges. **Assault** is intentionally attempting or threatening to touch a person's body without the person's consent. The person fears bodily harm. Threatening to "tie down" an uncooperative patient is an example of assault. **Battery** is the actual touching of a person's body without the person's consent. Consent is the important factor in assault and battery. The person must consent to any pro-

cedure, treatment, or other act that involves touching the body. The person has the right to withdraw consent at any time.

Consent is more than a person's verbal okay or signature on a form. For consent to be valid, it must be *informed consent* (see p. 29). Protect yourself from assault and battery by explaining to the person what is to be done and getting the person's consent. Consent may be verbal ("yes" or "okay") or a gesture (a nod, turning over for a back rub, or holding out an arm for a blood pressure measurement).

False imprisonment is the unlawful restraint or restriction of a person's freedom of movement. Threat of restraint or actual physical restraint is false imprisonment. Preventing a person from leaving the agency also is false imprisonment.

Every person has the right not to have his or her name, photograph, or private affairs exposed or made public without having given consent. Violating this right is an **invasion of privacy.** You must treat patients with respect and ensure their privacy. Only staff involved in the person's care should see, handle, or examine the person's body. The precautions listed in Box 2-7 help ensure the right to privacy.

Fraud is saying or doing something to trick, fool, or deceive another person. The act is fraud if it does or could cause harm to a person or the person's property. Telling a patient or family that you are an RN is fraud. So is giving incomplete or inaccurate information on a job application.

Informed Consent

Informed consent recognizes a person's right to decide what will be done to his or her body and who can touch his or her body. Consent is informed when the person clearly understands the reason for a treatment, what will

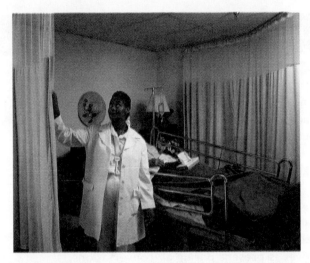

Fig. 2-3 *Pulling the curtain around the bed helps protect the person's privacy.*

be done, how it will be done, who will do it, and the expected outcomes. The person also must understand other treatment options and the effects of not having the treatment. The doctor is responsible for informing the person about all aspects of treatment.

Often consent is needed for persons under legal age (usually 18 years of age). A parent or legal guardian gives consent. Mentally incompetent persons also cannot give legal consent. Persons who are unconscious, sedated, or confused are not mentally competent to give legal consent. Persons with certain mental health disorders also are incompetent to give consent. Consent is given by a responsible party—a husband, wife, son, daughter, or a legal representative. As with consent given by the patient, consent by a responsible party must be informed consent.

Consent is given when the person enters the agency. A form is signed giving general consent to treatment. Special consent forms are required for surgery and other complex and invasive procedures. The doctor is responsible for informing the person about all aspects of the surgery or procedure. The RN may be given this responsibility. *You are never responsible for obtaining written consent.* However, you can be a witness to the signing of a consent. When you are a witness, you must be present when the person signs the consent.

REPORTING ABUSE

Abuse is more evident in today's society. Abuse has one or more of the following elements:
- Willful causing of injury
- Unreasonable confinement
- Intimidation (to make afraid with threats of force or violence)

- Punishment
- Deprivation of goods or services needed for physical, mental, or psychosocial well-being

With abuse, one or more of these elements result in physical harm, pain, or mental anguish. Protection against abuse extends to persons in a coma. With child and elderly abuse, the abuser is usually a family member or a caregiver. All states require the reporting of child abuse and elderly abuse. In domestic abuse (domestic violence), the abuser is a partner. The victim is responsible for reporting the abuse and filing criminal charges.

Elderly Abuse

There are different forms of elderly abuse:
- *Physical abuse* involves hitting, slapping, kicking, pinching, and beating. It also includes corporal punishment—punishment inflicted directly on the body, such as beatings, lashings, or whippings. Neglect is also physical abuse. It involves depriving the person of needed medical services or treatment. Neglect is also failure to provide food, clothing, hygiene, and other basic needs. In health care, neglect includes but is not limited to leaving persons lying or sitting in urine or feces, isolating persons in their rooms or other locations, and failing to answer call bells.
- *Verbal abuse* is the use of oral or written words or statements that speak badly of, sneer at, criticize, or condemn the person. Verbal abuse includes unkind gestures.
- *Involuntary seclusion* is confining the person to a specific area. Older people have been locked in closets, basements, attics, and other spaces.
- *Financial abuse* is when the elderly person's money is used by another person.
- *Mental abuse* includes humiliation, harassment, and threats of being punished or deprived of needs such as food, clothing, care, a home, or a place to sleep.
- *Sexual abuse* is when the person is harassed about sex or is attacked sexually. The person may be forced to perform sexual acts out of fear of punishment or physical harm.

There are many signs of elderly abuse. The abused person may show only some of the signs listed in Box 2-8 on p. 30.

Federal and state laws require the reporting of elderly abuse. If abuse is suspected, it must be reported. Where and how to report suspected abuse vary in each state. You may suspect that a person is being abused. If so, discuss the situation and your observations with the RN. Give as much information as possible. The RN then contacts the appropriate members of the health team. Community agencies that investigate elderly abuse also are contacted. They act

BOX 2-8

SIGNS OF ELDERLY ABUSE

- Living conditions are unsafe, unclean, or inadequate.
- Personal hygiene is lacking. The patient is unclean, and clothes are dirty.
- Weight loss—there are signs of poor nutrition and inadequate fluid intake.
- Frequent injuries—circumstances behind the injuries are strange or seem impossible.
- Old bruises and new bruises are seen.
- The patient seems very quiet or withdrawn.
- The patient seems fearful, anxious, or agitated.
- The patient does not seem to want to talk or answer questions.
- The patient is restrained or locked in a certain area for long periods. Toilet facilities, food and water, and other necessary items cannot be reached.
- Private conversations are not allowed. The caregiver is present during all conversations.
- The patient seems anxious to please the caregiver.
- Medications are not taken properly. Medications are not purchased, or too much or too little medication is taken.
- Visits to the emergency room may be frequent.
- The patient may go from one doctor to another. Some people do not have a doctor.

immediately if there is a life-threatening situation. Sometimes the help of police or the courts is necessary.

Helping abused elderly persons is not always easy or possible. The abuse may never be reported or recognized, or the investigating agency may be unable to gain access to the person. Sometimes elderly persons are abused by their children. A victim may want to protect the child. Some victims are embarrassed or believe the abuse is deserved. A victim may be afraid of what will happen. He or she may think that the present situation is better than no care at all. Some people fear not being believed if they report the abuse themselves.

Child Abuse

Child abuse occurs at every social level. It occurs in low-, middle-, and high-income families. The abuser may have little education or be highly educated. The abuser is usually a household member (parent, a parent's partner, brother or sister, nanny) or someone known to the family. Risk factors for child abuse include the following:

- Stress
- Family crisis (divorce, unemployment, relocation, poverty, crowded living conditions)
- Drug or alcohol abuse
- Abuser history of being abused as a child
- Discipline beliefs that include physical punishment
- Lack of emotional attachment to the child
- A child with birth defects or chronic illness
- A child with a personality or behaviors that the abuser considers "different" or unacceptable

- Unrealistic expectations for the child's behavior or performance
- Families that move frequently and do not have family or friends nearby

Types of child abuse

Abuse differs from neglect. *Physical neglect* involves depriving the child of food, clothing, shelter, and medical care. *Emotional neglect* involves not meeting the child's need for affection and attention.

Physical abuse is intentionally injuring the child. Death can occur from physical abuse. *Sexual abuse* is using, persuading, or forcing a child to engage in sexual conduct. It may take several forms:

- Rape—forced sexual intercourse without the person's consent.
- Molestation—sexual advances toward a child. Molesting includes kissing, touching, or fondling sexual areas. The abuser may kiss, touch, or fondle the child. Or the child is forced to kiss, touch, or fondle the abuser.
- Incest—sexual activity between family members. The abuser may be a parent, stepparent, brother or sister, stepbrother or stepsister, aunt or uncle, cousin, or grandparent.
- Child pornography—photographing or videotaping a child involved in sexual acts.
- Child prostitution—forcing a child to engage in sexual activity for money. Usually the child is forced to have many sexual partners.

BOX 2-9

SIGNS AND SYMPTOMS OF CHILD ABUSE

Physical Abuse
- Bruises on the face (lips, mouth, cheeks), back, buttocks, abdomen, chest, and inner thighs
- Welts on the face (lips, mouth, cheeks), back, buttocks, abdomen, chest, and inner thighs
  - The shape of the object causing the welt may be evident. The shape may be of a belt, belt buckle, wooden spoon, chain, clothes hanger, rope, or other object.
- Burns and scalds on the feet, hands, back, or buttocks
  - Intentional burns leave a pattern from the item causing the burn: cigarettes, irons, curling irons, ropes, stove burners, and radiators.
  - In scalds, the area immersed in the hot liquid is clearly marked. For example, with a scald to the hand, the hand looks like a glove. A scald to a foot looks like a sock.
- Fractures of the nose, skull, arms, or legs
- Bite marks

Sexual Abuse
- Bleeding, cuts, and bruises of the genitalia, anus, or mouth
- Stains or blood on underclothing
- Painful urination
- Vaginal discharge
- Genital odor
- Difficulty walking or sitting
- Pregnancy

Box 2-9 lists the signs of physical and sexual abuse in children. Behaviors of the child and parents may arouse suspicion that something is wrong. The child may be quiet and withdrawn and fear adults. Sometimes children are afraid to go home. Sudden behavior changes are common in sexual abuse. Bed-wetting, thumb-sucking, loss of appetite, poor grades, and running away from home are some examples.

Parents give different stories about what happened. Injuries are blamed on play accidents or other children. Frequent emergency room visits are common.

Child abuse is a complex syndrome. Many more behaviors, signs, and symptoms are present than discussed here. Health care professionals must be alert for signs and symptoms of child abuse. State laws require that suspected child abuse be reported. However, it is important not to falsely accuse someone. If you suspect child abuse, share your concerns with the RN. As with elderly abuse, give as much information as you can. The RN will contact appropriate members of the health team and child protection agencies.

Domestic Abuse

Domestic abuse occurs in relationships. One partner has power and control over the other. Such power and control occurs through abuse. Fear and harm occur. Types of abuse include physical, sexual, verbal, economic, or social abuse. Usually more than one type of abuse is present in the relationship:

- *Physical abuse* is unwanted punching, slapping, biting, pulling hair, or kicking. Other forms of violence include burns and the use of weapons. Physical injuries occur. Death is a constant threat.
- *Sexual abuse* is unwanted sexual contact.
- *Verbal abuse* involves unkind and hurtful remarks. The remarks leave the person feeling unwhole, unattractive, and with little value.
- *Economic abuse* involves controlling money. Having or not having a job, paychecks, money gifts from family and friends, and money for household expenses (food, clothing) are controlled by the abuser.
- *Social abuse* is controlling friendships and other relationships. The abuser controls phone calls, use of the car, leaving the home, and visits with family and friends.

Like child and elderly abuse, domestic abuse is complex. The victim often hides the abuse and protects the abusive partner. However, unlike child and elderly abuse, state laws do not require that health professionals report suspected domestic abuse. However, health professionals have an ethical responsibility to provide emotional support and to give information about safety and community resources. If you suspect that a person is a victim of domestic abuse, share your concerns with the RN. The RN will gather additional information as necessary to help the person.

Circle T *if the statement is true or* F *if the statement is false.*

1 T F A health care worker is guilty of negligence. The person can be sent to prison.

2 T F Assistive personnel are always responsible for their own actions.

3 T F Laws are ethical standards of what is right conduct and wrong conduct.

4 T F You are responsible for obtaining the person's informed consent in writing.

5 T F State laws require the reporting of child, elderly, and domestic abuse.

6 T F A child is deprived of food and clothing. This is physical abuse.

7 T F Domestic abuse always involves violence.

Circle the best *answer.*

8 Which health care trend moves patient services from departments to the bedside?
   a Managed care
   b Health care systems
   c Staffing mix
   d Patient-focused care

9 Nursing practice is regulated by
   a The Omnibus Budget Reconciliation Act of 1987
   b Medicare and Medicaid
   c Nurse practice acts
   d All of the above

10 What state law affects what assistive personnel can do?
   a The state's nurse practice act
   b The Omnibus Budget Reconciliation Act of 1987
   c Medicare
   d Medicaid

11 You perform a nursing task not allowed by your state. Which is *true?*
   a If an RN delegated the task, there is no legal problem.
   b You could be found guilty of practicing nursing without a license.
   c Performing the task is allowed if it is in your job description.
   d If you complete the task safely, there is no legal problem.

12 An RN asks you to give medications. Which is *true?*
   a Assistive personnel never give medications.
   b The RN must supervise your work.
   c OBRA allows you to give medications.
   d You must know how the medications affect the patient.

13 These statements are about delegation. Which is *false?*
   a RNs can delegate their responsibilities to you.
   b A delegated task must be safe for the patient.
   c The delegated task must be in your job description.
   d The delegating nurse is responsible for the safe completion of the task.

14 A task is in your job description. Which is *false?*
   a The RN must always delegate the task to you.
   b The RN delegates the task to you if the patient's circumstances are right.
   c The RN must make sure you have the necessary education and training.
   d You must have clear directions before you perform the task.

15 An RN delegates a task to you. You must
   a Complete the task
   b Decide if you can accept the task or if you must say "no"
   c Delegate the task to another assistive person if you are too busy to complete the task
   d Ignore the request if you do not know how to perform the task

16 You are responsible for

a Completing tasks safely
b Delegation
c The "five rights of delegation"
d Delegating tasks to assistive personnel

17 You can refuse to perform a task for the following reasons *except*

a The task is beyond the legal limits of your role
b The task is not in your job description
c You do not like the task
d An RN is not available to supervise you

18 You decide to refuse to perform a task. Your first action is to

a Delegate the task to another assistive person
b Communicate your concerns to the RN
c Ignore the request
d Talk to the RN's supervisor

19 The doctor orders several laboratory tests for a patient. The patient wants to know why. Who is responsible for telling the patient?

a The doctor
b You are
c The RN
d Any health team member

20 Which is *not* a crime?

a Negligence
b Murder
c Robbery
d Rape

21 These statements are about negligence. Which is *true*?

a It is an unintentional tort.
b The negligent person did not act in a reasonable manner.
c Harm was caused to a person or a person's property.
d All of the above.

22 The intentional attempt or threat to touch a person's body without the person's consent is

a Assault   c Defamation
b Battery   d False imprisonment

23 The illegal restraint of another person's movement is

a Assault
b Battery
c Defamation
d False imprisonment

24 Mr. Blue's photograph is made public without his consent. This is

a Battery
b Fraud
c Invasion of privacy
d Malpractice

25 Which will *not* protect the person's right to privacy?

a Getting the person's consent for treatment
b Screening the person when giving care
c Exposing only the body part involved in the treatment or procedure
d Asking visitors to leave the room when care is given

26 A patient asks if you are a nurse. You answer "yes." This is

a Negligence
b Fraud
c Libel
d Slander

27 Which is *not* a sign of elderly abuse?

a Stiff joints and joint pain
b Old bruises and new bruises
c Poor personal hygiene
d Frequent injuries

28 You suspect a patient has been abused. What should you do?

a Tell the family.
b Call a state agency.
c Tell an RN.
d Ask the patient if he or she has been abused.

Answers to these questions are on p. 850.

3 Work Ethics

- Define the key terms in this chapter
- Identify good health and personal hygiene practices
- Describe the practices for professional appearance
- Describe the qualities and characteristics of successful assistive personnel
- Explain what you should do to get a job
- Prepare for work by planning for childcare and transportation
- Describe ethical behavior on the job
- Explain what is meant by harassment and sexual harassment
- Explain how to resign from a job
- Identify the common reasons for losing a job

confidentiality Trusting others with personal and private information

courtesy A polite, considerate, or helpful comment or act

gossip Spreading rumors or talking about the private matters of others

harassment Troubling, tormenting, offending, or worrying a person by one's behavior or comments

work ethics Behavior in the workplace

As explained in Chapter 2, ethics deals with right conduct and wrong conduct. It involves making choices and judgments about what or what not to do. An ethical person does the right thing. In the workplace, certain behaviors (conduct), choices, and judgments are expected. Therefore **work ethics** deals with behavior in the workplace. Your conduct reflects your choices and judgments. Your appearance, what you say, how you behave, and how you treat and work with others are all part of work ethics. To get and keep a job, you must conduct yourself in the right way.

PERSONAL HEALTH, HYGIENE, AND APPEARANCE

The health team sets an example for others. Patients and families expect the team to look and act healthy. A patient has reason to question health team members who smoke, especially when the patient is told to stop smoking. If you look unclean or unhealthy, the patient and family wonder if you can give good care. You are a member of the health team. Therefore your personal health, appearance, and hygiene deserve careful attention.

Your Health

Patients and employers trust you. They believe you will give careful and effective care. To fulfill this trust you must be physically and mentally healthy. Otherwise you cannot function at your best.

- *Diet*—Good nutrition involves eating a balanced diet from the Food Guide Pyramid (see Chapter 19). Start your day with a good breakfast. To maintain your weight, the number of calories taken in must equal your energy needs. To lose weight, caloric intake must be less than energy needs. Avoid foods from the fats, oils, and sweets groups, salty foods, and crash diets.
- *Sleep and rest*—Adequate sleep and rest are needed to stay healthy and to do your job well. Most adults need about 7 hours of sleep daily. Fatigue, lack of energy, and irritability mean you need more rest and sleep.
- *Body mechanics*—You will bend, carry heavy objects, and lift, move, and turn patients. These activities place stress and strain on your body. You need to use your muscles effectively (see Chapter 12).

- *Exercise*—Exercise is needed for muscle tone, circulation, and weight control. Walking, running, swimming, and biking are good forms of exercise. You will feel better physically and mentally with regular exercise. Consult your doctor before starting a vigorous exercise program.
- *Your eyes*—Good vision is needed in your work. You will read instructions and measure blood pressures and temperatures. These involve fine measurements. Inaccurate readings can place patients in danger. Have your eyes examined, and wear glasses or contact lenses as prescribed. Make sure you have enough light when reading or doing fine work.
- *Smoking*—Smoking causes lung cancer, lung diseases, and many heart and circulatory disorders. Cigarette smoke can offend others. Smoke odors stay on a person's breath, hands, clothing, and hair. Therefore handwashing and good personal hygiene are essential.
- *Drugs*—Some drugs affect thinking, feeling, behavior, and functioning. They affect a person's ability to work effectively. A person who works under the influence of drugs places patients in danger. Take only those drugs that are prescribed by a doctor and only in the way prescribed.
- *Alcohol*—Alcohol is a drug that depresses the brain. It affects thinking, balance, coordination, and mental alertness. Never report to work under the influence of alcohol or drink alcohol while working. Otherwise you risk patient, co-worker, and your own safety.

Your Hygiene

You must pay careful attention to your personal cleanliness. Prevent offensive body odors by bathing daily and using a deodorant or antiperspirant. Brush your teeth after meals, and use a mouthwash regularly to prevent breath odors. Shampoo often, and style your hair in an attractive and simple way. Keep fingernails clean, short, and neatly shaped.

Special hygiene measures are needed during menstrual periods. Change tampons or sanitary napkins often, especially if flow is heavy. Wash your genital area with soap and water at least twice a day. Handwashing is necessary after going to the bathroom, changing tampons or sanitary napkins, and washing the genital area.

Your Appearance

Good health and personal hygiene practices help you look and feel well. Box 3-1 describes practices and suggestions to help you look neat, clean, and professional (Fig. 3-1).

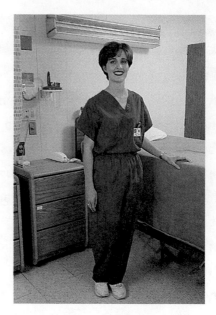

Fig. 3-1 *The assistive person is well groomed. Her uniform and shoes are clean. Her hair has a simple style and is out of her face and off of her collar. No jewelry is worn.*

GETTING A JOB

You may know where you want to work. If not, there are some simple ways to find out about job openings. One place is the *classified ad* sections of newspapers. The local *state employment service* is also a source. You may hear about jobs from *people you know*. You can also directly *contact the agencies* where you would like to work. Phone book yellow pages list health care agencies.

The agency for your student clinical experience is another place to look. The staff always looks at students as future employees. They watch how students treat patients and co-workers. They look for the qualities and characteristics described on page 38. So you are really being considered for a job while still a student. This is one more reason to always display good work ethics. If that agency is not hiring, the staff may know of places looking for assistive personnel.

What Employers Look For

Before applying for a job or interviewing, think about what employers want in those they hire. If you had your own business, who would you want to hire? Answering that question helps you better understand the employer's point of view.

Employers want employees who:
- Are well groomed
- Are dependable
- Have the skills and training needed to do the job
- Have the values and attitudes that fit with the agency

PRACTICES FOR A PROFESSIONAL APPEARANCE

- Uniforms fit well and are modest in length and style.
- Uniforms are clean, pressed, and mended. Wear a clean uniform daily.
- Wear your name badge or photo ID at all times when on duty.
- Underclothes are clean and fit properly. They are changed daily and are an appropriate color. Colored undergarments can be seen through white and light colored uniforms.
- Jewelry is not worn. Most agencies let employees wear wedding rings; some allow engagement rings. Large rings and bracelets can scratch patients. Confused or combative persons can easily pull off necklaces, bracelets, and earrings. Young children also like to pull on jewelry.
- Stockings or socks are clean, well-fitting, and changed daily.
- Shoes are comfortable, give needed support, and fit properly. Clean and polish shoes often. Wash laces, and replace them as necessary.
- Fingernails are clean, short, and neatly shaped. Long nails can scratch patients.
- Nail polish is not worn. Chipped nail polish provides a place for microorganisms to grow and multiply.
- Hairstyles are simple and attractive. Hair is off your collar and away from your face. Use simple pins, combs, barrettes, and bands to keep long hair up and in place.
- Makeup is modest in amount and moderate in color. Avoid a painted and severe appearance.
- Perfume, cologne, and after-shave lotions are not worn. They may offend, nauseate, or cause breathing problems in patients.

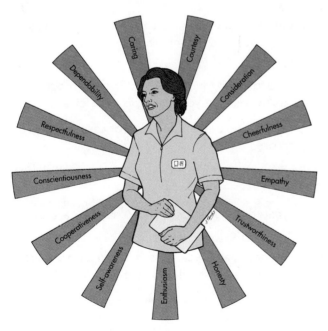

Fig. 3-2 *Good work ethics involves these qualities and characteristics.*

Caring about others is a common trait of health team members. Assistive personnel must care enough to want to make the life of a person happier, easier, or less painful. Good work ethics involves certain traits, attitudes, and manners. These qualities and characteristics are described in Box 3-2 on p. 38. They are necessary for you to function effectively in your role (Fig. 3-2). (See Focus on Home Care on p. 39.)

Applicants who look good communicate many things to the employer. You have only one chance to make a good first impression. A well-groomed person is likely to get the job over someone who is sloppy, has wrinkled or dirty clothes, and has body or breath odors. Proper dress for an interview is discussed later in this section.

Being dependable is important. Health care agencies provide services to people. Staff must be at work on time and when scheduled. Undependable people cause everyone problems. Other staff take on extra work. Fewer people give care. Quality of care can easily suffer. Supervisors spend time trying to find out if the person is coming to work. They also have to find someone else to cover for the absent employee. If you had your own business, you would want people to be at work when expected. Otherwise your business would be less efficient and productive.

Employers need to know that you can perform required job skills. The employer requests proof of the required training. A certificate of course completion or a high school, college, or technical school transcript documents your training. Some employers accept a copy of an official grade report (report card).

BOX 3-2

QUALITIES AND CHARACTERISTICS FOR GOOD WORK ETHICS

Caring   Have concern for patients. Help make the person's life happier, easier, or less painful.

Dependability   Report to work on time and when scheduled. Perform delegated tasks and keep obligations and promises.

Consideration   Respect the person's physical and emotional feelings. Be gentle and kind toward patients, families, and co-workers.

Cheerfulness   Greet and talk to people in a pleasant manner. Do not be moody, bad tempered, or unhappy while at work.

Empathy   Look at things from the person's point of view—put yourself in the person's position. Always ask yourself how you would feel if you had the person's problem.

Trustworthiness   Patients and staff members have confidence in you. They believe you will keep patient information confidential. They trust you not to gossip about patients, co-workers, doctors, or the health team.

Respectfulness   Patients have rights, values, beliefs, and feelings. If they differ from yours, do not criticize or condemn the person. Treat the person with respect and dignity at all times. Also show respect for supervisors and co-workers.

Courtesy   Be polite and courteous to patients, families, visitors, and co-workers. Address people by title and name (e.g., Mr. Tyler, Ms. Crane, Dr. Gilson). Other courtesies include explaining to the person what you are going to do, saying "please" and "thank you," and not interrupting others unnecessarily.

Conscientiousness   Be careful, alert, and exact in following instructions. Give thorough care with knowledge and skill. Always give your best possible effort.

Honesty   Truthfully and accurately report the amount and kind of care given, your observations, and any errors.

Cooperation   Willingly help and work with others. Also take that "extra step" during busy and stressful times.

Enthusiasm   Be eager, interested, and excited about your work. What you are doing is important.

Self-awareness   Know your own feelings, strengths, and weaknesses. You need to understand yourself before you can understand your patients.

HOME CARE

focus on

Home health care assistants also must be able to work alone and have self-discipline. You work alone in the home. An RN can be reached by phone. The RN makes some home visits. However, an RN is not immediately available to you at the bedside if problems occur. You must be able to perform procedures skillfully and safely.

Self-discipline also is essential. You must arrive at homes on time. Organize activities so personal care needs and housekeeping tasks are fulfilled. Avoid temptations. This includes watching TV, talking on the telephone, visiting, and stopping for an extra cup of coffee.

Honesty is very important. You may be asked to shop. You must be honest and thrifty with the person's money. Accurately report to the person or family the items purchased, their cost with receipts, total amount spent, and amount of money returned.

Respecting the person's property also is important. Assistive personnel handle valuables and personal property in health care settings. However, access to the person's property is greater in the home. Home furnishings, appliances, linens, and household items are used for personal care and housekeeping. Treat personal and family property with respect. Prevent damage. Read the manufacturer's instructions before using any appliance. Clean the appliance after use.

LONG-TERM CARE

focus on

The Omnibus Budget Reconciliation Act of 1987 (OBRA) requires that long-term centers hire nursing assistants who have completed a state-approved training and competency evaluation program. The employer requests proof of training and also checks your record in the state nursing assistant registry.

HOME CARE

focus on

Home care agencies receiving Medicare funds must meet OBRA requirements. Assistive personnel must meet the training and competency evaluation requirements outlined in OBRA. Some states have additional training requirements for assistive personnel employed by home care agencies.

Give the employer a copy of your certificate, transcript, or grade report. Never give the original to the employer. Keep the original for future use. The employer may request that a transcript be sent directly from the school or college. (See Focus on Long-Term Care and Focus on Home Care.)

Job Applications

The agency asks you to complete a job application (Fig. 3-3, pp. 40-42). You get the application from the *personnel office* or *human resources office*. You may be asked to complete the application in that office. Some agencies have you take the application home and return it by mail or in person. Make sure you are well groomed and behave pleasantly when seeking or returning a job application. It may be your first chance to make a good impression.

Refer to the guidelines in Box 3-3 on p. 43 when completing a job application. How you fill it out may mean the difference between getting or not getting the job. The application may also be your first chance to impress the employer. A neat, legible, and complete application gives a better image than one that is sloppy or incomplete. Remember, employers use applications to screen out unqualified applicants.

The Job Interview

A job interview is the employer's chance to get to know and evaluate you. It also lets you find out more about the agency. Remember, employers hire well-groomed, dependable, and skilled people.

The interview may be when you complete the job application. Some employers review the application first to

Text continued on p. 43

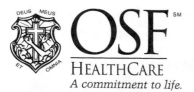

APPLICATION FOR EMPLOYMENT

OSF St. Francis Hospital
3401 Ludington Street, Escanaba, MI 49829

OSF Saint Joseph Hospital
1005 Julien Street, Belvidere, IL 61008

OSF Saint Anthony Medical Center
5666 E State Street, Rockford, IL 61108

OSF Saint James Hospital
610 E Water Street, Pontiac, IL 61764

OSF St. Joseph Medical Center
2200 E Washington Street, Bloomington, IL 61701

OSF Saint Francis Medical Center
530 NE Glen Oak Avenue, Peoria, IL 61637

OSF St. Mary Medical Center
3333 N Seminary, Galesburg, IL 61401

OSF St. Francis Continuation Care and Nursing Home Center
210 S Fifth Street, Burlington, IA 52601

OSF St. Anthony's Continuing Care Center
767 30th Street, Rock Island, IL 61201

OSF HEALTHPLANS, INC.
300 SW Jefferson Street, Peoria, IL 61602

OSF SAINT FRANCIS, INC.
4541 N Prospect, Peoria, IL 61614

OSF HEALTHCARE SYSTEM
800 NE Glen Oak Avenue, Peoria, IL 61603

OSF HealthCare is an equal opportunity employer and does not discriminate because of age, sex, race, creed, color, religion, national origin, marital status, disability, or other protected status.

PLEASE PRINT

LAST NAME	FIRST NAME	MIDDLE INITIAL	SOCIAL SECURITY NO.

STREET ADDRESS, CITY, STATE, ZIP

HOME PHONE
( )

ALTERNATE PHONE
( )

POSITION(S) DESIRED

DATE AVAILABLE

PAYRATE DESIRED

HAVE YOU EVER APPLIED AT OSF HEALTHCARE BEFORE? ☐ YES ☐ NO	WHEN?	WHERE?	WHAT POSITION?
WERE YOU EVER EMPLOYED BY OSF HEALTHCARE BEFORE? ☐ YES ☐ NO	IF YES, WHEN? / UNDER WHAT LAST NAME?	WHAT FACILITY?	WHAT CAPACITY?

IF UNDER AGE 18, GIVE BIRTHDATE.

ARE YOU A U.S. CITIZEN OR AN ALIEN LEGALLY AUTHORIZED TO WORK IN THE U.S.A.?
☐ YES   ☐ NO

DO YOU HAVE ANY RELATIVES WORKING AT THIS FACILITY? ☐ YES ☐ NO

IF YES, PLEASE LIST NAMES AND RELATIONSHIP

Have you ever pled guilty to or been convicted of any criminal offense (other than minor traffic violations)?   ☐ Yes ☐ No
If "yes," please explain. Note: A criminal conviction is not an automatic bar to employment.

EMPLOYMENT DATA

WHAT SHIFT(S) ARE YOU WILLING TO WORK?
1ST   2ND   3RD
OTHER: _____

CIRCLE DAYS YOU CAN WORK
MON.   TUES.   WED.   THURS.
FRI.   SAT.   SUN.
ARE YOU WILLING TO WORK OT IF REQUIRED? ☐ YES ☐ NO

ARE YOU WILLING TO WORK
WEEKENDS? ☐ YES ☐ NO
HOLIDAYS? ☐ YES ☐ NO

STATUS DESIRED
☐ FULL-TIME
☐ PART-TIME
☐ PRN
☐ TEMPORARY

IF APPLYING FOR PART-TIME, HOW MANY HOURS PER WEEK ARE YOU ABLE TO WORK? _____

WHAT PROMPTED YOUR APPLICATION? (PLEASE BE SPECIFIC)
☐ EMPLOYEE REFERRAL _____
☐ NEWSPAPER _____
☐ OWN ACCORD _____
☐ JOB LINE _____
☐ OTHER _____

Form No. Z8020 (Rev. 10/96) **MFI**

NAME   LAST   FIRST   MIDDLE INITIAL

POSITION DESIRED

DATE

Fig. 3-3 *A sample job application. (Courtesy OSF St. Joseph Medical Center, Bloomington, Ill.)*

EDUCATION

	NAME & ADDRESS OF SCHOOL	COURSE OF STUDY	CIRCLE LAST YEAR COMPLETED	DID YOU GRADUATE	LIST DEGREE OR DIPLOMA
HIGH SCHOOL			1 2 3 4	☐ YES ☐ NO	
COLLEGE			1 2 3 4	☐ YES ☐ NO	
POST GRADUATE			1 2 3 4	☐ YES ☐ NO	
OTHER					
IF NOW ATTENDING SCHOOL, PLEASE GIVE ANTICIPATED GRADUATION DATE.					

EMPLOYMENT HISTORY

PRESENT OR MOST RECENT EMPLOYER

NAME OF EMPLOYER	STREET ADDRESS, CITY, STATE, ZIP	PHONE NUMBER ( )
YOUR LAST NAME AT THAT TIME?	JOB TITLE	DATE OF EMPLOYMENT FROM: TO:
REASON FOR LEAVING?	SUPERVISOR'S NAME	ENDING SALARY
CONTACT FOR REFERENCE? IF NO, WHY? ☐ YES ☐ NO	DUTIES, SKILLS, EQUIPMENT USED:	

PREVIOUS EMPLOYERS LIST MOST RECENT FIRST

NAME OF EMPLOYER	STREET ADDRESS, CITY, STATE, ZIP	PHONE NUMBER ( )
YOUR LAST NAME AT THAT TIME?	JOB TITLE	DATE OF EMPLOYMENT FROM: TO:
REASON FOR LEAVING?	SUPERVISOR'S NAME	ENDING SALARY
CONTACT FOR REFERENCE? IF NO, WHY? ☐ YES ☐ NO	DUTIES, SKILLS, EQUIPMENT USED:	

NAME OF EMPLOYER	STREET ADDRESS, CITY, STATE, ZIP	PHONE NUMBER ( )
YOUR LAST NAME AT THAT TIME?	JOB TITLE	DATE OF EMPLOYMENT FROM: TO:
REASON FOR LEAVING?	SUPERVISOR'S NAME	ENDING SALARY
CONTACT FOR REFERENCE? IF NO, WHY? ☐ YES ☐ NO	DUTIES, SKILLS, EQUIPMENT USED:	

NAME OF EMPLOYER	STREET ADDRESS, CITY, STATE, ZIP	PHONE NUMBER ( )
YOUR LAST NAME AT THAT TIME?	JOB TITLE	DATE OF EMPLOYMENT FROM: TO:
REASON FOR LEAVING?	SUPERVISOR'S NAME	ENDING SALARY
CONTACT FOR REFERENCE? IF NO, WHY? ☐ YES ☐ NO	DUTIES, SKILLS, EQUIPMENT USED:	

I HEREBY GIVE PERMISSION TO OSF HEALTHCARE TO CONTACT THE EMPLOYERS LISTED ABOVE TO OBTAIN ANY INFORMATION DEEMED RELEVANT. I COMPLETELY RELEASE OSF HEALTHCARE AND THE PROVIDERS OF THE INFORMATION FROM ANY AND ALL LIABILITY ARISING OUT OF INQUIRIES MADE OR INFORMATION PROVIDED RELATIVE TO MY APPLICATION FOR EMPLOYMENT EVEN IF SUCH INFORMATION IS NEGATIVE AND/OR ADVERSELY AFFECTS MY APPLICATION FOR EMPLOYMENT.

_____   _____
DATE   APPLICANT SIGNATURE

Fig. 3-3, cont'd *For legend see opposite page.*

PROFESSIONAL LICENSES, REGISTRATIONS, AND/OR CERTIFICATIONS

ARE YOU CURRENTLY: ☐ REGISTERED   ☐ LICENSED   ☐ CERTIFIED

TYPE	STATE ISSUED	DATE	NO.
TYPE	STATE ISSUED	DATE	NO.
TYPE	STATE ISSUED	DATE	NO.

HAVE YOU EVER HAD YOUR LICENSES, REGISTRATION OR CERTIFICATION REVOKED, SUSPENDED OR PUT ON PROBATION?   ☐ YES ☐ NO
IF YES, PLEASE EXPLAIN.

IF THE JOB YOU ARE APPLYING FOR REQUIRES THE DRIVING OF A MOTOR VEHICLE WHILE ON DUTY, PLEASE PROVIDE THE FOLLOWING INFORMATION:

DRIVER'S LICENSE NO. _____ STATE _____

ADDITIONAL SKILLS

PLEASE CHECK ANY SKILLS BELOW IN WHICH YOU ARE PROFICIENT:

COMPUTER SKILLS: (SPECIFY SOFTWARE)

☐ TYPING _____ WPM

☐ SHORTHAND OR SPEEDWRITING

☐ MACHINE TRANSCRIPTION

☐ MEDICAL TERMINOLOGY

☐ FOREIGN LANGUAGE _____

☐ OTHER: _____

☐ WINDOWS

☐ WORD PROCESSING

☐ SPREADSHEET

☐ DATABASES

☐ GRAPHICS

☐ ALPHANUMERIC DATA ENTRY _____ SPH

PLEASE NOTE ANY ADDITIONAL SKILLS, EXPERIENCE, OR TRAINING THAT YOU FEEL IS IMPORTANT. PLEASE INCLUDE EQUIPMENT OR COMPUTER SOFTWARE USED.

I UNDERSTAND THAT IF I MAKE ANY FALSE STATEMENTS, MISREPRESENTATIONS, OR OMISSIONS ON THIS APPLICATION OR DURING THE HIRING PROCESS, I MAY BE REFUSED EMPLOYMENT OR, IF EMPLOYED, I MAY BE TERMINATED, REGARDLESS OF WHEN DISCOVERED. IN CONSIDERATION OF MY EMPLOYMENT, I AGREE TO CONFORM TO THE RULES, REGULATIONS AND PHILOSOPHY AND VALUES OF OSF HEALTHCARE. I UNDERSTAND THIS APPLICATION IS NOT INTENDED TO BE A CONTRACT OF EMPLOYMENT. I UNDERSTAND THAT MY EMPLOYMENT CAN BE TERMINATED AT ANY TIME AND FOR ANY REASON, AT THE OPTION OF EITHER OSF HEALTHCARE OR MYSELF. I UNDERSTAND THAT NO ONE OTHER THAN AN ADMINISTRATOR HAS ANY AUTHORITY TO ENTER INTO ANY AGREEMENT FOR EMPLOYMENT FOR ANY SPECIFIED PERIOD OF TIME OR TO MAKE ANY AGREEMENT CONTRARY TO THE FOREGOING AND THAT ANY SUCH AGREEMENT MUST BE IN WRITING, SIGNED BY AN ADMINISTRATOR, AND NOTARIZED. I ALSO UNDERSTAND THAT I WILL BE REQUIRED TO COMPLETE A MEDICAL EXAMINATION WHICH MAY INCLUDE A DRUG SCREEN AND A CRIMINAL BACKGROUND CHECK BEFORE BEGINNING EMPLOYMENT. I UNDERSTAND THIS APPLICATION AND ANY INFORMATION IN IT MAY BE SHARED WITH ANY OSF HEALTHCARE ENTITY.

_____   _____
APPLICANT SIGNATURE   DATE

Fig. 3-3, cont'd *A sample job application.* *(Courtesy OSF St. Joseph Medical Center, Bloomington, Ill.)*

BOX 3-3

GUIDELINES FOR COMPLETING A JOB APPLICATION

- Read the directions first, and then follow them. The directions may ask you to use black ink and to print. Following directions is important on the job. Employers look at job applications to see if you can follow directions.
- Write neatly. Your writing must be legible. A messy application gives a bad image. Legible writing lets the employer have the correct information. You will not be contacted if the employer cannot read your telephone number. You may miss getting the job.
- Complete the entire application. If something does not apply to you, write "N/A" for nonapplicable or draw a line through the space. This tells the employer that you read the section and that you did not skip the item on purpose.
- Report any felony arrests or convictions as directed. Write "no" or "none" as appropriate. Some states require criminal background checks.
- Provide information about employment gaps. If you did not work for a time, the employer wonders why. Provide this information to give the employer a good impression about your honesty. Some reasons include going to school, staying home to raise children, caring for an ill family member, or your own illness.
- Tell why you left a job, if asked. Be brief but honest. People leave jobs for one that pays better or for career advancement. Other reasons include those given above for employment gaps. If you were fired from a job, give an honest but positive response. However, do not talk badly about a former employer.
- Provide references as requested. Be prepared to give the names, titles, addresses, and telephone numbers of at least three references. You should have this information written down before completing an application. (Always ask references if an employer can contact them.) You may get the job faster or over another applicant if the employer can quickly check references. If references are missing or incomplete, the employer waits for all of the information. This wastes your time and the employer's time. Also, the employer wonders if you are hiding something with incomplete reference information.
- Be honest in all your responses. Lying on an application is fraud. It is grounds for being fired.

see if you are qualified. Box 3-4 on p. 44 lists common interview questions. Prepare your answers to these questions before the interview. Also prepare a typed list of your skills to give to the interviewer.

Your appearance is important. You must make a good impression. You need to be neat, clean, and well groomed (Fig. 3-4). The way you dress is also important. Box 3-5 on p. 44 gives guidelines on how to dress for an interview.

You must be on time. It shows you are dependable. If you have not been to the agency or do not know where it is, a *dry run* may be useful. Go to the agency some day before your interview. Note how long it takes to get there and where to park. Also ask where to find the personnel office. A dry run gives you an idea of the time it takes to get from your home to the personnel office.

When you arrive for the interview, give the receptionist your name and your purpose for being there. Also give

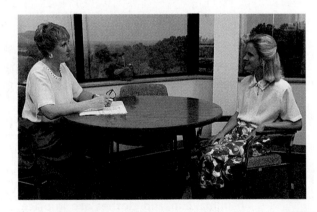

Fig. 3-4 *A simple skirt and blouse is worn for a job interview. Note that the applicant sits with her back straight and legs together.*

BOX 3-4

COMMON INTERVIEW QUESTIONS

- Tell me about yourself.
- Please tell me about your career goals.
- What are you doing currently to achieve these goals?
- Describe what you consider to be *professional* behavior.
- Tell me about your last job.
- What did you like the most about your last job? What did you like the least?
- Why did you leave your last job?
- What would your supervisor and co-workers tell me about your dependability? Your skills? Your ability to adapt?
- Of all your functions, which presented the most difficulty for you?
- How did you handle this difficulty?
- How do you set priorities?
- In what ways have your past experiences prepared you for this position?
- If there is one thing that you could change about your last job, what would it be?
- How do you handle problems with patients and co-workers?
- Why do you want to work here?
- Why should this agency hire you?

BOX 3-5

GROOMING AND DRESSING FOR AN INTERVIEW

- Take a bath, brush your teeth, and wash your hair.
- Use a deodorant or antiperspirant.
- Make sure your hands and fingernails are clean.
- Apply makeup in a simple, attractive manner.
- Style your hair so that it is neat and attractive. You may want to wear it as you would for work.
- Do not wear jeans, shorts, tank tops, halter tops, or other casual clothing.
- Women should wear a simple dress, skirt and blouse, or suit. Men should wear a suit or dark slacks, shirt and tie, and a jacket. A long-sleeved white or light blue shirt is best.
- Make sure clothing is pressed and in good repair. Sew on loose buttons, and mend garments as needed.
- Wear socks (men and women) or hose (women). Hose should be free of runs and snags.
- Make sure shoes are polished and in good repair.
- Avoid heavy perfumes, colognes, and aftershaves. A lightly scented fragrance is acceptable.
- Wear only simple jewelry that complements your clothes.
- Stop in the restroom when you arrive at the interview location. Check to make sure that your hair, makeup, and clothes are in place.

BOX 3-6

QUESTIONS TO ASK THE INTERVIEWER

- Which of the job functions do you think are the most important?
- What employee qualities and characteristics are most important to you?
- What nursing care pattern is used here? (see Chapter 1, p. 10).
- Who will I be working with?
- When are performance evaluations done? Who does them? How are they done?
- What performance factors are evaluated?
- How does the supervisor handle problems?
- What are the most common reasons that assistive personnel quit their jobs here?
- What are the most common reasons that assistive personnel lose their jobs here?
- How do you see this job in the next year? In the next 5 years?
- What is the greatest reward from this job?
- What is the greatest challenge of this job?
- What do you like the most about assistive personnel who work here?
- What do you like the least about assistive personnel who work here?
- Why should I work here rather than in another agency?
- Why are you interested in hiring me?
- May I have a tour of the agency and the unit I will be working on? Will you introduce me to the nurse manager and unit staff?
- Can I have a few minutes to talk with my nurse manager?

the interviewer's name. Then take a seat in the waiting area. Sit quietly in a professional manner. Do not smoke or chew gum. Use the time to review your answers to the common interview questions. Remember, waiting may be part of the interview. The interviewer may ask the receptionist about you—how you presented yourself when you arrived and what you did while waiting. You must be polite and friendly at all times. Remember to smile.

Greet the interviewer in a polite, courteous manner. A firm handshake is correct for both men and women. Address the interviewer as Mr., Mrs., Ms., Miss, or Doctor. Then remain standing until asked to take a seat. When sitting, use good posture and sit in a professional manner (see Fig. 3-4). If the interviewer offers you a beverage, it is correct to accept. Remember to thank the person.

Good eye contact with the interviewer is important. Look directly at the interviewer when answering or asking questions. Poor eye contact can communicate negative information. This negative information includes being shy, insecure, or dishonest or lacking interest. Also watch your body language (see Chapter 6). Body language relates to facial expressions, gestures, postures, and body movements. What you say is important. However, how you use and move your body also communicates a great deal. Avoid distracting habits such as biting your nails, playing with jewelry or clothing, crossing your arms, and

swinging your legs back and forth. Keep your mind on the interview. Do not touch or read things on the interviewer's desk.

The interview lasts 15 to 45 minutes. Answer honestly and to the best of your ability. Speak clearly and with confidence. Avoid short and long answers. "Yes" and "no" answers give little information. You generally want to give a brief explanation of "yes" and "no" responses.

The interviewer is likely to ask about your skills. Give him or her your skill list. The employer may ask about a skill not on your list. Explain that you are willing to learn the skill if your state allows assistive personnel to perform the task.

Whenever you look for employment, you want to find the right job for you. A right match is important. You do not want a job that is not right for you. Nor does the employer want to hire someone who will not be happy in the job or at the agency. At the end of the interview, you will have the chance to ask questions. Box 3-6 lists some questions to ask during your interview. The interviewer's answer will help you decide if the job is right for you.

You should also review the job description with the interviewer. If you have any questions, ask them at this time. Also advise the interviewer of any functions you cannot perform because of training, legal, ethical, or religious reasons. An honest talk with the interviewer prevents problems later.

Also ask questions about starting salary, work hours, your job description, uniform requirements, and the agency's new employee orientation program. Remember to ask about benefits such as health and disability insurance, vacation, and continuing education.

The interviewer signals when the interview is over. You will be thanked for coming for the interview. You may be offered a job at this time. Or the interviewer tells you when to expect a call. Follow-up is acceptable. Ask the interviewer when you can check on your application. Before leaving, thank the interviewer and tell the person that you look forward to hearing from him or her.

A written thank-you note is advised. Write this the day of or the day after the interview. Your writing must be neat and legible. Use a computer or typewriter if your writing is hard to read. The thank-you note should include:

- The date
- The interviewer's formal name using Mr., Mrs., Ms., Miss, or Dr.
- A statement thanking the person for the interview
- Comments about the interview, the agency, and your eagerness to hear about the job
- Your signature using your first and last names

Accepting a Job

Accept the job that is best for you. You can apply several places and have many interviews. Take time to think about any offers before accepting one. If you have more questions about the agency, ask them before accepting the job. Discussing the offer with a relative, friend, co-worker, or your instructor may help you with your decision.

When you accept a job, agree on a starting date and time. Find out where to report on your first day. Ask for the employee handbook and other agency information. Read all materials before you start working.

PREPARING FOR WORK

Having a job is a privilege. It is not a right or something due to you. You earned the job by getting the necessary education and training. You succeeded in a job interview. Now you must function well and work well with others to keep your job.

You must work when scheduled. This means getting to work on time and staying through the entire shift. Absences and tardiness (being late) are among the most common reasons for losing a job. Childcare and transportation issues often interfere with getting to work and getting to work on time. You need to plan in advance for childcare and transportation. Do not wait until it is time to leave for work.

Childcare

Someone needs to care for your children when you leave for work, while you are at work, and before you get home from work. Also plan for the following emergencies:

- Your childcare provider is ill or unable to care for your children that day
- A child becomes ill while you are at work
- You will be late getting home from work

Transportation

Plan for how you get to and from work. If you drive your own car, keep the car in good working order. Keep plenty of gas in the car, or leave early enough to get gas.

Car pooling is another option. Every member of the car pool has responsibilities to each other. If the driver is late leaving or picking one person up, everyone is late for work. If one person is not ready when the driver arrives, everyone in the car pool is late for work. Car pool with persons you trust to be ready and on time. When you drive, make sure you leave and pick others up on time. When a passenger, be ready when the driver arrives.

Public transportation (buses and trains) is common in large cities. Know your bus or train schedule. Know what other bus or train you can take if delays occur. Always make sure you have enough money for your fares to and from work.

Always have a back-up transportation plan. Your car may not start, the car pool driver may not be going to work, or public transportation may not be operating. If you have a back-up plan, you will be able to get to work on time.

ON THE JOB

You will have contact with patients, visitors, and co-workers. How you look, how you behave, and what you say affect everyone in the agency. Working when scheduled, being cheerful and friendly, performing delegated tasks, helping others, and being kind in what you do and say are part of good work ethics. The *Employee Handbook* of OSF Saint Francis Medical Center (Peoria, Ill.) says it best:

You are what people see when they arrive here; yours are the eyes they look into when they're frightened and lonely. Yours are the voices people hear when they ride the elevators, when they try to sleep, and when they try to forget their problems. You are what they hear on their way to appointments which could affect their destinies, and what they hear after they leave those appointments. Yours are the comments people hear when you think they can't.

Yours is the intelligence and caring that people hope they'll find here. If you're noisy, so is the medical center. If you're rude, so is the medical center. And if you're wonderful, so is the medical center.

Attendance

You must report to work when scheduled and on time. The entire unit is affected when just one person is late. You must call your supervisor if you will be late or cannot go to work. Agency attendance policies are explained in its employee handbook. You must follow these policies. Poor attendance can cause you to lose your job.

Being on time does not mean arriving at the agency when your shift begins. It means being ready to work when your shift starts. Remember, you need to store your coat, purse, backpack, and other personal items. You might need to use the restroom when you arrive at the agency. Plan to arrive on your nursing unit a few minutes early. This gives you time to greet others and settle yourself.

Attendance is more than getting to work when scheduled and on time. You must stay the entire shift. Preparing for childcare emergencies is important. Watching the clock so that you can leave as soon as the shift ends gives a bad image. Working overtime is sometimes necessary. You need to prepare to stay longer if necessary. (See Focus on Home Care.)

Your Attitude

You need to show a positive attitude about your job. Show that you are happy to be at the agency and that you enjoy your work. Listen to others, and be willing to learn. Stay busy, and use your time well. You must demonstrate the qualities and characteristics described in Box 3-2.

The work you do is very important. RNs and patients rely on you to give good care. You need to believe that you and your work are valuable to the agency.

Always think before you speak. The following statements signal a negative attitude:

- "I can't. I'm too busy."
- "I didn't do it."
- "It's not my fault."
- "Don't blame me."
- "It's not my turn. I did it yesterday."
- "Nobody told me."
- "I can't come to work today. I have a headache."
- "That's not my job."
- "You didn't tell me that you needed it right away."
- "I work harder than anyone else."
- "No one appreciates what I do."

Gossip

Gossip means spreading rumors or talking about the private matters of others. Gossiping is unprofessional. It

Focus on HOME CARE

Home care assignments must be completed. You must never leave in the middle of an assignment. Nor should you leave before someone from the next shift arrives. Unfortunately, conflicts or problems may occur. Make every effort to finish the assignment. Explain the problem to your supervisor. The supervisor will try to make any needed changes. You must not walk out on the person. That would leave the person in an unsafe situation. Walking out is a most unethical behavior.

can hurt others. The following guidelines will help you to avoid being a part of gossip:

- Remove yourself from a group or situation where gossip is occurring.
- Do not make or repeat any comment that can hurt a patient, family member, co-worker, or the agency.
- Do not make or repeat any comment that you do not know to be true. Remember, making or writing false statements about another person is defamation (see Chapter 2, p. 28).
- Do not talk about patients, visitors, family members, co-workers, or the agency at home or in social settings.

Confidentiality

Patient information is private and personal. **Confidentiality** means trusting others with personal and private information. Patient information is shared only among health team members involved in the person's care. Privacy and confidentiality are patient rights (see Chapter 2, p. 28. Agency and co-worker information also is confidential.

Avoid talking about patients, the agency, or co-workers where others are present. Share information only with the RN supervising your work. Avoid talking about patients, the agency, or co-workers in hallways, elevators, dining areas, or outside the agency. Others not involved in the situation may overhear you. Patients and visitors are very alert to what is said. Other patients or visitors can overhear you and think you are talking about them or their loved ones. Misinformation and the wrong impressions are given about the patient's condition. You can easily upset the patient or family. Therefore you must be very careful about what you say, how you say it, when you say it, and where you say it.

Avoid eavesdropping. To eavesdrop means to listen in or overhear the conversations of others. When you eavesdrop, you invade another person's privacy.

Intercom systems require special considerations (see Chapter 4, p. 10. Many agencies have intercom systems to allow communication between the bedside and the nurses' station.

Patients use the intercom to signal when they need help. The intercom is answered by a staff member at the nurses' station. The nursing team also uses the intercom to communicate with other team members. Be careful what you say over the intercom. It is like a loudspeaker. Others nearby can hear what you are saying.

Personal Hygiene and Appearance

How you look affects the way people think about you and the agency. If staff are clean and neat, people think the agency is clean and neat. They think the agency is unclean if staff are messy and unkempt. People also wonder about the quality of care given.

Attire that is accepted in home and social settings is often unacceptable in the work setting. You cannot wear jeans, halter tops, tank tops, or short skirts. Clothing must not be tight, revealing, or sexual in nature. That is, females cannot show cleavage, the tops of breasts, or the upper thigh. Males must avoid tight pants and exposing their chests. Only the top shirt button can be open.

Follow these guidelines for good personal hygiene and appearance in the work setting:

- Practice personal hygiene (see p. 36).
- Follow the guideline for professional appearance listed in Box 3-1.
- Follow the agency's dress code.
- Tend to grooming needs in private. Use the restroom to brush hair, freshen make-up, apply lipstick, floss, or brush your teeth.
- Do not smoke or chew gum or tobacco while on duty.
- Cover tattoos. They may offend patients, visitors, and co-workers.

Speech and Language

Your speech and language must be professional. Accepted speech and language in home and social settings may be unacceptable at work. The words you use when talking to family and friends may offend patients, visitors, and co-workers. Remember the following:

- Do not swear or use foul, vulgar, or abusive language.
- Do not use slang.
- Control the volume and tone of your voice. Speak softly and gently.
- Speak clearly. Persons with hearing problems may have difficulty hearing you (see Chapter 30).
- Do not shout or yell.
- Do not fight or argue with patients, families, or co-workers.

Courtesies

A **courtesy** is a polite, considerate, or helpful comment or act. Courtesies are easy. They require little time or energy. And they mean so much to people. Even the smallest act of kindness can brighten someone's day.

- Address others by Miss, Mrs., Ms., Mr., or Doctor. Call a person by first name only if he or she asks you to do so.
- Say "please." Begin or end each request with "please."
- Say "thank you" whenever someone does something for you.
- Apologize to others. Say "I'm sorry" whenever you make a mistake or hurt someone. Even little things—like bumping into someone in the hallway—require an apology.
- Be thoughtful of others. Compliment others as appropriate. Wish others a happy birthday, a happy day or weekend off, or a happy holiday.
- Wish patients and families well when they leave the agency. "Stay well" or "stay healthy" are good phrases to use.
- Hold doors open for others. If you are at the door first, open the door and let others pass through. In business, males and females hold doors open for each other.
- Hold elevator doors open for others coming down the hallway.
- Help others willingly when asked.
- Praise others. If you see a co-worker do or say something that impresses you, tell that person. Also tell your co-workers.
- Do not take credit for another person's deed. Give the person credit for the action.

Personal Matters

You are employed to do a job. Personal matters cannot interfere with the job. Otherwise patient care is neglected. You could lose your job for tending to personal matters while at work. Practice the following to keep personal matters separate from the work place:

- Make personal phone calls only during breaks and your meal break. Use public pay phones.
- Do not let family and friends visit you on the unit. If they must see you, arrange for them to meet you during your meal break.
- Arrange personal appointments (doctor, dentist, lawyer, beauty, and others) for times when you are not scheduled to work.
- Do not use agency computers, printers, fax machines, or photocopiers for your personal use.
- Do not take agency supplies (pens, paper, and others) for your personal use.
- Do not discuss personal problems at work.
- Control your emotions. If you need to cry or express anger, do so in a private place. Get yourself together quickly, and return to your work.
- Avoid borrowing money from or lending money to co-workers. This includes meal money and bus or train fares. Borrowing and lending can lead to problems with co-workers.
- Do not engage in selling or fund-raising activities at work. Do not sell your child's candy or raffle tickets to co-workers.
- Do not carry personal pagers or cellular phones while at work.

Meals and Breaks

Meal breaks are usually 30 minutes long. Other breaks are usually for 15 minutes. Meals and breaks are scheduled so that some staff are always on the unit. Staff remaining on the unit cover for the staff on break.

Staff members have responsibilities to each other. Leave for and return from your meal or break on time. That way other staff can have their breaks. Do not take longer than you are allowed. Also remember to tell the RN when you leave and return to the unit.

Job Safety

Safety involves protecting patients, visitors, co-workers, and yourself from harm. Every employee is responsible for job safety. Negligent behavior affects the safety of others (see Chapter 2). Safety practices are presented throughout this book. The following guidelines are important no matter what you are doing:

- Understand the roles, functions, and responsibilities in your job description.
- Be familiar with the contents and policies in personnel and procedure manuals.
- Know the difference between right and wrong.
- Know what you can and cannot do.

- Develop the desired qualities and characteristics of assistive personnel.
- Follow the RN's directions and instructions.
- Question unclear instructions and things you do not understand.
- Help others willingly when asked.
- Follow agency rules and regulations.
- Ask for any training that you might need.
- Report measurements, observations, the care given, patient complaints, and any errors accurately.
- Accept responsibility for your actions. Admit when you are wrong or make mistakes. Do not blame others. Do not make excuses for your actions. Learn what you did wrong and why. Always try to learn from your mistakes.

Planning and Organizing Your Work

Working well with others includes working in an organized and efficient way. You will give nursing care to patients. You also will perform routine tasks on the nursing unit. Some assignments must be completed by a certain time. Other tasks or functions are to be done by the end of the shift. You must plan and organize your work to give safe, thorough care and to make good use of your time. The guidelines in Box 3-7 on p. 50 will help you plan and organize your work.

HARASSMENT

Harassment means troubling, tormenting, offending, or worrying a person by one's behavior or comments. Harassment can be sexual. Or it can involve one's age, race, ethnic background, religion, or disability. What you say and do must be respectful of others. You must not offend others by your gestures, remarks, or use of touch. Nor can you offend others with jokes or pictures. Harassment is not legal in the workplace.

Sexual Harassment

Sexual harassment involves unwanted sexual behaviors by another. The behavior may be a sexual advance or request for a sexual favor. It can be in the form of a comment or touch. The behavior interferes with the person's work and comfort. In extreme cases, the person's job may be threatened if sexual favors are not granted.

Victims of sexual harassment may be men or women. Men harass women or men. Women harass men or women. If you feel that you are being harassed, you must report the situation to your supervisor and the human resource officer.

BOX 3-7

PLANNING AND ORGANIZING YOUR WORK

- Discuss priorities with the RN.
- Know the routine of your shift and nursing unit.
- List care or procedures that are on a schedule. Some persons are turned or offered the bedpan every 2 hours.
- Estimate how much time is needed for each person, procedure, and task.
- Identify which tasks and procedures can be done while patients are eating, visiting, or involved in activities or therapies.
- Plan care around meal times, visiting hours, and therapies. If working in a long-term care center, you must also consider daily recreation and social activities.
- Identify situations in which you will need help from a co-worker. Ask a co-worker to help you, and give the approximate time when you will need help.
- Schedule any equipment or rooms if necessary. Some agencies have only one shower or bathtub to a nursing unit. You will need to schedule the room for patient use.
- Review the procedures to be performed, and gather needed supplies beforehand.
- Do not waste time. Stay focused on your work.
- Do not leave a messy work area. Make sure patient rooms are neat and orderly. Also clean utility areas.
- Be a self-starter. That is, have initiative. Ask others if they need help, follow unit routines, stock supply areas, and clean utility rooms. Stay busy.

You must be careful about what you say or do. Even innocent remarks and behaviors can be viewed as harassment. Employee orientation programs include information about harassment. If you are not sure about your own or another person's remarks or behaviors, discuss the situation with the RN. You cannot be too careful.

RESIGNING FROM A JOB

A new job closer to home with better pay or with new opportunities may prompt you to leave your current job. Going to school, childcare responsibilities, and illness are other reasons. Or you may not like your job or the work setting. Whatever the reason, you need to inform your employer. Give a written notice. Prepare a letter of resignation, or complete a form in the human resources office. Giving 2 weeks' notice is a good practice. Include the following in your written notice:

- Your reason for leaving
- The last date you will work
- Comments thanking the employer for the opportunity to work in the agency

An exit interview is common practice. You and the employer talk before you leave the agency. Usually the employer asks what you liked about the agency and your job. Often employees are asked how the agency can improve.

LOSING A JOB

Remember, a job is a privilege. You must perform your job well and protect patients from harm. Not being awarded a pay raise or losing your job results from poor performance. Failure to follow an agency policy is often grounds for termination. So is failure to get along with others. Box 3-8 lists the many reasons why you can lose your job. Protect your job by performing to the best of your ability. Always practice good work ethics.

BOX 3-8

COMMON REASONS FOR LOSING A JOB

- Poor attendance—not showing up for work or excessive tardiness (being late)
- Abandonment—leaving the job during your shift
- Falsifying a record—application or patient record
- Violent behavior in the workplace
- Possessing weapons in the work setting—guns, knives, explosives, or other dangerous items
- Possessing, using, or distributing alcohol in the work setting
- Possessing, using, or distributing illegal/controlled drugs in the work setting (this excludes taking drugs ordered by a doctor)
- Taking a patient's drug for your own use or distribution to others
- Harassment—see p. 49
- Using offensive speech and language
- Stealing the agency's or a patient's property
- Destroying the agency's or a patient's property
- Showing disrespect to patients, visitors, co-workers, or supervisors
- Abusing or neglecting a patient
- Invading a person's privacy
- Failing to maintain patient, agency, or co-worker confidentiality (includes access to computer information)
- Using the employer's supplies and equipment for your own use
- Defamation—see Gossiping and p. 28 in Chapter 2
- Abusing meal breaks and break periods
- Sleeping on the job
- Violating agency dress code
- Violating any agency policy
- Tending to personal matters while on duty

REVIEW QUESTIONS

Circle T *if the statement is true or* F *if the statement is false.*

1 T F Uncorrected eye problems can affect the person's safety.

2 T F Childcare and transportation issues require planning before going to work.

3 T F Being on time for work means arriving at your agency when your shift begins.

4 T F Failure to maintain confidentiality is grounds for losing your job.

5 T F You must be careful what you say over the intercom system.

6 T F You do not follow the agency's dress code. You can lose your job.

7 T F You can use the agency's computer for your personal use.

8 T F You should carry a personal pager so family members can reach you.

9 T F You should be familiar with agency policy and procedure manuals.

10 T F Harassment is legal in the workplace.

Circle the best *answer.*

11 To perform your job well you need the following *except*

   a To get adequate sleep and rest
   b To exercise regularly
   c To use drugs and alcohol
   d To have good nutrition

12 Good personal hygiene for work involves the following *except*

   a Bathing daily
   b Using a deodorant or antiperspirant
   c Brushing teeth after meals
   d Keeping fingernails long and polished

13 You are getting ready for work. Which should you *not* do?

   a Press and mend your uniform
   b Wear your name badge or photo ID
   c Wear jewelry
   d Style your hair so it is up and off the collar

14 Linda Ames applied for a job at West Bay Hospital. When should she ask questions about the job description?

   a After she completes the application
   b Before she completes the application
   c When her interview is scheduled
   d During the interview

15 Lying on an employment application is

   a Negligence
   b Fraud
   c Libel
   d Slander

16 When completing a job application you should do the following *except*

   a Write neatly and clearly
   b Provide references
   c Give information about employment gaps
   d Leave spaces blank that do not apply to you

17 Which of these qualities and characteristics do employers look for the most?

   a Cooperation
   b Courtesy
   c Dependability
   d Empathy

18 Empathy is

   a Feeling sorry for patients
   b Seeing things from the other person's point of view
   c Being polite to others
   d All of the above

REVIEW QUESTIONS—cont'd

19 What should you wear to a job interview
   a   A uniform
   b   Party clothes
   c   A simple dress or suit
   d   What is most comfortable

20 Which behavior is inappropriate during a job interview?
   a   Good eye contact with the interviewer
   b   Shaking hands with the interviewer
   c   Asking the interviewer questions
   d   Crossing your arms and legs

21 Which response to an interview question is best?
   a   "Yes" or "no"
   b   Long answers
   c   Brief explanations
   d   A written response

22 Which statement reflects a positive work attitude?
   a   "It's not my fault."
   b   "Please show me how this works."
   c   "That's not my job."
   d   "I did it yesterday. It's her turn."

23 A co-worker tells you that a doctor and nurse are dating. This is
   a   Gossip
   b   Eavesdropping
   c   Confidential information
   d   Sexual harassment

24 Which is professional speech and language?
   a   Speaking clearly
   b   Using vulgar and abusive words
   c   Shouting
   d   Arguing

25 Which is *not* a courteous act?
   a   Saying "please" and "thank you"
   b   Expecting others to open doors for you
   c   Saying "I'm sorry"
   d   Complimenting others

26 You are on your meal break. Which is *false?*
   a   You can make personal phone calls.
   b   Family members can meet you.
   c   You can take a few extra minutes if necessary.
   d   The RN needs to know that you are off the unit.

27 You are organizing your work. You should do the following *except*
   a   Discuss priorities with the RN
   b   Ask others if they need help
   c   Stay busy
   d   Plan care so that you can watch the patient's TV

28 A letter of resignation should include the following *except*
   a   Your reason for leaving
   b   The last day you will work
   c   A thank-you to the employer
   d   What problems you had during your work

Answers to these questions are on p. 850.

4 Communicating With the Health Team

- Define the key terms in this chapter
- Explain why health team members need to communicate
- Describe the rules for effective communication
- Explain the purpose, parts, and information found in the medical record
- Describe the legal and ethical aspects of medical records
- Describe the purpose of the Kardex
- Explain your role in the nursing process
- Identify information to collect about a person using sight, hearing, touch, and smell
- List the information to include when reporting to the RN
- List the basic rules for recording
- Know how to use the 24-hour clock
- Use medical terminology and abbreviations
- Explain how computers are used in health care
- Explain how to protect the person's right to privacy when using computers
- Describe the rules for answering the telephone
- Explain how to deal with conflict

KEY TERMS

abbreviation A shortened form of a word or phrase

assessment Collecting information about the person

chart Another term for the medical record

communication The exchange of information—a message sent is received and interpreted by the intended person

conflict A clash between opposing interests and ideas

evaluation To measure if goals are met or if progress is made

goal That which is desired in or by the person as a result of nursing care

implementation To perform or carry out

Kardex A type of file that summarizes information found in the medical record—treatments, diagnosis, routine care measures, and special equipment used by the patient

medical diagnosis The identification of a disease or condition by a doctor

medical record A written account of a person's illness and response to the treatment and care given by the health team; chart

nursing care plan A written guide giving direction about the nursing care a patient should receive

nursing diagnosis A statement describing a health problem that can be treated by nursing measures

nursing intervention An action or measure taken by the nursing team to help the person reach a goal

nursing process The method used by RNs to plan and deliver nursing care; its five steps are assessment, nursing diagnosis, planning, implementation, and evaluation

objective data Information that can be seen, heard, felt, or smelled by another person; signs

observation Using the senses of sight, hearing, touch, and smell to collect information about a person

Key Terms continued on p. 56

prefix A word element placed at the beginning of a word to change the meaning of the word

recording Writing or charting patient care and observations

reporting A verbal account of patient care and observations

root A word element containing the basic meaning of the word

signs Objective data

subjective data That which is reported by a person and that you cannot observe through your senses; symptoms

suffix A word element placed at the end of a root to change the meaning of the word

symptoms Subjective data

word element A part of a word

Health team members communicate with each other for coordinated and effective patient care. Information is shared about what was done and what needs to be done for the person. Information about the person's response to treatment also is shared.

You need to understand the basic elements and rules of communication. Then you can learn how to communicate patient information to the nursing and health teams.

COMMUNICATION

Communication is the exchange of information—a message sent is received and interpreted by the intended person. Words must have the same meaning for both the sender and the receiver of the message. The words "small," "moderate," and "large" mean different things to different people. Is small the size of a dime or the size of a half dollar? In health care, different meanings can cause serious problems. Try to avoid words with more than one meaning.

Use familiar words when communicating. You will learn medical terminology as you study and gain experience in health care. If someone uses an unfamiliar term, ask for an explanation. If you do not understand the message sent to you, communication did not occur. Likewise, do not use terms unfamiliar to patients and families.

Try to be brief and concise. Do not add unrelated or unneeded information. Stay on the subject, avoid wandering in thought, and do not get wordy. Being brief and concise reduces the chance of omitting important details.

Give information in a logical and orderly manner. Organize your thoughts so you can present them logically and in sequence. Think about what happened step by step. Present information to the RN in that way.

Present facts and be specific when giving information. The receiver should have a clear picture of what you are communicating. Asking for clarification or for more information should not be necessary. Telling the RN that a person's temperature is 100.2° F is more specific and factual than saying the "temperature is up."

THE MEDICAL RECORD

The **medical record (chart)** is a written account of a person's illness and response to treatment and care. It provides a way for the health team to communicate information about the person. The record is permanent and can be retrieved years later if the person's health history is needed. The record is a legal document. It can be used in court as evidence of the person's problems, treatment, and care.

The record has many forms organized into sections for easy use. Each page is stamped with the person's name, room number, and other identifying information. This helps prevent errors and improper placement of records. The record includes the person's:

- History
- Physical examination results
- Doctor's orders
- Doctor's progress notes
- Graphic sheet
- Laboratory results
- X-ray examination reports
- IV therapy record
- Respiratory therapy record
- Consultation reports
- Surgery and anesthesia reports
- Admission sheet
- Special consents

Health team members record information on forms for their department and service. The information is read by other health team members who need to know the care provided and the person's response.

Each agency has policies about the contents of medical records and who has access to them. Policies state how often to make recordings and who records on the specific forms. Policies specify acceptable abbreviations, how to correct errors, the color of ink to use, and information about signing entries. You need to know your agency's policies.

All professional staff involved in the person's care have access to the medical record. Those not directly involved usually cannot review the person's record. Cooks, laundry and housekeeping personnel, and office clerks have no need to see medical records.

Remember, you have an ethical and legal responsibility to keep information confidential. Only health team members involved in the person's care need to read the chart. If someone you know is in the agency and you are not involved in that person's care, you have no right to review that person's chart. To do so is an invasion of privacy.

Many agencies let patients see their records if they so request. Know your hospital's policy about patients reading their charts. If a person asks you for the chart, report the request to the RN. The RN is responsible for dealing with the person's request.

The following parts of the medical record relate to your work.

The Admission Sheet

The admission sheet is completed when the person is admitted to the agency. It has identifying information about the person: legal name, birth date, age, gender (male or female), current address, marital status, and Social Security number. Other information includes known allergies, diagnosis, religion, church, and doctor's name. Occupation, employer, insurance coverage, relative or legal representative, and the name and number of the person to notify in an emergency also are found on the admission sheet. Advance directives (the person's wishes about resuscitation and life support measures) also are found here (see Chapter 36).

The admission sheet is useful for filling out other forms that require some of the same information. That way the person does not have to answer the same question several times.

Nursing History

An RN completes the nursing history (Fig. 4-1, pp. 58-59) when the patient is admitted. The RN interviews the person. The RN asks about why the person sought health care, signs and symptoms, medications, and prior illnesses. You can use the history to learn about the person's background and health history.

The Graphic Sheet

The graphic sheet is used to record measurements and observations made daily, every shift, or 3 or 4 times a day (Fig. 4-2, p. 60). Information includes the person's blood pressure, temperature, pulse, respirations, height, and weight. Some graphic sheets include places to record intake and output, routine care, bowel movements, and the time of the doctor's visit.

focus on LONG-TERM CARE

An activities-of-daily-living flow sheet is common in long-term care. The form contains information about hygiene, food and fluids, elimination, rest and sleep, activity, and social interactions.

focus on HOME CARE

A weekly client care record is used in home care. The form has boxes for each day of the week and for care activities. The form includes boxes for temperature, pulse, respirations, blood pressure, and weight. The home health care assistant checks the box for the day care was given or records the measurement on the day it was done.

Nurses' Notes

Nurses' notes are a written description of nursing care given, the person's response to care, and any observations about the person's condition (Fig. 4-3, p. 61). They are used to record information about special treatments and medications. Teaching, counseling, and procedures performed by the doctor also are recorded in the nurses' notes.

Flow Sheets

A flow sheet is used to record frequent measurements or observations. For example, a person's blood pressure, pulse, and respirations are taken every 15 minutes or more often. The graphic sheet does not have enough room to record frequent measurements. A flow sheet designed for this purpose does. The intake and output record kept at the bedside is another type of flow sheet (see Chapter 19). (See Focus on Long-Term Care and Focus on Home Care boxes above.)

THE KARDEX

The **Kardex** is a type of card file. For each person there is a card containing some of the information found in the medical record. The Kardex is a summary of the current

Text continued on p. 62

BARNES HOSPITAL			
ST. LOUIS, MISSOURI			

Person to Contact:	Emergency Phone:	

Why you came to the hospital?

Allergies (food, drugs, latex, environment)?

Items brought in from home?	Did you bring:
☐ Medications ☐ Dentures	☐ Money ☐ Jewelry ☐ Credit Cards ☐ Checkbook/Checks ☐ Other _____
☐ Contacts ☐ Glasses	*(These need to be locked up with security or sent home. Hospital will not be responsible*
☐ Hearing Aid	*for valuables left in room)*

MEDICINE NAMES	Dose & How Often Taken	Reason You Take Medicine	Time of Last Dose
Prescribed by a Doctor			
Non-Prescription			

Do you have any problems with your medicines?

Do you smoke? ☐ Yes ☐ No	Do you use "street" drugs? ☐ Yes ☐ No	How much caffeine do you drink or eat?
Do you chew tobacco? ☐ Yes ☐ No	How much alcohol do you drink? _____	

Medical History:
☐ Heart Disease	☐ Epilepsy	☐ Cancer	☐ Chicken Pox/Shingles	☐ Menstrual Disease
☐ Lung Disease	☐ Stroke	☐ Hepatitis	☐ Fainting/Dizzy Spells	☐ Circulation Problems
☐ Liver Disease	☐ Diabetes	☐ High Blood Pressure	☐ Stomach Problems	☐ Swelling
☐ Immune Disorders	☐ TB	☐ Rheumatic Disease	☐ Bladder Problems	☐ Bleeding
☐ Other _____		☐ Sexually Transmitted Disease: _____		

HISTORY COMMENTS:

Could you be pregnant? ☐ Yes ☐ No	When was your last Period? _____

What surgeries or procedures have you had? (Date)

Family Health History: ☐ Hypertension   ☐ Diabetes   ☐ Heart Disease   ☐ Stroke   ☐ Cancer   ☐ Other _____

Which of the following have you had in the past 12 months?
☐ Self Breast Exam	☐ Prostate Check	☐ Glaucoma Check	☐ Rectal Check (over 40)	☐ Dental Exam
☐ Mammogram (over 40)	☐ Testicular Check	☐ Pelvic Exam	☐ Hearing Check	☐ Vision Check

Are your immunizations current?   ☐ Yes   ☐ No   ☐ Unknown
(Call ID Specialist)

Fig. 4-1 *Nursing history form. (From Potter PA, Perry AG:* Fundamentals of nursing: concepts, process, and practice, *ed 4, St Louis, 1997, Mosby.)*

Are you on a special diet?	How is your appetite?
Any foods you can't eat, and why?	Any difficulty eating or swallowing?
Nutritional supplements/or diet substitutions (e.g., vitamins, artificial sweeteners, salt, substitutes)	Weight loss/gain (amount) in the last 12 months?

How often do you have a BM?
Do you have any difficulty having a bowel movement?
☐ use laxatives   ☐ hemorrhoids
☐ use stool softeners   ☐ black/tarry stools

Do you tire easily?   ☐ Yes   ☐ No

Have you fallen recently?   ☐ Yes   ☐ No

Do you have any difficulty urinating?

☐ burning   ☐ blood   ☐ leaking   ☐ frequency

Do you get regular exercise?   ☐ Yes   ☐ No
What kind?_____   How often?_____

What activities do you need help with?
☐ Feeding/eating   ☐ Meal preparation
☐ Dressing   ☐ Transportation
☐ Grooming/bathing   ☐ Housework
☐ Taking medications   ☐ Handling finances
☐ Toileting   ☐ Grocery shopping
☐ Moving/positioning

☐ Walking on level surfaces
☐ Walking on stairs
☐ Paying for Medicines

(RN consider appropriate consults)

Aides used at home:
☐ Eye glasses   ☐ Contact lenses
☐ Hearing aid   ☐ Cane
☐ Walker   ☐ Wheelchair
☐ Prosthesis: _____
DENTURES: ☐ Upper ☐ Lower
PARTIALS: ☐ Upper ☐ Lower

Is it difficult for you to carry out prescribed health care regimens (Diet, Activity, Medications)?   ☐ Yes   ☐ No
If YES, explain:

How much sleep do you normally get?

What helps you fall asleep?

Who do you live with?   ☐ Alone   ☐ Spouse only   ☐ Family   ☐ Friends   ☐ Nursing Home

Who helps you at home?   ☐ Spouse   ☐ Family   ☐ Friends   ☐ Home Health   ☐ Visiting Nurse

Do you have concerns about your family while you are in the hospital?

What major changes have you had in your life in the past 12 months?

Do you feel you deal successfully with stress? ☐ Yes ☐ No	Would you like additional resources? ☐ Yes ☐ No

Do you have concerns that your illness/hospitalization will affect:
☐ appearance   ☐ job   ☐ male/female roles   ☐ how you feel about yourself

Is religion important in your life? ☐ Yes ☐ No	Will this illness/hospitalization interfere with any religious beliefs/practices? ☐ Yes ☐ No

What do you expect from us while in the hospital?

Do you have a Living Will?   ☐ Yes   ☐ No   Do you have a Power of Attorney?   ☐ Yes   ☐ No
Do you have a copy with you?   ☐ Yes   ☐ No

Patient/Significant Other Signature: Relationship:	Date	Staff Signature Title:	Date

☐ REVIEWED BY REGISTERED NURSE   SIGNATURE: DATE:

TO BE COMPLETED BY STAFF ONLY

Patient provided: ☐ Admit kit   ☐ ID band   ☐ Sensitivity/Allergy band on patient   ☐ Allergy sticker on chart
Patient instructed: ☐ Valuables policy   ☐ Waiver signed   ☐ Smoking   ☐ Visitation
                     ☐ Nursing call/Emergency   ☐ TV/phone   ☐ Fall precautions/band on wrist
                     ☐ Patient's Rights/responsibilities   ☐ Received copy of Personal Directions for My Healthcare

Time patient arrived on Division:_____   SIGNATURE: _____

Fig. 4-1, cont'd *For legend see opposite page.*

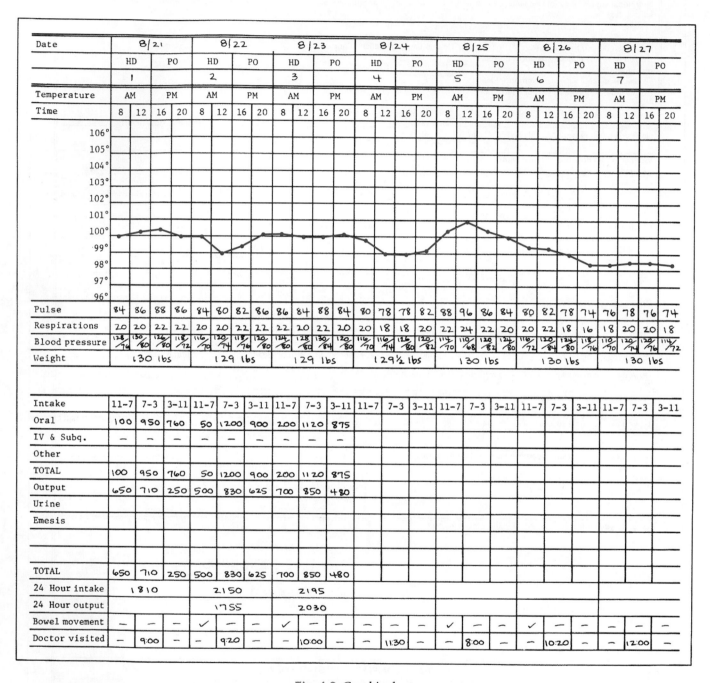

Fig. 4-2 *Graphic sheet.*

Date	Time		Signature
8/23	15⁴⁰/PM	Pt. complained of incisional pain. Pointed to incision and described pain as "throbbing." Holding pillow over incisional area. Skin warm and dry with perspiration noted on forehead. No new drainage noted on dressing; dressing intact.	S. Smith, R.N.
8/23	15⁴⁵/PM	BP 138/88, P 90, R 22. Demerol 100 mg IM in RVG for incisional pain. Pt. positioned in left side-lying position. Back massage given.	S. Smith, R.N.
8/23	16⁰⁰/PM	BP 132/84, P 84, R 20. Pt. stated pain "going away." Appears more relaxed and resting with more comfort.	S. Smith, R.N.

Nurses' Notes

NAME:
SOCIAL SECURITY NUMBER:
IDENTIFICATION NUMBER:
ROOM AND BED NUMBER:
PHYSICIAN NAME:

Fig. 4-3 *Nurses' notes.*

Medical Diagnosis and other pertinent medical information:				1083 13160 23-4 Smith, Phil
10/25 LBP c̄ RLE Sciatica				
10/26 Laminectomy L4-L5 c̄ Bone Graft				

Condition	Satis		PMH:	
Allergies (Drugs, food, other)	PCN, ASA, Codeine		DM	

Adm. Date	10/23	Age	64	Religion	Cath.	Mode of Travel	
Service	Ortho	Doctor	Ford		Resident	Kowalski	Intern

FREQUENTLY ORDERED ITEMS		Date	Specimens/Daily Lab	Date	Treatments
Temp.		10/25	Adm. Blood work	10/24	BR and Logroll q 2°
Pulse & Resp.	q 4°	10/25	UA c̄ Micro		
BP		10/25	BS		
I & O	q 8°				
Weights					
Spot Checks					
Chest P.T.					
Incentive Spirometer					
P.T.					

ACTIVITIES		NUTRITION				
Ad lib		Diet	Regular			
Ambulate	x 2					
Chair				Date	Diagnostic Procedures	
BRP						
Bedrest				10/25	Myelogram	
Bath		Feedings			CT Scan	
Self				10/25	CXR	
Tub		Assist c̄ meals		10/25	ECG	
Shower		FLUID BALANCE				
Bed	✓	Force				
Assist.		D E N				
		Restrict				
		D E N				
Orderlies Needed						
Family:						

NURSING CARE PLAN

Date	Nursing Diagnosis	Expected Outcomes	Nursing Plan/Orders
10/26	Pain related to incisional swelling	1. Client requests for pain med. decreases by 10/28. 2. Client respiratory expansion ↑ by 10/27.	1. Encourage client to Log Roll when turning. 2. Instruct client in relaxation exercizes.
10/27	Impaired physical mobility related to pain	1. Client increases ambulation from BID to QID or greater by 10/28. 2. Client assumes ADL by 10/29.	1. Ambulate in Hall c̄ client 20 min. after administration of analgesic. 2. Encourage family to walk client. 1. Allow client extra time to do self-care for hygiene needs.

Discharge Planning:	Destination:	Transportation:	Probable Date:	Referral Agencies:	Appointment:
				Supplies:	

| Patient Name | | | | | |

Fig. 4-4 *A sample Kardex. (From Potter PA, Perry AG:* Fundamentals of nursing: concepts, process, and practice, *ed 4, St Louis, 1997, Mosby.)*

treatments ordered by the doctor, the person's current diagnosis, routine care measures, and special equipment needs. The nursing care plan may be part of the Kardex. The Kardex is a quick, easy source of patient information (Fig. 4-4).

NURSING PROCESS

RNs must communicate with each other about the patient's problems, needs, and care. Information is communicated through the nursing process. The **nursing process** is the method used by RNs to plan and deliver nursing care. It has five steps: assessment, nursing diagnosis, planning, implementation, and evaluation. The purpose of the nursing process is to meet the patient's nursing needs. It requires good communication between the patient and the nursing team.

Each step is important. If done in order with good communication, the nursing process helps patients reach desired goals. Nursing care is organized and has purpose.

All members of the nursing team do the same things for the person and have the same goals. The person feels safe and secure with consistent care.

The nursing process is ongoing. That is, it constantly changes as new information is gathered and as the person's needs change. You will see the continuous nature of the nursing process as each step is explained.

Assessment

Assessment involves collecting information about the person. RNs gather information from many sources. A nursing history is taken to find out about current and past health problems. The family's health history also is important. Many diseases are genetic. That is, the risk for certain diseases is inherited from parents. For example, if a mother had breast cancer, her daughters are at risk. The RN reviews information collected by the doctor. If available, past medical records are reviewed. The RN also reviews laboratory and other test reports.

The RN performs a physical assessment. Information is collected about each body system. The RN also assesses the person's mental status. Information is gathered by observing the person. You play an important role in the assessment step. You make many observations as you give care and talk to patients.

Observation is using the senses of sight, hearing, touch, and smell to collect information. You see the way the person lies, sits, or walks. You see flushed or pale skin and reddened or swollen body areas. You *listen* to the person breathe, talk, and cough. You use a stethoscope to listen to the heartbeat and to measure blood pressure. When *touching* the person, you collect information about skin temperature and feel if the skin is moist or dry. You also use touch to take the person's pulse. *Smell* is used to detect body, wound, and breath odors and unusual kodors from urine and bowel movements.

Information observed about a person is called objective data. **Objective data (signs)** are seen, heard, felt, or smelled. You can feel a pulse, and you can see urine. However, you cannot feel or see the person's pain, fear, or nausea. **Subjective data (symptoms)** are things a person tells you that you cannot observe through your senses.

Box 4-1 on pp. 64-65 lists the basic observations you need to make and report to the RN. Make notes of your observations. They help when you report to the RN. They also help when recording observations. Carry a note pad and pen in your pocket to note observations as you make them.

The assessment step never ends. The nursing team collects new information with every patient contact. New observations are made, and patients share more information. Families often add more information. (See Focus on Long-Term Care.)

LONG-TERM CARE

OBRA requires the use of the minimum data set (MDS) for residents of long-term care centers. The MDS is an assessment and screening tool. The form is completed when the resident is admitted to the center. It provides extensive information about the person. Examples include the person's memory, communication, hearing and vision, physical function, and activities. The form is updated before each care conference. A new MDS is completed once a year and whenever the person's condition changes.

Nursing Diagnosis

The RN uses information from the assessment to make a nursing diagnosis. A **nursing diagnosis** is a statement describing a health problem that can be treated by nursing measures. The health problem may exist or may develop. Nursing diagnoses and medical diagnoses are different. A **medical diagnosis** is the identification of a disease or condition by a doctor. Medical diagnoses include cancer, pneumonia, chickenpox, stroke, heart attack, infection, AIDS, and diabetes. Medications, therapies, and surgery are ordered by doctors to cure, heal, or relieve pain.

A person may have many nursing diagnoses. Remember, nursing deals with the total person. Therefore nursing diagnoses involve the physical, emotional, social, and spiritual needs of patients. Nursing diagnoses may change, or new ones may be added as the RN gains more information about the person through assessment. Box 4-2 on pp. 68-69 lists the nursing diagnoses approved by the North American Nursing Diagnosis Association (NANDA).

Planning

Priorities and goals are set during planning. Nursing measures or actions are chosen to help the person meet the goals. The patient, family, and nursing team all help the RN plan. Other health workers may be involved.

Priorities relate to what is most important for the person. Maslow's theory of basic needs is useful for setting priorities (see Chapter 5). Maslow describes the needs that all humans have. The needs are arranged in order of importance. Some needs are required for life and survival,

Text continued on p. 68

BOX 4-1

BASIC PATIENT OBSERVATIONS

Ability to Respond

- Is the person easy or difficult to arouse?
- Is the person able to give his or her name, the time, and location when asked?
- Does the person identify others accurately?
- Does the person answer questions correctly?
- Does the person speak clearly?
- Are instructions followed correctly?
- Is the person calm, restless, or excited?
- Is the person conversing, quiet, or talking a lot?

Movement

- Can the person squeeze your fingers with each hand?
- Can the person move arms and legs?
- Are the person's movements shaky or jerky?
- Does the person complain of stiff or painful joints?

Pain or Discomfort

- Where is the pain located? (Ask the person to point to the pain.)
- Does the pain go anywhere else?
- When did the pain begin?
- What was the person doing when the pain began?
- How long does the pain last?
- How does the person describe the pain?
  - Sharp
  - Severe
  - Knifelike
  - Dull
  - Burning
  - Aching
  - Comes and goes
  - Depends on position

Pain or Discomfort—cont'd

- Was medication given?
- Did medication help relieve the pain? Is pain still present?
- Is the person able to sleep and rest?
- What is the position of comfort?

Skin

- Is the skin pale or flushed?
- Is the skin cool, warm, or hot?
- Is the skin moist or dry?
- What color are the lips and nails?
- Are sores or reddened areas present?
- Are bruises present? Where are they located?
- Does the person complain of itching?

Eyes, Ears, Nose, and Mouth

- Is there drainage from the eyes?
- Are the eyelids closed?
- Are the eyes reddened?
- Does the person complain of spots, flashes, or blurring?
- Is the person sensitive to bright lights?
- Is there drainage from the ears?
- Can the person hear? Is repeating necessary? Are questions answered appropriately?
- Is there drainage from the nose?
- Can the person breathe through the nose?
- Is there breath odor?
- Does the person complain of a bad taste in the mouth?

BOX 4-1

BASIC PATIENT OBSERVATIONS—cont'd

Respirations
- Do both sides of the person's chest rise and fall with respirations?
- Is breathing noisy?
- Does the person complain of difficulty breathing?
- What is the amount and color of sputum?
- What is the frequency of the person's cough? Is it dry or productive?

Bowels and Bladder
- Is the abdomen firm or soft?
- Does the person complain of gas?
- What is the amount, color, and consistency of bowel movements?
- Does the person have pain or difficulty urinating?
- What is the amount of urine?
- Is the person able to control the passage of urine?
- What is the frequency of urination?
- What is the frequency of bowel movements?
- Is the person able to control bowel movements?

Appetite
- Does the person like the diet?
- How much of the food on the tray is eaten?
- What are the person's food preferences?

Appetite—cont'd
- Is the person able to chew food?
- How much liquid was taken?
- What are the person's liquid preferences?
- How often does the person drink liquids?
- Is the person able to swallow food and liquids?
- Is the person experiencing nausea?
- What is the amount and color of material vomited?
- Does the person have hiccups?
- Is the person belching?

Activities of Daily Living
- Can the person perform personal care without help?
  - Bathing?
  - Brushing teeth?
  - Combing and brushing hair?
  - Shaving?
- Does the person use the toilet, commode, bedpan, or urinal?
- Is the person able to feed self?
- Is the person able to walk?
- What amount and kind of assistance is needed?

BOX 4-2

NURSING DIAGNOSES APPROVED BY THE NORTH AMERICAN NURSING DIAGNOSIS ASSOCIATION (NANDA)

- Activity Intolerance
- Activity Intolerance, Risk for
- Adaptive Capacity: Intracranial, Decreased
- Adjustment, Impaired
- Airway Clearance, Ineffective
- Anxiety
- Aspiration, Risk for
- Bathing/Hygiene Self-care Deficit
- Body Image Disturbance
- Body Temperature, Risk for Altered
- Breastfeeding, Effective
- Breastfeeding, Ineffective
- Breastfeeding, Interrupted
- Breathing Pattern, Ineffective
- Cardiac Output, Decreased
- Caregiver Role Strain
- Caregiver Role Strain, Risk for
- Communication, Impaired Verbal
- Community Coping, Ineffective
- Community Coping, Potential for Enhanced
- Confusion, Acute
- Confusion, Chronic
- Constipation
- Constipation, Colonic
- Constipation, Perceived
- Coping, Defensive
- Decisional Conflict (Specify)
- Denial, Ineffective
- Diarrhea
- Disuse Syndrome, Risk for
- Diversional Activity Deficit
- Dressing/Grooming Self-care Deficit
- Dysreflexia
- Energy Field Disturbance
- Environmental Interpretation Syndrome, Impaired

- Family Coping: Ineffective, Compromised
- Family Coping: Ineffective, Disabling
- Family Coping: Potential for Growth
- Family Processes, Altered: Alcoholism
- Family Processes, Altered
- Fatigue
- Fear
- Feeding Self-care Deficit
- Fluid Volume Deficit
- Fluid Volume, Risk for Deficit
- Fluid Volume Excess
- Gas Exchange, Impaired
- Grieving, Anticipatory
- Grieving, Dysfunctional
- Growth and Development, Altered
- Health Maintenance, Altered
- Health-seeking Behaviors (Specify)
- Home Maintenance Management, Impaired
- Hopelessness
- Hyperthermia
- Hypothermia
- Incontinence, Bowel
- Incontinence, Functional
- Incontinence, Reflex
- Incontinence, Stress
- Incontinence, Total
- Incontinence, Urge
- Individual Coping, Ineffective
- Infant Behavior, Disorganized
- Infant Behavior, Risk for Disorganized
- Infant Feeding Pattern, Ineffective
- Infection, Risk for
- Injury, Risk for
- Knowledge Deficit (Specify)
- Loneliness, Risk for

From North American Nursing Diagnosis Association: NANDA nursing diagnoses: definitions and classification 1997-1998, *Philadelphia, 1996.*

BOX 4-2

NURSING DIAGNOSES APPROVED BY THE NORTH AMERICAN NURSING DIAGNOSIS ASSOCIATION (NANDA)—cont'd

- Management of Therapeutic Regimen, Ineffective: Community
- Management of Therapeutic Regimen, Ineffective: Families
- Management of Therapeutic Regimen, Effective: Individual
- Management of Therapeutic Regimen, Ineffective (Individuals)
- Management of Therapeutic Regimen, Noncompliance (Specify)
- Memory, Impaired
- Neglect, Unilateral
- Neurovascular Dysfunction, Risk for Peripheral
- Nutrition, Altered: Less Than Body Requirements
- Nutrition, Altered: More Than Body Requirements
- Nutrition, Altered: Potential for More Than Body Requirements
- Oral Mucous Membrane: Altered
- Pain
- Pain, Chronic
- Parent/Infant/Child Attachment, Risk for Altered
- Parental Role Conflict
- Parenting, Altered
- Parenting, Risk for Altered
- Perioperative Positioning Injury, Risk for
- Personal Identity Disturbance
- Physical Mobility, Impaired
- Poisoning, Risk for
- Post-trauma Response
- Powerlessness
- Protection, Altered
- Rape-Trauma Syndrome
- Rape-Trauma Syndrome: Compound Reaction

- Rape-Trauma Syndrome: Silent Reaction
- Relocation Stress Syndrome
- Role Performance, Altered
- Self-esteem, Chronic Low
- Self-esteem Disturbance
- Self-esteem, Situational Low
- Self-mutilation, Risk for
- Sensory/Perceptual Alterations (Specify visual, auditory, kinesthetic, gustatory, tactile, olfactory)
- Sexual Dysfunction
- Sexuality Patterns, Altered
- Skin Integrity, Impaired
- Skin Integrity, Risk for Impaired
- Sleep Pattern Disturbance
- Social Interaction, Impaired
- Social Isolation
- Spiritual Distress
- Spiritual Well-Being, Potential for Enhanced
- Suffocation, Risk for
- Swallowing, Impaired
- Thermoregulation, Ineffective
- Thought Process, Altered
- Tissue Integrity, Impaired
- Tissue Perfusion, Altered (Specify renal, cerebral, cardiopulmonary, gastrointestinal, or peripheral)
- Toileting Self-care Deficit
- Trauma, Risk for
- Urinary Elimination, Altered
- Urinary Retention
- Ventilation, Inability to Sustain Spontaneous
- Ventilatory Weaning Response, Dysfunctional (DVWR)
- Violence, Risk for Self-directed or Directed at Others

such as oxygen, water, and food. The needs necessary for life and survival must be met before all other needs. They have priority and must be met first.

Goals are then set. A **goal** is that which is desired in or by a person as a result of nursing care. Goals are aimed at the person's highest level of well-being and functioning: physical, emotional, social, spiritual. Goals promote health and prevent health problems. They also promote the person's rehabilitation.

Then nursing interventions are chosen. An intervention is an action or measure. A **nursing intervention** is an action or measure taken by the nursing team to help the person reach a goal. In this book, nursing intervention, nursing action, and nursing measure mean the same thing. A nursing intervention does not need a doctor's order. However, some nursing measures come from a doctor's order. For example, a doctor orders that Mrs. Lange walk 50 yards two times a day. The RN includes this order in the care plan.

The **nursing care plan** is a written guide about the care a person should receive. The plan has the person's nursing diagnoses and goals. It also has the measures or actions for each goal. The nursing care plan is a communication tool. Nursing staff use the care plan to see what care to give. The plan helps ensure that the nursing team gives the same care. Some care plans are in the person's chart or on the Kardex (see Fig. 4-4). Others are on computer.

The RN may conduct a patient care conference to share information and ideas about the person's care. The purpose is to develop or revise a person's nursing care plan for effective care. Assistive personnel are usually included in the conference. You are encouraged to share your suggestions and observations. (See Focus on Long-Term Care.)

The plan must be carried out. The plan may change if the person's nursing diagnoses change. Remember, nursing diagnoses may change as new information is gained during assessment.

Implementation

Implementation means to perform or carry out. The **implementation** step is performing or carrying out nursing measures in the nursing care plan. Care is given in this step.

Nursing measures range from simple to complex. RNs delegate measures that are within your legal limits and job description. RNs often ask you to assist with complex measures.

You report the care given to the RN. Some agencies allow you to record care. Reporting and recording are done after giving care, not before. Also remember to report or record your observations. Observing is part of assessment. New observations may change the nursing

LONG-TERM CARE

focus on

OBRA requires regular interdisciplinary care planning (IDCP) conferences for each resident. It is attended by health team members (called the interdisciplinary health team by OBRA) involved in the person's care.

diagnoses, causing changes in the nursing care plan. You need to know about any changes in the nursing care plan so you can give the correct care.

Evaluation

Evaluation means to measure. The **evaluation** step involves measuring if the goals in the planning step were met. The RN evaluates the progress made. Goals may be met totally, in part, or not at all. Information from assessment is used for evaluation. Changes in nursing diagnoses, goals, and the care plan may result from evaluation.

The nursing process never ends. RNs constantly collect information about the person. As the person's needs change, the nursing process changes. Nursing diagnoses, goals, and the care plan may change. You play an important part in the nursing process. You make and report observations. The RN uses the information for nursing diagnoses, goals, and the care plan. You may help develop the care plan. In the implementation step, you perform nursing actions and measures written in the care plan. Your observations are used for the evaluation step.

REPORTING AND RECORDING OBSERVATIONS

Reporting and recording promote communication among health team members. Both are accounts of what was done for and observed about the person. **Reporting** is the verbal account of care and observations. **Recording** or charting is the written account of observations and care.

Reporting

You report patient care and observations to the RN. Reports must be prompt, thorough, and accurate. Always tell the RN the person's name, room and bed number, and the time your observations were made or the care was given. Report only those things that you observed or did yourself. Give reports as the person's condition requires or as often as requested by the RN. Immediately report

BOX 4-3

RULES FOR RECORDING

- Always use ink. Follow agency policy for the color of ink to use.
- Include the date and the time whenever a recording is made. Use conventional time (AM or PM) or 24-hour clock time according to agency policy.
- Make sure writing is legible and neat.
- Use only agency approved abbreviations (p. 70).
- Use correct spelling, grammar, and punctuation.
- Never erase or use correction fluid if you make an error. Cross out the incorrect part, write "error" over it, and rewrite the part. Follow agency policy for correcting errors.
- Sign all entries with your name and title as required by agency policy.
- Do not skip lines. Draw a line through the blank space of a partially completed line or to the end of a page. This prevents others from recording in a space with your signature.
- Make sure each form is stamped with the person's name and other identifying information.
- Record only what you observed and did yourself.
- Never chart a procedure or treatment until it has been completed.
- Be accurate, concise, and factual. Do not record judgments or interpretations.
- Record in a logical and sequential manner.
- Be descriptive. Avoid terms with more than one meaning.
- Use the person's exact words whenever possible. Use quotation marks to show that the statement is a direct quote.
- Chart any changes from normal or changes in the person's condition. Also chart that you informed the RN and the time you made the report (see Reporting, p. 68).
- Do not omit information.
- Record safety measures such as raising bed rails, assisting a person when up, or reminding someone not to get out of bed. This will help protect you if the person falls.

any changes from normal or changes in the person's condition. Use your written notes to give a specific, concise, and descriptive report (Fig. 4-5).

The RN gives a report at the end of the shift to the nursing team of the oncoming shift (called the end-of-shift report). Information is shared about the patient care given and the care that must be given. Information about the person's condition is also included. Some agencies have all nursing team members hear the end-of-shift report as they come on duty. Others have assistive personnel perform routine tasks while RNs and LPNs hear the report.

Recording

When recording on the person's chart, you must communicate clearly and thoroughly. You must follow the rules in Box 4-3. Anyone who reads your charting should know:

- What you observed
- What you did
- The person's response

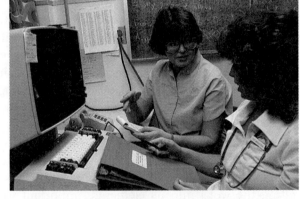

Fig. 4-5 *Write down your observations. Use the notes for reporting and recording.*

Recording time

The 24-hour clock (military time or international time) has four digits (Fig. 4-6, p. 70). The first two digits are for the hour: 0100 = 1:00 AM; 1300 = 1:00 PM. The last two digits are for minutes: 0110 = 1:10 AM. The AM and PM abbreviations are not used.

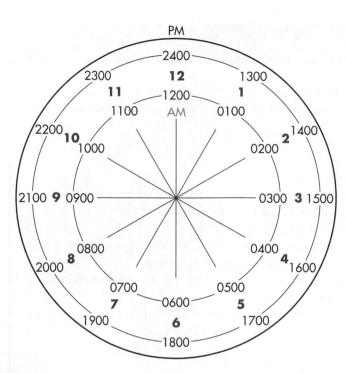

Fig. 4-6 *The 24-hour clock.*

24-HOUR CLOCK

Conventional Time	24-Hour Clock
1:00 AM	0100
2:00 AM	0200
3:00 AM	0300
4:00 AM	0400
5:00 AM	0500
6:00 AM	0600
7:00 AM	0700
8:00 AM	0800
9:00 AM	0900
10:00 AM	1000
11:00 AM	1100
12:00 noon	1200
1:00 PM	1300
2:00 PM	1400
3:00 PM	1500
4:00 PM	1600
5:00 PM	1700
6:00 PM	1800
7:00 PM	1900
8:00 PM	2000
9:00 PM	2100
10:00 PM	2200
11:00 PM	2300
12:00 midnight	2400 or 0000

As Box 4-4 shows, the hour is the same but AM is not used. For PM times, add 12 to the clock time. If it is 2:00 PM, add 12 and 2 for 1400. For 8:35 PM, add 12 and 835 for 2035.

MEDICAL TERMINOLOGY AND ABBREVIATIONS

Medical terminology and abbreviations are used to communicate in health care. They are presented throughout this book. If someone uses a word or phrase that you do not understand, ask an RN to explain its meaning. Otherwise, communication is not effective. You may also want to buy a medical dictionary so you can learn new words.

Like all words, medical terms are made up of parts or **word elements.** These elements are combined in various ways to form medical terms. A term is translated by separating the word into its elements. Important word elements are prefixes, roots, and suffixes.

Prefixes, Roots, and Suffixes

A **prefix** is a word element placed at the beginning of a word. A prefix changes the meaning of the word. The prefix *olig* (scant, small amount) is placed before the word *uria* (urine) to make *oliguria.* It means a scant amount of urine. Prefixes are always combined with other word elements. They are never used alone. Most prefixes are Greek or Latin. Box 4-5 lists commonly used prefixes.

The **root** contains the basic meaning of the word. It is combined with another root, with prefixes, and with suffixes to form a medical term. Roots are mainly from Greek and Latin. A vowel (an *o* or an *i*) is added when two roots are combined or when a suffix is added to a root. The vowel makes pronunciation easier. See Box 4-5 for the most common roots.

A **suffix** is placed at the end of a root to change the meaning of the word. Suffixes are not used alone. Like prefixes and roots, they are from Greek and Latin. When translating medical terms, begin with the suffix. For example, *nephritis* means inflammation of the kidney. It was formed by combining *nephro* (kidney) and *itis* (inflammation). See Box 4-5 for common suffixes.

Medical terms are formed by combining word elements. The important things to remember are that prefixes always come *before* roots and suffixes always come *after* roots. A root can be combined with prefixes, roots, or suffixes. The prefix *dys* (difficult) is combined with the root *pnea* (breathing). This forms the term *dyspnea,* meaning difficulty in breathing.

BOX 4-5

MEDICAL TERMINOLOGY

Prefixes

Prefix	Meaning
a-, an-	without, not, lack of
ab-	away from
ad-	to, toward, near
ante-	before, forward, in front of
anti-	against
auto-	self
bi-	double, two, twice
brady-	slow
circum-	around
contra-	against, opposite
de-	down, from
dia-	across, through, apart
dis-	apart, free from
dys-	bad, difficult, abnormal
ecto-	outer, outside
en-	in, into, within
endo-	inner, inside
epi-	over, on, upon
eryth-	red
eu-	normal, good, well, healthy
ex-	out, out of, from, away from
hemi-	half
hyper-	excessive, too much, high
hypo-	under, decreased, less than normal
in-	in, into, within, not
infra-	within
inter-	between
intro-	into, within
leuk-	white
macro-	large
mal-	bad, illness, disease
meg-	large
micro-	small
mono-	one, single
neo-	new
non-	not
olig-	small, scant
para-	beside, beyond, after
per-	by, through
peri-	around
poly-	many, much
post-	after, behind
pre-	before, in front of, prior to
pro-	before, in front of
re-	again, backward
retro-	backward, behind
semi-	half
sub-	under, beneath
super-	above, over, excess
supra-	above, over
tachy-	fast, rapid
trans-	across
uni-	one

Roots

Root (combining vowel)	Meaning
abdomin (o)	abdomen
aden (o)	gland
adren (o)	adrenal gland
angi (o)	vessel
arterio	artery
arthr (o)	joint
broncho	bronchus, bronchi
card, cardi (o)	heart
cephal (o)	head
chole, chol(o)	bile
chondr (o)	cartilage
colo	colon, large intestine
cost (o)	rib
crani (o)	skull
cyan (o)	blue
cyst (o)	bladder, cyst
cyt (o)	cell
dent (o)	tooth
derma	skin
duoden (o)	duodenum
encephal (o)	brain
enter (o)	intestines
fibr (o)	fiber, fibrous
gastr (o)	stomach
gloss (o)	tongue
gluc (o)	sweetness, glucose
glyc (o)	sugar
gyn, gyne, gyneco	woman
hem, hema, hemo, hemat (o)	blood
hepat (o)	liver
hydr (o)	water
hyster (o)	uterus

Continued

BOX 4-5

MEDICAL TERMINOLOGY—cont'd

Roots—cont'd

Root (combining vowel)	Meaning
ile (o), ili (o)	ileum
laparo	abdomen, loin, or flank
laryng (o)	larynx
lith (o)	stone
mamm (o)	breast, mammary gland
mast (o)	mammary gland, breast
meno	menstruation
my (o)	muscle
myel (o)	spinal cord, bone marrow
necro	death
nephr (o)	kidney
neur (o)	nerve
ocul (o)	eye
oophor (o)	ovary
ophthalm (o)	eye
orth (o)	straight, normal, correct
oste (o)	bone
ot (o)	ear
ped (o)	child, foot
pharyng (o)	pharynx
phleb (o)	vein
pnea	breathing, respiration
pneum (o)	lung, air, gas
proct (o)	rectum
psych (o)	mind
pulmo	lung
py (o)	pus
rect (o)	rectum
rhin (o)	nose
salping (o)	eustachian tube, uterine tube
splen (o)	spleen
sten (o)	narrow, constriction
stern (o)	sternum
stomat (o)	mouth
therm (o)	heat
thoraco	chest

thromb (o)	clot, thrombus
thyr (o)	thyroid
toxic (o)	poison, poisonous
toxo	poison
trache (o)	trachea
urethr (o)	urethra
urin (o)	urine
uro	urine, urinary tract, urination
uter (o)	uterus
vas (o)	blood vessel, vas deferens
ven (o)	vein
vertebr (o)	spine, vertebrae

SUFFIXES

Suffix	Meaning
-algia	pain
-asis	condition, usually abnormal
-cele	hernia, herniation, pouching
-centesis	puncture and aspiration of
-cyte	cell
-ectasis	dilation, stretching
-ectomy	excision, removal of
-emia	blood condition
-genesis	development, production, creation
-genic	producing, causing
-gram	record
-graph	a diagram, a recording instrument
-graphy	making a recording
-iasis	condition of
-ism	a condition
-itis	inflammation
-logy	the study of
-lysis	destruction of, decomposition
-megaly	enlargement
-meter	measuring instrument
-metry	measurement
-oma	tumor
-osis	condition
-pathy	disease
-penia	lack, deficiency
-phasia	speaking

BOX 4-5

MEDICAL TERMINOLOGY—cont'd

SUFFIXES—cont'd

Suffix	Meaning
-phobia	an exaggerated fear
-plasty	surgical repair or reshaping
-plegia	paralysis
-ptosis	falling, sagging, dropping, down
-rrhage, -rrhagia	excessive flow
-rrhaphy	stitching, suturing
-rrhea	profuse flow, discharge
-scope	examination instrument
-scopy	examination using a scope
-stasis	maintenance, maintaining a constant level
-stomy, -ostomy	creation of an opening
-tomy, -otomy	incision, cutting into
-uria	condition of the urine

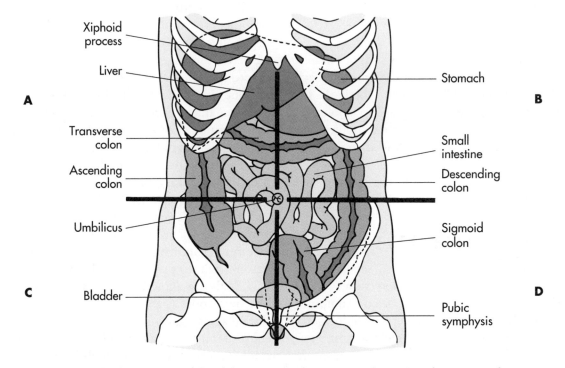

Fig. 4-7 *The four regions of the abdomen.* **A,** *Right upper quadrant.* **B,** *Left upper quadrant.* **C,** *Right lower quadrant.* **D,** *Left lower quadrant.*

Roots can be combined with suffixes. The root *mast* (breast) combined with the suffix *ectomy* (excision or removal) forms the term *mastectomy.* It means the removal of a breast.

Combining a prefix, root, and suffix is another way to form medical terms. *Endocarditis* consists of the prefix *endo* (inner), the root *card* (heart), and the suffix *itis* (inflammation). *Endocarditis* means inflammation of the inner part of the heart.

Abdominal Regions

The abdomen is divided into regions (Fig. 4-7) in order to help describe the location of body structures, pain, or discomfort. The regions are the:
- Right upper quadrant (RUQ)
- Left upper quadrant (LUQ)
- Right lower quadrant (RLQ)
- Left lower quadrant (LLQ)

Directional Terms

Certain terms describe the position of one body part in relation to another. These terms give the direction of the body part when a person is standing and facing forward. The following directional terms come from some of the prefixes listed in this chapter:

- *Anterior (ventral)*—located at or toward the front of the body or body part
- *Distal*—the part farthest from the center or from the point of attachment
- *Lateral*—relating to or located at the side of the body or body part
- *Medial*—relating to or located at or near the middle or midline of the body or body part
- *Posterior (dorsal)*—located at or toward the back of the body or body part
- *Proximal*—the part nearest to the center or to the point of origin

Abbreviations

Abbreviations are shortened forms of words or phrases. They save time and space in written communication. Each agency has a list of accepted abbreviations. Obtain the list when you are hired, and use only the abbreviations accepted by the agency. If you are unsure an abbreviation is acceptable, write the term out in full to communicate accurately.

Common abbreviations are listed on the inside of the back cover for easy reference.

COMPUTERS IN HEALTH CARE

Computer information systems collect, send, record, and store information. Information is retrieved when needed. Medical records and care plans are on computer in many agencies. Instead of recording on the person's chart, the nurse enters information into the computer (Fig. 4-8). Using a computer is easier, faster, and more efficient than writing on the chart. Recordings are more accurate, legible, and reliable.

Agency departments communicate with the nursing unit by computer. Instead of sending a typed report by messenger for the medical record, the medical records staff enters the information into the computer. The nurse accesses the information at the computer in the nurses' station or at the bedside. These computer communication links reduce clerical work and telephone calls. Information is communicated with greater speed and accuracy.

The computer is used for many other functions. For example, nurses use computers to monitor certain measurements such as blood pressures, temperatures, heart rates, and heart function. The computer recognizes nor-

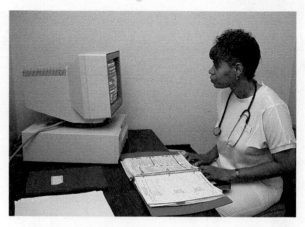

Fig. 4-8 *RN enters information into the computer.*

mal and abnormal measurements. When the abnormal is sensed, an alarm alerts the nursing staff. Monitoring by computer is accurate and promotes early detection of life-threatening events.

Doctors can use computers when diagnosing. Signs and symptoms are entered into the computer. The computer asks questions, and the doctor responds. Eventually the computer offers possible diagnoses. The doctor can use the computer also to prescribe medicines. The person's diagnosis is entered along with any requested information. The computer analyzes the information and suggests medicines and dosages.

Computers save time. Quality care and patient safety are increased. Fewer recording errors occur. Records are more complete and personnel more efficient.

Computer information is easy to access. Therefore the person's right to privacy must be protected. Only certain individuals are allowed to use the computer. They have their own codes (passwords) to access computer files. If allowed access, you will learn how to use the agency's system. You must follow the ethical and legal considerations relating to privacy, confidentiality, and defamation (see Chapter 2). Also follow the rules in Box 4-6.

TELEPHONE COMMUNICATIONS

Often it is necessary to answer phones at the nurses' station or in patient rooms. Good telephone communication skills are essential. The caller cannot see you. But you give much information by your tone of voice, how clearly you speak, and your attitude. When answering the phone, behave as if you are speaking to someone face-to-face.

Agencies have policies about answering telephones. You must be professional and courteous. Good work

BOX 4-6

RULES TO PROTECT PRIVACY WHEN USING THE COMPUTER

- Do not tell anyone your password. If someone has your password, that person can access the computer under your name. It will be hard to prove that entries were made by someone else.
- Change your password on a regular basis.
- Follow the rules for recording listed in Box 4-3 (see p. 69).
- Enter information carefully. Double-check your entries.
- Prevent others from seeing what is on the screen. Do not leave the computer unattended. Log off after making an entry.
- Position equipment so that the screen cannot be seen in the hallway.
- Do not leave printouts where others can read them or pick them up.
- Destroy or shred any computer-printed worksheets.

ethics apply when on the phone. Follow the guidelines in Box 4-7 on on p. 76. (See Focus on Home Care.)

DEALING WITH CONFLICT

People bring their own values, attitudes, opinions, experiences, and expectations to the work setting. Differences often lead to conflict. **Conflict** is described as a clash between opposing interests and ideas. Disagreements, misunderstandings, arguments, and unrest occur.

Conflicts arise over issues or events. Work schedules, absences, and the amount and quality of work performed are examples. The problems must be worked out. Otherwise, unkind words or actions may occur. The work environment becomes unpleasant, and patient care is affected.

Communication and good work ethics are essential for preventing and resolving conflicts. Identify and solve problems before they become major issues. The following guidelines can help you deal with conflict:

- Ask your supervisor for some time to talk privately. Explain the situation, and ask for advice in solving the problem. Give facts and specific examples.
- Approach the person with whom you have a conflict. Ask to talk privately. Be polite and professional in your approach.
- Agree on a time and place to talk.
- Talk in a private setting. Others should not be able to see or hear you and your co-worker.
- Explain the problem and what is bothering you. Give facts and specific behaviors. Focus on the problem, not on the person.
- Listen to the person's response. Do not interrupt the person.

focus on HOME CARE

When answering phones in patient homes, simply answer with "hello." This is for everyone's safety—the patient's, the family's, and your own. The caller has too much information when you give the patient's name ("Price residence") or your own name and title. People call homes for many reasons. They call to sell things or to obtain donations for charity. Others call with criminal intent. They want to know who is in the home. By saying that you are a home health assistant, you tell the caller that an ill, elderly, or disabled person is in the home. These people have difficulty defending themselves and are easy prey for criminals. Do not give your name or the patient's name until you know who is calling and why that person is calling. Give the information only when it is someone you are sure you want to talk to—the patient's family or friend, your supervisor, or a caller expected by the patient.

- Identify ways to solve the problem. Offer your own thoughts, and ask for the co-worker's ideas.
- Schedule a date and time to review the situation.
- Thank the person for meeting with you.
- Implement the solutions.
- Review the situation as scheduled.

BOX 4-7

GUIDELINES FOR ANSWERING TELEPHONES

- Answer the call after the first ring if possible. Business manners call for the phone to be answered by the fourth ring.
- Do not answer the phone in a rushed or hasty manner.
- Give a courteous greeting, identify the area, and give your name and title. For example: "Good morning. Three center. John Hayne, patient care assistant."
- Write the following information when taking a message: the caller's name and telephone number (include area code and extension number), the date and time, and the message.
- Repeat the message and telephone number back to the caller.
- Ask the caller to "Please hold" if necessary. However, find out who is calling first, and then ask if the caller can hold. Do not put callers with an emergency on hold.
- Do not lay the phone down or cover the receiver with your hand when not speaking to the caller. The caller may overhear confidential conversations.
- Return to a caller on hold within 30 seconds. Ask if the caller can wait longer or if the call can be returned.
- Do not give confidential information to any caller. Remember, information about patients and employees is confidential. Refer such calls to a RN.
- Transfer the call if appropriate. Tell the caller that you are going to transfer the call. Give the name of the department if appropriate. Give the caller the phone number in case the call gets disconnected or the line is busy.
- End the conversation politely. Thank the person for calling, and say good-bye.
- Give the message to the appropriate person.

REVIEW QUESTIONS

Circle T *if the statement is true or* F *if the statement is false.*

1 T F The health team communicates to provide effective and coordinated patient care.

2 T F Mrs. Reece was discharged from St. Jude's Medical Center. Her chart is destroyed to protect her right to privacy.

3 T F The medical record is not used in a lawsuit because of the right to privacy.

4 T F Assistive personnel generally have access to all medical records in the agency.

5 T F Information is collected about a person using the senses.

6 T F Subjective data are signs noted when observing a person.

7 T F The nursing care plan lists the medications and treatments ordered by the doctor.

Circle the best *answer.*

8 When communicating, you should do the following *except*

a Use terms that have more than one meaning
b Be brief and concise
c Present information logically and in sequence
d Give facts and be specific

9 These statements are about medical records. Which is *false*?

a The record is used to communicate information about the person.
b The record is a written account of the person's illness and response to treatment.
c The record is a written account of care given by the health team.
d Anyone working in the agency can read the medical record.

REVIEW QUESTIONS—cont'd

10 A person is weighed daily. The measurement is recorded on the

a Admission sheet

b Graphic sheet

c Flow sheet

d Nurses' notes

11 Where does the RN describe the nursing care given?

a Nursing care plan

b Nurses' notes

c Graphic sheet

d Kardex

12 Measures in the nursing care plan are carried out. What step of the nursing process is this?

a Nursing diagnosis

b Planning

c Implementation

d Evaluation

13 Which statement is *true?*

a The nursing process is done without the person's involvement.

b Assistive personnel are responsible for the nursing process.

c The nursing process is used to communicate the person's care.

d All of the above

14 The nursing care plan

a Is written by the doctor

b Consists of actions the nursing team takes to help a person

c Is the same for all persons

d Is also called the Kardex

15 When recording information, you should do the following *except*

a Use ink

b Include the date and time

c Erase if you make an error

d Sign all entries with your name and title

16 These statements are about recording. Which is *false?*

a Use the person's exact words when possible.

b Record only what you observed and did yourself.

c Do not skip lines.

d To save time, chart a procedure before it is completed.

17 In the evening you note that the clock says 9:26. In 24-hour clock time you record this as

a 9:26 PM   c 0926

b 926   d 2126

18 You are learning medical terminology. You know that a suffix is

a Placed at the beginning of the word

b Placed after a root

c A shortened form of a word or phrase

d Describes the body's position

19 These statements are about computers in health care. Which is *false?*

a Computers are used to collect, send, record, and store information.

b The person's privacy must be protected.

c All employees have the same password.

d Computers link one department to another.

20 You answer a person's phone in the hospital. How should you answer?

a "Good morning. Mrs. Reece's room."

b "Good morning. Third floor."

c "Hello."

d "Good morning. Mrs. Reece's room. John Hayne, patient care assistant, speaking."

21 A co-worker is often late for work. You have extra work in her absence. In resolving the conflict you should do the following *except*

a Explain the problem to your supervisor

b Discuss the matter during the end-of-shift report

c Give facts and specific instances

d Suggest ideas to solve the problem

Answers to these questions are on p. 850.

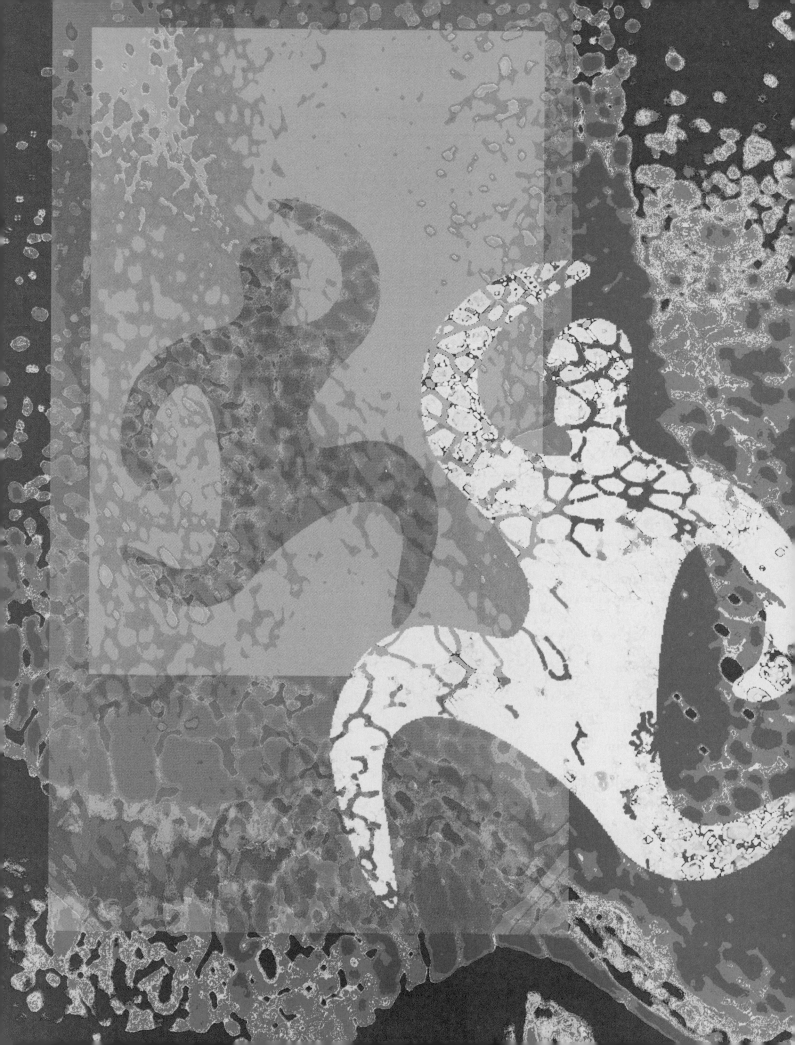

Unit II
Focusing on the Person

5 The Whole Person and Basic Needs

- Define the key terms in this chapter
- Identify the parts that make up the whole person
- Describe the basic needs identified by Abraham Maslow
- Explain how culture and religion influence health and illness
- Explain how patients are grouped in health care agencies
- Identify patient and resident rights
- Explain why family and visitors are important to patients
- Identify the courtesies given to patients and visitors

culture The values, beliefs, habits, likes, dislikes, customs, and characteristics of a group that are passed from one generation to the next

esteem The worth, value, or opinion one has of a person

geriatrics The branch of medicine concerned with the problems and diseases of old age and elderly persons

holism A concept that considers the whole person; the whole person has physical, social, psychological, and spiritual parts that are woven together and cannot be separated

involuntary seclusion Separating a person from others against his or her will; keeping the person confined to a certain area or away from his or her room without consent

need That which is necessary or desirable for maintaining life and mental well-being

obstetrics The branch of medicine concerned with the care of women during pregnancy, labor, and childbirth and during the 6 to 8 weeks after birth

pediatrics The branch of medicine concerned with the growth, development, and care of children ranging in age from the newborn to the adolescent

psychiatry The branch of medicine concerned with the diagnosis and treatment of people with mental health problems

religion Spiritual beliefs, needs, and practices

self-actualization Experiencing one's potential

self-esteem Thinking well of yourself and being thought well of by others

---

The patient is the most important person in your work. Age, religion, nationality, culture, education, occupation, and life-style are some factors that make each patient a unique person. The person is treated as a human being with value. The person is important and special. You must treat the person as someone who thinks, acts, and makes decisions.

Each person has fears, needs, and rights. This chapter focuses on understanding the persons you serve and help.

HOLISM

A person is someone who lives, works, loves, and has fun. When the person is ill or disabled, things are done to and for the person. The person is told when to eat, sleep, bathe, visit, sit in a chair, walk, and use the bathroom. It is easy to forget that the person once did these things without help. No wonder patients often complain that they are treated as things, not as people.

Too often the person is treated as a physical disease or problem: "the gallbladder in 310" rather than "Sally Jones in 310." Most patients have physical problems. However, to provide effective care, you must be aware of the whole person.

Holism means *whole*. With **holism,** the whole person has physical, social, psychological, and spiritual parts. The parts are woven together and cannot be separated (Fig. 5-1, p. 82). Each part relates to and depends on the others.

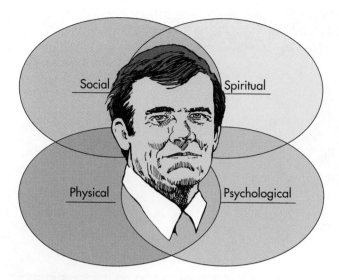

Fig. 5-1 *A person is a physical, psychological, social, and spiritual being. The parts overlap and cannot be separated.*

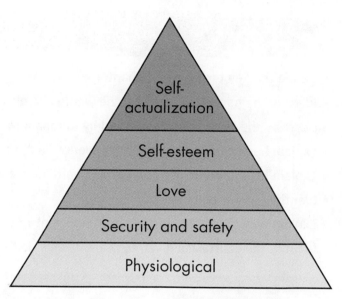

Fig. 5-2 *Basic needs for life as described by Maslow. These needs—from the lowest to the highest level—are physiological needs, the need for safety and security, the need for love and belonging, the need for self-esteem, and the need for self-actualization.*

As a social being, a person speaks and communicates with others. Physically, the brain, mouth, tongue, lips, and throat structures function for speech. Communication is also psychological. It involves the thinking and reasoning abilities of the mind. Considering only the physical part ignores the person's ability to think, make decisions, and interact with others. It also ignores the person's experiences, joys, sorrows, and needs.

In health care, the needs of the whole person are considered. A physical illness affects the person socially, psychologically, and spiritually. For example, Mr. Lund has lung cancer. He needs surgery. He is afraid of dying and asks for a priest. He also has fears about pain and losing his job. His wife is angry because he still smokes cigarettes. The RN plans care to help him with these problems.

BASIC NEEDS

A **need** is that which is necessary or desirable for maintaining life and mental well-being. According to Abraham Maslow, a famous psychologist, certain basic needs must be met for a person to survive and function. These needs are arranged in order of importance (Fig. 5-2). Lower-level needs must be met before the higher-level needs.

People normally meet their own needs every day. When they cannot, it is usually because of disease or injury. When ill, they usually seek health care.

- *Physiological needs*—Oxygen, food, water, elimination, rest, and shelter are required for life. These needs are the most important for survival. They must be met before higher-level needs. A person dies within minutes without oxygen. Without food or water, a person feels weak and ill within a few hours.

The kidneys and intestines must function normally. Otherwise poisonous wastes build up in the blood. If the problem is not corrected, the person dies. Without enough rest and sleep, a person becomes exhausted.

- *The need for safety and security*—Safety and security needs relate to protection from harm, danger, and fear. Many people are afraid of health care. Some procedures involve strange equipment and cause pain or discomfort. People feel safer and more secure if they understand the procedure. They should know why and how a procedure is to be done. The person also needs to know who will do it and what sensations or feelings to expect.

- *The need for love and belonging*—The need for love and belonging relates to love, closeness, affection, belonging, and meaningful relationships with others. There are many cases in which patients were slow to recover or died because of lack of love and belonging. This is particularly true of children and elderly persons. Love and belonging can be met by family, friends, and the health team.

- *The need for self-esteem*—**Esteem** is the worth, value, or opinion one has of a person. **Self-esteem** relates to thinking well of yourself and being thought well of by others. People often lack self-esteem when ill or injured. How does a father feel when he cannot work and support his family because of an illness? Does a woman feel pretty and whole after having a breast removed? Does a person with a leg amputation feel complete and attractive?

BOX 5-1

TOP TEN COUNTRIES OF ORIGIN OF IMMIGRANTS TO THE UNITED STATES*

Mexico	22.0%
Vietnam	8.0%
Philippines	6.3%
Former Soviet Union	4.5%
Dominican Republic	4.3%
Mainland China	4.0%
India	3.8%
El Salvador	2.7%
Poland	2.6%
United Kingdom	2.1%

*Information based on data gathered through the 1992 U.S. Department of Justice, Immigration and Naturalization Service.

- *The need for self-actualization*—**Self-actualization** means experiencing one's potential. It involves learning, understanding, and creating to the limit of a person's capacity. This is the highest need. Rarely, if ever, is it totally met. Most people constantly try to learn and understand more.

CULTURE AND RELIGION

Culture is the characteristics of a group of people—the language, values, beliefs, habits, likes, dislikes, and customs—passed from one generation to the next. The person's culture influences health beliefs and practices. Culture also influences behavior during illness.

You will care for people from different cultures. This includes Americans of various nationalities and people from other countries. These people have family practices, food preferences, hygiene habits, and clothing styles different from yours. The person may speak and understand another language. Some cultural groups have beliefs about the causes and cures of illnesses. They may perform certain rituals to rid the body of disease. Many have beliefs and rituals about dying and death.

Box 5-1 lists the top 10 countries of origin of persons who have immigrated to the United States. This list is based on data gathered through 1992 by the U.S. Department of Immigration and Naturalization Services. Box 5-2 on p. 84 gives general information about the health care beliefs of the people of these countries. Throughout this chapter and this book, information about the cultural beliefs and practices of these peoples will be given as appropriate.

Religion relates to spiritual beliefs, needs, and practices. Like culture, a person's religion influences health and illness practices. Religions have beliefs and practices for daily living habits, behaviors, relationships with others, diet, healing, days of worship, birth and birth control, medicine, and death.

Many people rely on religion for support and comfort during illness. They may want to pray and observe certain religious practices. A visit from their spiritual leader or adviser may be helpful. If a person asks to see a cleric, promptly report the request to the RN. Make sure the person's room is neat and orderly. Ensure privacy during the visit.

The nursing process reflects the person's culture and religion. The RN and the person plan measures that include the person's cultural and religious practices. You must show respect and accept the person's culture and religion. When you meet people from other cultures or religions, learn about their beliefs and practices. This helps you understand the person and give better care.

Individuals may not follow every belief and practice of their culture or religion. Remember, each person is unique. Do not judge patients by your own standards. (See Focus on Home Care below.)

focus on HOME CARE

Culture is reflected in the home. Homes vary in size, cleanliness, and furnishings. Some homes are expensive. Others reflect poverty. Whether rich or poor, treat each person and family with respect, kindness, and dignity. Do not judge the person's life-style, habits, religion, or culture.

BOX 5-2

TOP TEN COUNTRIES OF ORIGIN OF IMMIGRANTS TO THE UNITED STATES*: HEALTH CARE BELIEFS

Country	Health Care Beliefs
Mexico	Acute sick care only.
	Health is believed to be a matter of choice or God's will.
	Disease is influenced by hot and cold imbalances.
	Males are viewed as being healthier than females or children.
	Pain or the appearance of blood is used in determining severity of illness.
Vietnam	Acute sick care only.
	Practices such as pinching or scratching the area let the *bad winds* or the unhealthy air currents out of the body and restore health-producing marks or red lines.
	Medicine to restore the yin-yang balance and the hot-cold equilibrium is important.
Philippines	Health promotion is important.
	Mental illness is highly disgraceful.
	The evil eye can be cast upon someone through the eyes or the mouth.
Former Soviet Union	Health promotion is important.
	Maternal and child care are encouraged.
	Health care addresses acute problems.
	Rehabilitation is not emphasized.
Dominican Republic	Hot/cold balance theory is a factor in the cause of disease.
Mainland China	Health promotion is important.
	An upset in body energy is attributed to the cause of disease.
	Health is a state of spiritual and physical harmony with nature; health and illness are not separate but part of a lifelong continuum.
	Some resist surgery because of a religious belief that they do not own their physical bodies, that the soul or spirit will escape from the body and be lost forever if surgery is performed.
	Drawing blood may be resisted because of the belief that blood does not regenerate; blood is perceived as the source of life.
	Stigma is attached to mental illness.
India	Acute sick care only.
	Diseases are believed to be caused by an upset in body balance.
El Salvador	Fresh air, sleep, and good nutrition are important health practices.
Poland	Acute sick care.
United Kingdom	Acute sick care; health promotion is important.

From Geissler EM: Pocket guide to cultural assessment, St Louis, 1994, Mosby.

*Information based on data gathered through 1992 by the U.S. Department of Justice, Immigration and Naturalization Service.

BEING SICK

People cannot choose between health or illness. Illness and injury do occur. Besides physical problems, illness has some psychological and social effects.

Normal activities such as working, going to school, preparing meals, doing house or yard work, and taking part in sports or hobbies may be difficult or impossible. Daily activities bring personal satisfaction, worth, and contact with others. Most people are frustrated and angry when unable to perform them. These feelings may become even greater if others must perform routine functions for the person.

Sick people have many fears and anxieties. They fear death, disability, chronic illness, and loss of function. Some explain why they are afraid. Others keep their feelings to themselves. They fear being laughed at if afraid. A person with a broken leg may fear having a limp or not walking again. Persons having surgery are often afraid of cancer. These fears and anxieties are normal and expected. You must understand how people are affected by illness. Think about how you would feel if you had the person's illness and problems.

Sick people are expected to behave in a certain way. They need to see a doctor, stay in bed, and rely on others for care and comfort. These behaviors are accepted so the person can get well. When recovery is delayed or does not occur, the normal psychological and social effects of illness become greater.

Culture and religion are also factors in how people think and behave when ill. Box 5-3 on p. 86 lists the common sick care practices for persons from the top ten countries of origin of people who have immigrated to the United States. Remember, the information given in Box 5-3 is only general information.

PERSONS YOU WILL CARE FOR

Patients are grouped in health care agencies by their problems, needs, and age. Doctors and nurses have special knowledge and skills to care for certain patients.

- *Mothers and newborns*—**Obstetrics** is the branch of medicine concerned with the care of women during pregnancy, labor, and childbirth and during the 6 to 8 weeks after birth. Patients are seen in clinics or doctors' offices during pregnancy. When labor begins, these women usually are admitted to the obstetrical (maternity) department. Pregnancy, labor, and childbirth are normal and natural events. However, complications can occur at any time during pregnancy through the 6 to 8 weeks after childbirth.

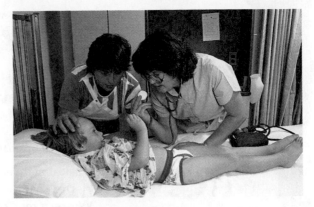

Fig. 5-3 *Care is given to a sick child.*

- *Children*—**Pediatrics** is the branch of medicine concerned with the growth, development, and care of children ranging in age from the newborn to the adolescent. When hospital care is needed, children are admitted to a pediatric unit. The unit is designed and equipped to meet the needs of children and parents. The nursing staff is concerned with the child's physical, safety, and emotional needs (Fig. 5-3).
- *Adults with medical problems*—Medical problems are illnesses, diseases, or injuries that do not need surgery. Patients may have acute, chronic, or terminal illnesses. Examples are infections, strokes, or heart attacks.
- *Persons having surgery*—Surgical patients are those being prepared for or who have had surgery. Surgeries range from simple to very complex. An appendectomy (removal of the appendix) is a simple surgery. Open-heart and brain surgeries are complex. Preoperative care involves preparing the person for what to expect after surgery. The person's fears and anxieties also are dealt with. Needs after surgery relate to relieving pain and discomfort, preventing complications, and adjusting to body changes.
- *Persons with mental health problems*—**Psychiatry** is the branch of medicine concerned with the diagnosis and treatment of people with mental health problems. Problems vary from mild to severe mental and emotional disorders. Some persons function normally but need help making decisions or coping with life stresses. Others are severely disturbed. They cannot do simple things such as eating, bathing, or dressing. Special precautions and treatments are necessary if patients are dangerous to themselves or others.

BOX 5-3

TOP TEN COUNTRIES OF ORIGIN OF IMMIGRANTS TO THE UNITED STATES*: SICK CARE PRACTICES

Country	Sick Care Practices
Mexico	Biomedical; magical and religious; and traditional. Common beliefs include: *mal ojo*—evil eye; *empacho*—bolus of food stuck to stomach wall; *susto*—result of a traumatic emotional experience; *mal puesto*—hex or illness imposed by another.
Vietnam	Magical and religious; Eastern medicine. Herbal medicine is important; most are classified as *cool,* whereas most Western medicines are considered *hot.* Traditionally, illness is dealt with through self-care and self-medication. Folk remedies include variations of acupuncture, massage, herbal remedies, and dermabrasive practices (cupping, pinching, rubbing, and burning).
Philippines	Biomedical; and magical and religious. Combination of home remedies, professional providers, and traditional healers. Fatalism accompanies beliefs that ghosts and spirits control life and death. Taking the powers of the gods is believed to have a cause-and-effect relationship to subsequent bad happenings.
Former Soviet Union	Biomedical; holistic, folk, and Western medical practices.
Dominican Republic	Magical and religious; traditional.
Mainland China	Holistic and traditional. Traditional health care includes cupping, acupuncture, and herbal medicine.
India	Biomedical and traditional. Spiritual values influence most aspects of life and death.
El Salvador	Biomedical.
Poland	Biomedical; magical and religious; folk. Older generations believe in the evil eye (*Szatan*) and in prayer and wearing religious medals and scapulars to help protect them against illness. Folk healers and miracle workers are also sought.
United Kingdom	Biomedical.

From Geissler EM: Pocket guide to cultural assessment, *St Louis, 1994, Mosby.*

*Information based on data gathered through 1992 by the U.S. Department of Justice, Immigration and Naturalization Service.

- *Elderly persons*—**Geriatrics** is the branch of medicine concerned with the problems and diseases of old age and elderly persons. Aging is a normal process. It is not an illness or disease. Many elderly people enjoy good health. Others suffer from acute or chronic illnesses. Some have degenerative diseases common in older persons. Body changes normally occur with the aging process. Social and psychological changes also occur.

- *Persons in special care areas*—Some patients have special problems or are seriously ill. They need special care and equipment. Special care units are designed and equipped to treat and prevent life-threatening problems and complications. These special care areas include intensive care units, coronary care units (Fig. 5-4), kidney dialysis units, burn units, and emergency rooms. RNs in these areas have special education and training. They are prepared to meet the patient's complex needs.

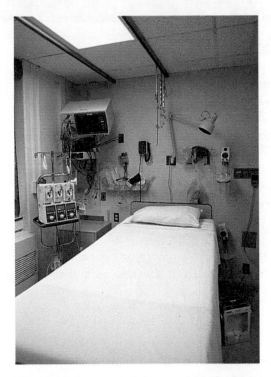

Fig. 5-4 *A general view of the design and equipment in a coronary care unit.*

LONG-TERM CARE

focus on

Residents have rights as citizens of the United States. They also have rights under OBRA (Box 5-5, pp. 89-91). These rights relate to their everyday lives and care in the center. The agency must protect and promote resident rights. Residents must be free to exercise their rights without agency interference (Fig. 5-5). Some residents are incompetent (not able) and cannot exercise their rights. Legal representatives exercise rights for them.

Agencies must inform residents of their rights. They must be informed orally and in writing. Such information is given before or during admission to the center. It must be given in the language used and understood by the resident.

- *Persons requiring rehabilitation*—As described in Chapter 1, rehabilitation is the process of restoring the disabled person to the highest level of functioning possible. The person may need to regain functions lost from surgery, illness, or accidents. Persons with birth defects need to learn skills using existing abilities.
- *Persons requiring subacute care*—Subacute care has a strong rehabilitation focus. Persons needing subacute care have a longer recovery period than persons with acute illnesses. However, long-term care or lengthy rehabilitation is not needed. Persons may need subacute care after joint replacement surgery. Persons with some lung and nervous system disorders may have longer recovery periods and need rehabilitation.

PATIENT RIGHTS

Patient rights came about when people demanded more information about their health problems and treatment. They also demanded better care at lower costs and greater involvement in treatment decisions. Patients were not willing to be helpless and to accept the doctor's advice without question.

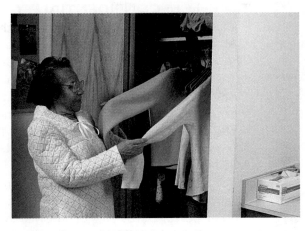

Fig. 5-5 *A resident chooses what to wear. This is based on the right to personal choice.*

A Patient's Bill of Rights was issued by the American Hospital Association (AHA). It has an ethical and legal basis. The right to privacy and informed consent are involved. Although the relationship between the doctor and the patient is stressed, there are important messages for the health team. The basic points of *A Patient's Bill of Rights* are presented in Box 5-4, p. 88. (See Focus on Long-Term Care above.)

Text continued on p. 92

BOX 5-4

PATIENT RIGHTS

The right to CONSIDERATION AND RESPECT
- The patient is treated as a person and given kind and thoughtful care.
- Personal values, beliefs, cultural practices, and personality are considered when planning and providing care.

The right to INFORMATION
- The patient receives information from the doctor about the diagnosis, treatment, and prognosis in terms the patient can understand.
- Unfamiliar medical terminology is avoided.
- An interpreter is needed if the patient does not understand or speak English.
- The nearest relative or legal representative is informed of the patient's diagnosis, treatment, and prognosis if it is unwise to tell the patient.

The right to INFORMED CONSENT
- The patient receives information and explanations about any treatments or procedures.
- The doctor provides information about a treatment's purpose, risks, alternatives, and the probable length of recovery.
- The patient is told who will perform the treatment or procedure.

The right to REFUSE TREATMENT
- The person can refuse treatment.
- The patient does not have to consent to each treatment or procedure recommended by the doctor.
- The doctor must inform the patient of the risks to life and health involved in refusing the treatment.

The right to PRIVACY
- The patient's body, record, care, and personal affairs are kept private.
- The right to privacy is still protected after death.

The right to CONFIDENTIALITY
- Information is shared with other health workers in a wise and careful manner.
- All health workers must recognize the confidential nature of patient information.

The right to HOSPITAL SERVICES
- The patient has the right to expect that the hospital can provide needed services.
- After immediate needs are met, the patient may be transferred to another agency better equipped to handle the patient's problems and needs.
- The patient is informed of the reason for the transfer and of other alternatives.

The right to INFORMATION ABOUT THE HOSPITAL'S RELATIONSHIP TO OTHER AGENCIES
- The patient is informed of any relationships with schools and other health care agencies.
- Patients have the right to know about these relationships and to know the names of students or other persons providing or involved in their care.

The right to INFORMATION ON RESEARCH AND HUMAN EXPERIMENTATION
- The patient receives information and explanations about research for making an informed decision about participating.
- The patient's consent is obtained before involvement in human experimentation or research.
- The patient may refuse to participate.

The right to CONTINUING CARE
- The patient is informed of the care needed after discharge.
- The patient is given written information about the times and locations of appointments with doctors.

The right to THE PATIENT'S BILL
- The patient has the right to examine bills and receive an explanation of the items in the bill.
- This right exists even if the bill is to be paid by an insurance company or the government.

The right to KNOW HOSPITAL RULES AND REGULATIONS
- The patient is informed of any rules and regulations applying to his or her conduct as a patient.
- The patient and family are given pamphlets that explain the rules and regulations.

BOX 5-5

RESIDENT RIGHTS

The right to INFORMATION

- The resident has the right to all records. This includes the medical record, contracts, incident reports, and financial records.
  - The request can be oral or written.
  - The record must be available within 24 hours of the request.
  - The agency has 2 working days to provide requested photocopies.
- The person must be fully informed of his or her total health condition.
  - Information is given in language the person can understand.
  - Interpreters are used for those speaking a language other than English.
  - Sign language or other aids are used for persons with hearing impairments.
- The person is given information about his or her doctor. This includes the doctor's name, specialty, and how to contact the doctor.

The right to REFUSE TREATMENT

- OBRA defines treatment as care provided to relieve symptoms, improve functional level, or maintain or restore health. A person who does not give consent or refuses treatment cannot be given the treatment.
- The agency must find out what the resident is refusing and why. The agency should try to educate the person about the treatment, problems from not having the treatment, and other treatment choices.
- Although the resident may refuse a specific treatment, the agency must provide all other services.
- Advance directives are part of the right to refuse treatment (see Chapter 36). They include living wills or other instructions about life support.
- The resident has the right to refuse to take part in research.

The right to PRIVACY

- The resident's body must not be exposed unnecessarily.
- Only those workers directly involved in care, treatments, or examinations should be present. The resident must give consent for others to be present.
- A resident has the right to use the bathroom in private.
- Privacy must be maintained for personal care activities.
- Residents have the right to visit with others in private.
  - They have the right to visit in an area where they cannot be seen or heard by others.
  - The agency must try to provide private space when it is requested. Offices, chapels, dining rooms, meeting rooms, activity rooms, and conference rooms can be used if available.
- Residents have the right to private telephone conversations.
- Residents have the right to send and receive mail without interference by others.
  - Letters sent and received by the resident are not opened by others without the resident's permission.
  - Mail must be delivered to the resident within 24 hours of its delivery to the center.

The right to CONFIDENTIALITY

- Information about the resident's care, treatment, and condition must be kept confidential.
- Medical and financial records are confidential.
- The resident must give consent for the release of any record to other agencies or persons.
  - Consent is not needed for the release of medical records when the resident is transferred to another agency.
  - Consent is not needed to release records when they are required by law or for insurance purposes.

Continued

BOX 5-5

RESIDENT RIGHTS—cont'd

The right to PERSONAL CHOICE

* Residents can choose their own doctors.
* Residents have the right to participate in planning their own care and treatment. This includes making decisions about their own care and treatment.
* Residents have the right to choose activities, schedules, and care based on their personal preferences. This includes choosing when to get up and go to bed, what to wear, how to spend their time, and what to eat (see Fig. 5-5).
* Residents are also free to choose companions and visitors inside and outside of the center.

The right to DISPUTES AND GRIEVANCES

* Residents have the right to voice concerns, questions, and complaints about treatment or care. The dispute or grievance may involve another resident. It may be about treatment or care that was not given.
* The agency must promptly try to correct the situation. The resident must not be punished in any way for voicing the dispute or grievance.

The right to NOT TO WORK

* The resident does not work to receive care, items, or other things or privileges.
* The resident *can* work or perform services if the desire or need for work is part of the resident's care plan.
  * The resident may like gardening, repairing things, building things, sewing, mending, cooking, or other work. The resident may want to work. Another resident may need to work for rehabilitation or activity purposes. In either case, the desire for work or the need for work should become part of the resident's care plan.
  * The care plan should specify the reason for the work (desire or need); what work will be done; if the services are paid or voluntary.

The right to PARTICIPATE IN RESIDENT AND FAMILY GROUPS

* Residents have the right to form groups.
* A resident's family has the right to meet with the families of other residents.
* Groups can discuss concerns and offer ideas to improve quality of life in the center. They can also plan activities for residents and families. Or the groups can provide support and reassurance for group members.
* Residents have the right to take part in social, religious, and community activities.
* Residents have the right to assistance in getting to and from activities of their choice.

The right to CARE AND SECURITY OF PERSONAL POSSESSIONS

* Residents have the right to keep and use personal items. This includes clothing and some furnishings.
* A person's property must be treated with care and respect. Although items may not have value to you, they are important to the resident. They also relate to personal choice, dignity, and quality of life.
* The agency must take reasonable measures to protect the person's property.
  * Items are labeled with the resident's name.
  * The agency must investigate reports of lost, stolen, or damaged items. Police help is sometimes needed.
* The resident and family are advised not to keep jewelry and other expensive items in the center.
* No one can go through a resident's closet, drawers, purse, or other space without the person's knowledge and consent. Have another worker with you and the resident or legal representative present if you must inspect closets and drawers. The worker serves as a witness to your activities.

BOX 5-5

RESIDENT RIGHTS—cont'd

The right to FREEDOM FROM ABUSE, MISTREATMENT, AND NEGLECT

- Residents must be free from verbal, sexual, physical, or mental abuse (see Chapter 2).
- Residents have the right to be free from involuntary seclusion. **Involuntary seclusion** is separating the resident from others against his or her will. It can also mean keeping the person confined to a certain area or away from his or her room without consent.
- No one can abuse, neglect, or mistreat the resident. This includes center staff, volunteers, staff from other agencies or groups, other residents, family, visitors, and legal guardians.
- Agencies must have policies and procedures for investigating suspected or reported cases of resident abuse.
- Long-term care centers cannot employ persons who were convicted of abusing, neglecting, or mistreating other individuals.

The right to FREEDOM FROM RESTRAINTS

- Residents have the right not to have body movements restricted.
  - Restraints (see Chapter 10) and some drugs restrict body movements. Some drugs restrain the person because they affect mood, behavior, and mental function.
- A doctor's order is necessary to use restraints.
  - Sometimes residents are restrained to protect them from harming themselves or others.
  - Restraints cannot be used for the convenience of the staff or to discipline a resident.

The right to QUALITY OF LIFE

- Residents must be cared for in a manner that promotes dignity, self-worth, and physical, psychological, and emotional well-being.
  - Personal choice, privacy, participation in group activities, having personal property, and freedom from restraint show respect for the person.
  - The resident is spoken to in a polite and courteous manner (see Chapter 6).
  - Good, honest, and thoughtful care enhances the resident's quality of life.
- The actions in Box 5-6 on p. 92 show concern for the person's dignity and privacy. These actions are required by OBRA.
- Long-term care centers must provide activity programs that meet the interests and physical, mental, and psychosocial needs of each resident.
- Activities must allow personal choice and promote physical, intellectual, social, and emotional well-being.
- The center's environment must promote quality of life.
- The environment must be clean and safe and be as homelike as possible.
- Residents are allowed to have personal possessions. This allows personal choice and promotes a homelike environment.

BOX 5-6

OBRA-REQUIRED ACTIONS TO PROMOTE THE RESIDENT'S DIGNITY AND PRIVACY

Courteous and dignified interactions with residents
- Use appropriate tone of voice (see Chapter 6).
- Use good eye contact when interacting with the resident (see Chapter 6).
- Stand or sit close enough to the resident as appropriate.
- Use the resident's proper name and title.
- Obtain the resident's attention before interacting with the resident.
- Use touch if approved by the resident (see Chapter 6).
- Respect the resident's social status, and listen with interest to what the resident is saying.
- Do not yell, scold, or embarrass the resident.

Courteous and dignified care to residents
- Groom hair, beards, and nails as the resident wishes.
- Assist with dressing in clothing appropriate to time of day and resident's personal choice.
- Promote the residents' independence and dignity in dining.
- Respect resident's private space and property.
- Assist with ambulation and transfer without interfering with independence.
- Assist with bathing and personal hygiene preferences without interfering with independence
  - The resident is neat and clean.
  - The resident is clean shaven or has groomed beard.
  - Nails are trimmed and clean.
  - Dentures, hearing aid, glasses, and other prostheses are used as appropriate.
  - Clothing fits, is clean, and is properly fastened.
  - Shoes and hose are properly applied and fastened.
  - Extra clothing is available for warmth (such as sweaters or lap blankets).

Privacy and self-determination of residents
- Resident is draped properly during personal care and procedures to avoid exposure and embarrassment.
- Resident is draped properly in chair.
- Use curtains or screens during personal care and procedures.
- Close door to the room during care and procedures or as resident desires.
- Knock on the door before entering, and wait to be asked in.
- Provide privacy during examinations with draping and curtains or screen.
- Close the bathroom door when the resident uses the bathroom.

Maintain personal choice and independence
- Resident smokes in designated areas.
- Resident participates in activities according to interests.
- Resident is involved in scheduling activities and care.
- Resident gives input into plan of care regarding preferences and independence.
- Resident is involved in a room or roommate change.

From Jaffe MS: The OBRA guidelines for quality improvement, *El Paso, 1993, Skidmore-Roth Publishing Co.*

THE FAMILY AND VISITORS

Family, relatives, and friends help meet the person's needs for safety and security, love and belonging, and self-esteem. They offer support and comfort and lessen loneliness. Some also help with the person's care—meals, bathing, brushing and combing hair, and other care. The presence or absence of significant family members or friends can affect recovery. Box 5-7 on p. 93 describes family roles in hospital care for some cultural groups.

BOX 5-7

TOP TEN COUNTRIES OF ORIGIN OF IMMIGRANTS TO THE UNITED STATES*: FAMILY ROLES IN HOSPITAL CARE

Country	Family Roles in Hospital Care
Mexico	The male should be consulted before health care decisions are made and should be included in any counseling sessions.
	Culturally, a mother is not allowed the authority to give consent for her child's treatment.
	Family decisions overrule decisions made by health care providers.
	Women may not give care at home if that care involves touching adult male genitalia.
Vietnam	The patient is considered a person who needs to be taken care of by all family members.
Philippines	A child may feel an obligation to the parent who is ill and spend hours giving care.
	The family may decide to give physical care.
Former Soviet Union	Family members usually bathe, feed, and comfort the patient, as well as change bed linen.
Dominican Republic	No information.
Mainland China	A family member may be given leave from work to care for an aged relative.
	The family traditionally remains with the patient during hospitalization.
	They supply food and assist with feeding, bathing, and keeping the patient comfortable.
India	No information.
El Salvador	No information.
Poland	Parents may wish to be involved in caring for their hospitalized child.
United Kingdom	No information.

From Geissler EM: Pocket guide to cultural assessment, St Louis, 1994, Mosby.

*Information based on data gathered through 1992 by the U.S. Department of Justice, Immigration and Naturalization Service.

The person should visit with family and friends in private and without unnecessary interruptions (Fig. 5-6). Sometimes care must be given when visitors are present. Politely ask them to leave the room and show them a comfortable waiting area. Do not expose the person's body in front of visitors. Promptly tell visitors when they may return to the room.

Family and visitors are treated with courtesy and respect. They have concerns and fears about the person's condition. They need support and understanding from the nursing team. However, do not discuss the person's condition with them. Refer their questions to the RN.

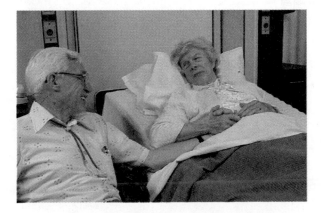

Fig. 5-6 *A patient visits with her husband.*

Visitors often have questions about visiting rules. The number of visitors allowed and the visiting hours vary among agencies. Often they depend on the person's age or condition. A child's parents can usually visit as often and as long as they want. Only short visits are allowed in special care units. Dying persons can usually have family members present constantly. Know your agency's visiting policies and the special needs of individual patients. Visitors may also have questions about where to find the chapel, gift shop, business office, lounge, or dining room. You must know the location, special rules, and hours of these facilities.

Sometimes a visitor can upset or tire a patient. Report your observations to the RN. The RN will speak with the visitor about the person's needs. (See Focus on Home Care and Focus on Older Persons.)

focus on HOME CARE

Family personalities and attitudes affect the mood in the home. Many families are happy and supportive. Others have poor relationships. Mental illness, alcoholism, drug addiction, unemployment, delinquency, and physical illness may affect the family. Some families have difficulty adjusting to or accepting the person's illness or disability.

Your supervisor explains the nature of any family problems to you. Do not get involved in family problems. Always maintain a professional manner and have empathy. However, do not give advice, take sides, or make judgments about family conflicts.

focus on OLDER PERSONS

Sometimes older brothers, sisters, and cousins live together. They provide companionship and share living expenses. They care for each other during illness or disability. One may be the caregiver if the other is ill or disabled.

Some elderly people live with their adult children. The elderly parent may be healthy, need some supervision, or be ill or disabled. The elderly parent (or parents) moves in with the child or the child moves into the parent's home. Living with a child can help the elderly person feel safe and secure. Often the adult child is a caregiver for an ill or disabled parent.

Adult children often need to work even though the elderly parent cannot be left alone. *Adult day care* centers provide meals, supervision, and activities for older persons. Activities include cards, board games, movies, crafts, dancing, walks, and lectures. Some provide bowling and swimming. All activities are supervised. Assistance is given as needed. Some provide transportation from home to the center.

Living with an adult child is a social change. The parent, adult child, and the child's family all need to adjust. The adult child's family still needs time alone. Other brothers, sisters, and family members may help give care. *Respite care* provides a break for the family. The older person enters a long-term care center for a few days or weeks. This gives caregivers a vacation, rest, or simply a break from the stress of giving care. Community and church groups often have volunteers who can help give care.

REVIEW QUESTIONS

Circle the best *answer.*

1 Sally Jones had gallbladder surgery. You must be concerned

   a Only with her nursing care plan

   b With her physical, safety and security and self-esteem needs

   c With her as a physical, psychological, social, and spiritual person

   d Only with her cultural and religious needs

2 Which basic need is the most essential?

   a Self-actualization

   b Esteem needs

   c Love and belonging

   d Safety and security

3 Based on Maslow's theory of basic needs, which person's needs must be met first?

   a Mr. Hart, who wants another blanket

   b Miss Parks, who asks you to read her mail to her

   c Ms. Street, who asks for more water

   d Mr. Hill, who is crying

4 Sally Jones said "I don't know what they are going to do to me." What basic need is not being met?

   a Physical needs

   b The need for safety and security

   c The need for love and belonging

   d Self-esteem needs

5 Which is *false?*

   a A person's cultural background influences health and illness practices.

   b Culture and religion influence dietary practices.

   c A person's religious and cultural practices are not allowed in the hospital.

   d A person may not follow all of the beliefs and practices of his or her religion or culture.

6 Geriatrics is the branch of medicine dealing with a disease commonly known as aging.

   a True

   b False

7 As a patient, Sally Jones has the right to

   a Considerate and respectful care

   b Information about her diagnoses, treatment, and prognosis

   c Refuse treatment

   d All of the above

8 The right to privacy is protected after death.

   a True

   b False

9 You are working in a long-term care center. You must

   a Open a resident's mail

   b Choose what the resident will wear

   c Provide for the resident's privacy

   d Search the resident's closet and drawers

10 Who decides how a resident's hair should be styled?

   a The resident

   b The nurse

   c The assistive person

   d The family

11 Which statement is *false?*

   a Residents can offer suggestions to improve the center.

   b Residents can be restrained to prevent them from leaving the center.

   c Residents must be free from abuse, neglect, and mistreatment.

   d Allowing personal choice is important for the resident's quality of life.

12 Sally Jones has many visitors. Which is *true?*

   a Family and friends can help meet her basic needs.

   b Privacy should be allowed.

   c Visitors should be politely asked to leave the room when care must be given.

   d All of the above

Answers to these questions are on p. 850.

6 Communicating With the Person

- Define the key terms in this chapter
- Identify the elements needed for effective communication
- Describe how verbal and nonverbal communication are used
- Explain the techniques and barriers to effective communication
- Explain how to deal with the angry person
- Explain how to admit, transfer, and discharge patients

KEY TERMS

admission Official entry of a person into an agency or nursing unit

body language Facial expressions, gestures, posture, and body movements that send messages to others

discharge Official departure of a person from an agency or nursing unit

nonverbal communication Communication that does not involve words

paraphrasing Restating the person's message in your own words

transfer Moving a person from one room, nursing unit, or agency to another

verbal communication Communication that uses the written or spoken word

Remember, communication involves sending and receiving messages. You communicate with patients every time you give care. You give information to the patient, and the patient gives information to you. Your body sends messages all the time—at the bedside, in the hallway, at the nurses' station, in the dining room, and everywhere else. Patients and families are aware of what you say. They also are aware of what you do. Good work ethics and understanding the person are necessary for good communication. What you say and do also are important.

EFFECTIVE COMMUNICATION

Several elements are necessary for effective communication between you and the patient.

- You must understand and respect the patient as a person.
- You must view the person as more than a disease or an illness. The person is a physical, psychological, social, and spiritual human being.
- You must appreciate the person's problems and frustrations from being sick.
- You must recognize and respect the person's rights.
- You must accept and respect the person's religion and culture.

Communication rules discussed in Chapter 4 apply when you communicate with patients.

- Use words that have the same meaning to both you and the person.
- Avoid medical terminology and other words that are unfamiliar to the person.
- Communicate in a logical and orderly manner. Do not wander in thought.
- Give specific and factual information.
- Be brief and concise

VERBAL AND NONVERBAL COMMUNICATION

Communication is what you say and do. You communicate verbally and nonverbally with patients. You must use both methods effectively.

Verbal Communication

Words are used in **verbal communication.** The words are spoken or written. Verbal communication is used to talk with patients, to find out how they are feeling, and to share information with them.

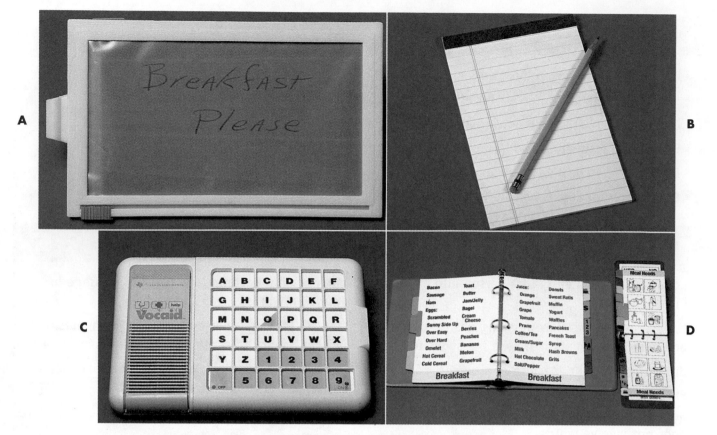

Fig. 6-1 A, *A Magic Slate.* **B,** *Paper and pencil.* **C,** *Electronic talking aid.* **D,** *Communication and picture board.*

Most verbal communication involves the spoken word. Shouting, whispering, and mumbling cause ineffective communication. You need to:

- Control the loudness and tone of your voice
- Speak clearly, slowly, and distinctly
- Avoid using slang or vulgar words
- Repeat information as needed
- Ask one question at a time, and wait for the answer; do not ask several questions at once

The written word is used when persons cannot speak or hear. If a person cannot speak, provide a way for the person to send messages. A Magic Slate, paper and pencil, an electronic talking aid, picture board, or a communication board are useful (Fig. 6-1). Write messages to communicate with deaf persons or those with severe hearing problems. Deaf persons may use speech reading and sign language to communicate (see Chapter 30).

Nonverbal Communication

Nonverbal communication does not use words. Gestures, facial expressions, posture, body movements, touch, and smell are examples of sending and receiving messages without words. Nonverbal messages more accurately reflect a person's feelings. They are usually involuntary and hard to control. A person may say one thing but act in a different way. Therefore you need to watch the person's eyes, hand movements, gestures, posture, and other actions.

Touch

Touch is a very important form of nonverbal communication. It conveys comfort, caring, love, affection, and reassurance. Touch means different things to different people. The meaning depends on the person's age, culture (Box 6-1), gender (male or female), and life experiences. Some people do not like being touched. However, do not be afraid to use touch to convey caring and warmth. Patients are often comforted by stroking or having their hands held. Touch should be gentle, not hurried or rough. Touch should not be sexual in nature.

BOX 6-1

TOP TEN COUNTRIES OF ORIGIN OF IMMIGRANTS TO THE UNITED STATES*: TOUCH PRACTICES

Country	Touch Practices
Mexico	Touch is used often.
	Touching people while complimenting them neutralizes the power of the evil eye in some believers.
Vietnam	The head is considered the seat of the soul and should not be touched.
	Only the older persons are allowed to touch the heads of young children.
	Touching persons of the same sex is acceptable.
	The female breast is accepted as the means of infant feeding.
	The lower torso is extremely private. The area between the waist and knees is kept covered, even in private.
	Handshaking has wide acceptance with men but not with women. A man will not extend his hand in handshake to a woman or a superior.
	Sisters and brothers do not touch or kiss each other.
Philippines	In some parts of the country, people believe that the evil eye can be neutralized on a child by putting a bit of saliva on the finger and making the sign of the cross on a child's forehead when giving a compliment.
	Touch is stressed.
Former Soviet Union	Three kisses on the cheek for greeting and for farewells are common.
	Touch is an important part of nonverbal communication.
Dominican Republic	No information.
Mainland China	Chinese do not like to be touched by strangers. Nod or slight bow is given when introduced.
India	Men may shake hands with other men but not with women. Instead, the man places his palms together and bows slightly
El Salvador	No information.
Poland	Hugging and kissing on the cheek are acceptable between sexes.
United Kingdom	The English have generally low touch practices.

From Geissler EM: *Pocket guide to cultural assessment*, St Louis, 1994, Mosby.

*Information based on data gathered through 1992 by the U.S. Department of Justice, Immigration and Naturalization Service.

Body language

People send messages through their **body language.** Body language includes:

- Posture
- Gait
- Facial expressions
- Eye contact
- Hand movements
- Gestures
- Body movements
- Appearance (dress, hygiene, and adornments such as jewelry, perfume, and cosmetics)

Patients send messages with their body language. Slumped posture may mean the person is not happy or not feeling well. A person may deny pain but protects the affected body part by standing, lying, or sitting in a certain way. Patients send many other messages with body language.

You also send messages by the way you act and move. Your facial expressions and how you stand, sit, walk, and look at a person all send messages. Your body language should show interest and enthusiasm about your work. It should also show caring and respect for the person. You need to control your body language in many instances. For example, do not react to odors from excretions or the person's body. Many odors are beyond the person's control. The person's embarrassment and humiliation increase if you react to the odor.

BOX 6-2

TOP TEN COUNTRIES OF ORIGIN OF IMMIGRANTS TO THE UNITED STATES*: EYE CONTACT PRACTICES

Country	Eye Contact Practices
Mexico	Sustained direct eye contact is rude, immodest, or dangerous for some. *Mal ojo* (evil eye) is the result of admiration. Women and children are thought to be more susceptible to *mal ojo;* therefore children may avoid direct eye contact.
Vietnam	Blinking means only that a message has been received. Looking directly into another's eyes when talking is considered disrespectful.
Philippines	Some may fear eye contact. However, if it is established, it is important to return and to maintain eye contact.
Former Soviet Union	Direct, sustained eye contact is the norm.
Dominican Republic	No information.
Mainland China	Gazing around and looking to one side when listening to another are polite. With older persons, direct eye contact is used.
India	No information.
El Salvador	No information.
Poland	Direct eye contact is made.
United Kingdom	Staring is believed to be a part of good listening. Understanding is indicated by blinking the eyes.

From Geissler EM: *Pocket guide to cultural assessment*, St Louis, 1994, Mosby.

*Information based on data gathered through 1992 by the U.S. Department of Justice, Immigration and Naturalization Service.

COMMUNICATION TECHNIQUES

Certain techniques help you communicate with patients and families. The techniques result in better relationships with these persons. You also gain more information for the nursing process. The following techniques also are helpful when communicating with staff and your own family

Listening

Listening means being attentive to the person's verbal and nonverbal communication. You use the senses of sight, hearing, touch, and smell. You must concentrate on what the person is saying. You also observe nonverbal clues. The person's nonverbal communication can support what the person says. Or it can show other feelings. For example, Mr. Hart says "I want to go to a nursing home. That way my daughter won't have to stay home to care for me." However, you see tears in his eyes and he looks away from you. His verbal says happy, but his nonverbal shows sadness.

Listening requires that you care and have interest. The following guidelines are important:

- Face the person.
- Have good eye contact with the person. See Box 6-2 for the eye contact practices of other cultures.
- Lean toward the person (Fig. 6-2). Do not sit back with your arms crossed.
- Respond to the person. Nod your head. Say "uh huh," "mmm," and "I see." Repeat what the person says, and ask questions.
- Avoid the barriers to effective communication (p. 101).

Paraphrasing

Paraphrasing is restating the person's message in your own words. You use fewer words than the person did to send the message. Paraphrasing serves three purposes:

- It shows you are listening.
- It lets the person see if you understand the message sent.
- It promotes further communication.

The person usually responds to your statement. For example:

Patient: My wife was crying after she spoke with the doctor. I don't know what he said to her.

You: You don't know why your wife was crying.

Patient: He must have told her that I have a tumor.

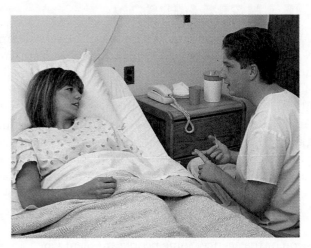

Fig. 6-2 *Listen by facing the person, having good eye contact, and leaning toward the person.*

Direct Questions

Direct questions focus on specific information. You ask the person something you need to know. Some direct questions have "yes" or "no" answers. Others require the person to give more information. For example:

You: Mr. Hart, do you want to shave this morning?

Patient: Yes.

You: Mr. Hart, when would you like to shave and have your bath?

Patient: Could we start in about 15 minutes? I'd like to call my son first.

You: Yes, we can start in 15 minutes. Did you have a bowel movement today, Mr. Hart?

Patient: No.

You: You said you didn't eat well this morning. Can you tell me what you ate?

Patient: I only had toast and coffee. I just don't feel like eating this morning.

Open-ended Questions

Open-ended questions lead or invite the person to share thoughts, feelings, or ideas. The person chooses what to talk about. Answers require more than a "yes" or "no." However, the person controls what is talked about and the information given. Consider these examples:

- "What do you like about living with your daughter?"
- "Tell me about your grandson."
- "What was your wife like?"
- "What do you like about being retired?"

The person chooses how to answer the question. Responses to open-ended questions generally are longer and give more information than direct questions.

Clarifying

Clarifying lets you make sure that you understand the message. You can ask the person to repeat the message, say you do not understand, or restate the message. For example:

- "Could you say that again?"
- "I'm sorry, Mr. Hart. I don't understand what you mean."
- "Are you saying that you want to go home?"

Focusing

Focusing is dealing with a specific topic. It is useful when a person rambles or wanders in thought. For example, Mr. Daley talks at length about his favorite foods and places to eat. You need to know why he did not eat breakfast. You focus the conversation on breakfast by saying: "Let's talk about today's breakfast. You said you didn't feel like eating."

Silence

Silence is a very powerful way to communicate. Sometimes, especially during sad times, you do not need to say anything. Just being there shows you care. At other times, silence gives you or the person time to think, organize thoughts, or choose words. Silence is useful when making difficult decisions. It is also useful when the person is upset and needs time to regain control. Silence on your part shows caring and respect for the person's situation and feelings.

Sometimes pauses or long silences are uncomfortable. Do not think you need to talk when the person is silent. The person may need silence. Dealing with silence gets easier as you gain experience in your role.

COMMUNICATION BARRIERS

Communication barriers prevent sending and receiving messages effectively. Communication fails. You must avoid the following barriers:

- Using unfamiliar language. You and the person must use and understand the same language. If not, messages are not accurately interpreted.
- Changing the subject. Either you or the person change the subject when the topic is uncomfortable. Avoid changing the subject whenever possible.
- Giving your opinion. This tells the person that you are judging his or her values, behavior, or feelings. Let others express their feelings and concerns without adding your opinion, making a judgment, or jumping to conclusions.

- Talking a lot when others are silent. Excessive talking is usually because of nervousness and discomfort with silence. Silences have meaning. They convey acceptance, rejection, fear, or the need for quiet and time to think.
- Failure to listen. Communication is blocked if you fail to listen with interest and sincerity. Do not pretend to listen. This causes inappropriate responses and conveys a lack of interest and caring. You can miss important complaints of pain, discomfort, or other abnormal sensations that must be reported to the RN.
- Pat answers. "Don't worry," "Everything will be okay," and "Your doctor knows best" block communication. These make patients feel that you are ridiculing their concerns, feelings, and fears. They think you do not care about what they think or feel.
- Illness. Some central nervous system disorders affect speech and body movements. The person may be unable to speak. Disorders that affect movement interfere with nonverbal communication.

THE ANGRY PERSON

Anger is a common emotion seen in patients and families. The many causes of anger include fear, pain, and death and dying. Loss of body function and lose of control of one's health and life also cause anger. So do long waits for treatment or to see the doctor.

Anger also is a symptom of diseases that affect thinking and behavior. Persons who abuse alcohol and drugs are likely to show anger. Also, some people are generally angry. Few things please them or make them happy.

Anger is communicated verbally and nonverbally. Verbal outbursts, shouting, raised voices, and rapid speech are common. The person tells you what to do or threatens you or the agency. Some people are silent when angry. Others are uncooperative and may refuse to answer questions. Nonverbal signs of anger include rapid movements, pacing, clenched fists, and a reddened face. Glaring and getting close to you when speaking are other signs. Violent behaviors can occur.

Good communication is important to prevent and deal with anger. Follow the guidelines in Box 6-3.

BOX 6-3

DEALING WITH THE ANGRY PERSON

- Recognize frustrating and frightening situations. Put yourself in the person's situation. How would you feel? How would you want to be treated?
- Treat the person with dignity and respect.
- Answer the person's questions clearly and thoroughly. Ask the RN to answer questions you cannot answer.
- Keep the person informed. Tell the person what you are going to do and when.
- Do not keep the person waiting for long periods. Answer call bells promptly. If you tell the person that you will do something for him or her, do it promptly.
- Explain the reason for long waits. Ask if there is something you can get or do for the person to increase his or her comfort.
- Stay calm and professional if the person directs anger and hostility toward you. Often the person is not angry at you, but at another person or situation.
- Do not argue with the person.
- Listen, and use silence. The person may feel better if able to express angry feelings.
- Report the person's behavior to the RN. Discuss how you should deal with the person.
- Protect yourself from violent behaviors (see Chapter 10, p. 189).

ADMITTING, TRANSFERRING, AND DISCHARGING PATIENTS

Your first communication with the person often occurs when the person is admitted to the nursing unit. The patient may be new to the agency or be transferred from another nursing unit within the agency. This is your first chance to make a good impression of yourself and the agency.

Patients leave your unit because of a transfer or discharge. That is your last chance to leave a good impression. You want the patient to leave feeling good about you, the nursing unit, the agency, and the care given.

All that you have learned in these first six chapters applies when admitting, transferring, and discharging patients. This includes privacy, confidentiality, reporting and recording, communicating with the health team, communication rules, and understanding and communicating with patients. Respect for the person and the person's property also apply.

Admissions

Admission is the official entry of a person into an agency or nursing unit. Admitting office staff or a nurse obtains identifying information (see Chapter 4). The information is recorded on the admission record. The person is given an identification (ID) number and an ID bracelet.

An RN usually greets and admits the person. It may be your responsibility if the person has no serious discomfort or distress (Fig. 6-3). The following are part of the admission process:

- Greet the person by name. Use the admission record to find out the person's name. Ask if he or she prefers a certain name.
- Introduce yourself to the person and relatives or friends who may be present. Give your title, and explain that you assist the nurses in giving care.
- Introduce the roommate.
- Provide for privacy. Ask family members or friends to leave the room. Tell them how much time you need and where they can wait comfortably. (Allow a family member or friend to stay if the person prefers.)

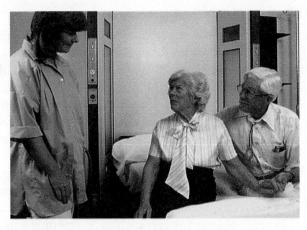

Fig. 6-3 *The assistive person introduces herself to the patient and family member.*

- Have the person put on a gown or pajamas. Assist as needed. Make sure the person is comfortable.
- Complete a clothing and valuables list (see Chapter 10).
- Hang clothes in the closet. Put personal items in the drawers and bedside stand.
- Measure vital signs (see Chapter 23). Weigh and measure the person (see Chapter 26).
- Obtain a urine specimen if ordered (see Chapter 17).
- Orient the person to furniture and equipment in the room. Also explain visiting hours, meal times, and the location of the nurses' station, lounge, chapel, dining room, and gift shop.
- Fill the water pitcher if oral fluids are allowed (see Chapter 20). Provide a drinking cup and straw.
- Place the call bell within reach (see Chapter 10). Place other controls and needed items within reach. Explain how to use the call bell and bed and TV controls.
- Keep the bed in its lowest position (see Chapter 10).
- Raise or bed side rails as instructed by the RN (see Chapter 10).

Transfers

A **transfer** is moving a person from one room, nursing unit, or agency to another. Reasons for the transfer are explained by the doctor or RN. The RN also notifies the family and business office. You may assist in the transfer. This involves transporting the patient and the patient's belongings. The patient is transferred by wheelchair, stretcher, or bed. The person's belongings are transported by utility cart.

The person needs support and reassurance during a transfer. The person is going to a new unit or agency and does not know the staff. Use good communication skills at this time. Avoid pat answers such as "everything will be OK." Touch is often comforting at this time. Also help the person by introducing him or her to new nursing team members. Wish the person well as you leave him or her.

Discharges

Discharge is the official departure of a person from an agency or nursing unit. This is a happy time if the person is going home. Some people are discharged to another hospital or to a long-term care center. Some need home care. The doctor, nurse, dietitian, social worker, and other health team members plan the person's discharge.

The doctor writes a discharge order allowing the person to leave. The RN tells you when the person can leave and how to transport him or her. You assist the person with dressing and packing. You also assist in transporting the person to the exit area. As with transfers, use good communication skills. Wish the person well as he or she leaves the agency.

REVIEW QUESTIONS

Circle the best *answer.*

1 Which is *false?*

a Verbal communication involves the written or spoken word.

b Verbal communication is the truest reflection of a person's feelings.

c Messages are sent by facial expressions, gestures, posture, body movements, appearance, and eye contact.

d Touch means different things to different people.

2 To communicate with Sam Long you should

a Use medical words and phrases

b Change the subject often to show you care about his interests and concerns

c Give your opinion when he shares fears and concerns

d Be quiet when he is silent

3 You and Sam Long are talking. Which might mean that you are not listening?

a You sit facing him.

b You have good eye contact with him.

c You sit with your arms crossed.

d You ask him questions.

4 You and Sally Jones are talking about her surgery. Which is a direct question?

a "Do you feel better now?"

b "Tell me what your plans are for home."

c "What will you do when you get home?"

d "You said that you will be off work for awhile."

5 Sally Jones wants to take a shower. You say "You would like a shower." This is

a Focusing

b Clarifying

c Paraphrasing

d An open-ended question

6 Focusing is a useful communication tool when

a A person is rambling

b You want to make sure you understand the message

c You want the person to share thoughts and feelings

d You need certain information

7 Which is not a barrier to communication?

a Using silence

b Giving your opinions

c Changing the subject

d Illness

8 A patient is angry. Which is *true?*

a The person probably has disease that affects thinking and behavior.

b Drug or alcohol abuse is likely.

c You can tell the person to calm down and that everything will be fine.

d Listening and the use of silence are important.

9 You are admitting a patient to the nursing unit. Your first action is to

a Greet the person by name

b Ask the person his or her name

c Tell the person that everything will be OK

d Introduce the roommate

10 A patient is discharged. You should

a Tell the person that everything will be OK

b Tell the person not to worry

c Wish the person well

d Introduce the patient to new nursing staff

Answers to these questions are on p. 850.

7 Body Structure and Function

- Define the key terms in this chapter
- Identify the basic structures of the cell, and explain how cells divide
- Describe four types of tissue
- Identify the structures of each body system
- Describe the functions of each body system

artery A blood vessel that carries blood away from the heart

capillary A tiny blood vessel; food, oxygen, and other substances pass from the capillaries to the cells

cell The basic unit of body structure

digestion The process of physically and chemically breaking down food so that it can be absorbed for use by the cells

hemoglobin The substance in red blood cells that carries oxygen and gives blood its color

hormone A chemical substance secreted by the glands into the bloodstream

immunity Protection against a disease or condition; the person will not get or be affected by the disease

menstruation The process in which the lining of the uterus breaks up and is discharged from the body through the vagina

metabolism The burning of food for heat and energy by the cells

organ Groups of tissues with the same function

peristalsis Involuntary muscle contractions in the digestive system that move food through the alimentary canal; the alternating contraction and relaxation of intestinal muscles

system Organs that work together to perform special functions

tissue A group of cells with the same function

vein A blood vessel that carries blood back to the heart

NOTE: Students are responsible for only those terms mentioned in the text. Additional terms used in labeling figures throughout this chapter are for illustrative purposes only.

You will help patients meet their basic needs. Their bodies do not work at peak efficiency because of illness, disease, or injury. You will provide care and perform procedures to promote comfort, healing, and recovery. A basic knowledge of the body's normal structure and function will help you understand certain signs and symptoms, reasons for care, and purposes of procedures. This knowledge should result in safer and more efficient patient care.

CELLS, TISSUES, AND ORGANS

The basic unit of body structure is the **cell.** Each cell has the same basic structure. However, the function, size, and shape of cells may be different. Cells are so small that a microscope is needed to see them. Cells need food, water, and oxygen to live and perform their functions.

The cell and its basic structures are shown in Figure 7-1 on p. 108. The *cell membrane* is the outer covering that encloses the cell and helps it hold its shape. The *nucleus* is the control center of the cell; it directs the cell's activities. The nucleus is in the center of the cell. The *cytoplasm* is the portion of the cell that surrounds the nucleus. Cytoplasm contains many smaller structures that perform cell functions. The *protoplasm,* which means "living substance," refers to all of the structures, substances, and water within the cell. Protoplasm is a semiliquid substance much like an egg white.

Chromosomes are threadlike structures within the nucleus. Each cell has 46 chromosomes. Chromosomes contain *genes*. Genes control the physical and chemical traits inherited by children from their parents. Inherited traits include height, eye color, and skin color.

Besides controlling cell activities, the nucleus is responsible for cell reproduction. Cells reproduce by

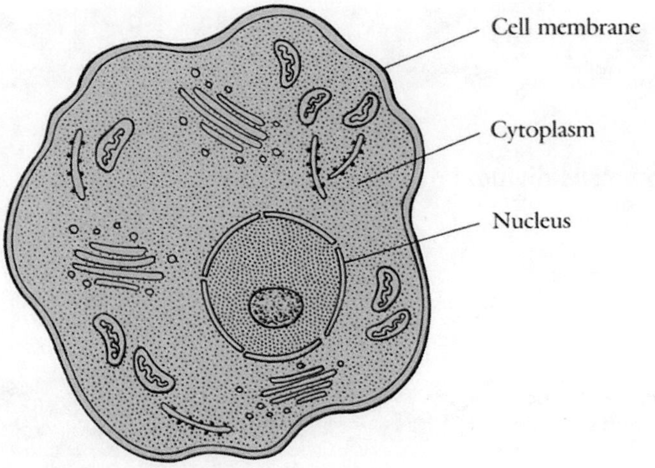

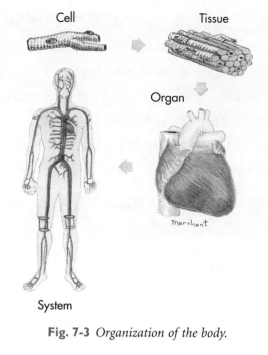

Fig. 7-3 *Organization of the body.*

Fig. 7-1 *Parts of a cell.*

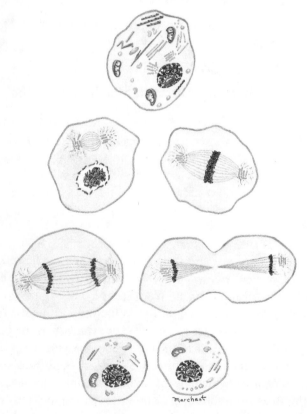

Fig. 7-2 *Cell division.*

dividing in half. The process of cell division is called *mitosis.* Cell division is needed for growth and repair of body tissues. During mitosis, the 46 chromosomes arrange themselves in 23 pairs. As the cell divides, the 23 pairs of chromosomes are pulled in half. The two new cells are identical, and each contains 46 chromosomes (Fig. 7-2).

The cells are the body's building blocks. Groups of cells with similar functions combine to form **tissues.** The body has four basic types of tissue:

- *Epithelial tissue* covers internal and external body surfaces. Tissue that lines the nose, mouth, respiratory tract, stomach, and intestines is epithelial tissue. So are the skin, hair, nails, and glands.
- *Connective tissue* anchors, connects, and supports other body tissues. Connective tissue is found in every part of the body. Bones, tendons, ligaments, and cartilage are connective tissue. Blood is a form of connective tissue.
- *Muscle tissue* allows the body to move by stretching and contracting. There are three types of muscle tissue (p. 111).
- *Nerve tissue* receives and carries impulses to the brain and back to body parts.

Groups of tissues form **organs.** An organ performs one or more functions. Examples of organs include the heart, brain, liver, lungs, and kidneys. **Systems** are formed by organs that work together to perform special functions (Fig. 7-3).

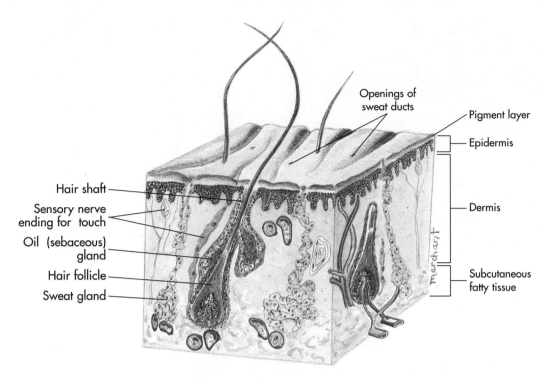

Fig. 7-4 *Layers of the skin.*

THE INTEGUMENTARY SYSTEM

The *integumentary system*, or skin, is the largest system of the body. *Integument* means covering. The skin is the body's natural covering. Skin is made up of epithelial, connective, and nerve tissues, as well as oil and sweat glands. There are two skin layers: the epidermis and the dermis (Fig. 7-4). The *epidermis* is the outer layer; it contains living cells and dead cells. The dead cells were once deeper in the epidermis and were pushed upward as other cells divided. Dead cells constantly flake off and are replaced by living cells. Living cells also die and flake off. Living cells of the epidermis contain *pigment*. Pigment gives skin its color. The epidermis has no blood vessels and few nerve endings. The *dermis* is the inner layer of the skin and is made up of connective tissue. Blood vessels, nerves, sweat and oil glands, and hair roots are found in the dermis.

Oil and *sweat glands, hair,* and *nails* are skin appendages. The entire body, except the palms of the hands and soles of the feet, is covered with hair. Hair in the nose, eyes, and ears protects these organs from dust, insects, and other foreign objects. Nails protect the tips of fingers and toes. Nails help fingers pick up and handle small objects. Sweat glands help the body regulate temperature. Sweat consists of water, salt, and a small amount of wastes. Sweat is secreted through pores in the skin. The body is cooled as sweat evaporates. Oil glands lie near hair shafts. They secrete an oily substance into the space near the hair shaft. Oil travels to the skin surface, helping to keep the hair and skin soft and shiny.

The skin has many important functions. It is the protective covering of the body. Bacteria and other substances are prevented from entering the body. The skin prevents excessive amounts of water from leaving the body and protects organs from injury. Nerve endings in the skin sense both pleasant stimulation and unpleasant stimulation. There are nerve endings over the entire body. The body is protected because cold, pain, touch, and pressure are sensed. The skin helps regulate body temperature. Blood vessels dilate (widen) when temperature outside the body is high. More blood is brought to the body surface for cooling during evaporation. When blood vessels constrict (narrow), the body retains heat because less blood reaches the skin.

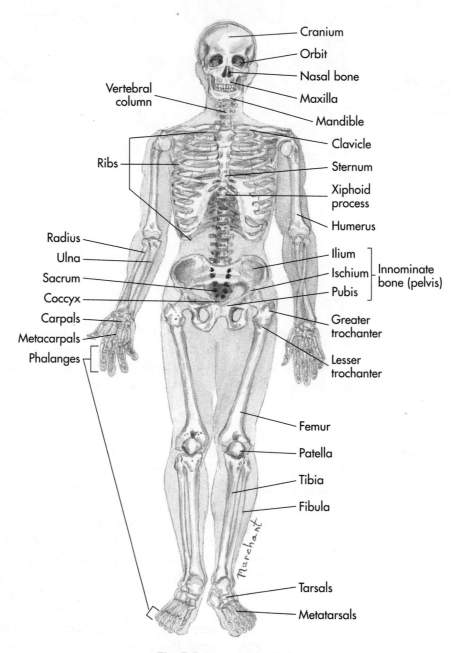

Cranium
Orbit
Nasal bone
Maxilla
Mandible
Clavicle
Sternum
Xiphoid process
Humerus
Ilium
Ischium   Innominate bone (pelvis)
Pubis
Greater trochanter
Lesser trochanter
Femur
Patella
Tibia
Fibula
Tarsals
Metatarsals

Vertebral column
Ribs
Radius
Ulna
Sacrum
Coccyx
Carpals
Metacarpals
Phalanges

Fig. 7-5 *Bones of the body.*

THE MUSCULOSKELETAL SYSTEM

The musculoskeletal system provides the framework for the body and allows the body to move. This system also protects and gives the body shape. Besides bones and muscles, the system has ligaments, tendons, and cartilage.

Bones

The human body has 206 bones (Fig. 7-5). There are four types of bones:

- *Long bones* bear the weight of the body. Leg bones are long bones.
- *Short bones* allow skill and ease in movement. Bones in the wrists, fingers, ankles, and toes are short bones.
- *Flat bones* protect the organs. Such bones include the ribs, skull, pelvic bones, and shoulder blades.
- *Irregular bones* are the vertebrae in the spinal column. They allow various degrees of movement and flexibility.

Bones are hard, rigid structures that are made up of living cells. They are covered by a membrane called *periosteum*. Periosteum contains blood vessels that supply bone cells with oxygen and food. Inside the hollow centers of the bones is a substance called *bone marrow*. Blood cells are manufactured in the bone marrow.

Joints

A *joint* is the point at which two or more bones meet. Joints allow movement (see Chapter 22). *Cartilage* is the connective tissue at the end of long bones. Cartilage cushions the joint so that bone ends do not rub together. The *synovial membrane* lines the joints. The membrane secretes *synovial fluid*. Synovial fluid acts as a lubricant so the joint can move smoothly. Bones are held together at the joint by strong bands of connective tissue called *ligaments*.

There are three types of joints (Fig. 7-6):

- *Ball-and-socket joint* allows movement in all directions. It is made up of the rounded end of one bone and the hollow end of another bone. The rounded end of one fits into the hollow end of the other. The joints of the hips and shoulders are ball-and-socket joints.
- *Hinge joint* allows movement in one direction. The elbow is a hinge joint.
- *Pivot joint* allows turning from side to side. The skull is connected to the spine by a pivot joint.

Muscles

There are more than 500 muscles in the human body (Figs. 7-7 and 7-8, pp. 112-113). Some are voluntary, and

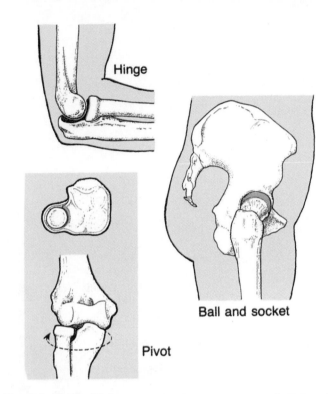

Fig. 7-6 *Types of joints. (Modified from Austrin M, Austrin H:* Learning medical terminology: a worktext, *ed 8, St Louis, 1995, Mosby.)*

others are involuntary. *Voluntary* muscles can be consciously controlled. Muscles attached to bones *(skeletal muscles)* are voluntary. Arm muscles do not work unless you move your arm; likewise for leg muscles. Skeletal muscles are *striated;* that is, they look striped or streaked. *Involuntary muscles* work automatically and cannot be consciously controlled. Involuntary muscles control the action of the stomach, intestines, blood vessels, and other body organs. Involuntary muscles are also called *smooth muscles.* They look smooth, not streaked or striped. *Cardiac muscle* is in the heart. Although it is an involuntary muscle, it appears striated like skeletal muscle.

Muscles perform three important body functions:

- Movement of body parts
- Maintenance of posture
- Production of body heat

Strong, tough connective tissues called *tendons* connect muscles to bones. When muscles contract (shorten), tendons at each end of the muscle cause the bone to move. The body has many tendons; the Achilles tendon is shown in Figure 7-8. Some muscles constantly contract to maintain the body's posture. When muscles contract, they burn food for energy, resulting in the production of heat. The greater the muscular activity, the greater the amount of heat produced in the body. Shivering is a way the body produces heat when exposed to cold. The shivering sensation is from rapid, general muscle contractions.

Text continued on p. 114

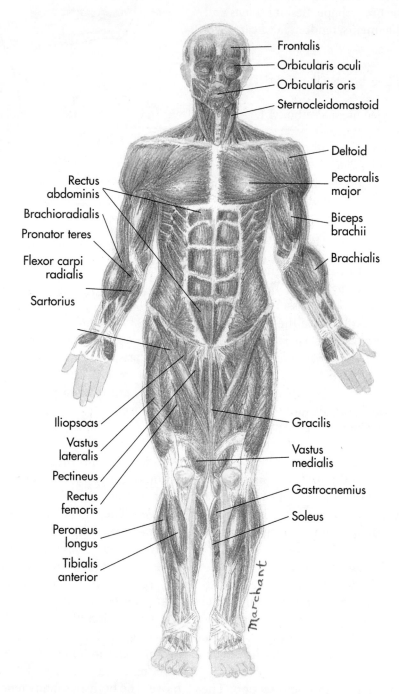

Frontalis

Orbicularis oculi

Orbicularis oris

Sternocleidomastoid

Deltoid

Pectoralis major

Biceps brachii

Brachialis

Rectus abdominis

Brachioradialis

Pronator teres

Flexor carpi radialis

Sartorius

Iliopsoas

Vastus lateralis

Pectineus

Rectus femoris

Peroneus longus

Tibialis anterior

Gracilis

Vastus medialis

Gastrocnemius

Soleus

Marchant

Fig. 7-7 *Anterior view of the muscles of the body.*

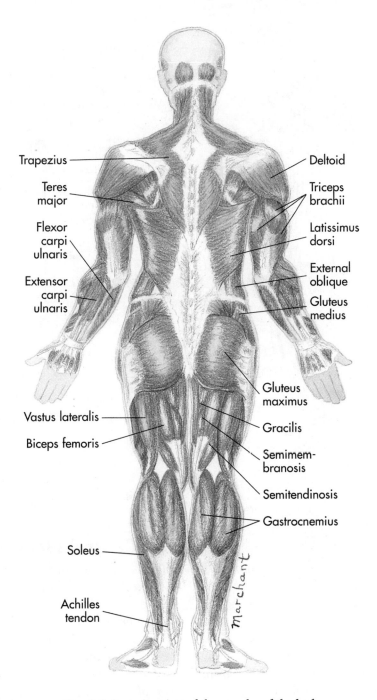

Fig. 7-8 *Posterior view of the muscles of the body.*

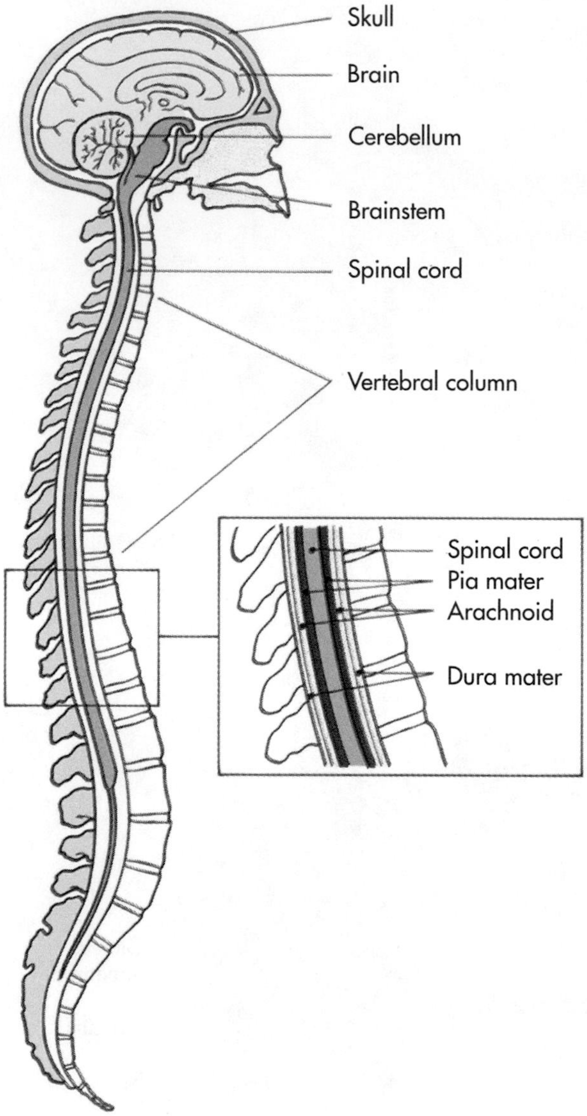

Fig. 7-9 *Central nervous system.*

THE NERVOUS SYSTEM

The nervous system controls, directs, and coordinates body functions. The two main divisions of the nervous system are the *central nervous system* (CNS) and the *peripheral nervous system*. The central nervous system consists of the *brain* and *spinal cord* (Fig. 7-9). The peripheral nervous system involves the *nerves* throughout the body (Fig. 7-10). Nerves carry messages or impulses to and from the brain. Nerves are connected to the spinal cord.

Nerves are easily damaged and take a long time to heal. Some nerve fibers have a protective covering called a *myelin sheath.* The myelin sheath also insulates the nerve fiber. Nerve fibers covered with myelin can conduct impulses faster than those fibers without the protective covering.

The Central Nervous System

The central nervous system consists of the brain and spinal cord. The brain is covered by the skull. The three main parts of the brain are the *cerebrum*, the *cerebellum*, and the *brainstem* (Fig. 7-11, p. 116).

The cerebrum is the largest part of the brain. It is the center of thought and intelligence. The cerebrum is divided into two halves called the *right hemisphere* and *left hemisphere.* The right hemisphere controls movement and activities on the body's left side. The left hemisphere controls the right side. The outside of the cerebrum is called the *cerebral cortex.* The cerebral cortex controls the highest functions of the brain. These include reasoning, memory, consciousness, speech, voluntary muscle movement, vision, hearing, sensation, and other activities.

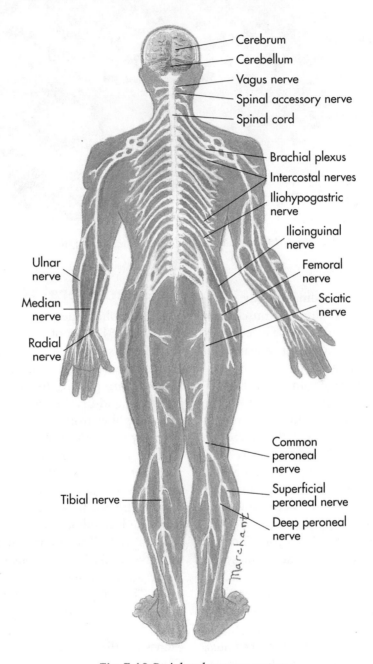

Fig. 7-10 *Peripheral nervous system.*

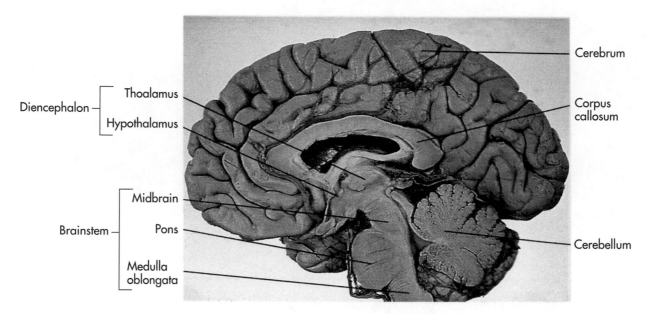

Diencephalon — Thoalamus / Hypothalamus

Brainstem — Midbrain / Pons / Medulla oblongata

Cerebrum

Corpus callosum

Cerebellum

Fig. 7-11 *The brain. (From Seeley RR, Stephens TD, Tate P:* Anatomy and physiology, *St Louis, 1992, Mosby.)*

The cerebellum regulates and coordinates body movements. The smooth movements of voluntary muscles and balance are possible because of control by the cerebellum. Injury to the cerebellum results in jerky movements, loss of coordination, and muscle weakness.

The brainstem connects the cerebrum to the spinal cord. Important structures within the brainstem are the *midbrain, pons,* and *medulla.* The midbrain and pons relay messages between the medulla and the cerebrum. The medulla is directly below the pons. Heart rate, breathing, blood vessel size, swallowing, coughing, and vomiting are some functions controlled by the medulla. The brain is connected to the spinal cord at the lower end of the medulla.

The spinal cord lies within the spinal column. The cord is about 18 inches long. Pathways that conduct messages to and from the brain are contained within the cord.

The brain and spinal cord are covered and protected by three layers of connective tissue called *meninges.* The outer layer lies next to the skull. It is a tough covering called the *dura mater.* The middle layer is called the *arachnoid.* The inner layer is the *pia mater.* The space between the middle layer and inner layer is the *arachnoid space.* The space is filled with fluid called *cerebrospinal fluid.* It circulates around the brain and spinal cord. Cerebrospinal fluid protects the central nervous system. It cushions shocks that could easily injure structures of the brain and spinal cord.

The Peripheral Nervous System

The peripheral nervous system has 12 pairs of *cranial nerves* and 31 pairs of *spinal nerves.* Cranial nerves conduct impulses between the brain and the head, neck, chest, and abdomen. They conduct impulses for smell, vision, hearing, pain, touch, temperature, pressure, and voluntary and involuntary muscle control. Spinal nerves carry impulses from the skin, extremities, and the internal body structures not supplied by cranial nerves.

Some peripheral nerves with special functions form the *autonomic nervous system.* This system controls involuntary muscles and certain body functions. The functions include the heartbeat, blood pressure, intestinal contractions, and glandular secretions. These functions occur automatically. The autonomic nervous system is divided into the *sympathetic nervous system* and the *parasympathetic nervous system.* These divisions balance one another. The sympathetic nervous system tends to speed up functions. The parasympathetic nervous system slows them down. When you are angry, frightened, excited, or exercising, the sympathetic nervous system is stimulated. The parasympathetic system is activated when you relax or when the sympathetic system is under stimulation for too long.

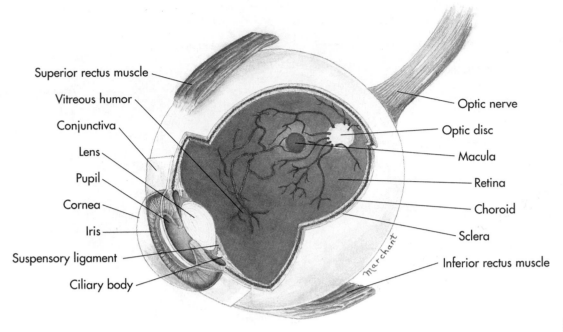

Fig. 7-12 *The eye.*

The Sense Organs

The five major senses are sight, hearing, taste, smell, and touch. Receptors for taste are in the tongue and are called *taste buds*. Receptors for smell are in the nose. Touch receptors are found in the dermis, especially in the toes and fingertips.

The eye

Receptors for vision are in the eyes. The eye is a delicate organ that can be easily injured. Bones of the skull, eyelids and eyelashes, and tears protect the eyes from injury. Eye structures are shown in Figure 7-12. The eye has three layers:

- The *sclera*, the white of the eye, is the outer layer. It is made of tough connective tissue.
- The *choroid* is the second layer. Blood vessels, the *ciliary muscle*, and the *iris* make up the choroid. The iris gives the eye its color. The opening in the middle of the iris is the *pupil*. Pupil size varies with the amount of light entering the eye. The pupil constricts (narrows) in bright light and dilates (widens) in dim or dark places.
- The *retina* is the inner layer of the eye. Receptors for vision and the nerve fibers of the optic nerve are contained in the retina.

Light enters the eye through the *cornea*. The cornea is the transparent part of the outer layer that lies over the eye. Light rays pass to the *lens*, which lies behind the pupil. The light is then reflected to the retina and carried to the brain by the optic nerve.

The *aqueous chamber* separates the cornea from the lens. The chamber is filled with a fluid called *aqueous humor*. The fluid helps the cornea keep its shape and position. The *vitreous body* is behind the lens. The vitreous body is a gelatin-like substance that supports the retina and maintains the eye's shape.

The ear

The ear is a sense organ that functions in hearing and balance. It is divided into the *external ear, middle ear,* and *inner ear*. Ear structures are shown in Figure 7-13, p. 118.

The external ear (outer part) is called the *pinna* or *auricle*. Sound waves are guided through the external ear into the *auditory canal*. Glands in the auditory canal secrete a waxy substance called *cerumen*. The auditory canal extends about 1 inch to the *eardrum*. The eardrum *(tympanic membrane)* separates the external ear and middle ear.

The middle ear is a small space that contains the *eustachian tube* and three small bones called *ossicles*. The eustachian tube connects the middle ear and the throat. Air enters the eustachian tube so that there is equal pressure on both sides of the eardrum. The ossicles amplify sound received from the eardrum and transmit the sound to the inner ear. The three ossicles are:

- The *malleus*, which looks like a hammer
- The *incus*, which resembles an anvil
- The *stapes*, which is shaped like a stirrup

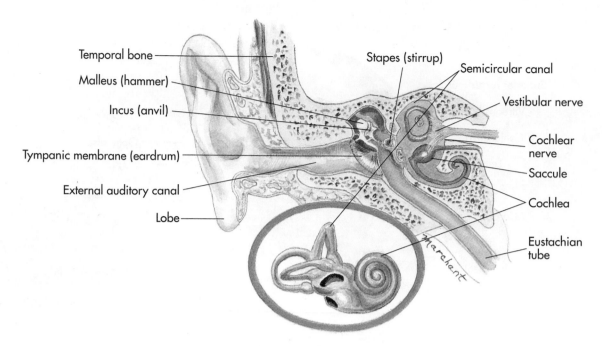

Fig. 7-13 *The ear.*

The inner ear consists of the *semicircular canals* and the *cochlea.* The cochlea, which looks like a snail shell, contains fluid. The fluid carries sound waves received from the middle ear to the *auditory nerve.* The auditory nerve then carries the message to the brain.

The three semicircular canals are involved with balance. They sense the head's position and changes in position and send messages to the brain.

THE CIRCULATORY SYSTEM

The circulatory system is made up of the blood, heart, and blood vessels. The heart pumps blood through the blood vessels. The circulatory system has many important functions. Blood carries food, oxygen, and other substances to the cells. Blood also removes waste products from cells. Regulation of body temperature is aided by the blood and blood vessels. Heat from muscle activity is carried by the blood to other body parts. Blood vessels in the skin dilate if the body needs to be cooled. They constrict if heat should be kept in the body. The circulatory system also produces and carries cells that defend the body from disease-causing microorganisms.

The Blood

The blood consists of blood cells and a liquid called *plasma.* Plasma is mostly water. It carries blood cells to other body cells. Plasma also carries other substances needed by cells for proper functioning. Food (proteins, fats, and carbohydrates), hormones (p. 126), chemicals, and waste products are among the many substances carried in the plasma.

Red blood cells are called *erythrocytes.* They give the blood its red color because of a substance in the cell called **hemoglobin.** As red blood cells circulate through the lungs, hemoglobin picks up oxygen. The hemoglobin carries oxygen to the cells. When the blood is bright red, hemoglobin in the red blood cells is saturated (filled) with oxygen. As blood circulates through the body, oxygen is given to the cells. The cells release carbon dioxide (a waste product), which is picked up by the hemoglobin. Red blood cells saturated with carbon dioxide make the blood look dark red.

There are about 25 trillion (25,000,000,000,000) red blood cells in the body. About 4½ to 5 million cells are in a cubic millimeter of blood (the size of a tiny drop). These cells live for 3 or 4 months. They are destroyed by the liver and spleen as they wear out. Bone marrow produces new red blood cells. About 1 million new red blood cells are produced every second.

White blood cells, called *leukocytes,* are colorless. They protect the body against infection. There are 5,000 to 10,000 white blood cells in a cubic millimeter of blood. At the first sign of infection, white blood cells rush to the site of the infection and begin to multiply rapidly. The number of white blood cells increases when there is an infection in the body. White blood cells also are produced by the bone marrow. They live about 9 days.

Platelets (thrombocytes) are necessary for the clotting of blood. They also are produced by the bone marrow. There are about 200,000 to 400,000 platelets in a cubic millimeter of blood. A platelet lives about 4 days.

The Heart

The heart is a muscle. It pumps blood through the blood vessels to the tissues and cells. The heart lies in the middle to lower part of the chest cavity toward the left side (Fig. 7-14). The heart is hollow and has three layers (Fig. 7-15):

- The *pericardium* is the outer layer. It is a thin sac covering the heart.
- The *myocardium* is the second layer. This layer is the thick, muscular portion of the heart.
- The *endocardium* is the inner layer. The endocardium is the membrane lining the inner surface of the heart.

The heart has four chambers (see Fig. 7-15). Upper chambers receive blood and are called the *atria*. The *right atrium* receives blood from body tissues. The *left atrium* receives blood from the lungs. Lower chambers are called ventricles. Ventricles pump blood. The *right ventricle* pumps blood to the lungs for oxygen. The *left ventricle* pumps blood to all parts of the body. *Valves* are located between the atria and ventricles. The valves allow blood to flow in one direction. They prevent blood from flowing back into the atria from the ventricles. The *tricuspid valve* is between the right atrium and right ventricle. The *mitral valve (bicuspid valve)* is between the left atrium and left ventricle.

There are two phases of heart action. During *diastole,* the resting phase, heart chambers fill with blood. During *systole,* the working phase, the heart contracts. Blood is pumped through the blood vessels when the heart contracts.

The Blood Vessels

Blood flows to body tissues and cells through the blood vessels. There are three groups of blood vessels: arteries, capillaries, and veins. **Arteries** carry blood away from the heart. Arterial blood is rich in oxygen. The *aorta* is the largest artery. The aorta receives blood directly from the left ventricle. The aorta branches into other arteries that carry blood to all parts of the body (Fig. 7-16, p. 120). These arteries branch into smaller parts within the tissues. The smallest branch of an artery is an *arteriole.* Arterioles connect with blood vessels called **capillaries.** Capillaries

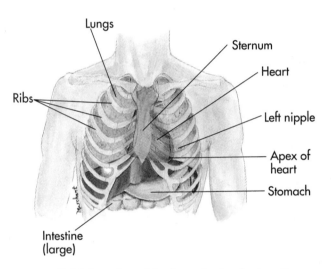

Fig. 7-14 *Location of the heart in the chest cavity.*

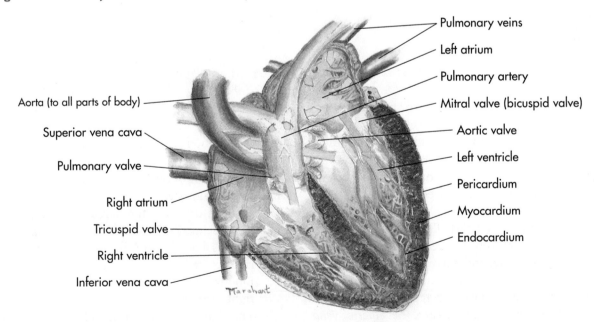

Fig. 7-15 *Structures of the heart.*

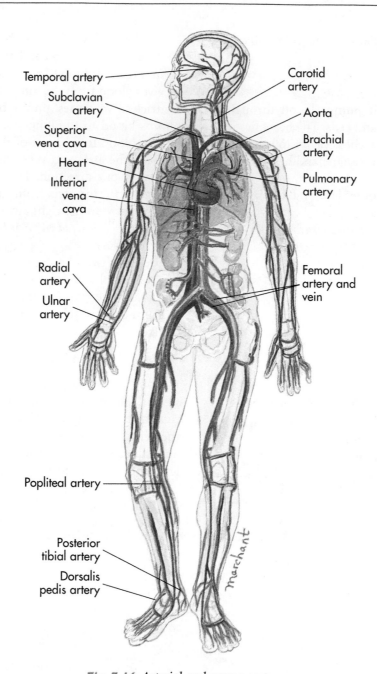

Fig. 7-16 *Arterial and venous systems.*

are very tiny vessels. Food, oxygen, and other substances pass from capillaries into the cells. Waste products, including carbon dioxide, are picked up from cells by the capillaries. Waste products are carried back to the heart by the veins.

Veins return blood to the heart. They are connected to the capillaries by *venules.* Venules are small veins. Venules begin branching together to form veins. The many branches of veins also branch together as they near the heart to form two main veins (see Fig. 7-16). The two main veins are the *inferior vena cava* and the *superior vena cava.* Both empty into the right atrium. The inferior vena

cava carries blood from the legs and trunk. The superior vena cava carries blood from the head and arms. Venous blood is dark red because it contains little oxygen and a lot of carbon dioxide.

Blood flow through the circulatory system is diagrammed in Figure 7-15 and can be summarized as follows:

1. Venous blood, poor in oxygen, empties into the right atrium.
2. Blood flows through the tricuspid valve into the right ventricle.
3. The right ventricle pumps blood into the lungs to pick up oxygen.

4. Oxygen-rich blood from the lungs enters the left atrium.
5. Blood from the left atrium passes through the mitral valve into the left ventricle.
6. The left ventricle pumps the blood to the aorta, which branches off to form other arteries.
7. The arterial blood is carried to the tissues by arterioles and to the cells by capillaries.
8. The cells and capillaries exchange oxygen and nutrients for carbon dioxide and waste products.
9. Capillaries connect with venules.
10. Venules carry blood that contains carbon dioxide and waste products.
11. The venules form veins.
12. Veins return blood to the heart.

THE RESPIRATORY SYSTEM

Oxygen is needed for survival. Every cell needs oxygen. Air contains about 20% oxygen, enough to meet body needs under normal conditions. The respiratory system brings oxygen into the lungs and eliminates carbon dioxide. The process of supplying the cells with oxygen and removing carbon dioxide from them is called *respiration*. Respiration involves *inhalation* (breathing in) and *exhalation* (breathing out). The terms *inspiration* (breathing in) and *expiration* (breathing out) also are used. The respiratory system is shown in Figure 7-17.

Air enters the body through the *nose*. The air then passes into the *pharynx* (throat), a tube-shaped passageway for both air and food. Air passes from the pharynx into the *larynx* (the voice box). A piece of cartilage called the *epiglottis* acts like a lid over the larynx. The epiglottis prevents food from entering the airway during swallowing. During inhalation the epiglottis lifts up to let air pass over the larynx. Air passes from the larynx into the *trachea* (the windpipe). The trachea divides at its lower end into the *right bronchus* and *left bronchus*. Each bronchus enters a lung. Upon entering the lungs, the bronchi further divide several times into smaller branches called *bronchioles*. Eventually the bronchioles subdivide and end in tiny one-celled air sacs called *alveoli*. Alveoli look like small clusters of grapes. They are supplied by capillaries. Oxygen and carbon dioxide are exchanged between the alveoli and capillaries. Blood in the capillaries picks up oxygen from the alveoli. Then the blood is returned to the left side of the heart and pumped to the rest of the body. Alveoli pick up carbon dioxide from the capillaries for exhalation.

The lungs are spongy tissues filled with alveoli, blood vessels, and nerves. Each lung is divided into lobes. The right lung has three lobes; the left lung has two. The lungs are separated from the abdominal cavity by a muscle

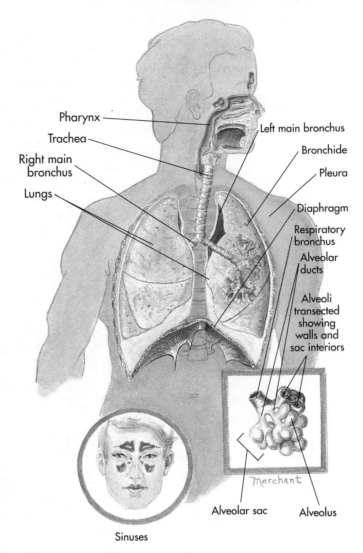

Fig. 7-17 *Respiratory system.*

Labels: Pharynx, Trachea, Right main bronchus, Lungs, Left main bronchus, Bronchide, Pleura, Diaphragm, Respiratory bronchus, Alveolar ducts, Alveoli transected showing walls and sac interiors, Sinuses, Alveolar sac, Alveolus

called the *diaphragm*. Each lung is covered by a two-layered sac called the *pleura*. One layer is attached to the lung and the other to the chest wall. The pleura secretes a very thin fluid that fills the space between the layers. The fluid prevents the layers from rubbing together during inhalation and exhalation. A bony framework consisting of the ribs, sternum, and vertebrae protects the lungs.

THE DIGESTIVE SYSTEM

The digestive system breaks down food physically and chemically so it can be absorbed for use by the cells. This process is called **digestion.** The digestive system is also called the *gastrointestinal system (GI system)*. The system also eliminates solid wastes from the body. The digestive system consists of the *alimentary canal (GI tract)* and the accessory organs of digestion (Fig. 7-18, p. 122). The alimentary canal is a long tube extending from the mouth to the anus. Its major parts are the mouth, pharynx,

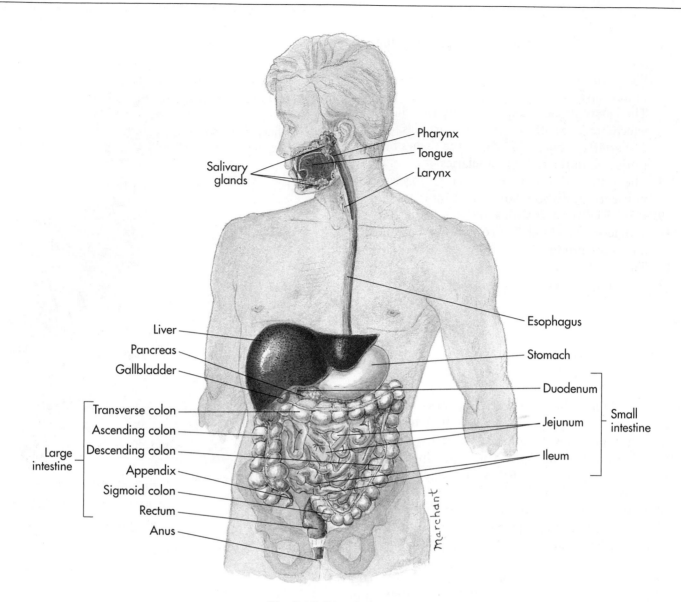

Fig. 7-18 *Digestive system.*

esophagus, stomach, small intestine, and large intestine. The accessory organs of digestion are the teeth, tongue, salivary glands, liver, gallbladder, and pancreas.

Digestion begins in the *mouth.* The mouth is also called the *oral cavity.* The oral cavity receives food and prepares it for digestion. Using chewing motions, the *teeth* cut, chop, and grind food into smaller particles for digestion and swallowing. The *tongue* aids in chewing and swallowing. *Taste buds* on the tongue's surface contain nerve endings. Taste buds allow sweet, sour, bitter, and salty tastes to be sensed. *Salivary glands* in the mouth secrete *saliva.* Saliva moistens food particles for easier swallowing and begins to digest food. During swallowing, the tongue pushes food into the pharynx.

The *pharynx* (throat) is a muscular tube. The act of swallowing is continued as the pharynx contracts. Contraction of the pharynx pushes food into the *esophagus.* The esophagus is a muscular tube about 10 inches long.

It extends from the pharynx to the stomach. Involuntary muscle contractions called **peristalsis** move food down the esophagus into the stomach.

The *stomach* is a muscular, pouchlike sac in the upper left portion of the abdominal cavity. Strong stomach muscles stir and churn food to break it up into even smaller particles. The stomach is lined with a mucous membrane containing glands that secrete *gastric juices.* Food is mixed and churned with the gastric juices to form a semiliquid substance called *chyme.* Through peristalsis, the chyme is pushed from the stomach into the small intestine.

The *small intestine* is about 20 feet long and has three parts. The first part is the *duodenum.* In the duodenum, more digestive juices are added to the chyme. One is called *bile.* Bile is a greenish liquid produced by the *liver* and stored in the *gallbladder.* Juices from the *pancreas* and small intestine also are added to the chyme. The diges-

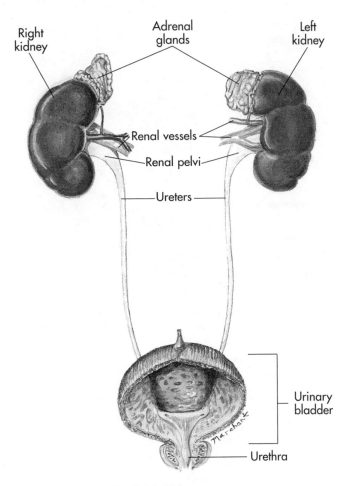

Fig. 7-19 *Urinary system.*

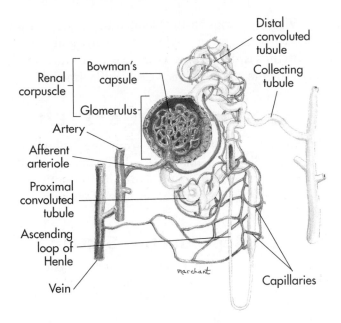

Fig. 7-20 *A nephron.*

tive juices chemically break down food so that it can be absorbed.

Peristalsis moves the chyme through the two remaining portions of the small intestine: the *jejunum* and the *ileum.* Tiny projections called *villi* line the small intestine. Villi absorb the digested food into the capillaries. Most of the absorption of food takes place in the jejunum and ileum.

Some chyme remains undigested. The undigested chyme passes from the small intestine into the *large intestine (large bowel or colon).* The colon absorbs most of the water from the chyme. The remaining semisolid material is called *feces.* Feces consist of a small amount of water, solid wastes, and some mucus and germs. These are the waste products of digestion. Feces pass through the colon into the *rectum* by peristalsis. Feces pass out of the body through the *anus.*

THE URINARY SYSTEM

Wastes are removed from the body through the respiratory system, the digestive system, and the skin. The digestive system rids the body of solid wastes. The lungs

rid the body of carbon dioxide. Water and other substances are contained in sweat. There are other waste products in the blood as a result of body cells burning food for energy. The functions of the urinary system are to remove waste products from the blood and to maintain water balance within the body. The structures of the urinary system are shown in Figure 7-19.

The *kidneys* are two bean-shaped organs in the upper abdomen. They lie against the muscles of the back on each side of the spine. They are protected by the lower edge of the rib cage.

Each kidney has over a million tiny *nephrons* (Fig. 7-20). The nephron is the basic working unit of the kidney. Each nephron has a *convoluted tubule,* which is a tiny, coiled tubule. Each convoluted tubule has a *Bowman's capsule* at one end. The capsule partially surrounds a cluster of capillaries called a *glomerulus.* Blood passes through the glomerulus and is filtered by the capillaries. The fluid portion of the blood is squeezed into the Bowman's capsule. The fluid then passes into the tubule. Most of the water and other necessary substances are reabsorbed by the blood and recirculated in the body. The rest of the fluid and the waste products form *urine* in the tubule. Urine flows through the tubule to a *collecting tubule.* All of the collecting tubules within the millions of nephrons drain into the *renal pelvis* within the kidney.

A tube, called the *ureter,* is attached to the renal pelvis of the kidney. Each ureter is about 10 to 12 inches long. The ureters carry urine from the kidneys to the *bladder.* The bladder is a hollow, muscular sac situated toward the front in the lower part of the abdominal cavity. Urine is stored in the bladder until the desire to urinate is felt. The need to urinate usually occurs when there is about half a pint (250 ml) of urine in the bladder. Urine passes from the bladder through the *urethra*. The opening at the end of the urethra is the *meatus*. Urine passes from the body through the meatus. Urine is a clear, yellowish fluid.

THE REPRODUCTIVE SYSTEM

Human reproduction results from the union of a female sex cell and a male sex cell. Structures of the male reproductive system and female reproductive system are different. The differences allow for the process of reproduction.

The Male Reproductive System

The structures of the male reproductive system are shown in Figure 7-21. The *testes (testicles)* are the male sex glands. Sex glands are also called *gonads*. The two testes are oval or almond-shaped glands. Male sex cells are produced in the testes. Male sex cells are called *sperm* cells. *Testosterone,* the male hormone, also is produced in the testes. This hormone is needed for the functioning of the reproductive organs and for the development of the male's secondary sex characteristics (see Chapter 8). The testes are suspended between the thighs in a sac called the *scrotum*. The scrotum is made of skin and muscle.

Sperm travel from the testis to the *epididymis*. The epididymis is a coiled tube on top and to the side of the testis. From the epididymis, sperm travel through a tube called the *vas deferens*. Eventually each vas deferens joins a *seminal vesicle*. The two seminal vesicles store sperm and produce *semen*. Semen is a fluid that carries sperm from the male reproductive tract. The ducts of the seminal vesicles unite to form the *ejaculatory duct*. The ejaculatory duct passes through the prostate gland.

The *prostate gland,* shaped like a doughnut, lies just below the bladder. The gland secretes fluid into the semen. As the ejaculatory ducts leave the prostate, they join the *urethra*, which also runs through the prostate. The urethra is the outlet for both urine and semen. The urethra is contained within the penis.

The *penis* is outside of the body and has *erectile* tissue. When a man becomes sexually excited, blood fills the erectile tissue. This causes the penis to become enlarged, hard, and erect. The erect penis can enter the vagina of the female reproductive tract. The semen, which contains sperm, is then released into the female vagina.

The Female Reproductive System

The structures of the female reproductive system are shown in Figure 7-22. The female gonads are two almond-shaped glands called *ovaries*. There is an ovary on each side of the uterus in the abdominal cavity. The ovaries contain *ova*, or eggs. Ova are the female sex cells. One

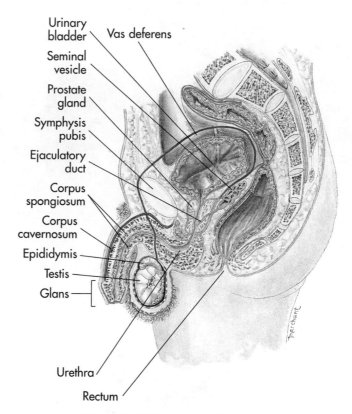

Urinary bladder
Vas deferens
Seminal vesicle
Prostate gland
Symphysis pubis
Ejaculatory duct
Corpus spongiosum
Corpus cavernosum
Epididymis
Testis
Glans
Urethra
Rectum

Fig. 7-21 *Male reproductive system.*

ovum (egg) is released monthly during the woman's reproductive years. Release of an ovum from an ovary is called *ovulation*. The ovaries also secrete the female hormones *estrogen* and *progesterone*. These hormones are needed for the functioning of the reproductive system and the development of secondary sex characteristics in the female (see Chapter 8).

When an ovum is released from an ovary, it travels through a *fallopian tube*. There are two fallopian tubes, one on each side. The tubes are attached at one end to the uterus. The ovum travels through the fallopian tube to the *uterus*. The uterus is a hollow, muscular organ shaped like a pear. The uterus is in the center of the pelvic cavity behind the bladder and in front of the rectum. The main part of the uterus is the *fundus*. The neck or narrow section of the uterus is the *cervix*. Tissue lining the uterus is called the *endometrium*. There are many blood vessels in the endometrium. If sex cells from the male and female unite into one cell, that cell implants into the endometrium, where it grows into a baby. The uterus serves as a place for the unborn baby to grow and receive nourishment.

The cervix of the uterus projects into a muscular canal called the *vagina*. The vagina opens to the outside of the body and is located just behind the urethra. The vagina receives the penis during sexual intercourse and serves as part of the birth canal. Glands in the vaginal wall keep it moistened with secretions. In young girls, the external

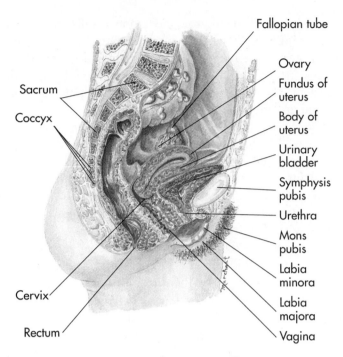

Fig. 7-22 *Female reproductive system.*

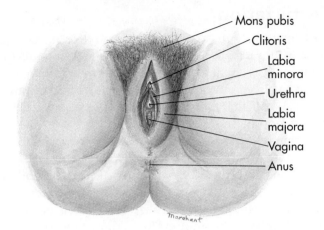

Fig. 7-23 *External female genitalia.*

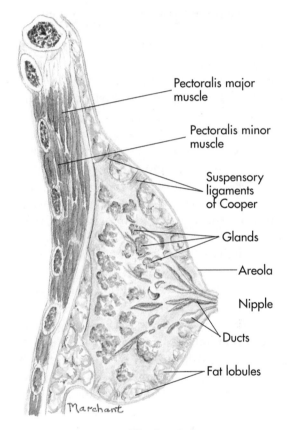

Fig. 7-24 *The female breast.*

vaginal opening is partially closed by a membrane called the *hymen.* The hymen ruptures when the female has intercourse for the first time.

The external genitalia of the female are referred to as the *vulva* (Fig. 7-23). The *mons pubis* is a rounded, fatty pad over a bone called the *symphysis pubis.* The mons pubis is covered with hair in the adult female. The *labia majora* and *labia minora* are two folds of tissue on each side of the vaginal opening. The *clitoris* is a small organ composed of erectile tissue. The clitoris becomes hard when sexually stimulated.

The *mammary glands (breasts)* are considered organs of reproduction because they secrete milk after childbirth. The glands are located on the outside of the chest. They are made up of glandular tissue and fat (Fig. 7-24). The milk drains into ducts that open onto the nipple.

Menstruation

The endometrium is rich in blood to nourish the cell that grows into an unborn baby *(fetus).* If pregnancy does not occur, the endometrium breaks up and is discharged through the vagina to the outside of the body. This process is called **menstruation.** Menstruation occurs about every 28 days. Therefore it is also called the *menstrual cycle.*

The first day of the cycle begins with menstruation. Blood flows from the uterus through the vaginal opening. Menstrual flow usually lasts 3 to 7 days. Ovulation occurs during the next phase of the cycle. An ovum matures in an ovary and is released. Ovulation usually occurs on or about day 14 of the cycle. Meanwhile, estrogen and progesterone (the female hormones) are secreted by the ovaries. These hormones cause the endometrium to thicken for possible pregnancy. If pregnancy does not occur, the hormones decrease in amount. Blood supply to the endometrium decreases because of the decrease in hormones. The endometrium breaks up and is discharged through the vagina. Another menstrual cycle begins.

Fertilization

For reproduction to occur, a male sex cell (sperm) must unite with a female sex cell (ovum). The uniting of the sperm and ovum into one cell is called *fertilization*. A sperm has 23 chromosomes, and an ovum has 23 chromosomes. When the two cells unite, the fertilized cell has 46 chromosomes.

During intercourse, millions of sperm are deposited in the vagina. Sperm travel up the cervix, through the uterus, and into the fallopian tubes. If a sperm and an ovum unite in a fallopian tube, fertilization occurs and results in pregnancy. The fertilized cell travels down the fallopian tube to the uterus. After a short time, the fertilized cell implants in the thick endometrium and grows during pregnancy.

THE ENDOCRINE SYSTEM

The endocrine system is made up of glands called the *endocrine glands* (Fig. 7-25). The endocrine glands secrete chemical substances called **hormones** into the bloodstream. Hormones regulate the activities of other organs and glands in the body.

The *pituitary gland* is called the *master gland*. About the size of a cherry, it is at the base of the brain behind the eyes. The pituitary gland is divided into the anterior pituitary lobe and the posterior pituitary lobe. The *anterior pituitary lobe* secretes important hormones. *Growth hormone* is needed for the growth of muscles, bones, and other organs. Adequate amounts of growth hormone are needed throughout life to maintain normal-size bones and muscles. Growth is stunted if a baby is born with deficient amounts of the growth hormone. Too much of the hormone causes excessive growth.

Thyroid-stimulating hormone (TSH) also is secreted by the anterior pituitary lobe. The thyroid gland requires thyroid-stimulating hormone for proper functioning. *Adrenocorticotropic hormone* (ACTH) is another hormone secreted by the anterior lobe. This hormone stimulates the adrenal gland. The anterior lobe also secretes hormones that regulate the growth, development, and function of the male and female reproductive systems.

The *posterior pituitary* lobe secretes *antidiuretic hormone* (ADH) and *oxytocin*. Antidiuretic hormone prevents the kidneys from excreting excessive amounts of water. Oxytocin causes the uterine muscles to contract during childbirth.

The *thyroid gland,* shaped like a butterfly, is in the neck in front of the larynx. *Thyroid hormone* (TH) is secreted by the thyroid gland. Thyroxine is another term for thyroid hormone. Thyroid hormone regulates **metabolism.** Metabolism is the burning of food for heat and energy by the cells. Too little thyroid hormone results in slowed body processes, slowed movements, and weight gain. Too much of the hormone causes increased metabolism, excess energy, and weight loss. If a baby is born with deficient amounts of thyroid hormone, physical and mental growth will be stunted.

The *parathyroid glands* secrete *parathormone.* There are four parathyroid glands. Two are located on each side of the thyroid gland. Parathormone regulates the body's use of calcium. Calcium is needed for the proper functioning of nerves and muscles. Insufficient amounts of calcium cause *tetany.* Tetany is a state of severe muscle contraction and spasm. If untreated, tetany can cause death.

There are two *adrenal glands.* An adrenal gland is on the top of each kidney. The adrenal gland has two parts: the *adrenal medulla* and the *adrenal cortex.* The adrenal medulla secretes *epinephrine* and *norepinephrine.* These hormones stimulate the body to quickly produce energy during emergencies. Heart rate, blood pressure, muscle power, and energy all increase. The adrenal cortex secretes three groups of hormones that are essential for life. The *glucocorticoids* regulate metabolism of carbohydrates. They also control the body's response to stress and inflammation. The *mineralocorticoids* regulate the amount of salt and water that is absorbed and lost by the kidneys. The adrenal cortex also secretes small amounts of male and female sex hormones.

The *pancreas* secretes *insulin.* Insulin regulates the amount of sugar in the blood available for use by the cells. Insulin is needed for sugar to enter the cells. If there is too little insulin, sugar cannot enter the cells. If sugar cannot enter the cells, excess amounts of sugar build up in the blood. This condition is called *diabetes mellitus.*

The *gonads* are the glands of human reproduction. Male sex glands (testes) secrete *testosterone.* Female sex glands (ovaries) secrete *estrogen* and *progesterone.*

THE IMMUNE SYSTEM

The immune system protects the body from disease and infection. Abnormal body cells can grow into tumors. Sometimes the body produces substances that cause the body to attack itself. Microorganisms (bacteria, viruses, and other germs) in the environment can lead to an infection. The immune system defends against threats inside and outside the body.

The immune system functions to provide the body with immunity. **Immunity** means that a person has protection against a disease or condition. The person will not get or be affected by the disease. *Specific immunity* is the body's reaction to a specific threat. *Nonspecific immunity* is the body's reaction to anything it does not recognize as a normal body substance.

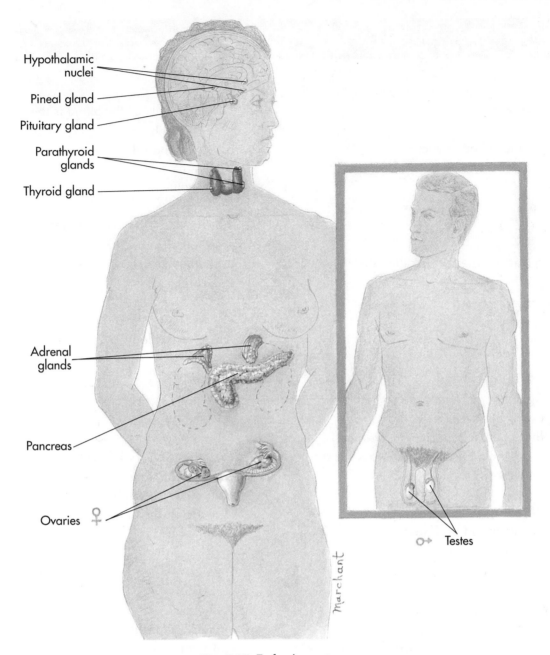

Fig. 7-25 *Endocrine system.*

Special cells and substances function to produce immunity:

- *Antibodies*—normal body substances that recognize abnormal or unwanted substances. They attack and destroy such substances.
- *Antigens*—an abnormal or unwanted substance. An antigen causes the body to produce antibodies. The antibodies attack and destroy the antigens.
- *Phagocytes*—types of white blood cells that digest and destroy microorganisms and other unwanted substances.
- *Lymphocytes*—types of white blood cells that produce antibodies. Lymphocyte production increases as the body responds to an infection.

- *B lymphocytes (B cells)*—cause the production of antibodies that circulate in the plasma. The antibodies react to specific antigens.
- *T lymphocytes (T cells)*—function to destroy invading cells. *Killer T cells* produce poisonous substances near the invading cells. Some T cells attract other cells; these other cells destroy the invaders.

When the body senses an antigen (an unwanted substance), the immune system is activated. Phagocyte and lymphocyte production increases. Phagocytes destroy the invaders through digestion. The lymphocytes produce antibodies that attack and destroy the unwanted substances.

REVIEW QUESTIONS

Circle the best *answer.*

1 The basic unit of body structure is the
a   Cell
b   Neuron
c   Nephron
d   Ovum

2 The outer layer of the skin is called the
a   Dermis
b   Epidermis
c   Integument
d   Myelin

3 Which is *not* a function of the skin?
a   Providing the protective covering for the body
b   Regulating body temperature
c   Sensing cold, pain, touch, and pressure
d   Providing the shape and framework for the body

4 Which part allows movement?
a   Bone marrow and periosteum
b   Synovial membrane
c   Joints
d   Ligaments

5 Skeletal muscles
a   Are under involuntary control
b   Appear smooth
c   Are under voluntary control
d   Appear striped and smooth

6 The highest functions of the brain take place in the
a   Cerebral cortex
b   Medulla
c   Brainstem
d   Spinal nerves

7 Besides hearing, the ear is involved with
a   Regulating body movements
b   Balance
c   Smoothness of body movements
d   Controlling involuntary muscles

8 The liquid part of the blood is the
a   Hemoglobin
b   Red blood cell
c   Plasma
d   Alveolus

9 Which part of the heart pumps blood to the body?
a   Right atrium
b   Right ventricle
c   Left atrium
d   Left ventricle

10 Which carry blood away from the heart?
a   Capillaries
b   Veins
c   Venules
d   Arteries

11 Oxygen and carbon dioxide are exchanged
a   In the bronchi
b   Between the alveoli and capillaries
c   Between the lungs and the pleura
d   In the trachea

12 The process of digestion begins in the
a   Mouth
b   Stomach
c   Small intestine
d   Colon

13 Most food absorption takes place in the
a   Stomach
b   Small intestine
c   Colon
d   Large intestine

14 Urine is formed in the
a   Jejunum
b   Kidneys
c   Bladder
d   Liver

REVIEW QUESTIONS—cont'd

15 Urine passes from the body through
- a The ureters
- b The urethra
- c The anus
- d Nephrons

16 The male sex gland is called the
- a Penis
- b Semen
- c Testis
- d Scrotum

17 The male sex cell is called the
- a Semen
- b Ovum
- c Gonad
- d Sperm

18 The female sex gland is called the
- a Ovary
- b Fallopian tube
- c Uterus
- d Vagina

19 The discharge of the lining of the uterus is called
- a The endometrium
- b Ovulation
- c Fertilization
- d Menstruation

20 The endocrine glands secrete substances called
- a Hormones
- b Mucus
- c Semen
- d Insulin

21 The immune system protects the body from
- a Low blood sugar
- b Disease and infection
- c Falling and loss of balance
- d Stunted growth and loss of fluid

Answers to these questions are on p. 850.

8 Growth and Development

- Define the key terms in this chapter
- Understand the principles of growth and development
- Identify the stages of growth and development and the normal age ranges for each stage
- Identify the developmental tasks for each age-group
- Describe the normal growth and development for each age-group

KEY TERMS

adolescence A time of rapid growth and psychological and social maturity

development Changes in a person's psychological and social functioning

developmental task That which the person must complete during a stage of development

ejaculation The release of semen

geriatrics The care of aging people

gerontology The study of the aging process

growth The physical changes that can be measured and that occur in a steady, orderly manner

menarche The time when menstruation first begins

menopause The time when menstruation stops

primary caregiver The person in the child's environment who is mainly responsible for providing or assisting with the child's basic needs

puberty The period when the reproductive organs begin to function and secondary sex characteristics appear

reflex An involuntary movement

You will care for people in different stages of development. A basic understanding of growth and development helps you give better care. Patient needs also are easier to understand. This chapter presents the basic changes that occur in normal, healthy persons from birth through old age.

Human growth and development are presented in nine stages. Age ranges and normal characteristics are given for each stage. Only basic descriptions are given. The stages overlap. Therefore it is hard to see clear-cut endings and beginnings of the stages. Also, the rate of growth and development varies with each person.

Growth and development theories generally involve the two-parent family. In our society, many households have only one parent. Often children are raised by a relative while the parent works or attends school. *Primary caregiver* is used in this chapter where *mother* or *father* would have been used. The **primary caregiver** is that person in the child's environment who is mainly responsible for providing or assisting with the child's basic needs. The primary caregiver may be a mother, father, grandparent, aunt, uncle, or court-appointed guardian. The words *parent* and *parents* are used in this chapter. However, another primary caregiver may have the parent role.

PRINCIPLES

Growth is the physical changes that are measured and that occur in a steady and orderly manner. Growth is measured in height and weight. Changes in physical appearance and body functions also are measures of growth.

Development relates to changes in psychological and social functioning. A person behaves and thinks in certain ways in different stages of development. A 2-year-old thinks in simple terms and needs a primary caregiver for many basic needs. A 40-year-old thinks in complex ways and meets most basic needs without help from others.

Growth and development affect the entire person. Although each is defined, growth and development:

- Overlap
- Depend on each other
- Occur at the same time

For example, an infant cannot say simple syllables (development) until the physical structures needed for speech are strong enough (growth). The basic principles of growth and development are:

- Growth and development occur from the moment of fertilization until death.
- The process proceeds from the simple to the complex. A baby learns to sit before standing, to stand before walking, and to walk before running.
- Growth and development occur in specific directions:
  - From the head to the foot—babies learn to hold up their heads before they learn to sit. After learning to sit, they learn to stand.
  - From the center of the body outward—babies control shoulder movements before they control hand movements.
- Growth and development occur in a sequence, order, and pattern. Certain **developmental tasks** must be completed during each stage. A stage cannot be skipped. Each stage lays the foundation for the next stage.
- The rate of growth and development is uneven, not at a set pace. Growth is more rapid during infancy. Also, children have growth spurts. Some children develop rapidly; others develop slowly.
- Each stage of growth and development has its own characteristics and developmental tasks.

INFANCY (BIRTH TO I YEAR)

Infancy is the first year of life. Rapid physical, psychological, and social growth and development occur during this time. The developmental tasks of infancy are:

- Learning to walk
- Learning to eat solid foods
- Beginning to talk and communicate with others
- Beginning to have emotional relationships with primary caregivers, brothers, and sisters
- Developing stable sleep and feeding patterns

The *neonatal period* of infancy is the first 4 weeks after birth. A baby is called a *neonate* or a *newborn* during this time.

The average newborn is 19 to 21 inches long and weighs 7 to 8 pounds at birth. Birth weight usually doubles by the age of 5 to 6 months and triples by the first birthday. Babies are usually 20 to 30 inches long at the end of the first year.

The newborn's head is large compared with the rest of the body. The skin is wrinkled, and the baby appears red. Arms and legs seem short compared with the trunk, and the abdomen is large and round. Eyes are a deep blue. The newborn has fat, pudgy cheeks, a flat nose, and a receding chin.

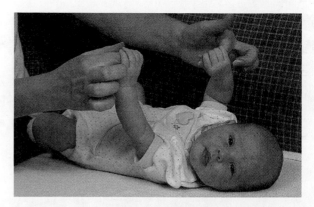

Fig. 8-1 *The grasping reflex.*

The central nervous system is not well developed. Movements are uncoordinated and lack purpose. Babies can see at birth, although vision is not clear. They seem attracted to patterns. As babies develop, they prefer colors. Babies hear well. They are startled by loud noises and soothed by soft sounds. Babies respond better to female than to male voices. Infants react to touch, and the senses of smell and taste are developed.

Newborns have certain **reflexes** (involuntary movements). These reflexes decline and then disappear as the central nervous system develops.

- The *Moro reflex (startle reflex)* occurs when a baby is frightened by a loud noise or sudden movement. The arms are thrown apart, the legs extend, and the head is thrown back.
- The *rooting reflex* is stimulated when the infant's cheek is touched at or near the mouth. The baby's head turns toward the touch. The rooting reflex is necessary for feeding; it helps guide the baby's mouth to the nipple.
- The *sucking reflex* is produced by touching the cheeks or side of the lips.
- The *grasping reflex* occurs when the infant's palm is stimulated, causing the fingers to close around the object (Fig. 8-1). This reflex begins to decline around the second month and disappears by the third month.

Infants sleep most of the time during the first few weeks of life. They awaken when hungry and fall asleep right after eating. The time between feedings lengthens as infants grow and develop. They stay awake more and sleep less as growth and development occur.

Body movements are uncoordinated and without purpose. They are generally involuntary. As the central nervous system and muscular system develop, infants develop specific, voluntary, and coordinated movements. Newborns cannot hold their heads up. At 1 month infants can hold their heads up when held and can lift and turn

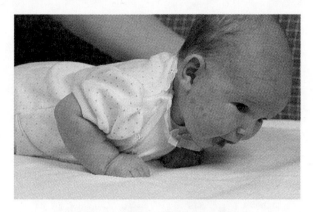

Fig. 8-2 *A 1-month-old infant can lift its head when lying on the stomach.*

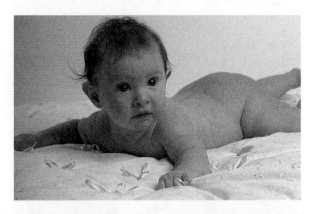

Fig. 8-4 *A 3-month-old child can raise its head and shoulders.*

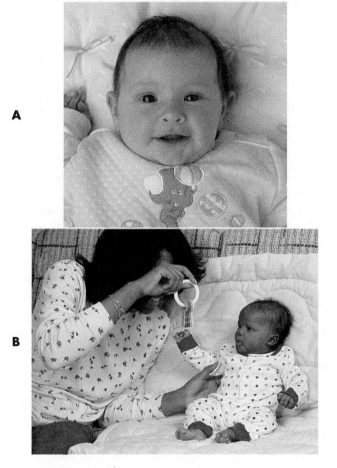

A

B

Fig. 8-3 *A 2-month-old child.* **A,** *Child smiles.* **B,** *Child follows objects with the eyes.*

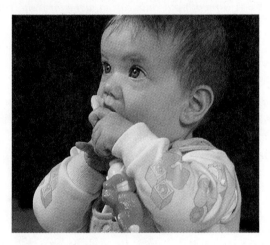

Fig. 8-5 *A 5-month-old child puts objects into the mouth as teeth begin to erupt.*

their heads when lying on their stomachs (Fig. 8-2). At 2 months they can smile and follow objects with their eyes (Fig. 8-3).

Three-month-old infants can raise their heads and shoulders when lying on their stomachs (Fig. 8-4). They can sit for a short while when supported and can hold a rattle. Infants 4 months of age should be able to roll over. They can sit up if supported and may sleep all night. The Moro and rooting reflexes have disappeared. Tears are shed when crying. A rattle is held with both hands, objects are put in the mouth, and the infant babbles when spoken to. At 5 months infants can grasp objects and play with their toes. Teeth start to come through (Fig. 8-5).

Six-month-old infants usually have two lower front teeth and start to chew and bite finger foods. They can hold a bottle for feeding and can sit alone for a short time (Fig. 8-6, p. 134). At 7 months the upper teeth start to erupt. Babies respond to their names, can say "dada," and show a fear of strangers. At 8 months infants may be able to stand when holding onto something. They react to the word "no." Infants at this age do not like to be dressed or have diapers changed. Nine-month-old infants crawl (Fig. 8-7, p. 134), and more upper teeth appear.

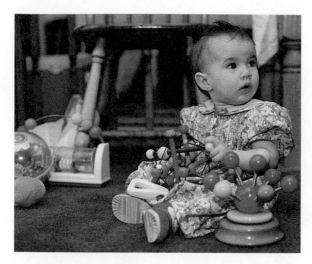

Fig. 8-6 *A 6-month-old child can sit alone for a short time.*

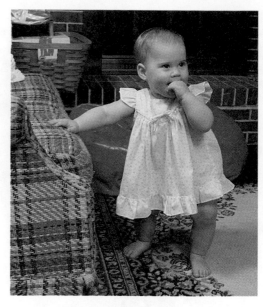

Fig. 8-8 *A 10-month-old child can walk while holding onto furniture.*

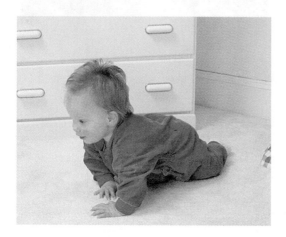

Fig. 8-7 *A 9-month-old child is able to crawl.*

At 10 months most infants can walk around while holding on to furniture (Fig. 8-8). They understand the words "bye-bye," "mama," and "dada." They smile when looking into a mirror. Infants at 11 months may begin to take steps and can hold a crayon. Many infants start to walk at 1 year of age. They can hold a cup for drinking. One-year-olds know more words, can say "no," and shake their heads for "no."

During the first 6 months the infant's diet is mainly breast milk or formula. Solid foods (strained fruits and vegetables) are usually added at 5 to 6 months. Junior foods are added during the eighth and ninth months. A 1-year-old can eat table foods.

TODDLERHOOD (1 TO 3 YEARS)

Physical growth during the second year of life is not as rapid as during infancy. The developmental tasks during this period are:

- Tolerating separation from the primary caregiver
- Gaining control of bowel and bladder function
- Using words to communicate with others
- Becoming less dependent on the primary caregiver

Because of the need to assert independence, the toddler years are known as the "terrible twos." The ability to move about and walk increases. So does the child's curiosity. Toddlers get into anything and everything. Whatever can be reached is touched, smelled, and tasted. As toddlers become more coordinated, they start to climb. The toddler's new and increasing skills allow exploration of the environment. The child ventures farther away from the primary caregiver. The toddler also discovers that some things can be done without the primary caregiver. By 3 years the toddler can run, jump, climb, ride a tricycle, and walk up and down stairs.

Increased hand coordination gives toddlers new skills. The need to feel, smell, and taste things is shown in their increasing ability to feed themselves. They progress from eating with fingers to using a spoon (Fig. 8-9). Toddlers can drink from cups. They can scribble, build towers with blocks, string beads, and turn book pages. Right- or left-handedness is seen during the second year.

Toilet training is a major developmental task for toddlers. Bowel and bladder control are related to central nervous system development. Children must be psychologically and physically ready for toilet training. The process starts with bowel control. Bowel control is easier because the frequency of bowel movements per day is less than urination. Bowel training usually is complete at about 2½ years of age. Bladder control during the day

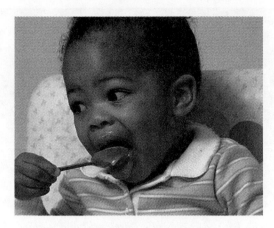

Fig. 8-9 *A toddler is able to use a spoon.*

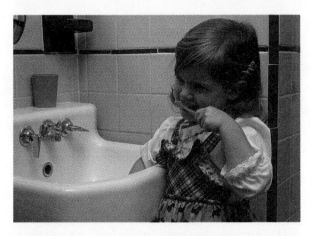

Fig. 8-10 *A 3-year-old has increased coordination.*

occurs before bladder control at night. Bladder training is usually complete at about 3 years of age.

Speech and language skills increase. Speech is clearer, and vocabulary increases. Words are learned by imitating others. Toddlers understand more words than they use. They are capable of 2- or 3-word sentences. By 3 years children speak in short sentences.

Play ability increases. The child plays alongside other children but does not play with them. There is no sharing of toys with others. The toddler is very possessive and does not understand sharing. The word "mine" is often used.

Temper tantrums and saying "no" are common during this stage. When disciplined the toddler often kicks and screams. The temper tantrum is the child's way of objecting to having independence challenged. The use of "no" can frustrate primary caregivers. Almost every request may be answered "no," even if the toddler is following the request.

Another developmental task is tolerating separation from the primary caregiver. As toddlers start to explore their environments, they tend to venture away from primary caregivers. When discomfort, frustration, or injury occurs, they quickly return to primary caregivers or cry for their attention. If the primary caregiver is consistently present whenever needed, a child learns to feel secure. Thus toddlers learn to tolerate brief periods of separation.

PRESCHOOL (3 TO 6 YEARS)

The preschool years (early childhood) are from the ages of 3 to 6 years. Children grow taller but gain little weight. Preschoolers are thinner, more coordinated, and more graceful than toddlers. The developmental tasks of the preschool years include:

- Increasing the ability to communicate and understand others
- Performing self-care activities
- Learning the differences between the sexes and developing sexual modesty
- Learning right from wrong and good from bad
- Learning to play with others
- Developing family relationships

The 3-Year-Old

Three-year-olds become more coordinated. They can walk on tiptoe, balance on one foot for a few seconds, and run, jump, and climb with ease. Personal care skills increase. They can put on shoes, dress themselves, manage buttons, wash their hands, and brush their teeth (Fig. 8-10). They can feed themselves, pour from a bottle, and help set the table without breaking dishes. Hand skills also include drawing circles and crosses.

Most 3-year-olds know about 1000 words, imitate new words, and talk and ask questions constantly. Sentences are brief—usually 3 or 4 words. Three-year-olds can name body parts, family members, friends, and animals. They like talking dolls and musical toys.

Play is important. Three-year-olds play in small groups with two or three other children and share toys. They play simple games and learn to follow simple rules. Imaginary playmates and imitating adults during play are common. They enjoy coloring books and crayons, scissors and paper, and playing "house" and "dress-up" (Fig. 8-11, p. 136).

At 3 years children know that there are two sexes. They know that male and female bodies are different. They also know their own sex. Little girls may wonder how the penis works and why they do not have one. Little boys may wonder how girls can urinate without a penis.

The concept of time develops. Children 3 years of age may speak of the past, present, and future. "Yesterday" and "tomorrow" are still confusing. Children may be afraid of the dark and need a night-light in the bedroom.

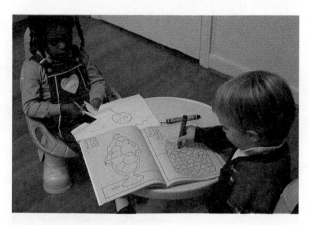

Fig. 8-11 *Three-year-olds enjoy cutting paper and using coloring books and crayons.*

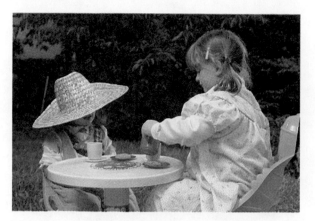

Fig. 8-12 *Four-year-olds play "dress-up" and imitate adults.*

Three-year-olds are less fearful of strangers. They tolerate separation from primary caregivers for short periods. They are less jealous than toddlers of a new baby. Things are done to please primary caregivers at this age.

The 4-Year-Old

Four-year-olds can hop, skip, and throw and catch a ball. They can lace shoes, draw faces, copy a square, and try to print letters. They can bathe with some help and usually tend to toileting needs with help.

Vocabulary increases to about 1500 words. The child continues to ask many questions and tends to exaggerate when telling stories. The 4-year-old can sing simple songs, repeat four numbers, count to three, and name a few colors.

Children 4 years of age may tend to attack others. They also tease, tattle, and tell fibs. They are more impatient and may blame an imaginary playmate when in trouble. Bragging, telling tales about family members, and showing off are common. They can play cooperatively with other children. Four-year-olds are proud of their accomplishments but have mood swings.

Children in this age-group enjoy playing "dress-up," wearing costumes, and telling and hearing stories. They like to draw and make things. Imagination, drama, and imitation of adults are seen during play (Fig. 8-12). They play in groups of two or three and tend to be bossy. Playing "doctor and nurse" is common as curiosity about the opposite sex continues.

Four-year-olds strongly prefer the primary caregiver of the other sex. Rivalries with brothers and sisters are seen, especially when younger children take the 4-year-old's possessions. Rivalries also occur when older children have more and different privileges. Family members are often the focus of the child's frustrations and aggressive behavior. Some 4-year-olds try to run away from home.

The 5-Year-Old

Coordination continues to develop. Five-year-olds can jump rope, skate, tie shoelaces, dress, and bathe. They can use a pencil and copy diamond and triangle shapes. They can print a few letters and numbers and their first names. Drawings of people include the body, head, arms, legs, and feet.

Communication skills also increase. Vocabulary consists of about 14,000 words. Sentences have six to eight words. They ask fewer questions than before, but questions have more meaning. They want definitions for unknown terms and take part in conversations. Four or more colors, coins, days of the week, and months can be named. They specify what they draw and give detailed descriptions of drawings.

Five-year-olds are more responsible and truthful, and they quarrel less than before. There is greater awareness of rules and an eagerness to do things the right way. They have manners, are independent, and can be trusted within limits. Five-year-olds have fewer fears but may have nightmares and dreams. They are also proud of their accomplishments.

Simple number and word games are enjoyed by 5-year-olds. Although they may cheat to win, they like rules and try to follow them. They imitate adults during play and have a greater interest in watching television. They also enjoy activities with the primary caregiver of the same sex (Fig. 8-13). Such activities include cooking, housecleaning, shopping, yard work, and sports.

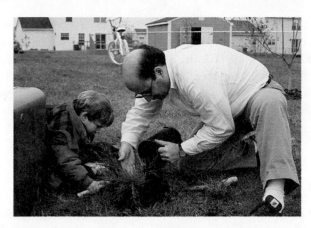

Fig. 8-13 *Five-year-olds enjoy doing things with the parent of the same sex.*

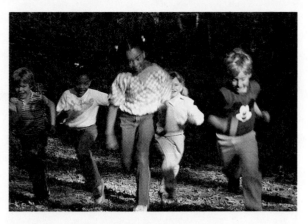

Fig. 8-14 *Six-year-olds play with children of both sexes but begin to prefer playing with children of the same sex.*

These children tolerate brothers and sisters well. Although younger children are considered a nuisance, 5-year-olds usually protect them.

MIDDLE CHILDHOOD (6 TO 8 YEARS)

Preschoolers often have nursery school and kindergarten experiences. However, middle childhood is the time for school. Children enter the world of peer groups, games, and learning. The developmental tasks of middle childhood are:

- Developing the social and physical skills needed for playing games
- Learning to get along with other children of the same age and background (peers)
- Learning behaviors and attitudes appropriate to one's own sex
- Learning basic reading, writing, and arithmetic skills
- Developing a conscience and morals
- Developing a good feeling and attitude about oneself

The 6-Year-Old

The 6-year-old grows about 2 inches taller and gains 3 to 6 pounds. Baby teeth are lost, and replacement with permanent teeth begins. Children are very active and are skilled at running, jumping, skipping, hopping, and riding a bicycle. They seem to have a need to be constantly on the go. Sitting is tolerated for only a short time.

Six-year-olds enter the first grade and the world of school, activities, and other children. Children this age are often described as bossy, opinionated, charming, argumentative, and "know-it-alls." They have set ways of doing things and like to have their own way. They may have temper tantrums. Six-year-olds play well with chil-

dren of both sexes. However, they begin to prefer playing with children of the same sex (Fig. 8-14). There is more sharing with others, and the child may have a "best friend." A child may cheat to win or leave a game before it is over to avoid losing. Tattling is common.

Six-year-olds have a vocabulary of about 16,500 words. They know the alphabet and begin to read and spell. They communicate thoughts and feelings better than before.

Play interests range from rough play to quiet activities such as playing with cards, paints, clay, and checkers. Collections are started of odds and ends rather than specific things like stamps, rocks, or butterflies. More active play includes tag, hide-and-seek, playing with balls, skating, and playing in mud or sand.

The 7-Year-Old

Seven-year-olds grow about 2 inches in height. The average 7-year-old weighs about 49 to 56 pounds and is 47 to 49 inches tall. Hand coordination increases. Children learn to write rather than print. They are quieter than 6-year-olds and spend much time alone. They are more serious, less stubborn, and more concerned about being well-liked. Seven-year-olds are more aware of themselves, their bodies, and the reactions of others. They do not like being teased or criticized and are sensitive about how others treat them. They like going to school, learning, and reading. There are concerns about grades and what the teacher thinks about them. Reading skills increase, and the child can tell time.

Play includes swimming, biking, collecting and trading objects, playing ball and games with rules, and working puzzles and magic tricks (Fig. 8-15, p. 138). They play in groups. However, boys prefer to play with boys and girls prefer to play with girls. They may join scouting groups, such as the Cub Scouts or Brownies.

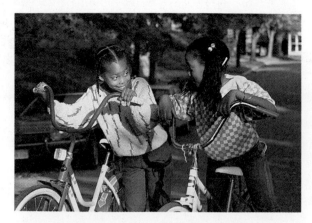

Fig. 8-15 *Seven-year-olds enjoy biking.*

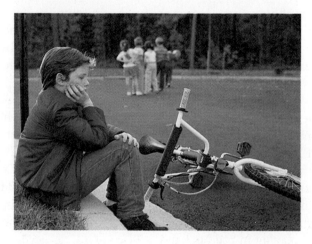

Fig. 8-16 *Belonging to a peer group is important to the 8-year-old.*

The 8-Year-Old

The 8-year-old enters the third grade. Growth in height and weight continues. More permanent teeth appear. Movements are faster and more graceful.

Peer group activities and opinions are important. Being accepted and included in peer groups are important for love and belonging and self-esteem (Fig. 8-16). Children this age get along with adults. However, they prefer peer group fads, opinions, and activities. Boys and girls play separately. Their interests relate to group games, collections, television, and movies.

Eight-year-olds have been described as defensive, opinionated, practical, and outgoing. Advice is freely given to others. However, they do not accept criticism well. They often do household tasks such as vacuuming, cooking, and yard work but expect to be paid. They expect more privileges than younger brothers and sisters.

Learning continues. They are curious about science, history, and other places and countries. School also provides social opportunities with peers. Eight-year-olds are daring in the classroom. They may pass notes and throw spitballs or paper airplanes when they think the teacher is not looking. Despite this mischief, they are mannerly, relate well to adults, and take part in adult conversations. They are also friendly and affectionate.

LATE CHILDHOOD (9 TO 12 YEARS)

Late childhood (preadolescence) is between leaving childhood and dependency on others and entering adolescence. Developmental tasks are similar to those of middle childhood. However, a preadolescent is expected to show more refinement and maturity in achieving the following tasks:

- Becoming independent of adults and learning to depend on oneself
- Developing and keeping friendships with peers
- Understanding the physical, psychological, and social roles of one's sex
- Developing moral and ethical behavior
- Developing greater muscular strength, coordination, and balance
- Learning how to study

Boys grow about 1 inch per year. Girls grow about 2 inches per year. Boys gain about 3½ to 4 pounds each year. Girls gain between 4 and 5 pounds each year. Girls are usually taller than boys during late preadolescence. Many permanent teeth erupt.

Body movements are more graceful and coordinated (Fig. 8-17). Muscular strength and physical skills increase. Skill in team sports is important.

Body changes occur as the onset of puberty nears. In girls the pelvis becomes broader, fat appears on the hips and chest, and the budding of breasts occurs. Boys show fewer signs of maturing sexually during this time. Genital organs begin to grow.

These children must have factual sex education. Information about sex is shared among friends, although the information is often incomplete and inaccurate. Parents and children may be uncomfortable discussing sex with each other and may avoid the subject. When children do ask questions, honest and complete answers must be given in terms the children can understand.

Peer groups are the center of preadolescent activities. The group begins to affect the child's attitudes and behavior. Preference for companions of the same sex continues. Boys need to show their strength and toughness and may give each other nicknames. Arguments between boys and girls are common, and boys often tease girls.

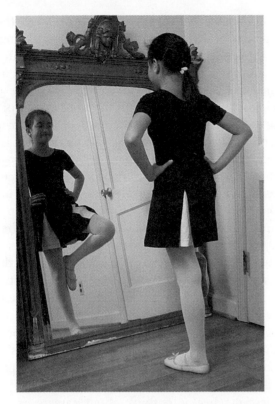

Fig. 8-17 *Movements are smooth and graceful in late childhood.*

Preadolescents are more aware of the mistakes and weaknesses of adults. They do not accept adult standards and rules without question. Rebellion against adults is common. Disagreements between parents and children increase, although the parents continue to be important for the child's development.

By the age of 12 years the child uses about 7000 words in conversation and understands about 50,000 words in reading. Dictionary, encyclopedia, and other reference book use increases. Interest in science, history, and geography continues. Girls often enjoy reading romantic books and stories. Boys usually prefer science fiction, mysteries, and adventure stories.

ADOLESCENCE (12 TO 18 YEARS)

Adolescence is a time of rapid growth and psychological and social maturity. The stage begins with puberty. **Puberty** is the period during which the reproductive organs begin to function and the secondary sex characteristics appear. Girls experience puberty between the ages of 10 and 14 years. Most boys reach puberty between the ages of 12 and 16 years.

Because the age of puberty varies, adolescence ranges from the ages of 12 to 18 years. The developmental tasks of adolescence include:

- Accepting changes in the body and appearance
- Developing appropriate relationships with males and females of the same age
- Accepting the male or female role appropriate for one's age
- Becoming independent from parents and adults
- Developing morals, attitudes, and values needed for functioning in society

Menarche, the beginning of menstruation, marks the onset of puberty in girls. Secondary sex characteristics appear. These include:

- Increase in breast size
- Appearance of pubic and axillary (underarm) hair
- Slight deepening of the voice
- Widening and rounding of the hips

During late childhood, male sex organs begin to increase in size. This growth continues during adolescence. **Ejaculation** (the release of semen) signals the onset of puberty in boys. Nocturnal emissions ("wet dreams") occur. During sleep (nocturnal) the penis becomes erect and semen is released (emission). Other secondary sex characteristics appear. These include:

- Appearance of facial hair and growth of a beard
- Pubic and axillary hair
- Hair on the arms, chest, and legs
- Deepening of the voice
- Increases in neck and shoulder size

A growth spurt occurs. Boys grow about 4 to 16 inches and gain 15 to 60 pounds. They usually stop growing between the ages of 18 and 21 years. Some continue to grow until about age 25. Girls grow about 2 to 9 inches and gain between 15 and 50 pounds. They usually stop growing between the ages of 17 and 18 years. Some continue to grow until about age 21.

Adolescence is described as the awkward stage. Awkwardness and clumsiness are the result of the uneven growth of muscles and bones. Coordination and graceful body movements develop as muscle and bone growth even out.

Changes in appearance are often hard to accept. Some girls are embarrassed about breast development, especially very large or small breast size. Some are embarrassed about wearing a bra. Others wear tight sweaters so the breasts are noticed. Genital size may be a concern of boys. Height is a problem for both boys and girls. Being short limits play in some sports. Boys do not like being much shorter than their peers. Tall girls may feel embarrassed about being different and taller than other girls and boys.

Emotional reactions vary from high to low. Adolescents can be happy one moment and sad the next. Predicting a reaction to a comment or event is difficult. Teenagers can

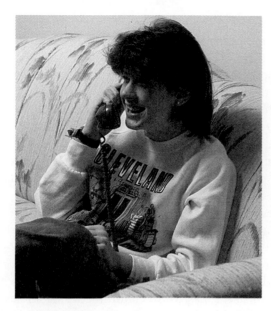

Fig. 8-18 *Adolescents enjoy talking on the phone.*

control their emotions better later in this stage. Older adolescents (15- to 18-year-olds) can still become sad and depressed. However, they can better control the time and place of their emotional reactions.

Adolescents need to become independent of adults, especially their parents. They must learn to function, make decisions, and act in a responsible manner without adult supervision. Many teenagers work toward this independence with part-time jobs, babysitting, going to dances and parties, dating, taking part in school clubs and organizations, shopping without an adult, and staying home alone.

Judgment and reasoning are not always sound. Guidance, discipline, and emotional and financial support are still needed from parents. Disagreements with parents are common, especially about behavior and activity restrictions and limitations. Teenagers would rather be with peers than do things with parents and other family members. Adolescents tend to confide in and seek advice from adults other than their parents.

Teenage interests and activities reflect the need to become independent, to develop relationships with the opposite sex, and to act like males or females. Both sexes are interested in parties, dances, and other social activities. Clothing, makeup, and hairstyles are important. A teenager may babysit or get a part-time job to have extra money for clothes, makeup, and hair-care and skin-care products. Parents and teenagers rarely agree about clothing styles. Teenagers may spend a lot of time experimenting with makeup and hairstyles. They may also spend a lot of time talking to friends on the phone, listening to music, and reading teen magazines (Fig. 8-18).

Dating begins during adolescence. Although the age when dating begins varies, there is usually a dating pattern. "Crowd" dates are common in the seventh and eighth grades. They are usually related to school activities, such as a dance or basketball game. The same group of girls just happens to be with the same group of boys during these social events. In the ninth grade, pairing off is common during crowd dating. The tenth grade is usually when boy-girl couples go to social events together and then join other couples. Double dating occurs in the eleventh grade. Dates involve one couple during the twelfth grade, although there is some double dating.

Many difficult decisions and conflicts result as the adolescent matures physically, psychologically, and emotionally. Parents and teenagers often disagree about dating. Parents worry that dating will lead to sexual activities, pregnancy, and sexually transmitted diseases. Teenagers usually do not understand or appreciate these concerns. "Going steady" helps meet the teenager's need for security, love and belonging, and self-esteem. Teenagers sometimes have difficulty controlling sexual urges and considering the consequences of sexual activity.

Adolescents begin to think about careers and what to do after high school graduation. Interests, skills, and talents are some factors that influence the choice of further education and getting a job. Adolescents also need to develop morals, values, and attitudes for living in society. They need to develop a sense about what is good and bad, right and wrong, and important and unimportant. Parents, peers, culture, religion, television, school, and movies are among the many factors influencing teenagers. Drug abuse, unwanted pregnancy, alcoholism, and criminal acts are common problems of troubled adolescents.

YOUNG ADULTHOOD (18 TO 40 YEARS)

Psychological and social development continue during young adulthood. There is little physical growth. Adult height has been reached. Body systems are fully developed. Developmental tasks of young adulthood include:

- Choosing education and an occupation
- Selecting a marriage partner
- Learning to live with a partner
- Becoming a parent and raising children
- Developing a satisfactory sex life

Education and occupation are so closely related that they can rarely be separated. Most jobs require specific knowledge and skills. The amount and kind of education needed depends on the career choice. Most adults find that job choices are greater with adequate educational preparation. Employment is necessary for economic independence and for supporting a family.

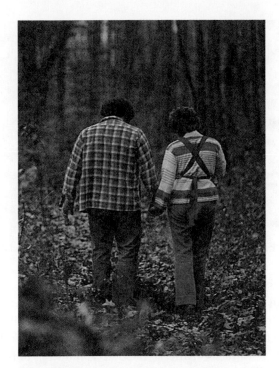

Fig. 8-19 *Communication is necessary for a successful partnership and a satisfactory sex life.*

Most adults marry at least once. Others choose to remain single. They may live alone, with friends of the same sex, or with a person from the opposite sex. Gay and lesbian persons may commit to a partner.

The many reasons for marriage include love, emotional security, wanting a family, sex, wanting to leave an unhappy home life, social status, companionship, and money. Some marry to feel wanted, needed, and desirable. Many factors also affect selecting a marriage partner. They include age, religion, interests, education, race, personality, and, of course, love. Some marriages are happy and successful, whereas others are not. There are no guarantees that a marriage will work. Therefore the two people must work together to build a marriage based on trust, respect, caring, and friendship.

Couples (married or unmarried) must learn to live together. Habits, routines, meal preparation, and pastimes are changed or adjusted to "fit" the other person's needs. They must learn how to solve problems and make decisions together. They need to work toward the same goals. Open and honest communication helps create a successful partnership (Fig. 8-19).

Adults also need to develop a satisfactory sex life. Sexual frequency, desires, practices, and preferences vary. Understanding and accepting the partner's needs are necessary for a satisfying and intimate relationship.

Most couples decide to have children. Modern birth control methods allow planning about the number of children and when to have them. However, many pregnancies are unplanned. Most couples have a child during the first few years of marriage; some wait several years before starting a family. Other couples decide not to have children. Some have difficulty or cannot have children because of physical problems in the husband or wife. Those couples having children need to agree on child-rearing practices and discipline methods. They need to adjust to the child and to the child's need for time, energy, and parental attention.

MIDDLE ADULTHOOD (40 TO 65 YEARS)

This stage of development is more stable and comfortable. Children are usually grown and have moved away. Husbands and wives now have time to spend alone together. There are fewer worries about children and money. The developmental tasks of middle adulthood relate to:
- Adjusting to physical changes
- Having grown children
- Developing leisure-time activities
- Relating to aging parents

Several physical changes occur. Many are gradual and go unnoticed; others are seen early. People in their early forties may feel energetic and able to function as they did in their twenties. However, energy and endurance begin to slow down. Weight control becomes a problem as metabolism and physical activities slow down. Facial wrinkles and gray hair appear. The need for eyeglasses is common. Hearing loss may begin. Menstruation stops between the ages of 42 and 55; this is called **menopause.** Ovaries stop secreting hormones, and the woman can no longer have children. Many diseases and illnesses can develop. The disorders can become chronic or life threatening.

Children leave home for college, marry, move to homes of their own, and start their own families. Adults have to cope with letting children go, being in-laws, and becoming grandparents. Parents must let children lead their own lives. However, they need to be available for emotional support in times of need.

Middle-age adults often discover spare time when the demands of parenthood decrease. Hobbies and pastimes such as gardening, fishing, painting, golfing, volunteer work, and membership in clubs and organizations are sources of pleasure (Fig. 8-20, p. 142). Hobbies and pastimes become even more important after retirement and during late adulthood.

Some middle-age adults have parents who are aging and developing poor health. Responsibility for aging parents may begin during this stage. Middle-age adults often have to deal with the death of parents.

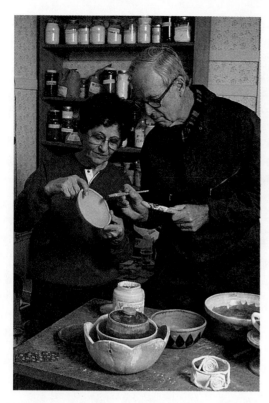

Fig. 8-20 *Middle-age adults usually have more time for hobbies.*

LATE ADULTHOOD (65 YEARS AND OLDER)

People live longer and are healthier than ever before. Today most people can expect to live into their 70s. Earlier in this century, most people died in their 50s. There also have been steady increases in the number of 70-, 80-, 90-, and 100-year-olds. Many of these persons continue to live healthy and happy lives. Late adulthood is broken down into the following age ranges:

- The young-old—65 to 74 years
- The middle-old—75 to 84 years
- The old-old—over 85 years

The developmental tasks of late adulthood are:

- Adjusting to decreased physical strength and loss of health
- Adjusting to retirement and reduced income
- Coping with the death of a partner
- Developing new friends and relationships
- Preparing for one's own death

Gerontology is the study of the aging process. **Geriatrics** is the care of aged persons. Aging, or growing old, is a normal process. Normal changes occur in body structure and function. Because of these changes, older persons have special needs. They are also at greater risk for illness, chronic diseases, and injuries.

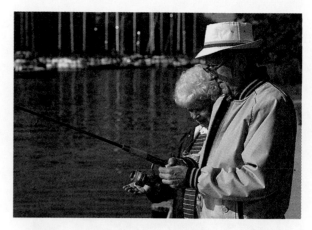

Fig. 8-21 *A retired couple enjoying fishing together.*

Physical, psychological, and social changes occur as a person grows older. Graying hair, wrinkles, and slow movements are physical reminders of growing old. Retirement and death of a partner, relatives, and friends are social reminders. American society values youth and beauty. This emphasis can make aging a painful process physically, socially, and psychologically.

Certain physical changes are a normal part of aging and occur in everyone (Table 8-1). The rate and degree of change vary with each person. Influencing factors include diet, general health, exercise, stress, environment, and heredity. The physical changes of aging result in a slowing down of body processes. Energy level and body efficiency decline. The normal changes of aging may be accompanied by changes caused by disease, illness, or injury.

People usually retire between the ages of 65 and 70 years. Some retire earlier. Retirement is a reward for a lifetime of working. The person can relax and enjoy life (Fig. 8-21). Travel, leisure, and doing whatever one wants are retirement "benefits." Retirement is often a person's first real experience with aging. Some must retire because of chronic disease or disability. Poor health and medical expenses can make enjoying retirement very difficult.

Retirement income is often less than one half of the person's working income. Social Security may provide the only income. However, retirement and aging do not mean fewer expenses. Rent or mortgage payments, food, clothing, utility bills, and taxes are usual expenses. Car expenses, home repairs, medicine, and health care are other costs. So are entertainment and gifts for children, grandchildren, and other family and friends.

Reduced income may force certain changes. Some retirees limit social and leisure activities. A move to cheaper housing may be necessary. Some older persons rely on children or other relatives for housing and money. Some cannot afford health care or needed medicines.

TABLE 8-1 PHYSICAL CHANGES DURING THE AGING PROCESS

System	Changes	System	Changes
Integumentary	Skin becomes less elastic Fatty tissue layer is lost Skin thins and sags Skin is fragile and easily injured Folds, lines, and wrinkles appear Decreased secretion of oil and sweat glands Dry skin develops Itching Increased sensitivity to cold Nails become thick and tough Whitening or graying hair Loss or thinning of hair Facial hair in some women	Cardiovascular	Heart pumps with less force Arteries narrow and are less elastic Less blood flows through narrowed arteries Weakened heart has to work harder to pump blood through narrowed vessels
Musculoskeletal	Muscle atrophy Decreasing strength Bones become brittle; can break easily Joints become stiff and painful Gradual loss of height Decreased mobility	Respiratory	Respiratory muscles weaken Lung tissue becomes less elastic Difficulty breathing Decreased strength for coughing
		Digestive	Decreased saliva production Difficulty in swallowing Decreased appetite Decreased secretion of digestive juices Fried and fatty foods difficult to digest Indigestion Loss of teeth Decreased peristalsis causing flatulence and constipation
Nervous	Vision and hearing decrease Decreased senses of taste and smell Reduced sense of touch Reduced sensitivity to pain Reduced blood flow to the brain Progressive loss of brain cells Shorter memory Forgetfulness Slowed ability to respond Confusion Dizziness Changes in sleep patterns	Urinary	Reduced blood supply to kidneys Kidneys atrophy Kidney function decreases Poisonous substances can build up in the blood Urine becomes concentrated Urinary frequency and urgency may occur Urinary incontinence may occur The need to urinate at night may occur

Many people plan for retirement through savings, investments, retirement plans, and insurance. Their retirement years are financially comfortable.

Social relationships change throughout life. Children grow up, leave home, and have their own families. Many live far away from parents. Older friends and relatives move away, die, or are disabled. Yet most older people have regular contact with children, grandchildren, brothers and sisters, nieces and nephews, and other relatives and friends. Some do not. Separation from children and

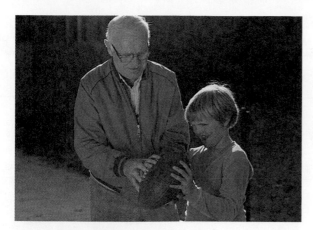

Fig. 8-22 *An older man plays with his grandchild.*

lack of companionship are common causes of loneliness in older persons.

Hobbies, church and community activities, and new friends help prevent loneliness. Being a grandparent can be a source of great love and enjoyment (Fig. 8-22). Being included in family activities helps the older person to feel useful and wanted.

Some older persons speak and understand a foreign language. Communication occurs with family and friends who speak the same language. These relatives and friends may move away or die. Greater loneliness and isolation for the foreign-speaking person may result. The person may not have anyone to talk to and may not be understood by others. In addition, the person's cultural values and practices may not be understood or recognized.

Children often care for older parents. Instead of the parent caring for the child, the child cares for the parent. This role change and dependency on a child can make the older person feel more secure. However, others feel unwanted, in the way, and useless. Some feel a loss of dignity and self-respect. Tensions may develop between the child, parent, and other family members in the household. Lack of privacy, disagreements, criticisms about housekeeping, childrearing, cooking, and friends are common causes of tension.

Adult day care centers are options when working children cannot leave parents alone. Meals, supervision, and activities are provided. Some provide transportation to and from the center.

Sometimes older brothers, sisters, and cousins live together. They provide companionship for each other. They can also share living expenses. They care for each other during illness or disability.

Some older persons need the type of care provided by nursing centers. Such care may be temporary for recovery from injury, illness, or surgery. For others, it is permanent.

A person may try to psychologically prepare for a partner's death. However, losing a partner is devastating. No amount of preparation is ever enough for the emptiness and changes that result. The person loses more than a partner. A friend, lover, companion, and confidant are also lost. The grief felt by the survivor may be very great. Serious physical and mental health problems can result.

REVIEW QUESTIONS

Circle the best *answer.*

1 Changes in psychological and social functioning are called

   a Growth   c A reflex

   b Development   d A stage

2 Which is *false?*

   a Growth and development occur from the simple to the complex.

   b Growth and development occur in an orderly pattern.

   c Growth and development occur at specific rates.

   d Each stage has its own characteristics.

3 The stage of infancy is the first

   a 4 weeks of life   c 6 months of life

   b 3 months of life   d Year of life

4 Which reflexes are needed for feeding in the infant?

   a The Moro and startle reflexes

   b The rooting and sucking reflexes

   c The grasping and Moro reflexes

   d The rooting and grasping reflexes

5 Crawling occurs at about

   a 6 months   c 8 months

   b 7 months   d 9 months

6 Solid foods are usually given to a baby during the

a Fifth or sixth month

b Seventh or eighth month

c Ninth or tenth month

d Eleventh or twelfth month

7 Toilet training begins

a During infancy

b During the toddler years

c When the primary caregiver is ready

d At the age of 3

8 The toddler can

a Use a spoon and cup

b Ride a bike

c Help set the table

d Name parts of the body

9 Playing with other children begins during

a Infancy

b The toddler years

c The preschool years

d Middle childhood

10 Loss of baby teeth usually begins at the age of

a 4   c 6

b 5   d 7

11 Peer group activities become more important at the age of

a 6   c 8

b 7   d 9

12 Reproductive organs begin to function and secondary sex characteristics appear during

a Late childhood   c Puberty

b Preadolescence   d Early adulthood

13 Which is *false?*

a Boys reach puberty earlier than girls.

b Most girls reach puberty between the ages of 12 and 13.

c Menarche marks the onset of puberty in girls.

d A growth spurt occurs during adolescence.

14 Dating usually begins

a During late childhood

b With "crowd" dating

c With "pairing off"

d During late adolescence

15 Adolescence is a time when parents and children

a Talk openly about sex

b Express love and affection

c Disagree

d Do things as a family

16 Which is *not* a developmental task of young adulthood?

a Adjusting to changes in the body and in physical appearance

b Selecting a partner

c Choosing an occupation

d Becoming a parent

17 Middle adulthood is from about

a 25 to 35 years   c 40 to 50 years

b 30 to 40 years   d 40 to 65 years

18 Middle adulthood is a time when

a Families are started

b Physical energy and free time are gained

c Children are grown and leave home

d People need to prepare for death

19 The physical changes of aging include the following *except*

a Dry skin

b Stiff and painful joints

c Shorter memory

d Greater blood flow

20 Retirement usually results in

a Lowered income

b Physical changes from aging

c Companionship and usefulness

d Financial security

21 Older people may experience loneliness because

a Children may have moved away

b Friends and relatives may have died or moved

c Of difficulties in communicating with others

d All of the above

22 Death of a partner results in the loss of a

a Friend   c Companion

b Lover   d All of the above

Answers to these questions are on p. 851.

9 Sexuality

- Define the key terms in this chapter
- Describe the differences between sex and sexuality
- Explain the importance of sexuality throughout life
- Describe five types of sexual relationships
- Explain how injury and illness can affect sexuality
- Explain how aging affects sexuality in older persons
- Explain how the nursing team can promote a person's sexuality
- Explain why some persons become sexually aggressive
- Describe how to deal with sexually aggressive persons

KEY TERMS

bisexual A person who is attracted to both sexes

heterosexual A person who is attracted to people of the other sex

homosexual A person who is attracted to members of the same sex

impotence The inability of the male to have an erection

menopause The time when menstruation stops; it marks the end of the woman's reproductive years

sex The physical activities involving the organs of reproduction; the activities are done for pleasure or to produce children

sexuality The physical, psychological, social, cultural, and spiritual factors that affect a person's feelings and attitudes about his or her sex

transsexual A person who believes that he or she is really a member of the other sex

transvestite A person who becomes sexually excited by dressing in the clothes of the other sex

Another part of the person involves the physical, psychological, social, and spiritual. That part is sexuality. Illness and injury can affect a person's sexuality. This chapter describes the effects of illness, injury, and aging on sexuality. You must view patients, young and old, as total persons. Total persons have sexuality.

SEX AND SEXUALITY

Sex and sexuality are different. Sex is the physical activities involving the reproductive organs. The activities are done for pleasure or to produce children. **Sexuality** involves the personality and the body. A person's attitudes and feelings are involved. Physical, psychological, social, cultural, and spiritual factors influence sexuality. It affects how a person behaves, thinks, dresses, and responds to others.

Sexuality is present when a baby's sex is known. Names, colors, and toys reflect sexuality. Blue is used for boys and pink for girls. Dolls are for girls. Trains are for boys. By the age of 2 years, children know their own sex. Three-year-olds know the sex of other children. Children learn male and female roles from their parents (Fig. 9-1, p. 148). Children learn early that there are certain behaviors for boys and certain ones for girls.

As children grow older, interest increases about the human body and how it works. Body changes during adolescence bring more interest about sex and the body. Their bodies respond to stimulation. Teenagers engage in sexual behaviors. They kiss, embrace, pet, or have intercourse. Pregnancy and sexually transmitted diseases (p. 151) are great risks for sexually active teenagers.

Sex has more meaning as young adults mature. Attitudes and feelings are important. Sexual partners are selected. Sex before marriage and birth control are other decisions.

Sexuality is important into adulthood and old age. Attitudes and sex needs change as a person grows older. Life circumstances change. These include divorce, death of a partner, injury, and illness.

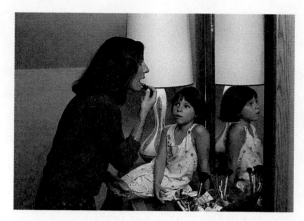

Fig. 9-1 *This little girl is learning female roles from her mother.*

SEXUAL RELATIONSHIPS

Sex and sexuality usually involve a partner. A **heterosexual** is a person who is attracted to people of the other sex. Men are attracted to women, and women are attracted to men. Sexual behavior is male-female.

A **homosexual** is attracted to members of the same sex. Men are attracted to men, and women are attracted to women. *Gay* refers to homosexuality. Homosexual men are referred to as *gay men. Lesbian* refers to a female homosexual.

Homosexuality has existed for centuries. Prior to the 1960s and 1970s, many gay persons were secret about their sexual orientation. Now many gay men and lesbians are more open about their sexual preference and relationships.

Bisexuals are attracted to both sexes. Some alternate between same-gender and male-female behaviors. Bisexuals often are married and have children. They may seek a same-gender relationship or experience outside of marriage.

Some people believe that they are really members of the other sex. These people are **transsexuals.** A male believes he is really a female in a man's body. A female believes she is really a male in a woman's body. Transsexual persons often describe feeling "trapped" in the wrong body. Most have had these feelings for as long as they can remember. As children they usually show behaviors of the other sex. Many seek psychiatric treatment. Some have sex-change operations. Psychiatric treatment and sex-change operations do not always help these people.

Transvestites become sexually excited by dressing in clothes of the other sex. Most are male. They are usually married and heterosexual. They dress normally as men most of the time. Dressing as a woman is usually done in private. Some dress completely as women. Others focus on bras and panties. The sex partner may not know about the practice. Some partners take part in transvestite activities. Some transvestites have same-gender friends with similar interests.

INJURY AND ILLNESS

Sexuality and sex involve the mind and body. Injury and illness can affect sexual function. A person may feel unclean, unwhole, unattractive, or mutilated after surgery or injury. Attitudes about sex may change. The person may feel unfit for closeness and love. Therefore the person may develop sexual problems that are psychological. Time, understanding, and a caring partner are very helpful. Counseling or psychiatric help may be needed.

Many illnesses, injuries, and surgeries affect the nervous, circulatory, and reproductive systems. If one or more of these systems are involved, the person's sexual ability may change. Most chronic illnesses affect sexual function.

Impotence is the inability of the male to have an erection. Diabetes mellitus, spinal cord injuries, multiple sclerosis, and alcoholism are common causes. Circulatory disorders and medications can interfere with achieving an erection. Impotence is a side effect of some medications that control high blood pressure.

Heart disease, stroke, chronic obstructive pulmonary disease, and nervous system disorders can affect sexual ability. Some reproductive system surgeries have physical and psychological effects. Prostate or testes removal affects erections. Removal of the uterus, ovaries, or a breast may affect a woman psychologically.

Changes in sexual functioning greatly impact the person. Fear, anger, worry, and depression are common. You see these in the person's behavior and comments. The person's feelings are very normal and expected.

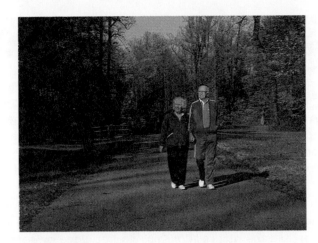

Fig. 9-2 *Love and affection are important to older persons.*

SEXUALITY AND OLDER PERSONS

Sexual relationships are important to older persons (Fig. 9-2). They fall in love, hold hands, embrace, and have sex. They need sex, love, and affection. Many have sexual intercourse.

Love, affection, and intimacy are needed throughout life. As other losses occur, feeling close to another person is more important. Children leave home. Friends and relatives die. People retire. Health problems may develop. Decreasing strength and a changing appearance add to these losses.

Reproductive organs change with aging. In men, the hormone testosterone decreases. The hormone affects strength, sperm production, and reproductive tissues. These changes affect sexual activity. It takes longer for an erection to occur. The phase between erection and orgasm is also longer. Orgasm is less forceful than in the younger years. After orgasm, the erection is lost quickly. The time between erections is also longer. Older men may need the penis stimulated for sexual arousal. These changes result in decreased frequency of sexual activity.

Mental and physical fatigue, overeating, and excessive drinking affect erections. Some men fear performance problems. Therefore they may avoid sexual activity.

Physical changes occur in women. Menopause occurs around 50 years of age. **Menopause** is when a woman stops menstruating. Her reproductive years end. Female hormones (estrogen and progesterone) decrease. Reduced hormone levels affect reproductive tissues. The uterus, vagina, and external genitalia atrophy (shrink). Intercourse may be uncomfortable or painful. This is from thin vaginal walls and vaginal dryness. Older women also have changes in sexual excitement. Arousal takes longer. The time between excitement and orgasm is longer. Orgasm is less intense. The pre-excitement state returns more quickly.

Frequency of sexual activity decreases for many men and women. Reasons relate to weakness, mental and physical fatigue, pain, and reduced mobility. The normal aging process or chronic illness are common causes. Pain and reduced mobility from illness and aging can affect frequency. One or both partners may have a chronic illness. It may lead to decreased frequency or no sexual activity.

Some older people do not have sexual intercourse. This does not mean sexual needs or desires are lost. They can express their needs in other ways. Hand holding, touching, caressing, and embracing bring closeness and intimacy.

Having a sexual partner is also important. Death and divorce result in loss of a sexual partner. The partner may also be in a hospital or nursing center. These situations occur in adults of all ages.

MEETING THE PERSON'S SEXUAL NEEDS

Sexuality is part of the total person. Some people are so ill that sexual activity is impossible. Others want and are capable of sexual activity. Sexual activity does not always mean intercourse. It may be expressed in other ways. The nursing team has an important role in sexuality. They allow and promote the meeting of sexual needs. Patients appreciate the measures listed in Box 9-1 on p. 150. They are carried out in cooperation with the nurse supervising your work. (See Focus on Long-Term Care and Focus on Older Persons on p. 150.

BOX 9-1

PROMOTING SEXUALITY

- Let the person practice grooming routines. This includes applying makeup, nail polish, and body lotion and wearing cologne. Hair care is important. Women may want to shave their legs and underarms and pluck eyebrows. Men may use after-shave lotion. Patients need help with these activities.
- Let the person choose clothing. Hospital gowns embarrass both men and women. Street clothes are worn if the person's condition permits.
- Protect the right to privacy. Avoid exposing the person. Drape and screen the person appropriately.
- Accept the person's sexual relationships. The person may not share your sexual attitudes, values, or practices. Do not expect the person to follow your standards. The person may have a homosexual, premarital, or extramarital relationship. Do not judge or gossip about relationships.
- Allow privacy. You can usually tell when two people want to be alone. If the person has a private room, close the door for privacy. Some agencies have *Do Not Disturb* signs for doors. Let the person and partner know how much time they have alone. For example, remind them about meal times, medications, or treatments. Tell other staff members that the person wants time alone.
- Knock before you enter any room. This is a simple courtesy that shows respect for privacy.
- Consider the patient's roommate. Privacy curtains provide little privacy. Arrange for privacy when the roommate is out of the room. Sometimes roommates volunteer to leave for a while. If the roommate cannot leave, other areas on the nursing unit are used for privacy.
- Allow privacy for masturbation. It is a normal form of sexual expression and release. Close the privacy curtain and the door. Knock before you enter any room to save you and the person embarrassment. Sometimes confused persons masturbate in public areas. Lead the person to a private area or engage his or her interest in some other activity.

focus on LONG-TERM CARE

Married couples in nursing centers are allowed to share the same room. This is a requirement of the Omnibus Budget Reconciliation Act of 1987 (OBRA). The couple has lived together for many years. Long-term care is no reason to keep them apart in rooms for men and women. They can share the same bed if their conditions permit. A double, queen-size, or king-size bed is provided by the couple or the agency.

Sexual partners are lost through death and divorce. A single resident may develop a relationship with another single resident. Instead of keeping them apart, they should be allowed time together (Fig. 9-3).

focus on OLDER PERSONS

Older persons have the right to be sexual. The measures described in Box 9-1 apply to older persons.

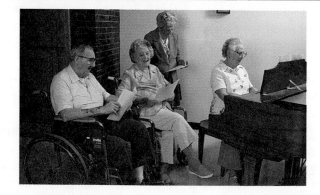

Fig. 9-3 *Intimate relationships occur in nursing centers.*

THE SEXUALLY AGGRESSIVE PERSON

Some persons want their sexual needs met by the health team. They flirt, make sexual advances or comments, expose themselves, masturbate, or touch staff. The staff member is usually angry or embarrassed when this happens. These reactions are normal. Often there are reasons for the person's behavior. Understanding this helps you deal with the situation.

Illness, injury, surgery, or aging often threaten a male's sense of manhood. He tries to prove to himself that he is still attractive and able to perform sexually. Therefore he may behave sexually toward a staff member.

Some sexually aggressive behaviors are from confusion or disorientation. Common causes are nervous system disorders, medications, fever, dementia (see Chapter 32), and poor vision. The person may confuse a staff member with his or her partner. Or the person cannot control behavior because of changes in mental function. The healthy person is able to control sexual urges. However, changes in the brain can make control difficult. Sexual behavior in these cases is usually innocent on the person's part.

Some persons do touch workers inappropriately. Their purpose is sexual. However, sometimes touch is the only way the person can get someone's attention. For example, Mr. Green had a stroke. His right side is paralyzed, and he cannot speak. Your back is to him, and you are bending over. Your buttocks are the closest part of your body to him. To get your attention, he touches your buttocks. You should not consider his behavior as sexual.

Often masturbation is viewed as a sexually aggressive behavior. It could indeed be touching and manipulating the genitals for sexual pleasure. However, urinary or reproductive system disorders can cause genital soreness or itching. Poor hygiene is another cause of itching. So is being wet or soiled from urine or a bowel movement. The nursing team must remember that touching the genitals could be a sign of a health problem.

Sexual advances may be intentional. You need to be professional about the matter. These suggestions may help:

- Ask the person not to touch you. State the places where you were touched.
- Tell the person that you will not do what he or she wants.
- Tell the person that those behaviors make you uncomfortable. Politely ask the person not to act in that way.
- Allow privacy if the person is becoming sexually aroused. Provide for safety; for example, raise bed rails if ordered for the person, place the call bell within reach (see Chapter 10). Tell the person when you will return.
- Discuss the situation with the RN. The RN can help you understand the person's behavior.

SEXUALLY TRANSMITTED DISEASES

Some diseases are spread by sexual contact. They are grouped under the heading of sexually transmitted diseases (STDs). STDs are presented in Chapter 30.

REVIEW QUESTIONS

Circle the best *answer.*

1 Sex involves

 a The organs of reproduction
 b Attitudes and feelings
 c Cultural and spiritual factors
 d All of the above

2 Sexuality is important to

 a Small children
 b Teenagers and young adults
 c Middle-age adults
 d Persons of all ages

3 Impotence is

 a When menstruation stops
 b A psychological reaction to disfigurement
 c The inability of the male to achieve an erection
 d The complete absence of sexual activity

4 Reproductive organs change with aging.

 a True
 b False

5 Mr. and Mrs. Green live in the same nursing center. Which will *not* promote their sexuality?

 a Allowing their normal grooming routines
 b Having them wear hospital gowns
 c Allowing them privacy
 d Accepting their relationship

6 An older lady and an older gentleman live in a nursing center. They are holding hands. Nursing staff should keep them apart.

 a True
 b False

7 Mr. Green wants time alone with his wife. The RN tells you this is okay. You should

 a Close the door to the room
 b Put a *Do Not Disturb* sign on the door
 c Tell other staff that Mr. and Mrs. Green want some time alone
 d All of the above

REVIEW QUESTIONS—cont'd

8 Mr. and Mrs. Green should be assigned to separate rooms.

   a True

   b False

9 A male patient is being sexually aggressive. The behavior may be

   a An attempt to prove he is still attractive and able to perform sexually

   b Caused by confusion or disorientation

   c Done on purpose

   d All of the above

10 A patient makes sexual advances to you. You should do the following *except*

   a Discuss the situation with the RN

   b Do what the person asks

   c Explain to the person that the behaviors make you uncomfortable

   d Ask the person not to touch you in places where you were touched

Answers to these questions are on p. 851.

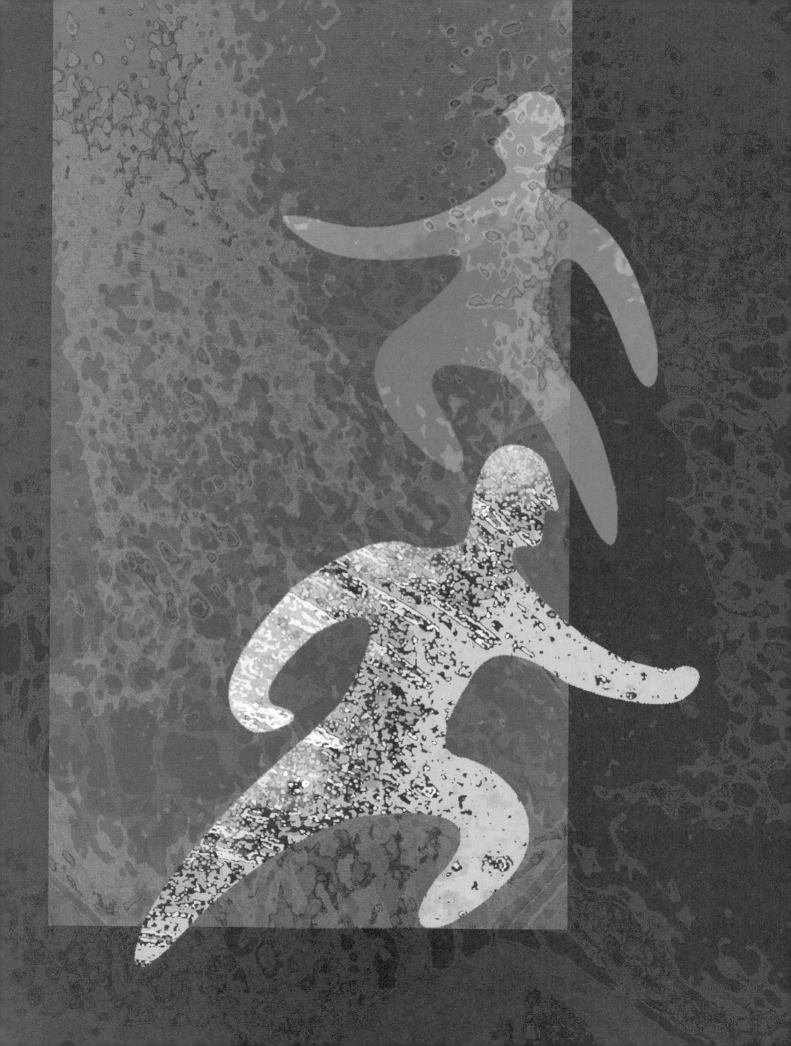

Unit III
Assisting With Protection Needs

10 Safety

OBJECTIVES

- Define the key terms in this chapter
- Describe accident risk factors
- Identify safety precautions for infants and children
- Describe the safety measures for preventing falls, burns, poisoning, and suffocation
- Explain why patients are identified before receiving care and how to accurately identify patients
- Explain how to prevent equipment accidents
- Explain the purpose and complications of restraints and how to use them safely
- Identify restraint alternatives
- Explain how to handle hazardous substances
- Describe the safety measures related to fire prevention and the use of oxygen
- Know what to do if there is a fire
- Give examples of natural and man-made disasters
- Explain how to protect yourself from workplace violence
- Describe your role in risk management
- Perform the procedures described in this chapter

KEY TERMS

active physical restraint A restraint attached to the person's body and to a stationary (nonmovable) object; movement and access to one's body are restricted

coma A state of being unaware of one's surroundings and being unable to react or respond to people, places, or things

disaster A sudden catastrophic event in which many people are injured and killed and property is destroyed

ground That which carries leaking electricity to the earth and away from an electrical appliance

hazardous substance Any chemical that presents a physical hazard or a health hazard in the workplace

hemiplegia Paralysis on one side of the body

paraplegia Paralysis from the waist down

passive physical restraint A restraint near but not directly attached to the person's body; it does not totally restrict freedom of movement and allows access to certain body parts

quadriplegia Paralysis from the neck down

restraint Any item, object, device, garment, material, or chemical that restricts a person's freedom of movement or access to one's body

suffocation When breathing stops from the lack of oxygen

Safety is a basic need. In a safe environment a person has little risk of illness or injury. The person feels safe and secure physically and mentally. Risk of falling, burns, poisoning, or other injuries is low. The person and the person's property are safe from fire and intruders. The person is not afraid and has few worries and concerns.

ACCIDENT RISK FACTORS

Certain factors increase a person's risk for injury. Age, poor vision, and loss of hearing are some examples. Some people cannot protect themselves. They rely on others for safety.

- *Awareness of surroundings*—People must be aware of their surroundings to protect themselves from injury. Some persons are unconscious or in a **coma**. A person in a coma cannot react or respond to people, places, or things. Other people must protect the person. Confused and disoriented persons may not understand what is happening to and around them. They can be dangerous to themselves and others.
- *Vision*—People who have difficulty seeing are at risk for falls. They also can trip on toys, rugs, furniture, or electrical cords. They also may have problems reading labels on medicines, cleaners, and other containers. Taking the wrong medicine or the wrong dose or poisoning can result.
- *Hearing*—Hearing-impaired persons have problems hearing explanations and instructions. For example, a person does not hear well and takes the wrong medicine or takes it the wrong way. Fire alarms, sirens, weather warnings, car horns, and oncoming cars may not be heard. The person does not know to move to safety.
- *Smell and touch*—Illness and aging affect the senses of smell and touch. The person may have problems smelling smoke or gas. Persons with a reduced sense of touch are easily burned. They have problems sensing heat and cold.
- *Paralysis*—**Paraplegia** is paralysis from the waist down. **Quadriplegia** is paralysis from the neck down. Those with **hemiplegia** are paralyzed on one side of the body. Paralyzed persons may not sense pain, heat, or cold. They may be aware of danger but unable to move to safety.
- *Medications*—Medications have side effects. Loss of balance, dizziness, light-headedness, difficulty concentrating, vision changes, reduced awareness, confusion, disorientation, drowsiness, and loss of coordination are some examples. The person may be fearful or uncooperative or act in unusual ways as a result. (See Focus on Children and Focus on Older Persons.)

focus on CHILDREN

Infants are helpless. Other people must protect them. Young children have not learned the difference between safety and danger. They normally explore their surroundings, put objects in their mouths, and touch and feel new things. Therefore they are at risk for falls, poisoning, choking, burns, and other accidents. Practice the safety measures listed in Box 10-1 when caring for infants and children. Also practice the safety measures to prevent falls (p. 161), burns (p. 164), poisoning (p. 164), and suffocation (p. 165).

focus on OLDER PERSONS

The physical changes of aging increase the older person's risk for injury. Movements are slower and less steady. Balance may be affected. Decreased sensitivity to heat and cold, poor vision, hearing problems, and a decreased sense of smell are common in older persons. Confusion, poor judgment, memory problems, and disorientation may occur.

SAFETY MEASURES

Common sense and simple safety measures can prevent most accidents. You must protect patients, yourself, and co-workers from accidents and injuries. The safety measures in this section apply to everyday activities. They also apply to hospital, long-term care, and home settings. The nursing care plan lists other safety measures needed by the person.

Preventing Falls

Most falls occur in bedrooms and bathrooms. They are caused by throw rugs, poor lighting, cluttered floors, furniture that is out of place, and pets underfoot. Slippery floors, bathtubs, and showers are other causes. The need to urinate also is a major cause of falls. For example, Mrs. Ford urgently needs to urinate. She falls trying to get out of bed quickly and without help.

BOX 10-1

SAFETY MEASURES FOR INFANTS AND CHILDREN

- Do not leave infants or young children unattended. They need supervision when in strollers, walkers, high chairs, infant seats, bathtubs, infant swings, playpens, and wading pools and when playing outside.
- Use the safety strap to fasten a child in a high chair.
- Lock the high chair tray after putting the child in the chair.
- Keep high chairs away from stoves, tables, and counters.
- Do not leave children unattended while they are eating.
- Check children in cribs often.
- Make sure crib rails are up and locked in place.
- Keep one hand on a child lying in a crib, on a scale, or on a table if you must look away for a moment (Fig. 10-1, p. 160).
- Keep electrical appliances away from sinks, tubs, toilets, and other water sources.
- Unplug all appliances when not in use.
- Place safety plugs in electrical outlets (Fig. 10-2, p. 160). The plugs prevent children from sticking their fingers or small objects into the openings.
- Keep cords and electrical equipment out of the reach of children.
- Keep childproof caps on medicine containers, cleaners, and other hazardous substances.
- Store cleaners, medicines, and hazardous substances in their original containers.
- Store cleaners, medicines, and hazardous substances in locked storage areas that are beyond the reach of children.
- Supervise any child who is in or near water. Keep bathroom doors closed to prevent drowning in toilets or bathtubs.
- Keep sinks and tubs empty when not in use.
- Keep buckets empty and upside down when not in use.
- Keep toilet lids down. Use safety locks that prevent children from lifting the lid.
- Keep diaper pails locked.
- Do not prop baby bottles on a rolled towel or blanket. Hold the baby and bottle during feedings.
- Keep plastic bags and wraps away from children. They can cause suffocation.
- Use guardrails at the top and bottom of stairs to prevent small children from climbing up and down stairs. Make sure the child cannot get caught in the guardrails.
- Do not use pins on children's clothing.
- Remove drawstrings from jackets, coats, sweaters, and other clothing. This includes drawstrings on the hood, at the neckline, and at the waist. Drawstrings can get tangled or caught in play equipment, furniture, handrails, car or bus doors, escalators, and other moving devices.
- Do not let children play on curbs or behind parked cars. They should not play in piles of leaves or snow near heavy traffic.
- Read all warning labels on toys.
- Check age recommendations on toys. Give children only age-appropriate toys.
- Check toys and other play equipment regularly.
- Use federally approved car restraints.
- Follow seat-belt laws.
- Protect the child from falls (Box 10-3, p. 161).
- Protect the child from burns (Box 10-4, p. 164).
- Protect the child from poisoning (Box 10-5, p. 164).
- Protect the child from choking and suffocating (Box 10-6, p. 165).

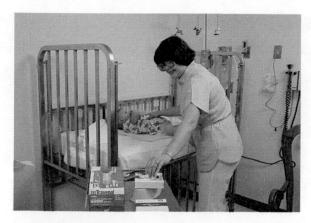

Fig. 10-1 *Keep one hand on the child if you need to look away momentarily.*

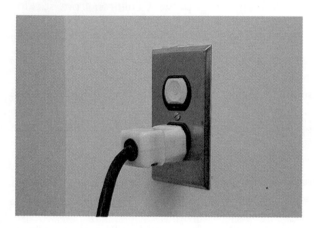

Fig. 10-2 *Safety plug in an electrical outlet.*

FACTORS INCREASING THE RISK OF FALLS

- A history of falls
- Weakness
- Slow reaction time
- Poor vision
- Confusion
- Disorientation
- Decreased mobility
- Foot problems
- Shoes that fit poorly
- Elimination needs
- Urinary incontinence
- Dizziness and lightheadedness
- Dizziness on standing
- Joint pain and stiffness
- Muscle weakness
- Low blood pressure
- Balance problems
- Medication side effects
  - Low blood pressure when standing or sitting
  - Drowsiness
  - Fainting
  - Dizziness
  - Poor muscle coordination
  - Unsteadiness
  - Frequent urination
  - Confusion and disorientation
  - Visual impairment
- Excessive alcohol use
- Depression
- Strange surroundings
- Poor judgment
- Memory problems
- Care equipment (e.g., IV poles, drainage tubes and bags)
- Improper use of wheelchairs, walkers, canes, and crutches

The risk of falling increases with age. Most falls are in persons between the ages of 65 and 85. A history of falls increases a person's risk of falling.

Most falls occur in the evening, between 1800 (6:00 PM) and 2100 (9:00 PM). Falls also are more likely during shift changes. Shift changes occur between 0600 (6:00 AM) and 0800 (8:00 AM) and between 1400 (2:00 PM) and 1600 (4:00 PM).

Besides the accident risk factors (see p. 158), patients have other problems that increase their risk of falling (Box 10-2). Therefore agencies have fall prevention programs. Box 10-3 lists safety measures that prevent falls. These are part of the agency's fall prevention program and the person's nursing care plan. The nursing care plan also lists measures for the person's specific risk factors.

Bed rails

Bed rails (side rails) on hospital beds are raised and lowered. They lock in place with levers, latches, or buttons. Bed rails are half, three quarters, or the full length

BOX 10-3

SAFETY MEASURES TO PREVENT FALLS

- Good lighting is provided in rooms, hallways, and bathrooms.
- Light switches (including those in bathrooms) are within reach and easy to find.
- Night-lights are placed in bedrooms, hallways, and bathrooms.
- Hand rails are on both sides of stairs and in bathrooms.
- Safety rails and grab bars are in showers and tubs and by the toilet.
- Floors have wall-to-wall carpeting or carpeting that is tacked down. Avoid scatter, area, and throw rugs.
- Floor coverings are one color. Bold designs can cause dizziness in older persons.
- Floors have nonglare, nonslip surfaces.
- Nonskid wax is used on hardwood, tiled, or linoleum floors.
- Floors and stairs are uncluttered. They are free of toys, electrical cords, and other items that can cause tripping.
- Floors are free of spills and excess furniture.
- Electric and extension cords are out of the way.
- Furniture is arranged for easy movement.
- Rearranging furniture is avoided.
- Chairs have armrests that give support when sitting and standing.
- A telephone and lamp are at the bedside.
- Tubs and showers have nonslip surfaces or nonslip bath mats.
- Nonskid shoes and slippers are worn. Long shoelaces are avoided.
- Clothing fits properly. Clothing is not loose and does not drag on the floor. Belts are tied or secured in place.
- Fluid needs are met.
- Glasses and hearing aids are worn as needed. Reading glasses are not worn when up and about.
- The person is taught how to use the call bell (p. 166).
- The call bell is always within the person's reach.
- The person is asked to call for assistance when help is needed in getting out of bed or a chair or when walking.
- Call bells are answered promptly. The person may need immediate assistance or may not wait for help.
- Frequent checks are made on persons with poor judgment or memory.
- Persons at risk for falling are in rooms close to the nurses' station.
- Family and friends are asked to visit during busy times and during the evening and night shifts.
- Companionship is provided. Arrangements are made for sitters, companions, or volunteers to be with the person at risk for falling.
- Electronic warning devices are used. Weight-sensitive alarms for beds and chairs sense when the person tries to get up (Fig. 10-3, p. 162).
- Explanations are given often about medical devices and treatments.
- Pillows or wedge pads or seats keep the person correctly positioned (see Chapter 12).
- Nonslip strips are on the floor next to the bed and in the bathroom.
- The person is assisted to the bathroom as soon as requested. Or the bedpan, urinal, or commode is provided.
- The person is assisted to the bathroom, or the bedpan, urinal, or commode is offered at regular times.
- The bedpan or urinal is kept within easy reach of persons able to use the device without assistance.
- A warm drink, soft lights, or a back massage is used to calm the agitated person.
- Barriers are used to prevent wandering (Fig. 10-4, p. 162).

Continued

BOX 10-3

SAFETY MEASURES TO PREVENT FALLS—cont'd

- The bed is in the lowest horizontal position except when giving bedside nursing care. The distance from the bed to the floor is reduced if the person falls or gets out of bed.
- Bed rails are kept up, if ordered. They are in the up position when the bed is raised.
- Crutches, canes, and walkers have nonskid tips.
- Wheelchair brakes are in working order.
- Wheels of beds, wheelchairs, and stretchers are locked when transferring persons.
- Caution is used when turning corners, entering corridor intersections, and going through doors. A person coming from the other direction could be injured.
- A safety check is made of the room after visitors leave. They may have lowered a bed rail, removed the call bell, moved a walker out of reach, or brought an item that could present dangers to the person.

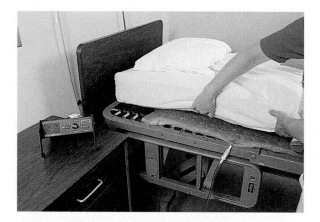

Fig. 10-3 *Weight-sensitive alarm.*

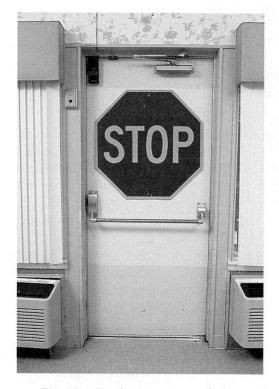

Fig. 10-4 *Barriers prevent wandering.*

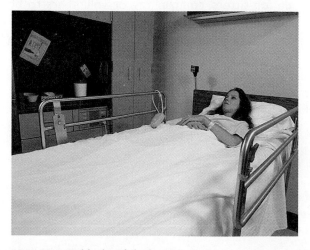

Fig. 10-5 *Hospital bed with bed rails locked in the raised position.*

of the bed (Fig. 10-5). When half-length rails are used, usually two rails are on each side. One is for the upper part of the bed and the other for the lower part.

The RN tells you when to raise bed rails. They are usually necessary for persons who are unconscious or sedated with medication. Some confused or disoriented patients require them. If a patient requires bed rails, the rails are kept up at all times except when giving bedside nursing care.

Bed rails are hazards for patients trying to get out of bed without help. A person can get caught or entangled in the rail. They can also get caught or entangled in bed rail gaps. Gaps occur between half-length rails and between the rail and the head or foot of the bed. These hazards are great risks for confused, disoriented, and restrained persons (p. 168).

Many people are embarrassed by the use of bed rails. They feel like children. RNs decide if rails are needed for physically and mentally stable adults. If a person objects to bed rails, tell the RN. Patients are protected physically. However, their self-esteem and dignity also are protected.

Bed rails prevent persons from getting out of bed. Therefore they are considered restraints under the Omnibus Budget Reconciliation Act of 1987 (OBRA). This law applies to nursing centers and hospital long-term care units. Under OBRA, the person or the person's legal representative must give consent for raised bed rails (p. 168).

The Joint Commission on Accreditation of Healthcare Organizations (JCAHO) has standards for bed rail use in hospitals (including mental health hospitals). Bed rails are allowed when the person's clinical condition requires them. Bed rails must be in the best interest of the patient.

The procedures in this book include using bed rails. This helps you to remember their importance and how to use them correctly. The RN tells you which patients require bed rails. *However, whenever the bed is raised to give care or perform a procedure, the bed rails are raised to prevent the person from falling. The right not to use bed rails applies only when the bed is in its lowest position. Always explain to the person why the bed rails are being used. Check persons with raised bed rails often.*

Hand rails and grab bars

Hand rails are in hallways, stairways, and bathrooms (Fig. 10-6). They provide support for persons who are weak or unsteady when walking. They also provide support for sitting down on or getting up from a toilet. Grab bars are along bathtubs for use in getting into and out of the tub.

Wheel locks

Bed legs have wheels or casters. A caster is a small wheel that lets the bed move easily. Each wheel or caster has a lock to prevent the bed from moving (Fig. 10-7). Lock the bed wheels when giving bedside care. Also lock them when you transfer a person to and from the bed. Wheelchair and stretcher wheels also are locked during transfers. You or the patient can be injured if the bed, wheelchair, or stretcher moves.

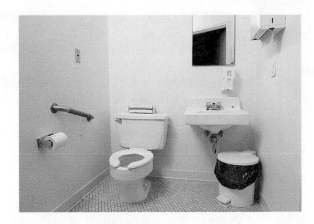

Fig. 10-6 *Hand rail in a bathroom.*

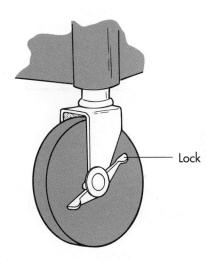

Lock

Fig. 10-7 *Lock on a bed wheel.*

Preventing Burns

Burns are a leading cause of death, especially among children and older persons. Common causes of burns are smoking in bed, spilling hot liquids, children playing with matches, charcoal grills, fireplaces, and stoves. Box 10-4 on p. 164 lists safety measures to prevent burns.

Preventing Poisoning

Poisoning also is a major cause of death. Children are often victims. Aspirin and household products are common poisons. Poisoning in adults may be from carelessness or poor vision when reading labels. Taking too much medicine is another cause. Confused or disoriented persons can forget taking medicine. Or they take more medicine than the amount ordered. Sometimes poisoning is a suicide attempt. Box 10-5 on p. 164 lists the safety measures that prevent poisoning.

BOX 10-4

SAFETY MEASURES TO PREVENT BURNS

- Keep matches out of the reach of children.
- Supervise the play of children.
- Never leave children at home alone.
- Teach children fire safety, fire prevention measures, and the dangers of fire.
- Turn pot and pan handles so they point inward. The must point away from where people stand and walk.
- Supervise the smoking of adults who cannot protect themselves.
- Do not allow smoking in bed.
- Keep space heaters and materials that can catch fire away from children.
- Measure the temperature of bath water (see Chapter 14).
- Do not leave children unattended in bathtubs. They may turn on the hot water.
- Position the child facing away from faucets when bathing a child in a tub or at a sink.
- Place knob covers over faucets to prevent children from turning on the water.
- Supervise children who are eating to prevent spills of hot foods. Also supervise persons who are eating in bed and older persons who are at risk for spilling.
- Apply hot applications correctly (see Chapter 29).
- Use electrical appliances correctly.

BOX 10-5

SAFETY MEASURES TO PREVENT POISONING

- Keep childproof caps on all medicine containers, household products, and hazardous substances.
- Label all medicine containers and household products clearly. Make sure hazardous substances are labeled.
- Store medicines and poisonous materials in places that are high, locked, and out of the reach of children. Store hazardous substances as directed by the manufacturer (p. 182).
- Store medicines, poisonous materials, and hazardous substances in their original containers. Do not store them in food containers.
- Keep medicines out of purses where children may find them.
- Provide good lighting for reading labels.
- Keep poisonous houseplants out of the reach of children.
- Teach children not to eat plants, unknown foods, or leaves, stems, seeds, berries, nuts, or bark.
- Place poison warning stickers ("Mr. Yuk") on household cleaners and toxic substances (Fig. 10-8).
- Never call medicine candy.
- Read labels and follow directions on household products and other toxic or hazardous substances.
- Keep all baby products and diaper-changing supplies out of the child's reach.
- Keep emergency phone numbers by the telephone: poison control center, police, ambulance, hospital, and doctor.

Fig. 10-8 *The "Mr. Yuk" warning sticker is placed on poisonous products. (Courtesy Children's Hospital, Pittsburgh Poison Center, Pittsburgh, Penn.)*

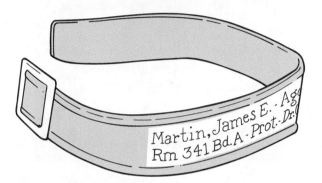

Fig. 10-9 *Patient identification bracelet.*

Preventing Suffocation

Suffocation is when breathing stops from the lack of oxygen. Death occurs if the person does not start breathing. Common causes of suffocation include choking on an object, drowning, inhaling gas or smoke, strangulation, and electrical shock. Carbon monoxide poisoning also results in the lack of oxygen. The person breathes in air filled with carbon monoxide rather than oxygen. Faulty exhaust systems on cars and damaged furnaces and chimneys are common causes of carbon monoxide poisoning. Safety measures to help prevent suffocation are listed in Box 10-6.

Identifying the Patient

Safety also means giving the right care to the right person. Patients have different treatments, therapies, and activity limits. A person's life and health are threatened if the wrong care is given.

Patients receive identification (ID) bracelets when admitted to the agency (Fig. 10-9). Information on the

---

BOX 10-6

SAFETY MEASURES TO PREVENT SUFFOCATION

- Dispose of plastic bags (including those from dry cleaners) properly.
- Do not place a pillow under an infant's head.
- Position infants on their back or sides. Do not lay infants on their stomachs.
- Do not use pillows to position infants or to prevent them from falling off beds.
- Check blankets, sheets, and comforters for loose threads or edging. An infant or child could choke on or become entangled in loose threads or edging.
- Do not leave rattles or toys in an infant's crib.
- Place cribs away from windows. This prevents the child from reaching blinds, shades, and drapes.
- Keep cords for blinds, shades, and drapes out of a child's reach.
- Check children's clothes and toys for loose buttons, decals, and other adornments.
- Take small bites of food. Chew food slowly and thoroughly.
- Make sure dentures fit properly.
- Have exhaust systems on cars checked regularly.
- Have gas odors promptly investigated by competent repairmen.
- Have furnaces and chimneys inspected when persons in the same dwelling have signs and symptoms of carbon monoxide poisoning. Signs and symptoms include headache, confusion, difficulty breathing, dizziness, sleepiness, or cherry-pink skin.
- Open doors and windows if you notice gas odors or signs and symptoms of carbon monoxide poisoning.
- Rest for at least 1 hour after eating and before strenuous activity or swimming.
- Keep all electric cords and appliances in good repair.

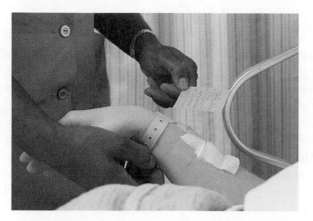

Fig. 10-10 *The patient's ID bracelet is compared with a treatment card to accurately identify the patient.*

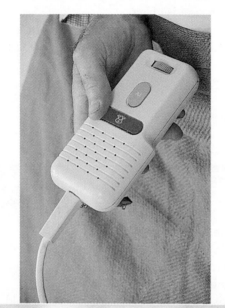

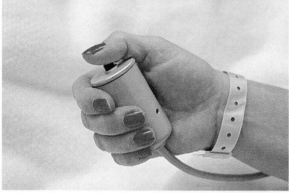

Fig. 10-12 *The patient presses the button on the call bell when help is needed.*

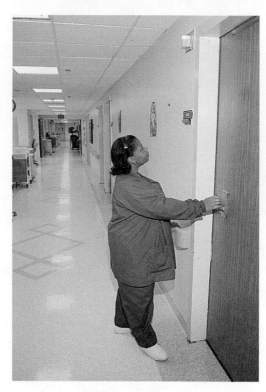

Fig. 10-11 *The call light is on above the person's room door.*

bracelet includes the person's name, room and bed numbers, age, gender (male, female), and doctor. Known allergies and the agency's name also are included.

You use the ID bracelet to identify the person before giving care. Assignment sheets or treatment cards state the treatment or therapy ordered by the doctor. To identify the person, compare the identifying information on the assignment sheet or treatment card with that on the ID bracelet (Fig. 10-10). This comparison helps ensure that you give the right care to the right person.

Also call the person by name when checking the ID bracelet. Calling the person by name is a courtesy given as you touch the person and before giving care. However, calling the person by name is not a safe way to identify the person. Confused, disoriented, drowsy, hearing-impaired, or distracted persons may answer to any name.

Using the Call System

The call system lets the person signal when help is needed. A common call system involves a call bell at the bedside that is connected to a light above the room door (Fig. 10-11). The call bell also is connected to a light panel or intercom system at the nurses' station. The call bell is at the end of a long cord or is part of the side rail (Fig. 10-12). It attaches to the bed or chair so it is always within the person's reach and vision. The person presses the call bell when help is needed. The staff member turns off

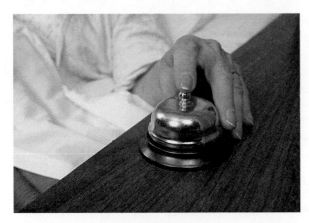

Fig. 10-13 *Tap bell.*

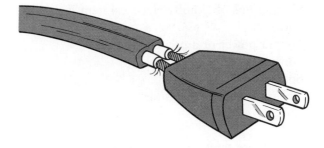

Fig. 10-14 *A frayed electric wire.*

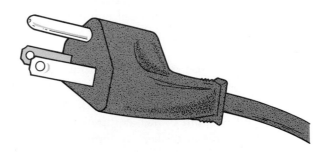

Fig. 10-16 *A three-pronged plug.*

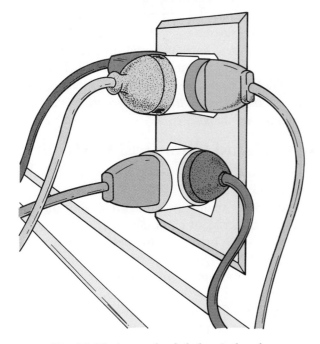

Fig. 10-15 *An overloaded electrical outlet.*

the call bell at the bedside when responding to the call for help.

An intercom system lets a nursing team member talk with the person from the nurses' station. It also allows the light to be turned off from the station. Be careful when using intercom systems. Remember patient confidentiality. Persons nearby can overhear what you say.

Different types of call systems exist. The call system may be part of the bed rail or involve personal pagers. Sometimes a tap bell is used in home care (Fig. 10-13). *The call system must always be within the person's reach. Therefore patient controls must be on the person's good side.*

Patients are shown how to use the call system when ad-

mitted to the agency. Some people cannot use the call bell. Check them often to make sure their needs are met.

Preventing Equipment Accidents

All equipment is unsafe if broken, not used correctly, or not functioning properly. Inspect all equipment before use. Check glass and plastic items for cracks, chips, and sharp or rough edges. All these can cause cuts, stabs, or scratches. Follow the Bloodborne Pathogen Standard (see Chapter 11). Do not use or give damaged equipment to patients.

Electric equipment must function properly and be in good repair. Frayed cords (Fig. 10-14) and overloaded electrical outlets (Fig. 10-15) can cause electrical shocks. Such shocks can cause death and fires. Frayed cords and broken equipment must be repaired by a trained person.

Three-pronged plugs (Fig. 10-16) are used on all electrical equipment. Two prongs carry electrical current. The third prong is the ground. A **ground** carries leaking electricity to the earth and away from the item. If a ground is not used, leaking electricity can be conducted to a person and cause electrical shocks and possible death. Immediately report any shock received while using a piece of equipment. Send the item for repair immediately.

Warning signs of a faulty electrical item include:
- Shocks
- Loss of power or a power outage
- Dimming or flickering lights
- Sparks
- Sizzling or buzzing sounds
- Burning odor
- Loose plugs

Practice these safety measures when using equipment:
- Follow the manufacturer's instruction.
- Read all caution and warning labels.
- Do not use unfamiliar equipment. Ask for needed training. Also ask the RN to supervise you the first time you use the item.
- Use equipment only for its intended purpose.
- Make sure the item is working before you begin.
- Make sure you have all needed equipment. For example, if you need to plug in an item, an outlet must be available.
- Place a "do not use" sticker on broken equipment. Complete a repair request form and explain the problem.
- Notify the RN about broken equipment.
- Do not try to repair broken equipment yourself.

An incident report (p. 193) is completed if a patient, visitor, or staff member has an equipment-related accident. The Safe Medical Devices Act requires that agencies report equipment related illnesses, injuries, and deaths.

APPLYING RESTRAINTS

A **restraint** is any item, object, device, garment, material, or chemical that restricts a person's freedom of movement or access to one's body. Restraints are used only as a last resort to protect persons from harming themselves or others.

Indications for Use

Restraints can cause serious injury and even death. Therefore OBRA has guidelines about using restraints. So does the Joint Commission on Accreditation of Health Care Organizations (JCAHO) and the Food and Drug Administration (FDA).

Restraints are not used to discipline a person or for staff convenience. Discipline is any action that punishes or penalizes a person. Convenience is any action that:
- Controls the person's behavior
- Requires less effort by the agency
- Is not in the person's best interests

Restraints are used only to ensure the physical safety of the patient or other persons. That is, persons are protected from harming themselves or others. Certain behaviors can be harmful to the person or to others in the area. They include:
- Getting out of bed, a chair, or a wheelchair or off of a stretcher when help is needed
- Crawling over bed rails or the foot of the bed
- Interfering with treatment (pulling out tubes, removing dressings, or disconnecting equipment)
- Wandering in or away from the agency
- Behaving in an agitated or combative way toward staff, family, or other persons

Restraints were once used to prevent falls. However, research shows that restraints cause falls. Falls occur when persons try to get free of the restraints. More serious injuries occur from falls in restrained persons than in nonrestrained persons.

Restraints were commonly used for persons who were confused, showed poor judgment, or had behavior problems. Older persons were restrained more often than younger persons. *Now, all other alternatives must be tried before using restraints.*

Physical and Chemical Restraints

The legal definition of *physical restraints* includes the following key points:
- May be any manual method, physical or mechanical device, material, or equipment
- Is attached to or next to the person's body
- Cannot be easily removed by the person
- Restricts freedom of movement or access to one's body

A restraint confines the person to a bed or chair or prevents movement of a body part. Restraints are applied to the chest, waist, elbows, wrists, hands, or legs. Certain furniture or barriers also prevent free movement. Geriatric chairs (Geri-chairs) or chairs with attached trays are examples (Fig. 10-17). Such chairs are often used for persons who need support to sit up. Placing any chair so close to a wall that the person cannot move is another form of restraint. Bed rails are also restraints. So are sheets tucked in so tightly that they restrict movement.

Chemical restraints are drugs used for discipline or for staff convenience. Drugs are chemical restraints if they:
- Are not required to treat the person's medical symptoms
- Affect the person's physical function
- Affect the person's mental function

BOX 10-7 RISKS OF RESTRAINT USE

- Agitation
- Anal incontinence (see Chapter 18)
- Anger
- Bruises
- Cuts
- Dehydration
- Depression
- Embarrassment
- Fractures
- Humiliation
- Mistrust
- Nerve injuries
- Nosocomial infection (see Chapter 11)
- Pneumonia
- Pressure ulcers (see Chapter 14)
- Strangulation
- Urinary incontinence (see Chapter 17)
- Urinary tract infection

BOX 10-8 ALTERNATIVES TO RESTRAINTS

- Diversion activities: for example, television, videos, music, games, books, relaxation tapes
- Pillows and positioning aids
- Keeping the call bell within reach
- Meeting food, fluid, and elimination needs
- Visits by family, friends, and volunteers
- Arranging for companions and sitters
- Spending time with the person
- Reminiscing with the person
- A calm, quiet environment
- Allowing wandering in a safe area
- Exercise programs
- Outdoor time
- Jobs or tasks the person consents to
- Electronic warning devices on beds and doors
- Measures to prevent falls (see Box 10-3)
- Reclining chairs
- Frequent observation
- Moving the person closer to the nurses' station
- Explaining all procedures and care measures
- Frequent explanations about required medical equipment or devices
- Orienting confused individuals to person, time, and place; providing calendars and clocks
- Good lighting
- Consistent staff assignments
- Promoting uninterrupted sleep

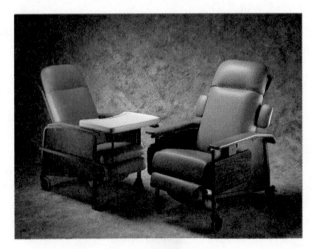

Fig. 10-17 *A Geri-chair with attached tray is considered to be a restraint (Courtesy Invacare Corporation, Elyria, Ohio).*

Complications of Restraint Use

Box 10-7 list the many complications from restraint use. Injuries occur as the person tries to get free of the restraint. Cuts, bruises, and fractures are common injuries. Injuries also occur from using the wrong restraint, applying it wrong, or keeping it on too long. *The most serious risk from restraints is death from strangulation.* There are also mental effects. Being restrained affects a person's dignity and self-esteem. Depression, anger, and agitation are common in restrained persons. So are embarrassment, humiliation, and mistrust.

Restraints are medical devices. The Safe Medical Device Act applies if a restraint causes illness, injury, or death.

Restraint Alternatives

OBRA, JCAHO, and the FDA do not forbid the use of restraints. Restraints are allowed only after trying all other alternatives. Box 10-8 lists some restraint alternatives. The RN selects alternatives for the person's nursing care plan.

Safety Guidelines

If a restraint is used, the least restrictive method is used. Remember the following about using restraints:

- *Restraints are used to protect the person, not for staff convenience.* Restraining a person is thought to be easier for the staff than properly supervising and observing the person. Actually, a restrained person requires more staff time for care, supervision, and observation. A restraint is used only when it is the best safety precaution for the person. It is not used to punish uncooperative persons.

- *Restraints require a doctor's order.* OBRA, JCAHO, state laws, and FDA warnings protect persons from unnecessary restraint. Agencies must have policies and procedures about restraint use. If a person needs restraining for medical reasons, a written doctor's order is required. The doctor gives the reason for the restraint, what to use, and how long to use the restraint. This information is on the person's Kardex and nursing care plan. You need to know the laws and policies about using restraints where you work.

- *The least restrictive method is used.* An **active physical restraint** attaches to the person's body and to a stationary (nonmovable) object. It restricts the person's movement or body access. Vest, leg, arm, wrist, hand, and some belt restraints are active physical restraints. A **passive physical restraint** is near but not directly attached to the person's body. It does not totally restrict freedom of movement and allows access to certain body parts. Passive physical restraints are the least restrictive.

- *Restraints are used only after trying other methods to protect the person.* Some people can harm themselves or others. The nursing care plan must include measures to protect the person and to prevent the person from harming others. Restraints lessen the person's dignity. They are allowed only after other measures fail to provide needed protection (see Box 10-8). Many fall prevention measures are restraint alternatives (see Box 10-3).

- *Unnecessary restraint is false imprisonment (see Chapter 2).* If told to apply a restraint, you must clearly understand the need. If not, politely ask about its use. If you apply a restraint unnecessarily, you face false imprisonment charges.

- *Restraints require informed consent.* The person must understand the reason for the restraint. The person is told how the restraint will help the planned medical treatment. The person also is told about risk of restraint use. If the person cannot give informed consent, the person's legal representative is given the information. Either the person or legal representative must give consent. Restraints cannot be used without consent. The doctor or RN provides the necessary information and obtains informed consent.

- *The manufacturer's instructions are followed.* The manufacturer gives specific instructions about applying and securing the restraint. Failure to follow the instructions could affect the person's safety. You could be negligent for improperly applying or securing a restraint.

- *The restrained person's basic needs are met by the nursing team.* The restraint must be snug and firm, but not tight. Tight restraints interfere with circulation and breathing. The person must be comfortable and able to move the restrained part to a limited and safe extent. Check the person at least every 15 minutes. Meet food, fluid, and elimination needs.

- *Restraints are applied with enough help to protect the person and staff from injury.* Persons in immediate danger of harming themselves or others are restrained quickly. Combative and agitated people can hurt themselves and the staff when restraints are applied. Enough staff members are needed to complete the task safely and efficiently.

- *Restraints can increase a person's confusion and agitation.* Whether confused or alert, people are aware of restricted body movements. They may try to get out of the restraint or struggle or pull at it. Many restrained persons beg anyone who passes by to set them free or to help release them. These behaviors are often viewed as signs of confusion. Confusion increases in some persons because they do not understand what is happening to them. Restrained persons need repeated explanations and reassurance. Spending time with them has a calming effect.

- *The person's quality of life is protected.* Restraints are used for as short a time as possible. The person's care plan shows how restraint use is slowly reduced. The goal is to meet the person's needs using as little restraint as possible. Besides meeting physical needs, you must meet the person's psychosocial needs. These needs are met by visiting with the person and explaining the purpose of the restraints.

Restraints are dangerous. The person is observed often. Complications from restraints such as interferences with breathing and circulation are prevented. Practice the safety measures in Box 10-9 when caring for a restrained person.

Text continued on p. 174

BOX 10-9

SAFETY MEASURES FOR USING RESTRAINTS

- Use the restraint specified by the RN and the care plan. The least restrictive device is used.
- Apply a restraint only after receiving instruction about its proper use. Demonstrate proper application to the RN before using it on any person.
- Use the correct size as instructed by the RN. Small restraints are tight. They cause discomfort, agitation, restricted breathing, or reduced circulation. Strangulation is a risk from big or loose restraints.
- Use only restraints that have manufacturer instructions. Read the manufacturer's warning labels. Note the front and back of the restraint.
- Follow the manufacturer's instructions. Some restraints are safe for bed, chair, and wheelchair use. Others are used only with certain equipment.
- Do not use sheets, towels, tape, rope, straps, bandages, or other items to restrain a person.
- Use intact restraints. Look for tears, frayed edges, missing loops or straps, or other damage.
- Do not use restraints to position a person on a toilet.
- Follow agency policies and procedures when applying restraints.
- Position the person in good body alignment before applying the restraint (see Chapter 12).
- Pad bony areas and skin to prevent pressure and injury from the restraint.
- Secure the restraint. It should be snug but allow some movement of the restrained part. If the restraint is applied to the chest, make sure that the person can breathe easily. A flat hand should slide between the restraint and the person's body (Fig. 10-18, p. 172).
- Criss-cross vest restraints in front (Fig. 10-19, p. 172). Do not criss-cross restraints in the back unless part of the manufacturer's instructions. Criss-crossing vests in the back can cause death from strangulation.
- Tie restraints according to agency policy. The policy should follow the manufacturer's instructions. The knot must be easily released in an emergency. Quick-release knots often are used (Fig. 10-20, p. 172). Some restraints have quick-release buckles.
- Secure straps out of the person's reach.
- Secure the restraint to the movable part of the bed frame or to the bed springs (see Fig. 10-20). Never secure restraints to the bed rails. The person can reach bed rails to release knots or buckles. Also, injury to the person is likely when raising or lowering bed rails. For chairs, secure straps to the wheelchair or the chair frame (Fig. 10-21, p. 173).
- Pad the bed rails as in Figure 10-22, p. 173. Padded bed rails prevent the person from getting caught between the rails (Fig. 10-23, p. 173).
- Keep full bed rails up when using a vest or belt restraint. If the bed rails are not up, the person could fall off the bed and strangle on the restraint. If half-length bed rails are used, the person could get caught between them.
- Position the person in a chair so the hips are well to the back of the chair. If using a belt restraint, apply it at a 45-degree angle over the hips (Fig. 10-24, p. 173).
- Do not use back cushions when a person is restrained in a chair. If the cushion moves out of place, slack occurs in the straps. Strangulation could result if the person slides forward or down because of the extra slack (Fig. 10-25, p. 174).
- Check the person's circulation every 15 minutes if wrist or leg restraints are applied. You should feel a pulse at a pulse site below the restraint. Fingers or toes should be warm and pink. Notify the RN immediately if:
  - You cannot feel a pulse
  - Fingers or toes are cold, pale, or blue in color
  - The person complains of pain, numbness, or tingling in the restrained part
  - The skin is red or damaged

Continued

BOX 10-9

SAFETY MEASURES FOR USING RESTRAINTS—cont'd

- Check the person every 15 minutes for safety and comfort. Also check the position of the restraint, especially in the front and back.
- Keep scissors in your pocket. In an emergency, cutting the tie may be faster than untying the knot. Never leave scissors at the bedside or where the person can reach them.
- Remove the restraint and reposition the person every 2 hours. Give skin care and perform range-of-motion exercises at this time.
- Meet the person's basic needs. The person must have food and fluids. Offer water often to prevent dehydration. Help the person meet elimination needs at least every 2 hours. Injuries often occur when restrained persons try to get up to go to the bathroom.
- Make sure the call bell is always within the person's reach.
- Report to the RN every time the restraint is released. Report your observations made and the care given. Follow agency policy for recording.

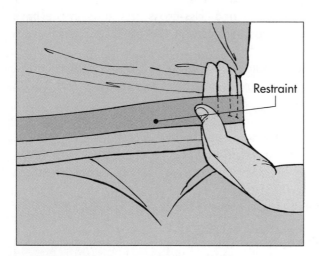

Fig. 10-18 *A flat hand should be able to slide between the restraint and the person.*

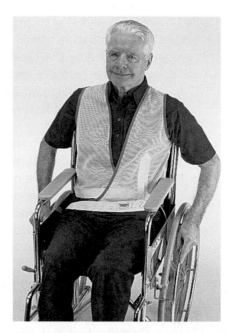

Fig. 10-19 *Vest restraint criss-crosses in front.* (Courtesy J. T. Posey Co, Arcadia, Calif.)

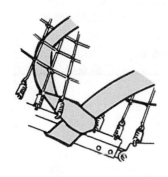
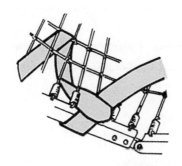
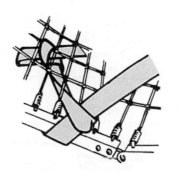
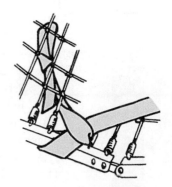

Fig. 10-20 *The Posey quick-release tie.* (Courtesy J. T. Posey Co, Arcadia, Calif.)

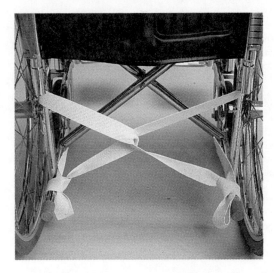

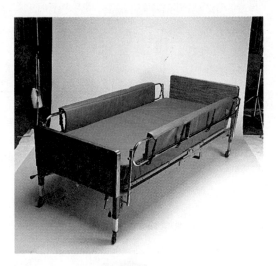

Fig. 10-21 *The restraint straps are secured to the wheelchair frame using a quick-release tie. (Courtesy J. T. Posey Co, Arcadia, Calif.)*

Fig. 10-22 *Padded bed rails. (Courtesy J. T. Posey Co, Arcadia, Calif.)*

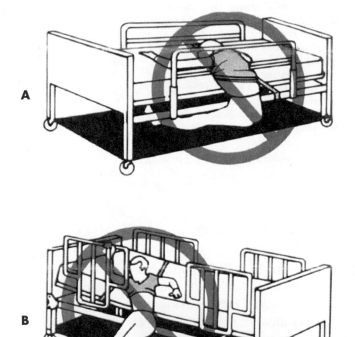

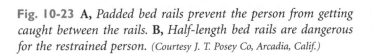

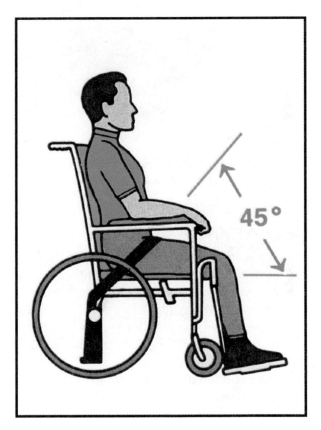

Fig. 10-23 A, *Padded bed rails prevent the person from getting caught between the rails.* **B,** *Half-length bed rails are dangerous for the restrained person. (Courtesy J. T. Posey Co, Arcadia, Calif.)*

Fig. 10-24 *The safety belt is at a 45-degree angle over the person's hips. (Courtesy J. T. Posey Co, Arcadia, Calif.)*

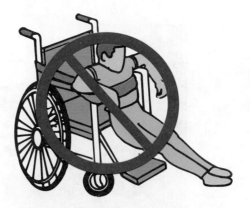

Straps to prevent sliding should always be over the thighs—NOT around the waist or chest. Straps should be at a 45° angle and secured to the chair under the seat, not behind the back. They should be snug but comfortable and not restrict breathing. If a belt or vest is too loose or applied around the waist, the patient may slide partially off the seat—resulting in the possible suffocation and death.

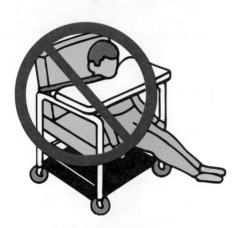

Tray tables (with or without a belt or vest) pose potential danger if the patient should slide partly under the table and become caught. This could result in suffocation and death. Make sure the patient's hips are positioned at the back of the chair—this may necessitate the use of an anti-slide material (Posey Grip), a pommel cushion, or a restrictive device if the patient shows any tendency to slide forward.

Fig. 10-25 *Strangulation could result if the person slides forward or down because of the extra slack in the restraint. (Courtesy J. T. Posey Co, Arcadia, Calif.)*

Reporting and Recording

Information about restraints is recorded in the person's medical record. You might apply restraints or care for a restrained person. Report and record the following:

- The type of restraint applied
- The reason for the application
- Safety measures taken (e.g., bed rails padded and up)
- The time you applied the restraint
- The time you removed the restraint
- The care given when the restraint was removed
- The color and condition of the person's skin
- The pulse felt in the restrained extremity
- Complaints of a tight restraint, difficulty breathing, and pain, numbness, or tingling in the restrained part

Types of Restraints

Restraints are made of cloth or leather. Cloth restraints (soft restraints) are belts, straps, and vests. They are applied to the wrists, ankles, hands, elbows and forearms, waist, and chest. Leather restraints are applied to the wrists and ankles. They are used in extreme cases of patient agitation and combativeness.

✦ *Wrist restraints and ankle restraints*

Wrist restraints limit the movement of arms and legs. They are often described by their application points.

- *2-point restraints* are applied to two extremities. The wrists are common sites.
- *3-point restraints* are applied to three extremities. They are usually applied to both wrists and one ankle.
- *4-point restraints* are applied to all four extremities. They are applied to both wrists and both ankles.

The RN tells you where to apply the restraints.

APPLYING WRIST AND ANKLE RESTRAINTS

PRE-PROCEDURE

1 Get the number of restraints you need.

2 Wash your hands.

3 Identify the person. Check the ID bracelet, and call the person by name.

4 Explain the procedure to the person.

5 Provide for privacy.

PROCEDURE

6 Make sure the person is comfortable and in good body alignment (see Chapter 12).

7 Apply the restraint following the manufacturer's instructions. Place the soft part toward the skin (Fig. 10-26, p. 176).

8 Secure the restraint so it is snug but not tight. Make sure that you can slide two fingers under the restraint (Fig. 10-27, p. 176).

9 Tie the ends to the movable part of the bed frame or to the bed springs. Use an agency approved knot.

10 Repeat steps 7, 8, and 9 for a 2-point, 3-point, or 4-point application.

POST-PROCEDURE

11 Place the call bell within the person's reach.

12 Unscreen the person.

13 Wash your hands.

14 Check the person and the restraints at least every 15 minutes. Check the pulse, color, and temperature of the restrained parts. Report your observations to the RN.

15 Do the following at least every 2 hours:

- Remove the restraints.

- Reposition the person.

- Meet the person's food, fluids, and elimination needs.

- Give skin care.

- Perform range-of-motion exercises.

- Reapply the restraints.

16 Report and record your observations and the care given.

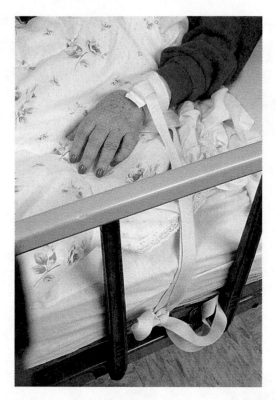

Fig. 10-26 *The soft part of the restraint is toward the skin.*

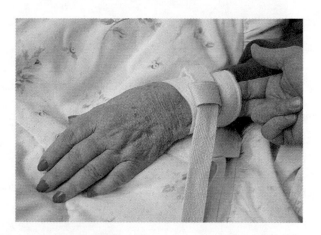

Fig. 10-27 *Two fingers should be able to fit between the restraint and the wrist.*

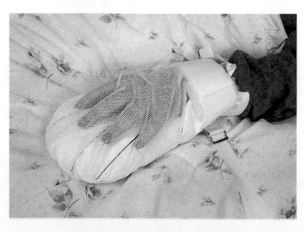

Fig. 10-28 *Padded mitt restraint.*

✦ *Mitt restraints*

Hands are placed in mitt restraints. They prevent finger use but do not prevent hand, wrist, or arm movements. Mitt restraints are thumbless and prevent the person from scratching, pulling out tubes, or removing dressings. The person holds a hand roll to keep the fingers in a normal position. Hand rolls are not needed with padded mitts (Fig. 10-28).

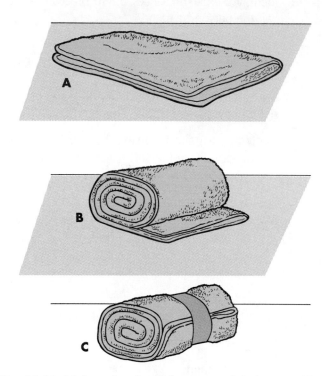

Fig. 10-29 *Make a hand roll from a washcloth.* **A,** *Fold the washcloth in half.* **B,** *Roll up the washcloth.* **C,** *Tape the rolled washcloth.*

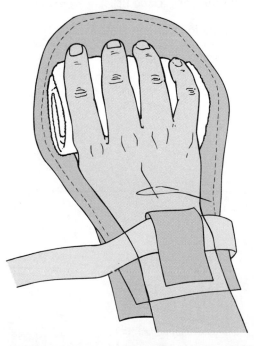

Fig. 10-30 *Mitt restraint. Person is holding a handroll.*

APPLYING MITT RESTRAINTS

PRE-PROCEDURE

1 Collect the following equipment:

- Two mitt restraints
- Two washcloths or two commercial hand rolls if the mitts are not padded
- Tape if washcloths are used

2 Make the hand rolls as in Figure 10-29, or use commercial ones.

3 Wash your hands.

4 Identify the person. Check the ID bracelet, and call the person by name.

5 Explain the procedure to the person.

6 Provide for privacy.

PROCEDURE

7 Make sure the person's hands are clean and dry. Fingernails should be short so they don't cut into the person's palm.

8 Give the person a hand roll to hold if a padded mitt is not used.

9 Apply the mitt restraint (Fig. 10-30). Follow the manufacturer's instructions.

10 Tie the ends to the movable part of the bed frame or to the bed springs. Use an agency-approved knot.

11 Repeat steps 8, 9, and 10 for the other hand.

POST-PROCEDURE

12 Place the call bell within the person's reach.

13 Unscreen the person.

14 Wash your hands.

15 Check the person and the restraints at least every 15 minutes.

16 Do the following at least every 2 hours:

- Remove the restraints.
- Reposition the person.

- Meet the person's food, fluids, and elimination needs.
- Give skin care.
- Perform range-of-motion exercises.
- Reapply the restraints.

17 Report and record your observations and the care given.

✦ *Vest restraints*

Vest restraints are applied to the chest. The person cannot get out of bed or out of a chair. The person's arms are put through the sleeves so the vest crosses in front (see Fig. 10-19). *Vest restraints always cross in the front.* The vest must *never* cross in the back. If it crosses in the back, there is only a small neck opening at the front. Strangulation can occur from the small neck opening if the person slides down in the bed or chair. The restraint is always applied over a gown, pajamas, or clothes.

Vest restraints carry great risks to the person's life. Death can occur from strangulation. If the person becomes caught in the restraint, it can become so tight that the person's chest cannot expand to inhale air. The person quickly suffocates and dies. Correct application of a restraint is always important. In the case of vest restraints it is critical. Therefore you are advised to only assist the RN in its application. It is best that the RN assume full responsibility for the application of a vest restraint.

✦ APPLYING A VEST RESTRAINT

PRE-PROCEDURE

1 Collect the following:

 • Vest restraint (the RN tells you the size)

 • Pads for the bed rails

2 Get assistance if needed.

3 Wash your hands.

4 Identify the person. Check the ID bracelet, and call the person by name.

5 Explain the procedure to the person.

6 Provide for privacy.

PROCEDURE

7 Put the pads on the bed rails if the person is in bed.

8 Assist the person to a sitting position.

9 Apply the restraint with your free hand. Follow the manufacturer's instructions. Remember, the vest crosses in front.

10 Make sure the vest is free of wrinkles in the front and back.

11 Help the person lie down if he or she is in bed.

12 Bring the ties through the slots.

13 Make sure the person is comfortable and in good body alignment (see Chapter 12).

14 Secure the straps to the movable part of the bed frame, the bed springs, or to the chair or wheelchair. Use an agency-approved knot.

15 Slide a flat hand under the restraint (see Fig. 10-18). Adjust the straps as needed so the restraint is snug but not tight.

POST-PROCEDURE

16 Place the call bell within the person's reach.

17 Raise the bed rails.

18 Unscreen the person.

19 Wash your hands.

20 Check the person and the restraint at least every 15 minutes.

21 Do the following at least every 2 hours:

 • Remove the restraint.

 • Reposition the person.

 • Meet the person's food, fluids, and elimination needs.

 • Give skin care.

 • Perform range-of-motion exercises.

 • Reapply the restraint.

22 Report your observations to the RN. Include the care given when the restraint was removed.

✦ *Belt restraints*

The belt restraint (Fig. 10-31) is used for the same reasons as the vest restraint. The belt is applied around the waist and secured to the bed or chair. It is applied over clothes, a gown, or pajamas. The person can release the quick-release type. It is less restrictive than those that are released only by a staff member.

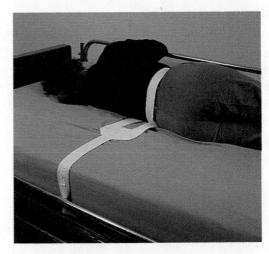

Fig. 10-31 *Roll belt. (Courtesy J. T. Posey Co, Arcadia, Calif.)*

✦ APPLYING A BELT RESTRAINT

PRE-PROCEDURE

1 Obtain a belt restraint. The RN tells you the size.

2 Get help if needed.

3 Wash your hands.

4 Identify the person. Check the ID bracelet, and call the person by name.

5 Explain the procedure to the person.

6 Provide for privacy.

PROCEDURE

7 Assist the person to a sitting position.

8 Apply the restraint with your free hand. Follow the manufacturer's instructions.

9 Remove wrinkles or creases from the front and back of the restraint.

10 Bring the ties through the slots in the belt.

11 Help the person lie down if he or she is in bed.

12 Make sure the person is comfortable and in good body alignment (see Chapter 12).

13 Secure the straps to the movable part of the bed frame, the bed springs, or to the chair or wheelchair. Use an agency-approved knot.

POST-PROCEDURE

14 Place the call bell within the person's reach.

15 Unscreen the person.

16 Wash your hands.

17 Check the person and the restraint at least every 15 minutes.

18 Do the following at least every 2 hours:

- Remove the restraint.

- Reposition the person.

- Meet the person's food, fluids, and elimination needs.

- Give skin care.

- Perform range-of-motion exercises.

- Reapply the restraint.

19 Report and record your observations and the care given.

✦ *Elbow restraints*

Elbow restraints prevent infants and small children from bending their elbows. They prevent children from scratching and touching incisions or pulling out tubes. A long-sleeved shirt is worn. The restraint is secured to the shirt with safety pins or tape. Both arms are restrained to achieve the desired effect.

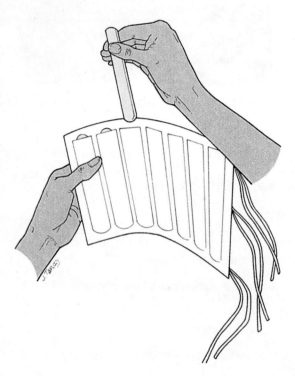

Fig. 10-32 *Tongue depressors keep the elbow restraint rigid.*

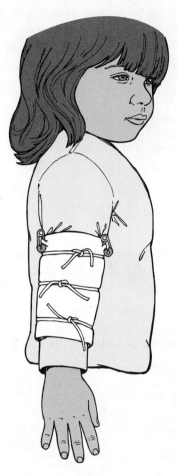

Fig. 10-33 *An elbow restraint is secured to the shirt with safety pins. The pins should point down and away from the child.*

APPLYING ELBOW RESTRAINTS

PRE-PROCEDURE

1 Collect the following:

- Two elbow restraints

- Tongue depressors

- Safety pins

2 Insert the tongue depressors into the slots (Fig. 10-32).

3 Wash your hands.

4 Identify the child. Check the ID bracelet, and call the child by name.

5 Explain the procedure to the child and parents.

6 Provide for privacy.

PROCEDURE

7 Wrap the restraint around the child's elbow.

8 Tie the strings around the arm.

9 Pin the restraint to the child's shirt. Point pins down and away from the child (Fig. 10-33).

10 Repeat steps 7, 8, and 9 to apply the other restraint.

POST-PROCEDURE

11 Place the call bell within the child's or parents' reach.

12 Unscreen the child.

13 Wash your hands.

14 Check the child and the restraints often.

15 Do the following at least every 2 hours:

- Remove the restraint.

- Reposition the child.

- Meet the child's food, fluids, and elimination needs.

- Give skin care.

- Perform range-of-motion exercises.

- Reapply the restraint.

16 Report and record your observations and the care given.

HANDLING HAZARDOUS SUBSTANCES

The Occupational Safety and Health Administration (OSHA) requires that health care employees understand the risk of hazardous substances and how to handle them safely. A **hazardous substance** is any chemical that presents a physical hazard or a health hazard in the workplace.

Physical hazards can cause fires or explosions. Health hazards are chemicals that can cause acute or chronic health problems. Acute problems occur rapidly and are of short duration. They usually occur from a short-term exposure. Chronic problems usually result from long-term exposure and occur over a long period. Health hazards can cause cancer and affect the formation and function of blood cells. They also can damage the kidneys, nervous system, lungs, skin, eyes, or mucous membranes. Birth defects, miscarriages, and fertility problems result from damage to the reproductive system.

Exposure to hazardous substances can occur under normal working conditions or during foreseeable emergencies. Such emergencies include equipment failures, container ruptures, or the uncontrolled release of a hazard into the workplace. Hazardous substances include:

- Drugs used in cancer therapy (chemotherapy, anti-cancer drugs)
- Gases used to give anesthesia
- Gases used to sterilize equipment
- Oxygen
- Disinfectants and cleaning solutions
- Radiation used for x-rays and cancer treatments

To protect employees, OSHA requires a hazard communication program. The program includes container labeling, material safety data sheets, and employee training about hazards and protective measures.

Labeling

Hazardous substance containers include bags, barrels, bottles, boxes, cans, cylinders, drums, and storage tanks. All hazardous substance containers need warning labels (Fig. 10-34). The manufacturer applies the labels. Warning labels always identify physical hazards and health hazards. Health hazards include the organs affected and potential health problems. Warning labels may include:

- Precaution measures (e.g., "do not use near open flame" or "avoid skin contact")
- What personal protective equipment to wear (see Chapter 11)
- Directions about using the substance safely
- Storage and disposal information

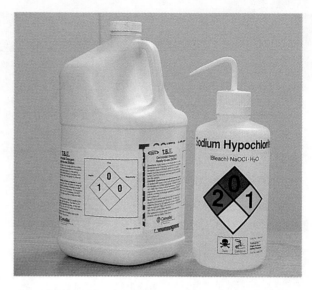

Fig. 10-34 *Warning label on a hazardous substance.*

Words, pictures, and symbols communicate the warnings. A container must always be labeled. Warning labels must not be removed or damaged in any way. If a warning label is removed or damaged, do not use the chemical. Take the container to the RN, and explain the problem. Do not leave the container unattended.

Material Safety Data Sheets

Every hazardous substance has a material safety data sheet (MSDS). An MSDS provides detailed information about each hazardous chemical.

- The chemical name and any common names
- The ingredients contained in the substance
- Physical and chemical characteristics (appearance, color, odor, boiling point, and others)
- Potential physical effects (fire, explosion)
- Conditions that could cause a chemical reaction
- How the chemical enters the human body (inhalation, ingestion, skin contact, or absorption)
- Health hazards including signs and symptoms
- Protective measures (how to use, handle, and store the substance)
- Emergency and first aid procedures
- Explosion information and firefighting measures (including what type of fire extinguisher to use—p. 185).
- How to clean up a spill or leak
- Personal protective equipment needed during clean up
- How to dispose of the hazardous material
- Manufacturer information (name, address, and a telephone number for information)

BOX 10-10

SAFETY MEASURES FOR HANDLING HAZARDOUS SUBSTANCES

- Read all warning labels.
- Follow the safety precautions on the warning label and material safety data sheets (MSDSs).
- Make sure each container has a warning label that is not damaged.
- Use a leak-proof container to carry or transport a hazardous substance.
- Wear personnel protective equipment to clean spills and leaks. The warning label or MSDS tells you what to wear (mask, gown, gloves, eye protection, safety boots).
- Clean up spills immediately. Work from clean to dirty using circular motions.
- Dispose of hazardous waste in sealed bags or containers.
- Stand behind a lead shield during x-ray or radiation therapy procedures.
- Do not enter a room while a person is having x-rays or radiation therapy.
- Wash your hands after handling hazardous substances.
- Work in well-ventilated areas to avoid inhaling gases.
- Store hazardous substances according to the MSDS.

Employees must have ready access to the MSDSs. They are in a binder at the nurses' station or on computer. Check MSDSs before using a hazardous substance, cleaning up a leak or spill, or disposing of the substance. Also, immediately notify the RN of a spill or leak. Do not leave a spill or leak unattended.

Employee Training

Your employer provides hazardous substance training. Information is given about the hazards, exposure risks, and protection measures. You also learn to read and use warning labels and the MSDSs.

Each hazardous substance requires specific protection measures. Box 10-10 lists general guidelines for the safe handling of hazardous substances.

FIRE SAFETY

Faulty electrical equipment and wiring, overloaded electrical circuits, and smoking are major causes of fire. Fire is a constant danger. The entire health team must prevent fires. They must act quickly and responsibly if a fire occurs.

Fire and the Use of Oxygen

Three things are needed for a fire:
- A spark or flame
- A material that will burn
- Oxygen

Air has some oxygen. However, some people need extra oxygen. Doctors order supplemental oxygen for these persons. Supplemental oxygen is supplied in oxygen tanks or through wall outlets (Chapter 21). Oxygen is needed for fires. Therefore special safety precautions are practiced where oxygen is used and stored.

- "No Smoking" signs are placed on the person's door and near the bed.
- Patients and visitors are politely reminded not to smoke in the person's room.
- Smoking materials (cigarettes, cigars, and pipes), matches, and lighters are removed from the room.
- Electrical equipment is turned off *before* being unplugged. Sparks occur when electrical appliances are unplugged while turned on.
- Wool blankets and synthetic fabrics that cause static electricity are removed from the person's room. The person wears a cotton gown or pajamas. Health team members wear cotton uniforms.
- Electrical equipment is removed from the person's room. This includes electric razors, heating pads, and radios.
- Materials that ignite easily are removed from the person's room. These include oil, grease, alcohol, nail polish remover, and other hazardous substances that ignite easily.

Many agencies have no smoking policies and are smoke-free environments. No smoking is allowed inside the buildings. Signs are posted on all entry doors. However, some people ignore such policies. If a person is receiving supplemental oxygen, remind the person, family, and any visitors about the need for no smoking. (See Focus on Home Care on p. 184.)

BOX 10-11

FIRE PREVENTION MEASURES

- Follow the fire safety precautions involved in the use of oxygen.
- Smoke only in areas where smoking is allowed. Do not smoke in patient homes.
- Be sure all ashes, cigars, and cigarettes are extinguished before emptying ashtrays.
- Provide ashtrays to persons who are allowed to smoke.
- Empty ashtrays into a metal container partially filled with sand or water. Do not empty ashtrays into plastic containers or wastebaskets lined with paper or plastic bags.
- Supervise the smoking of persons who cannot protect themselves. This includes persons who are confused, disoriented, or sedated.
- Follow safety practices when using electrical equipment.
- Supervise the play of children, and keep matches out of their reach.
- Do not leave cooking unattended on stoves, in ovens, or in microwave ovens.
- Store flammable liquids in their original containers. Keep the containers out of children's reach.
- Do not light matches or lighters or smoke around flammable liquids or materials.

focus on

HOME CARE

Home care patients may require supplemental oxygen. Remind the patient, family, and visitors about necessary safety precautions.

Preventing Fires

Fire prevention measures were described in relation to children, burns, equipment-related accidents, and the use of oxygen. These and other fire safety measures are summarized in Box 10-11. (See Focus on Home Care at top left on p. 185.)

What to Do if a Fire Occurs

Every agency has policies and procedures for fire emergencies. You must know your agency's policies and procedures. Also know the location of fire alarms, fire extinguishers, and emergency exits. Agencies conduct fire drills to practice emergency fire procedures.

Remember the word *RACE* when a fire occurs. That will help you remember what to do first:

- *R* stands for *rescue*. Rescue persons in immediate danger. Move them to a safe place.
- *A* stands for *alarm*. Sound the nearest fire alarm, and notify the switchboard operator.
- *C* stands for *confine*. Confine the fire by closing doors and windows. Turn off oxygen or electrical equipment being used in the general area of the fire.
- *E* stands for *extinguish*. Use a fire extinguisher on a small fire that has not spread to a larger area.

Also clear equipment from all regular and emergency exists. *Remember, do not use elevators if there is a fire.* (See Focus on Home Care at top right on p. 185.)

HOME CARE

Smoke detectors are important for fire safety. Always locate smoke detectors in patient homes. Make sure they are working. Notify the RN and the family if a smoke detector does not work.

Space heaters present additional fire hazards in the home. Electric and kerosene heaters are common. These safety measures are important:

- Follow the manufacturer's instructions when using space heaters.
- Keep space heaters at least 3 feet away from curtains, drapes, and furniture.
- Do not place the heater on stairs, in doorways, or where people walk.
- Protect yourself and others from burns. Heaters are hot. Do not touch them. Keep them away from children and persons who cannot protect themselves.
- Prevent electrocution. Keep electric heaters away from water (water conducts electricity). Make sure the cord is in good repair.
- Do not leave space heaters unattended.
- Store kerosene in its original container. Keep the container outside.

✦ Using a fire extinguisher

Agencies require that all employees demonstrate use of a fire extinguisher. Fire departments give fire extinguisher demonstrations once or twice a year.

Different extinguishers are used for different kinds of fires: oil and grease fires; electrical fires; and paper and wood fires. A general procedure for using a fire extinguisher follows. (See Focus on Home Care at bottom right.)

HOME CARE

Know the exit routes from the home or apartment building. If a fire occurs, get the patient, family, and yourself out as fast as possible. In an apartment building, notify others of the fire. Use the fire alarm system and yell FIRE in the hallways. Call 911 or the local fire department from a nearby phone. Do not go back into the building.

If your clothing is on fire, do not run. Drop to the floor or ground. Roll to smother the flames. If another person's clothing is on fire, get the person to the floor or ground. Roll the person, or cover the person with a blanket or coat. This smothers the flames.

If smoke is present, cover your nose and mouth with a damp cloth. Do the same for the patient and family. Have everyone crawl to the nearest exit.

Do the following if you cannot get out of the building because of flames or smoke:

- Call 911 or the fire department. Tell the operator where you are. Give precise information: address, phone number, and where you are in the home.
- Cover your nose and mouth with a damp cloth. Do the same for the patient and family.
- Move away from the fire. Go to a room with a window. Close the door to the room and place wet towels and blankets at the bottom of the door.
- Open the window.
- Hang something from the window (towel, sheet, blanket, clothing). This helps the firefighters find you.

HOME CARE

Locate fire extinguishers in the patient's home. Read the manufacturer's instructions. Make sure the fire extinguisher works. Notify the RN and the family if a fire extinguisher does not work.

USING A FIRE EXTINGUISHER

PROCEDURE

1 Pull the fire alarm.

2 Get the nearest fire extinguisher.

3 Carry the extinguisher upright.

4 Take the extinguisher to the fire.

5 Remove the safety pin (Fig. 10-35, *A*).

6 Push the top handle down (Fig. 10-35, *B*).

7 Direct the hose at the base of the fire (Fig. 10-35, *C*).

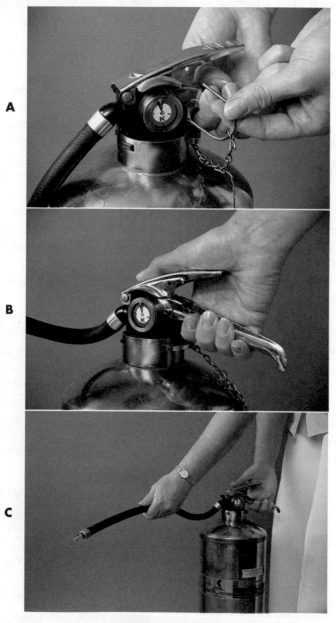

Fig. 10-35 A, *The safety pin of the fire extinguisher is removed.* **B,** *The top handle is pushed down.* **C,** *The hose is directed at the base of the fire.*

Evacuating patients

Agency policies and procedures specify evacuation procedures. If evacuation is necessary, persons closest to the danger are evacuated first. Ambulatory patients are given blankets to wrap around themselves. They are escorted to a safe place by a staff member. Figures 10-36 and 10-37 on p. 188 show how to rescue nonambulatory patients Once firefighters arrive, they direct rescue efforts.

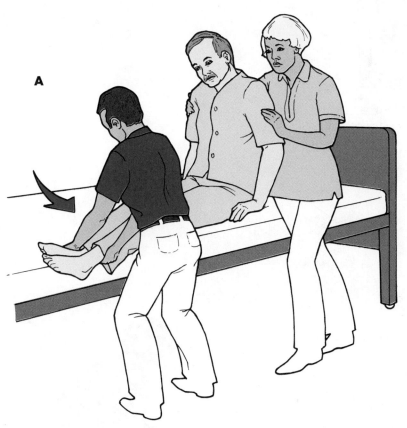

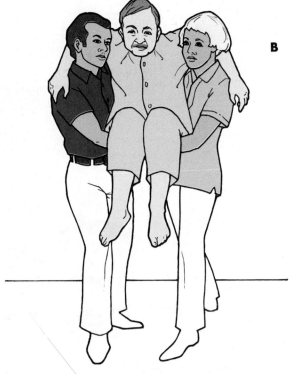

Fig. 10-36 *Swing-carry technique.* **A,** *Assist the person to a sitting position. A co-worker grasps the person's ankles as you both turn the patient so that he sits on the side of the bed.* **B,** *Pull the person's arm over your shoulder. With one arm, reach across the person's back to your co-worker's shoulder. Reach under the person's knees, and grasp your co-worker's arm. Your co-worker does the same.*

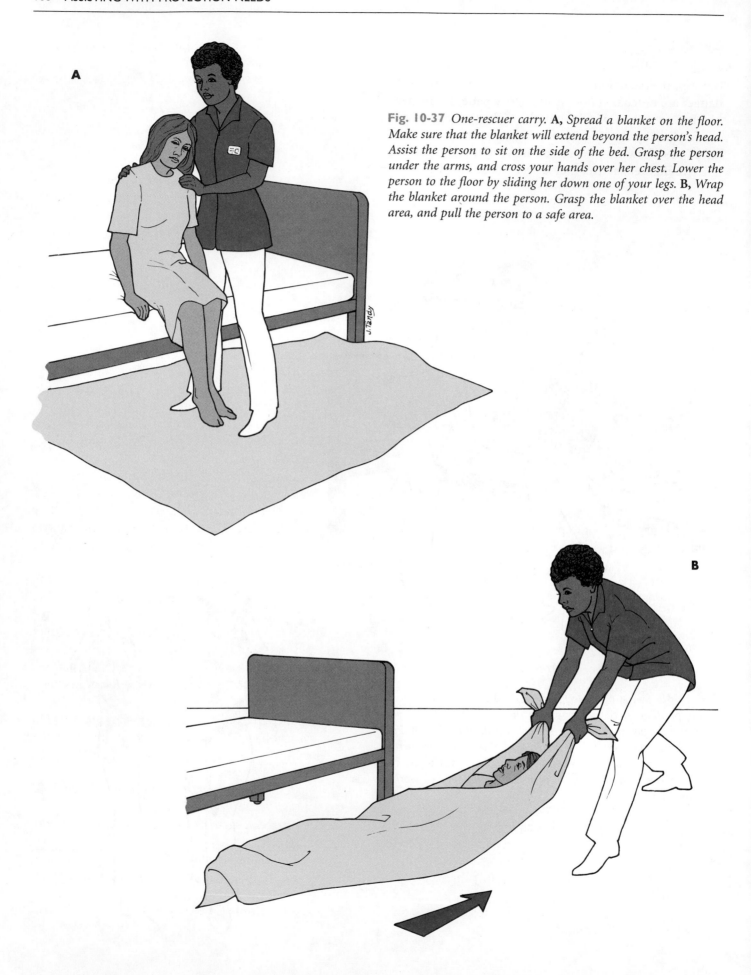

Fig. 10-37 *One-rescuer carry.* **A,** *Spread a blanket on the floor. Make sure that the blanket will extend beyond the person's head. Assist the person to sit on the side of the bed. Grasp the person under the arms, and cross your hands over her chest. Lower the person to the floor by sliding her down one of your legs.* **B,** *Wrap the blanket around the person. Grasp the blanket over the head area, and pull the person to a safe area.*

DISASTERS

A **disaster** is a sudden catastrophic event. Many people are injured and killed, and property is destroyed. Natural disasters include tornadoes, hurricanes, blizzards, earthquakes, volcanic eruptions, floods, and some fires. Human-made disasters include auto, bus, train, and airplane accidents. They also include fires, nuclear power plant accidents, riots, explosions, and wars.

Local communities, fire and police departments, and agencies have disaster plans. You should know the disaster plan where you work. Also know the disaster plan of the community where you live and work.

Disaster plans include policies and procedures to deal with great numbers of people needing treatment. The plan generally provides for the discharge of patients who can go home. Certain personnel are assigned to the emergency department. Others are assigned to take equipment to the emergency area and to transport persons from the initial treatment area. Off-duty personnel may be called in to work.

A disaster may damage the agency. Therefore the disaster plan includes policies and procedures for evacuating the agency.

WORKPLACE VIOLENCE

According to the Occupational Safety and Health Administration (OSHA), more assaults occur in health care settings than in other industries. Between 1980 and 1990, 106 pharmacists, doctors, nurses, assistive personnel, and other health team members were killed at work.

Risk factors for work-related assaults in health care agencies include:

- Handguns in the possession of patients, families, and friends
- Patients as police holds (persons arrested or convicted of crimes)
- Acutely disturbed and violent persons seeking health care
- Mentally ill persons who do not take medicine, do not receive follow-up care, and are not hospitalized unless they are an immediate threat to themselves or others
- Agency pharmacies being a source of drugs and therefore a target for robberies
- Gang members and substance abusers having access to agencies as patients or visitors
- Upset, agitated, and disturbed family members and visitors
- Long emergency room waits that increase a person's agitation and frustration

- Being alone with patients during care or transport to other agency areas
- Low staff levels during meals, emergencies, and at night
- Poorly lighted parking areas
- Lack of training in recognizing and managing potentially violent situations

OSHA has guidelines for violence prevention programs. The goal is to eliminate or reduce employee exposure to situations that can cause death or injury. The work site is analyzed for hazards. Prevention strategies are developed and implemented. Also, employees receive safety and health training. Your responsibilities in violence prevention programs include:

- Understanding and following the workplace violence prevention program
- Understanding and following safety and security measures
- Voicing safety and security concerns
- Reporting violent incidents promptly and accurately
- Serving on health and safety committees that review incidents of workplace violence
- Taking part in training programs that focus on recognizing and managing agitation, assaultive behavior, and criminal intent

Box 10-12 on p. 190 lists some of the many measures that can prevent or control workplace violence. Box 10-13 on p. 191 lists personal safety practices to follow in everyday activities. In addition, you can practice the following safety measures when dealing with agitated or aggressive persons:

- Stand away from the person. Judge the length of the person's arms and legs. Stand far enough away that the person cannot hit or kick you.
- Position yourself close to the door. Do not become trapped in the room.
- Note the location of panic buttons, call bells, alarms, closed-circuit monitors, and other security devices.
- Keep your hands free.
- Stay calm. Talk to the person in a calm manner. Do not raise your voice or argue, scold, or interrupt the person.
- Do not touch the person.
- Tell the person that you will get an RN to speak to the person.
- Leave the room as soon as you can. Make sure the person is safe.
- Notify the RN or security officer of the situation.
- Complete an incident report according to agency policy (see p. 193).

(See Focus on Home Care on p. 190.)

Text continued on p. 193

BOX 10-12

MEASURES TO PREVENT OR CONTROL WORKPLACE VIOLENCE

- Alarm systems, closed-circuit video monitoring, panic buttons, hand-held alarms, cellular phones, two-way radios, and telephone systems that have a direct line to police are installed.
- Metal detectors are at entrances to identify guns, knives, or other weapons.
- Curved mirrors are at hallway intersections and hard-to-see areas.
- Bullet-resistant, shatter-proof glass is at the nurses' stations, reception areas, and admitting areas.
- Waiting rooms are comfortable and reduce stress.
- Family and visitors receive information in a timely manner.
- Furniture is arranged to prevent entrapment.
- Pictures, vases, and other items that can serve as weapons are few in number.
- Staff restrooms lock and prevent access to visitors.
- Unused doors are locked, in keeping with local fire codes.
- Bright lights are inside and outside buildings.
- Burned-out lights are replaced or repaired.
- Broken lights, windows, and door locks are replaced or repaired.
- Security escort services are used for walking to cars, bus stops, or train stations.
- Vehicles are locked and in good repair.
- Security officers deal with agitated, aggressive, or disruptive patients and visitors.
- Patients and visitors are restrained if they are a threat to themselves or others.
- Visitors sign in and receive a pass to access patient areas.
- Visiting hours and policies are enforced.
- A list of "restricted visitors" is made for patients with a history of violence or who are victims of violence.
- Psychiatric patients are supervised as they move throughout the hospital.
- Access to the pharmacy and drug storage areas is controlled.
- The RN assesses the behavioral history of new and transferred patients.
- Aggressive and agitated patients are treated in open areas. Privacy and confidentiality are maintained.
- Staff is not alone when caring for persons with agitated or aggressive behaviors.
- Jewelry that can serve as weapons is not worn (grabbing earrings and bracelets, strangulating with necklaces).
- Keys, scissors, pens, or other items that can serve as weapons are not visible.
- Tools or items left by maintenance personnel or visitors are removed if they can serve as weapons.
- Staff wear ID badges (without last names) that verify employment.
- A "buddy system" is used when using elevators, restrooms, and low-traffic areas.
- Uniforms fit well. Tight uniforms limit your ability to run. An attacker can grab loose uniforms.
- Shoes have good soles. Shoes that cause slipping limit your ability to run.

HOME CARE

Other measures are needed for home safety. Always keep doors locked. Do not let strangers into the home or into apartment buildings. Also remember not to give information over the phone (see p. 76). Do not let any stranger know that you are with an ill or disabled person.

BOX 10-13

PERSONAL SAFETY PRACTICES

- Know the area you will visit. Ask questions about the area.
- Make a "dry run" of the area. Know the route in advance. The shortest route is not always the safest.
- Have plenty of gas in your car.
- Keep your car in good working order.
- Keep a flashlight with working batteries, flares, a fire extinguisher, and a first aid kit in your car.
- Raise the hood and use the flares if the car breaks down. Stay in the car and call the police if you have a cellular phone. If someone stops by to help, ask that person to call the police.
- Check for places to park. Choose a well-lit area. If using a parking garage, park near entrances, exits, and on the lower level. Try to get close to the attendant if possible. Remember, the closest space to your destination is not always the safest for parking.
- Park your car so that you can leave quickly and easily. Park at street corners so no one can park in front of you. In parking lots, back in. You can see more from your front windshield than from the back window.
- Lock your car. However, there are times you may consider leaving your car unlocked. If you need to get in the car fast, you do not want to fumble with keys. Use your judgment. Do not leave anything in the car if you leave it unlocked.
- Have your car key ready so you can get into the car quickly. Do not fumble for keys on the way to or at the car.
- Check the back seat before getting into the car. Make sure no one is in the car. Leave immediately if someone is in the car.
- Check under the car. A person hiding under the car can grab your ankle or leg. Leave immediately if someone is under the car.
- Lock car doors when you get in the car, and keep windows rolled up.
- Keep purses and other valuables under the seat or near your side. Do not leave them on the seat. They are an easy target for smash-and-grab robberies.
- Use well-lit and busy streets if you have to walk. Avoid vacant lots, alleys, wooded areas, and construction sites. Again, the shortest way is not always the safest.
- Note the location of phone booths, or carry a cellular phone. Know your location, and keep phone calls simple.
- Go to a police or fire station or a store if you think someone is following you.
- Carry money for phone calls and for bus, train, or taxi fares. Have money in your pocket to avoid fumbling with a purse or wallet.
- Stand with others and near the ticket booth if using public transportation. Sit near the driver or conductor.
- Do not hitchhike or pick up hitchhikers.
- Let someone know where you are at all times. Let someone know when you leave and when you arrive at your destination. If you do not call in when expected, the person knows something is wrong.
- Make it known that you do not carry drugs, needles, or syringes.
- Do not carry valuables with you. Leave them at home or in the car trunk. If someone wants what you have, give it. The only thing of value is you.
- Carry wallets and purses safely. A wallet should be in an inside coat or pants pocket. Never carry a wallet in the rear pocket. Keep a firm grip on a purse, and keep it close to your body.
- Do not wear headphones when walking. They keep you from hearing cars and people around you.
- Carry a whistle or shriek alarm.
- Scream as loud and as long as you can. Keep screaming. Both men and women should scream.

Modified from McLean County Sheriff's Department, Bloomington, Ill, and the Illinois Criminal Justice Information Authority, Chicago, Ill.

Continued

BOX 10-13

PERSONAL SAFETY PRACTICES—cont'd

- Use your car keys as a weapon. Carry them in your strong hand, and have one key extended (Fig. 10-38). Hold the key firmly. If you are attacked, go for the person's face. Use the key to slash the person's face. Do not use poking motions. Also, do not try for a specific target because you might miss. Do not be shy because your attacker will not be.
- Remember, you have two arms, two hands, two feet, and two knees. This means that you can attack from four directions at once. Do not be shy—your attacker will not be. Push, pull, yank, and so on. You can attack the genital area of either a man or woman.
- Use your thumbs as weapons. Go for the eyes and push hard.
- Carry a travel size of aerosol hair spray. Go for the face.

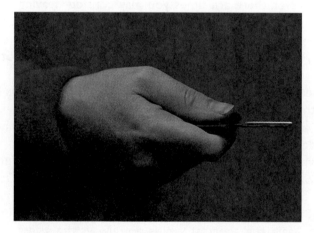

Fig. 10-38 *Car keys are held to use a car key as a weapon.*

RISK MANAGEMENT

Risk management involves identifying and controlling risk and safety hazards affecting the agency. The intent is to protect everyone in the agency (patients, visitors, and staff) and all agency property from harm or danger. The person's valuables also are protected. Safety, accident and fire prevention, negligence and malpractice, and federal and state requirements are among the many issues within the scope of risk management.

Risk managers work with all agency departments to prevent accidents and injuries. They study incident reports, patient and staff complaints, and accident and injury investigations for patterns and trends. Risk managers also look for and correct unsafe situations. They also make policy and procedure changes and training recommendations as needed.

Clothing and Valuables

The person's valuables must be kept safe. Often they are sent home with the family. A clothing list is completed. Each item is identified and described. The staff member and person sign the completed list.

A valuables envelope is used for money and jewelry. Each jewelry item is listed and described on the envelope. Describe what you see. For example, describe a ring as having a white stone with six prongs in a yellow setting. Do not assume the stone is a diamond in a gold setting. Place each jewelry item in the envelope while the person watches. Count money with the person. Then put it in the envelope. The envelope is sealed and signed like the clothing checklist. Give the envelope to the RN. The RN takes it to the safe or sends it home with the family.

Dentures, eyeglasses, contact lenses, watches, and radios are kept at the bedside. Valuables kept at the bedside are listed in the person's record. Some persons keep money for newspapers and gift cart items. The amount of money kept by the person is noted in the person's record. (See Focus on Long-Term Care.)

focus on

LONG-TERM CARE

Clothing and shoes are labeled with the person's name. Radios, blankets, and other items brought from home also are labeled.

Reporting Accidents and Errors

Accidents and errors are reported immediately to your supervisor. This includes accidents involving patients, visitors, or staff. You must report errors in care. Such errors include giving a person a wrong treatment, giving a treatment to the wrong person, or forgetting to give a treatment. Broken items owned by the person, such as dentures or eyeglasses, are reported. Lost money or clothing is also reported. So are hazardous substance accidents and workplace violence incidents.

An *incident report* is completed. The report is completed as soon as possible after the incident. The following information is required:
- Names of those involved
- Date and time of the accident or error
- Location of the accident or error
- A complete description of what happened
- Names of witnesses
- Any other requested information

Incident reports are reviewed by risk management and a committee of health care workers. They look for patterns and trends of accidents or errors. For example, are falls occurring on the same shift and on the same unit? Are patients reporting lost or missing items on the same shift or same unit? The committee may recommend new policies or procedures to prevent future incidents.

REVIEW QUESTIONS

Circle T *if the statement is true or* F *if the statement is false.*

1 T F Only medicine containers need childproof caps.

2 T F Household cleaners are kept in locked storage areas out of the reach of children.

3 T F Safety plugs in electrical outlets protect children from electrical shocks.

4 T F The "Mr. Yuk" sticker indicates a poisonous substance.

5 T F Keeping electrical cords and appliances in good repair prevents suffocation.

6 T F The person is called by name to accurately identify the person before giving care.

7 T F Persons between the ages of 65 and 85 are at risk of falling.

8 T F Falls are more likely to occur during the evening hours.

9 T F Restraints prevent falls.

10 T F The need to urinate is a major cause of falls.

11 T F Bed rails are restraints.

12 T F Bed rails are always raised when the bed is raised.

13 T F The call bell must always be within the person's reach.

14 T F A patient is in a coma. Bed rails are required for safety.

15 T F A restraint restricts freedom of movement or access to one's body.

16 T F Restraints require a nurse's order.

17 T F Restraints are used only to prevent persons from harming themselves or others.

18 T F Some drugs are chemical restraints.

19 T F Unnecessary restraint is false imprisonment.

20 T F Restraints are applied so that they are tight.

21 T F Restraints are removed every 2 hours to reposition the person and give care.

22 T F Elbow restraints prevent children from scratching and touching incisions.

23 T F Hazardous substances must have warning labels.

24 T F Many people are injured and killed and property is destroyed in a disaster.

Circle the best *answer.*

25 Why is age a factor in safety?
   a Young children have not learned what is safe and what is dangerous.
   b Infants are helpless.
   c Physical changes from aging can affect balance and movements.
   d All of the above

26 Which is not a risk for accidents?
   a The need for eyeglasses
   b Hearing impairment
   c Memory problems
   d Oriented to person, time, and place

27 You are assigned to the pediatric unit. Which measure is unsafe?
   a Checking children in cribs often
   b Keeping one hand on a child in a crib if you need to look away
   c Propping a baby bottle on a rolled towel or blanket
   d Keeping plastic bags away from children

28 A paraplegic is paralyzed
   a From the waist down
   b From the neck down
   c On the right side of the body
   d On the left side of the body

29 Safety measures are needed so Mrs. Ford does not fall. Which is unsafe?
   a Nonglare, waxed floors
   b One-color floor coverings
   c Safety rails and grab bars in the bathroom
   d Nonskid shoes

30 Burns can be caused by

   a Smoking in bed and space heaters

   b Leaving children unattended or home alone

   c Bath water that is too hot and applying warm applications incorrectly

   d All of the above

31 Mrs. Ford often tries to get up without help. You should do the following *except*

   a Remind her to use her call bell when she needs help

   b Check on her often

   c Help her to the bathroom at regular intervals

   d Place her chair by a wall

32 The following can occur because of restraints. Which is the most serious?

   a Fractures

   b Strangulation

   c Pressure ulcers

   d Urinary tract infection

33 A belt restraint is applied to a person in bed. Where should you tie the straps?

   a To the bed rails

   b To the head board

   c To the movable part of the bed frame

   d To the foot board

34 A vest restraint is ordered. Which statement is *false?*

   a The vest should criss-cross in back.

   b You should be able to slide a flat hand under the restraint.

   c The restraint is tied according to agency policy.

   d The bed rails must be padded.

35 Mrs. Ford has a restraint. How often should you check her and the position of the restraint?

   a Every 15 minutes   c Every hour

   b Every 30 minutes   d Every 2 hours

36 To prevent equipment accidents, you should

   a Fix broken equipment

   b Use two-pronged plugs to ground electrical equipment

   c Check glass and plastic items for damage

   d All of the above

37 You gave Mrs. Ford the wrong treatment. Which is *true?*

   a The error is reported to the RN at the end of the shift.

   b Action is taken only if Mrs. Ford was injured.

   c You will be found guilty of negligence.

   d An incident report must be completed.

38 All the following are needed to start a fire *except*

   a A spark or flame

   b A material that will burn

   c Oxygen

   d Carbon monoxide

39 You spilled a hazardous substance. You should do the following *except*

   a Read the material safety data sheet

   b Cover the spill and go tell the RN

   c Wear any needed personnel protective equipment to clean up the spill

   d Complete an incident report

40 The fire alarm sounds. The following are done *except*

   a Turning off oxygen

   b Using elevators

   c Closing doors and windows

   d Moving patients to a safe place

41 Your agency has a violence prevention program. You need to do the following *except*

   a Follow safety and security measures

   b Take part in training programs

   c Wear personnel protective equipment

   d Report safety and security concerns

42 A patient is agitated and aggressive. You should do the following *except*

   a Stand away from the person

   b Stand close to the door

   c Use touch to show you care

   d Talk to the person without raising your voice

Answers to these questions are on p. 851.

Infection Control

OBJECTIVES

- Define the key terms in this chapter
- Identify what microbes need to live and grow
- List the signs and symptoms of infection
- Explain the chain of infection
- Describe nosocomial infection and the persons at risk
- Describe the practices of medical asepsis
- Describe common disinfection and sterilization methods
- Explain how to care for equipment and supplies
- Carry out Standard Precautions and Transmission-Based Precautions
- Explain the Bloodborne Pathogen Standard
- Explain the principles and practices of surgical asepsis
- Perform the procedures described in this chapter

KEY TERMS

asepsis Being free of disease-producing microbes

autoclave A pressure steam sterilizer

biohazardous waste Items contaminated with blood, body fluids, secretions, and excretions and that may be harmful to others; *bio* means life, and *hazardous* means dangerous or harmful

carrier A human or animal that is a reservoir for microbes but does not have signs and symptoms of infection

clean technique Medical asepsis

communicable disease A disease caused by pathogens that spread easily; a contagious disease

contagious disease Communicable disease

contamination The process of becoming unclean

disinfection The process of destroying pathogens

germicide A disinfectant applied to skin, tissues, or nonliving objects

immunity Protection against a certain disease

infection A disease state resulting from the invasion and growth of microorganisms in the body

medical asepsis The practices used to remove or destroy pathogens and to prevent their spread

from one person or place to another person or place; clean technique

microbe A microorganism

microorganism A small *(micro)* living plant or animal *(organism)* seen only with a microscope; a microbe

nonpathogen A microbe that does not usually cause an infection

normal flora Microbes that usually live and grow in a certain location

nosocomial infection An infection acquired after admission to a health care agency

pathogen A microbe that is harmful and can cause an infection

spore A bacterium protected by a hard shell that forms around the microbe

sterile The absence of all microbes

sterile field A work area free of all pathogens and nonpathogens (including spores)

sterile technique Surgical asepsis

sterilization The process of destroying *all* microbes

surgical asepsis The practices that keep equipment and supplies free of all microbes; sterile technique

Infection is a major safety and health hazard. Some infections are minor and cause short illnesses. Others are serious and can cause death. Infections are serious for infants and older persons. The health team protects patients and themselves from infection. They prevent the cause of the infection from spreading.

MICROORGANISMS

A **microorganism (microbe)** is a small (micro) living plant or animal (organism) seen only with a microscope. Microbes are everywhere. They are in the air, food, mouth, nose, respiratory tract, stomach, intestines, skin, soil, water, and animals. They are on clothing and furniture. Some microbes cause infections and are harmful. They are called **pathogens**. **Nonpathogens** are microbes that usually do not cause an infection.

Types of Microbes

There are five types of microbes:
- *Bacteria*—microscopic plant life that multiply rapidly. Often called *germs,* they consist of one cell.
- *Fungi*—plants that live on other plants or animals. Mushrooms, yeasts, and molds are common fungi.
- *Protozoa*—microscopic one-celled animals.
- *Rickettsiae*—microscopic forms of life found in fleas, lice, ticks, and other insects. They are transmitted to humans by insect bites.
- *Viruses*—extremely small microscopic organisms that grow in living cells.

Requirements of Microbes

The *reservoir* or *host* is the environment where the microbe lives and grows. People, plants, animals, the soil, food, and water are common reservoirs. Microbes must get *water* and *nourishment* from the reservoir. They also need *oxygen* to live. A *warm* and *dark* environment is needed. Most microbes grow best at body temperature and are destroyed by heat and light.

Normal Flora

Normal flora are microbes that usually live and grow in a certain area. Certain microbes are found in the respiratory tract, in the intestines, and on the skin. They are nonpathogens when in or on a natural reservoir. When a nonpathogen is transmitted from its natural site to another site or host, it becomes a pathogen. *Escherichia coli* is normally found in the large intestine. If the *E. coli* enters the urinary system, it can cause an infection.

INFECTION

An **infection** is a disease state resulting from the invasion and growth of microbes in the body. A *local infection* is in a body part. A *systemic infection* involves the whole body. The person has certain signs and symptoms of infection. Some or all of the signs and symptoms listed in Box 11-1 are present. Pathogens do not always cause an infection. The development of an infection depends on many factors.

The Chain of Infection

The chain of infection (Fig. 11-1) is a process involving a:
- Source
- Reservoir
- Portal of exit
- Method of transmission
- Portal of entry
- Susceptible host

The *source* is a pathogen. The pathogen must have a *reservoir* where it can grow and multiply. Humans and animals are common reservoirs for microbes. If they do not have signs and symptoms of infection, they are **carriers**. Carriers can pass the pathogen to others. The pathogen must leave the reservoir. That is, it needs a *portal of exit*. Exits are the respiratory, gastrointestinal, urinary, and reproductive tracts, breaks in the skin, and the blood.

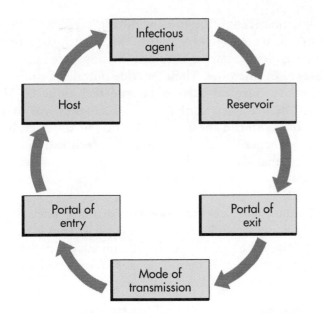

Fig. 11-1 *The chain of infection. (From Potter PA, Perry, AG: Funda-mentals of nursing: concepts, process, and practice, ed 4, St Louis, 1997, Mosby.)*

When a pathogen leaves the reservoir, it must be *trans-mitted* to another host. Methods of transmission include direct contact, air (airborne droplets from coughing or sneezing), food, water, animals, and insects. Microbes are also transmitted by eating and drinking utensils, dress-ings, and personal care items (Fig. 11-2). The pathogen must enter the body through a *portal of entry*. Portals of entry and exit are the same. A *susceptible host* (a person at risk for infection) is needed for the microbe to grow and multiply. The human body can protect itself from infection. A person's ability to resist infection relates to age, nutritional status, stress, fatigue, general health, medi-cations, and the presence of disease or injury.

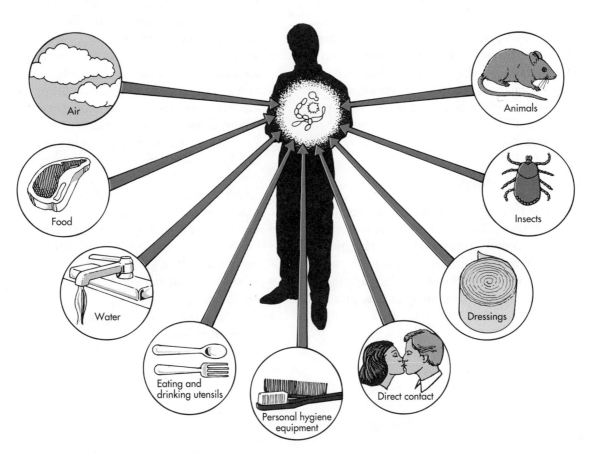

Fig. 11-2 *Methods of spreading microbes.*

Nosocomial Infection

Patients can develop infections in health care settings. A **nosocomial infection** is an infection acquired after admission to an agency. (*Nosocomial* comes from the Greek word for hospital.)

Nosocomial infections are caused by normal flora or by microbes transmitted to the patient from another source. Remember, normal flora become pathogens when transmitted from their natural location to another site or host. For example, *E. coli* is normally in the large intestine. Feces (bowel movements) contain *E. coli*. Poor wiping after bowel movements can cause *E. coli* to enter the urinary system. The hands can also transmit *E. coli* to other body areas. If handwashing is poor, *E. coli* spreads to any body part or anything the hands touch.

Microbes can enter the body through equipment used in treatments, therapies, and diagnostic tests. Therefore equipment must be free of microbes (see p. 205). Staff also can transfer microbes from one patient to another and from themselves to patients. The urinary and respiratory systems, wounds, and the bloodstream are common sites for nosocomial infections.

Patients are already weak from disease or injury. Surgical wounds or open skin areas are often present. Infants and older persons cannot fight infections like other persons. Therefore the health team must prevent the spread of infection. Medical and surgical asepsis, isolation precautions, and the Bloodborne Pathogen Standard all help prevent nosocomial infections.

MEDICAL ASEPSIS

Asepsis is being free of disease-producing microbes. Microbes are everywhere. Therefore practices are needed to achieve asepsis. **Medical asepsis (clean technique)** is the practices used to remove or destroy pathogens and to prevent their spread from one person or place to another person or place. The number of pathogens is reduced.

Microbes cannot be present during surgery or when instruments are inserted into the body. Also, open wounds (cuts, burns, surgical incisions) require the absence of microbes. These provide portals of entry for microbes. **Surgical asepsis (sterile technique)** is the practices that keep equipment and supplies free of all microbes. **Sterile** means the absence of *all* microbes, both pathogenic and nonpathogenic. **Sterilization** is the process that destroys *all* microbes. Both pathogens and nonpathogens are destroyed. Surgical asepsis is discussed on p. 219.

Contamination is the process of becoming unclean. In medical asepsis, an item or area is *clean* when it is free of pathogens. The item or area is contaminated if pathogens are present. A sterile item or area is contaminated when pathogens or nonpathogens are present.

Common Aseptic Practices

Aseptic practices break the chain of infection. To prevent the spread of microbes:

- Wash your hands after urinating or having a bowel movement. Also wash your hands after changing tampons or sanitary pads.
- Wash your hands after contact with your own or another person's blood, body fluids, secretions, or excretions. This includes saliva, vomitus, urine, feces, vaginal discharge, mucus, semen, wound drainage, pus, and respiratory secretions.
- Provide all persons with their own toothbrush, drinking glass, towels, washcloths, and other personal care items.
- Cover your nose and mouth when coughing, sneezing, or blowing your nose.
- Bathe, wash hair, and brush your teeth regularly.
- Wash your hands before and after handling, preparing, or eating food.
- Wash fruits and raw vegetables before eating or serving them.
- Wash cooking and eating utensils with soap and water after use.

(See Focus on Home Care p. 201.)

HOME CARE

focus on

You must prevent the spread of microbes in the home. Also protect the person from microbes brought into the home. Besides the measures just listed, other infection control measures are needed in the home setting:

- Handle meat and poultry safely as instructed on safe-handling labels (Fig. 11-3, p. 202).
- Cook meats and poultry adequately.
- Protect leftover food. Place leftover food in small containers. Cover containers with lids, foil, or plastic wrap. Date and refrigerate containers as soon as possible. Use the food within the next 2 to 3 days.
- Wash dishes and other eating and cooking utensils. Use liquid detergent and hot water. Wash glasses and cups first. Follow with silverware, plates, bowls, and then pots and pans. Rinse items well with hot water, and place them in a drainer to dry. Air drying is more aseptic than towel drying. If using a dishwasher, rinse dishes before loading them into the dishwasher (Fig. 11-4, p. 202). Use dishwasher soap. Do not wash pots and pans and cast iron, wood, and most plastic items in a dishwasher.
- Clean kitchen appliances, counters, tables, and other surfaces after each meal. Use a sponge or dishcloth moistened with warm water and detergent. Thoroughly remove grease, spills, and splashes. Use a liquid surface cleaner. Clean sinks with scouring powder.
- Dispose of garbage, leftover food, and other soiled supplies after each meal. Place paper, boxes, and cans in a paper or plastic bag or in recycle bins. A garbage disposal is preferred for food and liquid garbage. Otherwise, put food or wet items in a container lined with a plastic bag. Do not put bones in the garbage disposal. Some homes have trash compactors that crush garbage. Some cities recycle paper, glass, plastic, and other substances. Follow required recycling procedures.
- Empty garbage at least once a day.

- Dust furniture and vacuum and mop floors. Damp-mop uncarpeted floors at least weekly. Wipe up spills right away. Use a dust mop or broom for sweeping and a dustpan to collect dust and crumbs. Sweep daily or more often if needed.
- Wash clothes and linens.

Bathrooms need special attention. Microbes easily grow and spread in bathrooms. Every family member must help keep the bathroom clean. Aseptic measures are needed whenever the bathroom is used. These include:

- Flushing the toilet after each use
- Rinsing the sink after washing, shaving, or oral hygiene
- Wiping out the tub or shower after each use
- Removing and disposing of hair from the sink, tub, or shower
- Hanging towels out to dry or placing them in a hamper
- Wiping up water spills

Your job may include cleaning bathrooms every day. Use a disinfectant or water and detergent to clean all surfaces:

- The toilet bowl, seat, and outside areas
- The floor
- The sides, walls, and curtain or door of the shower or tub
- Towel racks
- Toilet tissue, toothbrush, and soap holders
- The mirror
- The sink
- Windowsills

Cleaning the bathroom also includes:

- Mopping uncarpeted floors. Vacuuming carpeted floors.
- Emptying wastebaskets.
- Putting out clean towels and washcloths.
- Opening bathroom windows for a short time and using air fresheners. These help eliminate odors and give a fresh smell to the bathroom.
- Washing bath mats, the wastebasket, and the laundry hamper every week.
- Replacing toilet and facial tissue as needed.

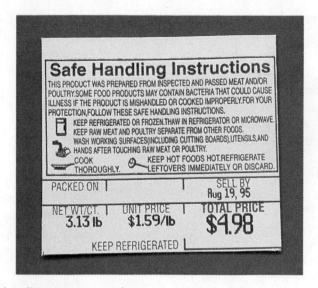

Fig. 11-3 *Safe-handling instructions for meat and poultry. These are required by the U.S. Department of Agriculture.*

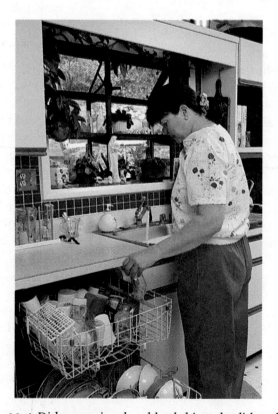

Fig. 11-4 *Dishes are rinsed and loaded into the dishwasher.*

✦ Handwashing

Handwashing with soap and water is the easiest and most important way to prevent the spread of infection. You use your hands in almost every task. They are easily contaminated. Without handwashing, microbes on the hands spread to other persons or items. *Wash your hands before and after giving care.* The rules for handwashing are in Box 11-2.

BOX 11-2

RULES OF HANDWASHING

- Wash your hands under warm running water.
- Hold your hands and forearms lower than your elbows throughout the procedure. Your hands are dirtier than your elbows and forearms. If you hold your hands and forearms up, dirty water runs from hands to elbows. Those areas become contaminated.
- Pay attention to areas often missed during handwashing: thumbs, knuckles, sides of the hands, little fingers, and under the nails. Use a nail file or orange stick to clean under fingernails (Fig. 11-5).
- Check agency policy for how long to wash your hands. At least a 10- to 15-second hand wash is required. Wash your hands longer if they are visibly soiled with blood, body fluids, secretions, or excretions. Your judgment is important.
- Use a clean paper towel for each faucet to turn water off (Fig. 11-6). Faucets are contaminated. Using paper towels prevents clean hands from becoming contaminated again.
- Use a lotion after handwashing to prevent skin chapping and drying. Skin breaks can occur in chapped and dry skin. Remember, skin breaks are portals of entry for microbes.

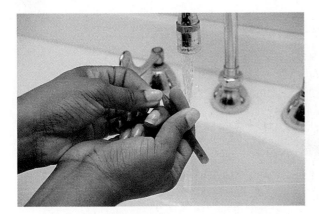

Fig. 11-5 *A nail file is used to clean under the fingernails.*

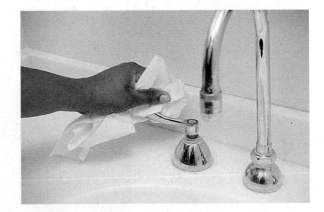

Fig. 11-6 *A paper towel is used to turn the faucet off.*

HANDWASHING

PROCEDURE

1 Make sure you have soap, paper towels, orange stick or nail file, and a wastebasket. Collect missing items.

2 Push your watch up 4 to 5 inches. Also push up uniform sleeves.

3 Stand away from the sink so your clothes do not touch the sink. Stand so the soap and faucet are easy to reach (Fig. 11-7).

4 Turn on the faucet. Adjust the water until it feels warm and comfortable.

5 Wet your wrists and hands thoroughly under running water. Keep your hands lower than your elbows during the procedure (see Fig. 11-7).

6 Apply about 1 teaspoon of soap to your hands.

7 Rub your palms together, and interlace your fingers to work up a good lather (Fig. 11-8). This step should last at least 10 seconds.

8 Wash each hand and wrist thoroughly. Clean well between the fingers. Clean under the fingernails by rubbing the tips of your fingers against your palms (Fig. 11-9).

9 Use a nail file or orange stick to clean under the fingernails (see Fig. 11-5). This step is necessary for the first hand washing of the day and when your hands are highly soiled.

10 Rinse your wrists and hands well. Water should flow from the arms to the hands.

11 Repeat steps 6 through 10, if needed.

12 Dry your wrists and hands with paper towels. Pat dry.

13 Discard the paper towels.

14 Turn off faucets with clean paper towels to avoid contaminating your hand. Use a clean paper towel for each faucet.

15 Discard paper towels.

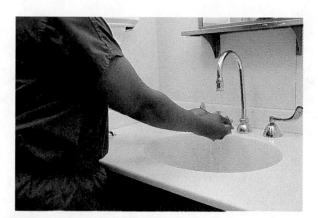

Fig. 11-7 *The uniform does not touch the sink. Soap and water are within reach. Hands are lower than the elbows.*

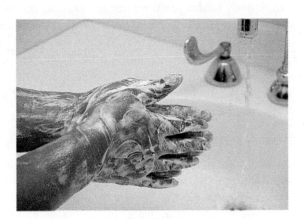

Fig. 11-8 *The palms are rubbed together to work up a good lather.*

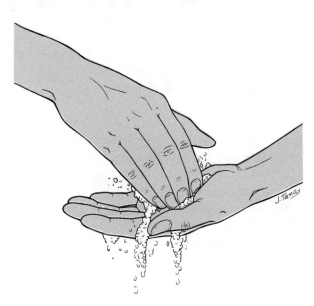

Fig. 11-9 *The tips of the fingers are rubbed against the palms to clean underneath the fingernails.*

Care of Supplies and Equipment

Supply departments disinfect, sterilize, and distribute equipment. Many items are disposable. They help reduce the spread of infection. Single-use disposable items are discarded after use. The same patient uses multi-use disposable items many times. Multi-use items include bedpans, urinals, wash basins, water pitchers, and drinking cups.

Large and costly equipment is not disposable. It is disinfected or sterilized before reuse. Before disinfection or sterilization, equipment is cleaned.

Cleaning

Cleaning removes debris and organic material. It also reduces the number of microbes present. Organic material includes blood, body fluids, secretions, and excretions. Follow these guidelines when cleaning equipment:

- Wear personal protective equipment (gloves, a mask, a gown, and protective eyewear) when cleaning items contaminated with blood, body fluids, secretions, or excretions.
- Rinse the item in cold water first. Rinsing removes organic material. Heat causes organic matter to become thick, sticky, and hard to remove.
- Wash the item with soap and hot water.
- Scrub thoroughly. Use a brush if necessary.
- Rinse the item in warm water.
- Dry the item.
- Disinfect or sterilize the item.
- Disinfect equipment and the sink used in the cleaning procedure.
- Discard personal protective equipment.

Disinfection

Disinfection is the process of destroying pathogens. However, spores are not destroyed. **Spores** are bacteria protected by a hard shell. Spores are killed by extremely high temperatures.

Germicides are disinfectants applied to skin, tissues, and nonliving objects. Alcohol is a common germicide.

Chemical disinfectants are used to clean nondisposable items. Such items include glass thermometers, metal bedpans, blood pressure cuffs, commodes, chairs, counter tops, wheelchairs, stretchers, and room furniture. Chemical disinfectants can burn and irritate the skin. Wear utility gloves or rubber household gloves to prevent skin irritation. These gloves are *waterproof.* Do not wear disposable gloves when using disinfectants. Some chemical disinfectants have special precautions for use or storage. Check the material safety data sheet (MSDS) (see p. 182) before handling a disinfectant.

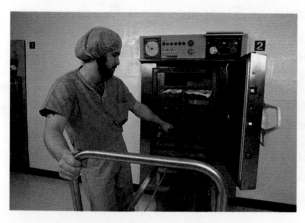

Fig. 11-10 *An autoclave.*

Sterilization

Sterilization procedures destroy all nonpathogens and pathogens, including spores. Very high temperatures are used. Remember, microbes grow best at body temperature. They are destroyed by heat.

Boiling water, radiation, liquid or gas chemicals, dry heat, and *steam under pressure* are sterilization methods. An **autoclave** (Fig. 11-10) is a pressure steam sterilizer. Glass, surgical linens, and metal objects (such as surgical instruments and basins) are autoclaved. High temperatures destroy plastic and rubber items. Therefore they are not autoclaved. Steam under pressure usually sterilizes objects in 30 to 45 minutes.

Other Aseptic Measures

Handwashing, cleaning, disinfection, and sterilization are important aseptic measures. However, other aseptic measures also prevent the spread of infection and microbes. These measures are listed in Box 11-3. The measures are useful in home, work, and everyday activities.

BOX 11-3

ASEPTIC MEASURES

- Hold equipment and linens away from your uniform (Fig. 11-11).
- Prevent dust movement. Do not shake linens or equipment. Use a damp cloth for dusting.
- Clean from the cleanest area to the dirtiest. This prevents soiling a clean area.
- Clean away from your body. If you dust, brush, or wipe toward yourself, you transmit microbes to your skin, hair, and clothing.
- Flush urine and feces down the toilet.
- Pour contaminated liquids directly into sinks or toilets. Avoid splashing onto other areas.
- Avoid sitting on a person's bed. You will pick up microbes and transfer them to the next surface that you sit on.
- Make sure all persons have their own personal hygiene equipment.
- Do not take equipment from one person's room to use for another person. Even if the item is unused, do not take it from one room to another.
- Use leakproof plastic bags for soiled tissues, linen, and other materials.
- Keep tables, counter tops, wheelchair trays, and other surfaces clean and dry.
- Label bottles with the person's name and the date the bottle was opened.
- Keep bottles and fluid containers tightly capped or covered.
- Provide for the person's hygiene needs (see Chapter 14). Wash contaminated areas with soap and water. Feces, urine, blood, pus, and other body fluids, secretions, or excretions may contain microbes.
- Wear personal protective equipment as needed (pp. 211-216).

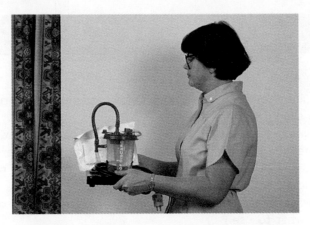

Fig. 11-11 *Hold equipment away from your uniform.*

ISOLATION PRECAUTIONS

Sometimes barriers are needed to prevent the escape of pathogens. The pathogens are kept within a certain area, usually the person's room. This requires isolation procedures.

The Centers for Disease Control and Prevention (CDC) has guidelines for isolation precautions. The guidelines recognize that all body fluids (including blood), secretions, and excretions can transmit pathogens. Two tiers of precautions are practiced—Standard Precautions and Transmission-Based Precautions.

Standard Precautions and Transmission-Based precautions prevent the spread of a **communicable** or **contagious disease.** Communicable diseases are caused by pathogens that are spread easily. Common communicable diseases are measles, mumps, chickenpox, syphilis, gonorrhea, and acquired immunodeficiency syndrome (AIDS) (see Chapter 30). Persons may have respiratory, wound, skin, gastrointestinal, or blood infections that are highly contagious.

Isolation precautions are based on *clean* and *dirty.* *Clean* areas or objects are not contaminated. Uncontaminated areas are free of pathogens. *Dirty* areas or objects are contaminated. If a *clean* area or object has contact with something *dirty,* the clean item is now dirty. *Clean* and *dirty* also depend on how the pathogen is spread.

Standard Precautions

Standard Precautions (Box 11-4, pp. 208-209) reduce the risk of spreading pathogens and known and unknown infections. *Standard Precautions are used in the care of all persons.* They prevent the spread of infection from:
- Blood
- All body fluids, secretions, and excretions (except sweat) even if blood is not visible
- Nonintact skin (skin with open breaks)
- Mucous membranes

Transmission-Based Precautions

Some infections require precautions in addition to the Standard Precautions. Transmission-Based Precautions (Table 11-1, p. 210) depend on how the pathogen is spread. You must understand how certain infections are spread (see Fig. 11-2). This helps you understand the different types of Transmission-Based Precautions.

Protective Measures

Agency policies may differ from those in this text. The rules in Box 11-5 on p. 211 are a guide for giving safe care when isolation precautions are used.

Isolation precautions involve wearing gloves, a gown, a mask, or protective eyewear. Removing linens, trash, and equipment from the room may require double-bagging. Special measures are needed to collect specimens and to transport persons on isolation precautions.

Text continued on p. 211

BOX 11-4

STANDARD PRECAUTIONS

Handwashing

- Wash your hands after touching blood, body fluids, secretions, excretions, and contaminated items. Wash your hands even if you wore gloves.
- Wash your hands immediately after removing gloves and between patient contacts. Also wash your hands whenever needed to avoid transferring microbes to other persons or environments.
- Wash your hands between tasks and procedures on the same person. This prevents cross-contamination of different body sites.
- Use plain soap for routine hand washing. (The RN tells you when other agents are needed. The RN also tells you what to use.)

Gloves

- Wear gloves when touching blood, body fluids, secretions, excretions, and contaminated items.
- Put on clean gloves just before touching mucous membranes and nonintact skin.
- Change gloves between tasks and procedures on the same person. Also change gloves after contacting material that may be highly contaminated.
- Remove gloves promptly after use. Remove gloves before touching uncontaminated items and surfaces. Also remove gloves before going to another person.
- Wash your hands immediately after removing gloves. This prevents the transfer of microbes to other persons or environments.

Masks, Eye Protection, and Face Shields

- Wear masks, eye protection, and face shields during procedures and tasks that are likely to cause splashes or sprays of blood, body fluids, secretions, and excretions. Masks, eye protection, and face shields protect the mucous membranes of the mouth, eyes, and nose from splashes or sprays (Fig. 11-12).

Gowns

- Wear a gown during procedures and care activities that are likely to cause splashes or sprays of blood, body fluids, secretions, or excretions. The gown protects the skin and prevents soiling of clothing.
- Remove a soiled gown as promptly as possible.
- Wash your hands after gown removal. This prevents transferring microorganisms to other persons or environments.

Patient-Care Equipment

- Handle used patient-care equipment carefully. Equipment may be soiled with blood, body fluids, secretions, and excretions. Prevent skin and mucous membrane exposure and clothing contamination. Also prevent the transfer of microbes to other persons and environments.
- Do not use reusable equipment for another person. The item must be cleaned and disinfected or sterilized.
- Discard disposable (single-use) items properly.

Environmental Control

- Follow agency procedures for the routine care, cleaning, and disinfection of surfaces. This includes environmental surfaces, bed rails, bedside equipment, and other frequently touched surfaces.

BOX 11-4

STANDARD PRECAUTIONS—cont'd

Linen
- Follow agency policy for used linen that is soiled with blood, body fluids, secretions, or excretions. The policy describes how to handle, transport, and process soiled linen. Prevent skin and mucous membrane exposures and clothing contamination. Also prevent the transfer of microbes to other persons and environments.

Occupational Health and Bloodborne Pathogens
- Prevent injuries handling needles, scalpels, and other sharp instruments or devices.
- Prevent injuries when handling sharp instruments after procedures and when cleaning used instruments.
- Prevent injuries when disposing of used needles.
- Never recap used needles. Do not manipulate them with both hands. Do not use any technique that involves directing the needle point toward any body part. Use a one-handed "scoop" technique or a mechanical device that holds the needle sheath.
- Do not remove used needles from disposable syringes by hand.
- Do not bend, break, or otherwise manipulate used needles by hand.
- Place used disposable syringes and needles, scalpel blades, and other sharp items in puncture-resistant containers.
- Place reusable syringes and needles in a puncture-resistant container for transport to the reprocessing area.
- Use resuscitation devices for mouth-to-mouth resuscitation (see Chapter 35).

Patient Placement
- A private room is used if the person:
  - Contaminates the environment
  - Does not or cannot assist in maintaining hygiene or environmental control
- Follow the RN's instructions if a private room is not available.

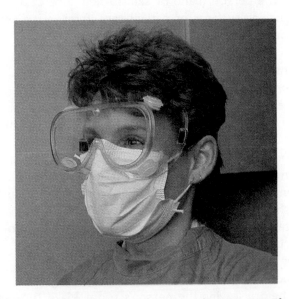

Fig. 11-12 *Goggles and a face mask protect the eyes and mucous membranes of the mouth.*
(From Potter PA, Perry, AG: Fundamentals of nursing: concepts, process, and practice, *ed 4, St Louis, 1997, Mosby.)*

TABLE 11-1

TRANSMISSION-BASED PRECAUTIONS

Airborne Precautions

For known or suspected infections involving microbes transmitted by airborne droplets—measles, chickenpox, tuberculosis

Practices:

- Standard Precautions are followed.
- A private room is preferred.
- Keep the room door closed and the person in the room.
- Wear respiratory protection (tuberculosis respirator, see p. 214) when entering the room of a person with known or suspected tuberculosis.
- Do not enter the room of a person with known or suspected measles or chickenpox if you are susceptible to these diseases.
- Wear respiratory protection (mask) if you must enter the room of a person with known or suspected measles or chickenpox if you are susceptible to these diseases. (Respiratory protection is not needed for persons immune to measles or chickenpox.)
- Limit moving and transporting the person from the room. The person wears a mask if moving or transporting from the room is necessary.

Droplet Precautions

For known or suspected infections involving microbes transmitted by droplets produced by coughing, sneezing, talking, or procedures—meningitis, pneumonia, epiglottitis, diphtheria, pertussis (whooping cough), influenza, mumps, rubella, streptococcal pharyngitis, scarlet fever

Practices:

- Standard Precautions are followed.
- A private room is preferred.
- Wear a mask when working within 3 feet of the person. (Wear a mask on entering the room if required by agency policy.)
- Limit moving and transporting the person from the room. The person wears a mask if moving or transporting from the room is necessary.

Contact Precautions

For known or suspected infections involving microbes transmitted by:

- Direct contact with the person (hand or skin-to-skin contact that occurs during care activities)
- Indirect contact (touching surfaces or patient-care items in the person's room)—gastrointestinal, respiratory, skin, wound infections

Practices:

- Standard Precautions are followed.
- A private room is preferred.
- Wear gloves when entering the room.
- Change gloves after having contact with infective material that may contain high concentrations of microbes.
- Remove gloves before leaving the person's room.
- Wash your hands immediately with an agent specified by the RN.
- Make sure your hands do not touch potentially contaminated surfaces or items after removing gloves and handwashing.
- Wear a gown on entering the room if you will have substantial contact with the person, environmental surfaces, or items in the room.
- Wear a gown on entering the room if the person is incontinent or has diarrhea, an ileostomy, a colostomy, or wound drainage not contained by a dressing.
- Remove the gown before leaving the person's room. Make sure your clothing does not contact potentially contaminated surfaces in the person's room.
- Limit moving or transferring the person from the room. Maintain precautions if the person is moved or transferred from the room.

BOX 11-5 RULES FOR ISOLATION PRECAUTIONS

- Collect all needed equipment before entering the room.
- Prevent contamination of equipment and supplies. Floors are contaminated. So is any object on the floor or that falls to the floor.
- Use mops wetted with a disinfectant solution to clean floors. Floor dust is contaminated.
- Prevent drafts. Pathogens are carried in the air by drafts.
- Use paper towels to handle contaminated items.
- Remove items from the room in sturdy, leakproof plastic bags.
- Double bag items if the outer part of the bag is or can be contaminated (p. 216).
- Follow agency policy for removing and transporting disposable and reusable items.
- Return reusable dishes, eating utensils, and trays to the food service department. Discard disposable dishes, eating utensils, and trays in the waste container in the person's room.
- Do not touch your hair, nose, mouth, eyes, or other body parts when caring for a person in isolation.
- Do not touch any clean area or object if your hands are contaminated.
- Wash your hands if they become contaminated.
- Place clean items or objects on paper towels.
- Do not shake linen.
- Use paper towels to turn faucets on and off.
- Tell the RN if you have any cuts, open skin areas, a sore throat, vomiting, or diarrhea.

✦ Wearing gloves

The skin is a natural barrier. It prevents microbes from entering the body. Small skin breaks on the hands and fingers are common. Some are very small and hard to see. Disposable gloves give added protection. They protect you from pathogens in the person's blood, body fluids, secretions, and excretions. They also protect the person from microbes on your hands.

Wear gloves whenever contact with blood, body fluids, secretions, excretions, mucous membranes, and nonintact skin is likely. Contact may be direct. Or contact may be with items or surfaces contaminated with blood, body fluids, secretions, or excretions.

Do not tear gloves when putting them on. Carelessness, long fingernails, and rings can tear gloves. Blood, body fluids, secretions, and excretions can enter the glove through the tear. This contaminates the hand. Remember the following about wearing gloves:

- You need a new pair for every person.
- Remove and discard torn, cut, or punctured gloves immediately. Wash your hands and put on a new pair.
- Wear gloves only once. Discard them after use.
- Put on clean gloves just before touching mucous membranes or nonintact skin.
- Put on new gloves whenever gloves become contaminated with blood, body fluids, secretions, or excretions. You may need more than one pair of gloves for a task.
- Make sure gloves cover your wrists. If you wear a gown, gloves must cover the cuffs (Fig. 11-13).
- Remove gloves so the inside part is on the outside. The inside is considered *clean*.
- Wash your hands after removing gloves.

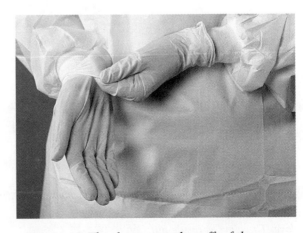

Fig. 11-13 *The gloves cover the cuffs of the gown.*

REMOVING GLOVES

PROCEDURE

1   Make sure that glove touches only glove. Do not let gloves touch skin on your wrists or arms.

2   Grasp a glove just below the cuff (Fig. 11-14, *A*).

3   Pull the glove down over your hand so it is inside out (Fig. 11-14, *B*).

4   Hold the removed glove with your other gloved hand.

5   Reach inside the other glove with the first two fingers of your ungloved hand (Fig. 11-14, *C*).

6   Pull the glove down (inside out) over your hand and the other glove (Fig. 11-14, *D*).

7   Discard the gloves. Follow agency policy.

8   Wash your hands.

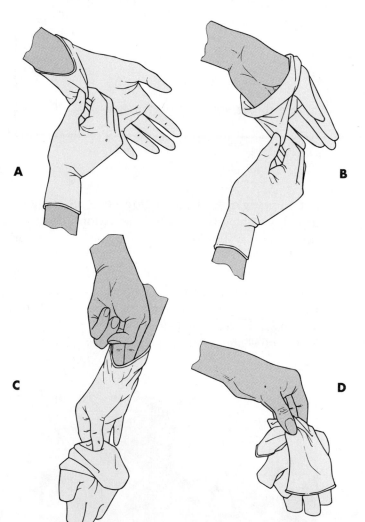

Fig. 11-14 *Removing gloves.* **A,** *The glove is grasped below the cuff.* **B,** *The glove is pulled down over the hand. The glove is inside out.* **C,** *The fingers of the ungloved hand are inserted inside the other glove.* **D,** *The glove is pulled down and over the hand and glove. The glove is inside out.*

✦ *Wearing protective apparel*

Gowns, plastic aprons, shoe covers, boots, and leg coverings are barriers that prevent the transmission of microbes. They protect your clothes, wrists, and arms from contact with blood, body fluids, secretions, or excretions. They also protect against splashes and sprays.

Gowns must be long and large enough to completely cover clothing. The sleeves are long with tight cuffs. The gown opens at the back. It is tied at the neck and waist. The inside and neck are *clean*. The outside and waist strings are contaminated.

Gowns are used once. A wet gown is contaminated. A wet gown is removed and a dry one put on. Disposable gowns are made of paper. They are discarded after use. Reusable gowns are made of cloth. Laundering is necessary before reuse.

DONNING AND REMOVING A GOWN

PROCEDURE

1 Remove your watch and all jewelry.

2 Roll up uniform sleeves.

3 Wash your hands.

4 Put on a face mask if required.

5 Pick up a clean gown. Hold it out in front of you, and let it unfold. Do not shake the gown.

6 Put your hands and arms through the sleeves (Fig. 11-15, *A*).

7 Make sure the gown covers the front of your uniform. It should be snug at the neck.

8 Tie the strings at the back of the neck (Fig. 11-15, *B*).

9 Overlap the back of the gown. Make sure the gown covers your uniform. The gown should be snug and not hang loosely (Fig. 11-15, *C*).

10 Tie the waist strings at the back.

11 Put on the gloves.

12 Provide necessary patient care.

13 Remove and discard the gloves.

14 Remove the gown.

   a Untie the waist strings.

   b Wash your hands.

   c Untie the neck strings. Do not touch the outside of the gown.

   d Pull the gown down from the shoulder.

   e Turn the gown inside out as it is removed. Hold the gown at the inside shoulder seams, and bring your hands together (Fig. 11-15, *D*).

15 Roll up the gown away from you. Keep it inside out.

16 Discard the gown. Follow agency policy.

17 Wash your hands.

18 Remove the face mask. Discard it following agency policy.

19 Wash your hands.

20 Open the door using a paper towel. Discard it as you leave.

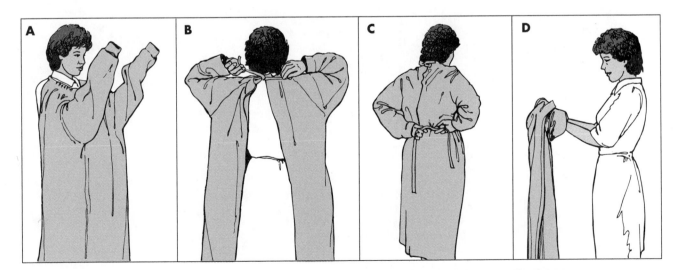

Fig. 11-15 *Gowning technique.* **A,** *The arms and hands are put through the sleeves.* **B,** *The strings are tied at the back of the neck.* **C,** *The gown is overlapped in the back to cover the entire uniform.* **D,** *The gown is turned inside out as it is removed.*

✦ *Wearing masks and respiratory protection*

Masks prevent the spread of microbes from the respiratory tract. They are used for Airborne and Droplet Precautions. Masks are worn by patients, visitors, or staff. Disposable masks are used. A wet or moist mask is contaminated. Breathing can cause masks to become wet or moist. Apply a new mask when contamination occurs.

A mask should fit snugly over your nose and mouth. Wash your hands before putting on a mask. To remove the mask, first remove your gloves. Touch only the ties during removal. The front of the mask is contaminated.

Tuberculosis respirators (Fig. 11-16) are worn when caring for persons with tuberculosis (TB). Such protection is used for Airborne Precautions.

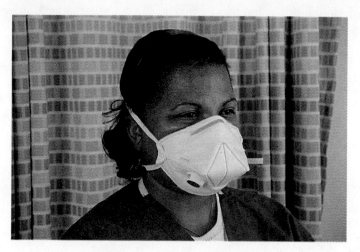

Fig. 11-16 *Tuberculosis respirator.*

WEARING A MASK

PROCEDURE

1 Wash your hands.

2 Pick up the mask by its upper ties. Do not touch the part that will cover your face.

3 Place the mask over your nose and mouth.

4 Place the upper strings over your ears. Tie the strings in the back toward the top of your head (Fig. 11-17, *A*).

5 Tie the lower strings at the back of your neck (Fig. 11-17, *B*). The lower part of the mask must be under your chin.

6 Pinch the metal band around your nose if you wear glasses. The top of the mask must be snug over your nose and under the bottom edge of the glasses.

7 Wash your hands.

8 Provide necessary care. Avoid coughing, sneezing, and unnecessary talking.

9 Change the mask if it becomes moist or contaminated.

10 Remove the mask as follows:

   a Remove the gloves.

   b Untie the lower strings.

   c Untie the top strings.

   d Hold the top strings, and remove the mask.

   e Bring the strings together. The inside of the mask folds together. Do not touch the inside of the mask.

11 Discard the mask. Follow agency policy.

12 Wash your hands.

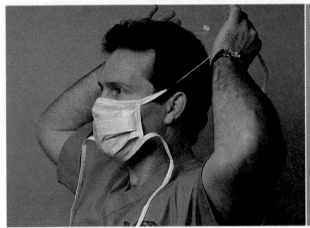 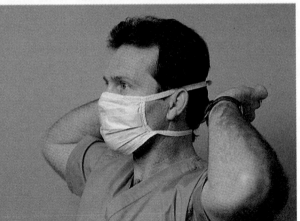

Fig. 11-17 A, *The upper strings are tied on the back of the head.* **B,** *The lower strings are tied at the neck.* (From Potter PA, Perry, AG: Fundamentals of nursing: concepts, process, and practice, *ed 4, St Louis, 1997, Mosby.)*

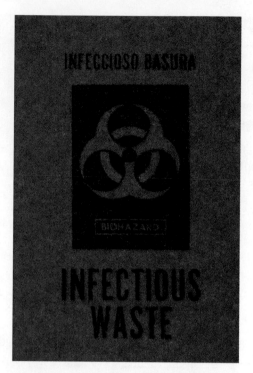

Fig. 11-18 *BIOHAZARD symbol.*

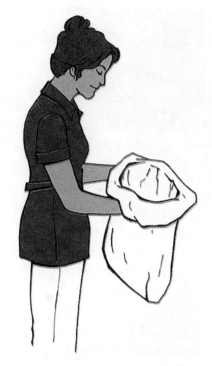

Fig. 11-19 *A cuff is made on a clean bag.*

Wearing eye protection and face shields

Goggles and face shields protect the mucous membranes of your eyes, mouth, and nose from the person's pathogens. You wear goggles or face shields with face masks (see Fig. 11-12). Together they protect your eyes, nose, and mouth from splashing or spraying of blood, body fluids, secretions, or excretions. You may need such protection when giving care, cleaning instruments, or disposing of contaminated fluids.

Discard disposable eyewear after use. Reusable eyewear is cleaned before reuse. After being washed with soap and water, a disinfectant is used.

Bagging items

Contaminated items are bagged to remove them from the person's room. Leakproof plastic bags are used.

Trash is placed in a container labeled with the *BIO-HAZARD* symbol (Fig. 11-18). **Biohazardous waste** is items contaminated with the person's blood, body fluids, secretions, or excretions. (*Bio* means life, and *hazardous* means dangerous or harmful.) Linen is bagged and transported following agency policy. Also follow agency policy for bagging and transporting equipment and supplies.

One bag is usually adequate. Double bagging involves two bags. The CDC does not recommend double bagging unless the outside of the bag is soiled. Two staff members are needed for double bagging. One is inside the room. The other is at the doorway outside the room. The person in the room places contaminated items into a bag.

Then the bag is sealed securely. The person outside the room holds open another bag. This bag is clean. A wide cuff is made on the clean bag to protect the hands from contamination (Fig. 11-19). The contaminated bag is placed in the clean bag at the doorway.

Collecting specimens

Specimen containers are labeled following agency policy. Then the container and lid are placed on a paper towel in the person's bathroom. Gloves are worn. Do not contaminate the outside of the container when collecting the specimen. Also avoid contamination when transferring the specimen from the collecting vessel to the container. Put the lid on securely. Some agencies bag specimens for transport to the laboratory. Check agency policy about applying warning labels.

Transporting persons

Persons on isolation precautions usually do not leave their rooms. However, special treatments or tests may require transporting the person to another area. Transporting procedures vary among agencies. Some require transport by bed. This prevents contaminating wheelchairs and stretchers. Other agencies use wheelchairs and stretchers.

A safe transport means that other patients, staff, and visitors are protected from the infection. Follow these guidelines for safely transporting persons on isolation precautions:

- The person wears a clean gown or pajamas and an isolation gown.
- The person wears a mask if on Airborne or Droplet Precautions.
- Cover any draining wounds.
- Give the person tissues and a leakproof bag. Used tissues are placed in the bag.
- Wear a gown, mask, and gloves as required by the isolation precaution.
- Place an extra layer of sheets and absorbent pads on the stretcher or wheelchair. This protects against draining body fluids.
- Do not let anyone else on the elevator. This reduces exposure to the infection.
- Alert staff in the receiving area about the isolation precautions. They wear gowns, masks, protective eyewear, and gloves as needed.
- Disinfect the stretcher or wheelchair after use.

Psychological Impact of Isolation Precautions

The person has love, belonging, and self-esteem needs. Too often these needs are unmet when isolation precautions are used. Visitors and staff often avoid the person. They may need to wear gowns, masks, protective eyewear, and gloves. This takes extra effort before entering the room. Some are unsure about what to touch. Fears about getting the disease are common. Loneliness, feeling unloved and unwanted, and rejection can occur.

Self-esteem easily suffers. The person knows the disease can be spread to others. The person may feel dirty and undesirable. Sometimes visitors and staff unknowingly make the person feel ashamed and guilty about having a contagious disease.

The RN helps the person, visitors, and staff understand the need for isolation precautions and how they affect the person. You can help meet the person's need for love, belonging, and self-esteem. The following actions are helpful. Remember to disinfect or discard objects that become contaminated with infected material:

- Remember, the pathogen is undesirable, not the person.
- Treat the person with respect, kindness, and dignity.
- Provide newspapers, magazines, and other reading matter.
- Provide hobby materials if possible.
- Place a clock in the room.
- Encourage the person to telephone family and friends.
- Provide a current television schedule.
- Organize your work so you can stay to visit with the person.
- Say hello from the doorway often.

(See Focus on Children, Focus on Older Persons, and Focus on Home Care.)

focus on CHILDREN

Infants and young children do not understand isolation. Goggles, masks, and gowns may frighten them. Parents and staff look different. Gloves and personal protective equipment prevent skin-to-skin contact with parents. Because of likely contamination, toys and comfort items (blankets and stuffed animals) may be kept from the child. This adds to the child's distress.

The RN prepares the child and family for isolation. Simple explanations are given to the child. If appropriate for the child's age, the child is given a mask, goggles, and a gown to touch and play with. Children need to see the faces of persons entering the room. Always let the child see your face before putting on a mask and goggles. Say hello to the child, and tell the child your name.

focus on OLDER PERSONS

Older persons also need to see your face. This helps persons with poor vision know who you are. Personal protective equipment may increase confusion in confused and demented persons. Always let the person see your face before you put on personal protective equipment. Also tell the person who you are and what you are going to do. Report signs and symptoms of confusion to the RN.

focus on HOME CARE

Standard Precautions are always practiced in home care. Sometimes Transmission-Based Precautions are needed. The RN tells you what measures are needed.

BLOODBORNE PATHOGEN STANDARD

The AIDS (human immunodeficiency virus [HIV]) and hepatitis B virus (HBV) are found in blood (see Chapter 30). Therefore they are bloodborne pathogens. The viruses exit the body through blood and are transmitted to others by blood. *Potentially infectious materials* also transmit the viruses. Such materials are contaminated with blood or with a body fluid that may contain blood. Potentially infectious materials also include needles, suction equipment, soiled linens, dressings, and other items used in the person's care.

The Bloodborne Pathogen Standard is a regulation of the Occupational Safety and Health Administration (OSHA). The standard is intended to protect the health team from exposure to the viruses.

Exposure Control Plan

Employers must have a written exposure control plan. The plan identifies employees at risk for exposure to blood or other potentially infectious materials. Staff at risk includes nurses, patient caregivers, surgical staff, central supply staff, laundry and housekeeping staff, and laboratory staff. The plan includes actions to take when an exposure incident occurs.

Staff at risk for exposure must receive free information and training. Training occurs upon employment and yearly. Training is required also for new or changed tasks involving exposure to bloodborne pathogens.

Preventive Measures

Preventive measures reduce the risk of occupational exposure. Such measures include hepatitis B vaccination and Standard Precautions (formerly called *universal precautions*).

Hepatitis B vaccination

Hepatitis B is a liver disease caused by the hepatitis B virus (HBV). HBV is transmitted by blood and sexual contact. The hepatitis B vaccine is given to produce immunity against hepatitis B. **Immunity** means that a person has protection against a certain disease. The immune person will not get the disease.

The hepatitis B vaccination is available to employees within 10 working days of being hired. The employer pays the cost. An employee can refuse the vaccination. The employee signs a statement refusing the vaccine. The employee can have the vaccination at a later date.

Methods of Control

The Occupational Safety and Health Administration (OSHA) requires engineering and work practice controls and personal protective equipment. Guidelines also are given for handling equipment and laundry.

Engineering and work practice controls

Engineering controls reduce employee exposure in the workplace. Special containers for contaminated sharps (needles, broken glass) and specimens remove and isolate the hazard from staff. Containers are puncture-resistant, leakproof, and color coded in red. Or they are labeled with the *BIOHAZARD* symbol (see Fig. 11-18).

Work practice controls also reduce exposure risks. All tasks involving blood or other potentially infectious materials are done in ways that limit splattering, splashing, and spraying. Producing droplets also is avoided. OSHA requires these work practice controls:

- Do not eat, drink, smoke, apply cosmetics or lip balm, or handle contact lenses in areas of occupational exposure.
- Do not store food or drinks in refrigerators or other areas where blood or potentially infectious materials are kept.
- Wash hands after removing gloves. Wash hands as soon as possible after skin contact with blood or other potentially infectious materials.
- Never recap, bend, or remove needles by hand. When a medical procedure requires recapping, bending, or removing contaminated needles, use mechanical means (forceps) or a one-handed method.
- Never shear or break contaminated needles.
- Discard contaminated needles and sharp instruments in containers that are closable, puncture-resistant, and leakproof. Containers are color coded red or have the *BIOHAZARD* symbol. Containers must be upright and not overfilled.

Personal protective equipment

Such equipment includes gloves, goggles, face shields, masks, laboratory coats, gowns, shoe covers, and surgical caps. Blood or other potentially infectious material must not pass through the equipment. The equipment protects clothes, undergarments, skin, eyes, mouth, and other mucous membranes.

Personal protective equipment is free to employees. Correct sizes are available. The employer makes sure that equipment is properly cleaned, laundered, repaired, replaced, or discarded. OSHA requires these measures for safely handling and using personal protective equipment:

- Remove protective equipment before leaving the work area and when a garment becomes contaminated.
- Place used protective equipment in marked areas or containers when being stored, washed, decontaminated, or discarded.
- Wear gloves when you expect contact with blood or other potentially infectious materials. Also wear gloves when handling or touching contaminated items or surfaces. Replace worn, punctured, or contaminated gloves.
- Never wash or decontaminate disposable gloves for reuse.
- Discard utility gloves that show signs of cracking, peeling, tearing, or puncturing. Utility gloves are decontaminated for reuse if the process will not ruin them.

Equipment

Contaminated equipment is cleaned and decontaminated. Decontaminate work surfaces with an appropriate disinfectant:

- Upon completing tasks
- Immediately when there is obvious contamination
- After any spill of blood or other potentially infectious material
- At the end of the work shift when surfaces became contaminated since the last cleaning

Use a brush and dustpan or tongs to clean up broken glass. Never pick up broken glass with your hands, not even if wearing gloves. Discard broken glass into a puncture-resistant container.

Laundry

OSHA requires these precautions for contaminated laundry:

- Handle contaminated laundry as little as possible.
- Wear gloves or other needed personal protective equipment when handling contaminated laundry.
- Bag contaminated laundry where it was used.
- Mark laundry bags or containers with the *BIOHAZARD* symbol for laundry sent offsite.
- Place wet, contaminated laundry in leakproof containers before transporting. The containers are color coded in red or labeled with the *BIOHAZARD* symbol.

Exposure Incidents

An *exposure incident* is any eye, mouth, other mucous membrane, nonintact skin, or parenteral contact with blood or other potentially infectious materials. *Parenteral* means piercing the mucous membranes or the skin barrier. Piercing occurs through needlesticks, human bites, cuts, and abrasions.

Report exposure incidents at once. Medical evaluation and follow-up are free. This includes required laboratory tests. The employee's blood is tested for HBV and HIV. If the employee refuses testing, the blood sample is kept for at least 90 days. Testing is done later if the employee changes his or her mind.

Confidentiality is important. The employee is told of evaluation results. The employee is also told of any medical conditions that may need further treatment. The employee receives a written opinion of the medical evaluation within 15 days after its completion.

The source individual's blood is tested for HIV or HBV. The *source individual* is the person whose blood or body fluids are the source of an exposure incident. State laws vary about releasing the results. The employer informs the employee about any laws affecting the source's identity and test results.

SURGICAL ASEPSIS

Surgical asepsis (sterile technique) is the practices that keep equipment and supplies free of all microbes. **Sterile** means the absence of *all* microbes, including spores. Surgical asepsis is required any time the skin or sterile tissues are penetrated. The operating room and labor and delivery areas require surgical asepsis. So do many tests and nursing procedures. If any break occurs in sterile technique, pathogens and nonpathogens can enter the body. An infection can develop.

Some states allow assistive personnel to perform selected sterile procedures. Examples include urinary catheterizations, sterile dressing changes, suctioning, and collecting blood specimens. In other states, assistive personnel can only assist RNs with sterile procedures. Do not perform any sterile procedure unless:

- Your state allows assistive personnel to perform the procedure.
- The procedure is in your job description.
- You received the necessary education and training.
- You review the procedure with the RN.
- An RN is available for questions and guidance.

HOME CARE

focus on

You may need to clean a work surface before you practice surgical asepsis. Use soap and water, and practice Standard Precautions. Always clean from the cleanest area to the dirtiest. Also clean away from your body and uniform. Dry the surface after cleaning.

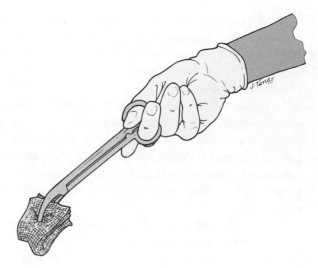

Fig. 11-20 *Sterile forceps are used to handle sterile items.*

Principles of Surgical Asepsis

Operating room and labor and delivery staff must follow certain procedures. They wear masks and surgical caps for handwashing. This handwashing is called a surgical "scrub." It takes at least 5 minutes. Then the staff put on sterile gowns and sterile gloves. For sterile nursing procedures, regular handwashing and sterile gloves are needed. You also wear personal protective equipment as needed to prevent contact with blood, body fluids, secretions, and excretions.

For a sterile procedure, all items in contact with the person are kept sterile. If any item is contaminated, the person is at risk for infection. Therefore you must maintain a sterile field. A **sterile field** is a work area free of pathogens and nonpathogens (including spores). Box 11-6 lists the principles and practices of surgical asepsis. Follow them to maintain a sterile field and when performing a sterile procedure. (See Focus on Home Care.)

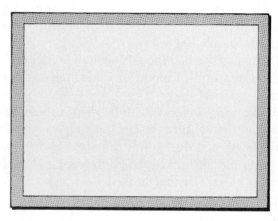

Fig. 11-21 *A 1-inch (2.5 cm) margin around the sterile field is considered contaminated.*

BOX 11-6

PRINCIPLES AND PRACTICES FOR SURGICAL ASEPSIS

- A sterile item can touch only another sterile item.
  - If a sterile item touches a clean item, the sterile item is contaminated.
  - If a clean item touches a sterile item, the sterile item is contaminated.
  - A sterile package that is open, torn, punctured, wet, or moist is contaminated.
  - A sterile package is contaminated after the expiration date on the package.
  - Place only sterile items on a sterile field.
  - Use sterile gloves or sterile forceps to handle other sterile items (Fig. 11-20).
  - Consider any item as contaminated if you are unsure of its sterility.
  - Do not use contaminated items. They are discarded or resterilized.
- Sterile items or a sterile field are always kept within your vision and above your waist.
  - If you cannot see an item, the item is contaminated.
  - If the item is below your waist, the item is contaminated.
  - Keep sterile gloved hands above your waist and within your sight.
  - Do not leave a sterile field unattended.
  - Do not turn your back on a sterile field.
- Airborne microorganisms can contaminate sterile items or a sterile field.
  - Prevent drafts by closing the door and avoiding extra movements. Ask other staff in the room to avoid extra moving.
  - Avoid coughing, sneezing, talking, or laughing over a sterile field. Turn your head away from the sterile field if you must talk.
  - Wear a mask if you need to talk during the procedure.
  - Do not perform sterile procedures if you have a respiratory infection.
  - Do not reach over a sterile field.
- Fluid flows downward, in the direction of gravity.
  - Hold wet items down (see Fig. 11-20). If wet items are held up, fluid flows down into a contaminated area. The contaminated fluid flows back into the sterile field when the item is held down.
  - Hold your hands higher than your elbows during a surgical scrub. Water from your elbows will not flow onto your clean hands and fingers.
- The sterile field is kept dry, unless the area below it is sterile.
  - The sterile field is contaminated if it gets wet and the area below it is not sterile.
  - Avoid spilling and splashing when pouring sterile fluids into sterile containers.
- The edges of a sterile field are contaminated.
  - A 1-inch (2.5 cm) margin around the sterile field is contaminated (Fig. 11-21).
  - Place all sterile items inside the 1-inch (2.5 cm) margin of the sterile field.
  - Items outside the 1-inch (2.5 cm) margin are contaminated.
- Honesty is essential to sterile technique.
  - You know when you contaminate an item or sterile field. Be honest with yourself even if other staff members are not present.
  - Remove the contaminated item and correct the situation. If necessary, start over with sterile supplies.
  - Report the contamination to the RN.

Sterile Equipment and Supplies

Sterile equipment and supplies are wrapped in cloth, paper, or plastic. Sterile liquids are sealed in containers. Labeling shows that the item is sterile. Some items have a chemical tape that changes color when sterilized. Sterile items are marked with expiration dates. If the date is past, do not use the item. If a container's seal is broken, do not use the solution. When handling sterile equipment and supplies, follow the principles and practices listed in Box 11-6. Also, wash your hands before opening sterile items and setting up a sterile field.

✦ Opening sterile packages

Some sterile packages are wrapped and have four flaps or corners. Other packages are peel-back. Different methods are used to open wrapped and peel-back packages.

The inside of a sterile package is sterile and is a sterile field. Before opening a sterile package, make sure the package is intact. The package must be dry and free of tears, punctures, holes, and watermarks. *Do not open sterile packages while wearing sterile gloves. The outside of the package is unsterile. You will contaminate your gloves.*

Text continued on p. 226

OPENING A STERILE PACKAGE

PROCEDURE ALERT

- Does your state allow assistive personnel to perform the procedure?

- Is the procedure in your job description?

- Do you have the necessary training and education?

- Is an RN available to answer questions and to supervise you?

PRE-PROCEDURE

1 Explain the procedure to the person.

2 Wash your hands.

3 Collect all needed supplies and equipment.

4 Inspect the package for sterility.

   a Check the label and chemical tape.

   b Check the expiration date.

   c See if the package is dry.

   d Check for tears, holes, punctures, and watermarks.

5 Prepare the person for the procedure.

   a Explain the procedure to the person.

   b Check ID bracelet. Identify the person with the assignment sheet.

   c Provide for privacy. Close the door, and pull the privacy curtain.

   d Assist the person to meet elimination needs.

   e Wash your hands.

   f Drape the person for the procedure and for privacy.

6 Arrange a work surface.

   a Make sure you have enough room.

   b Arrange the work surface at waist level and within your vision.

   c Clean and dry the work surface.

   d Do not reach over or turn your back on the work surface.

OPENING A STERILE PACKAGE—cont'd

PROCEDURE

7 Opening a wrapped sterile package on a surface:

  a Place the sterile package in the center of your work surface.

  b Position the package so the top flap points toward you.

  c Reach around the package and grasp the outside of the top flap with your thumb and index finger (Fig. 11-22, *A*, p. 224).

  d Pull the flap open, and lay it flat.

  e Grasp the outside of the first side flap with your thumb and index finger. Use your right hand if the flap is on your right and your left hand if it is on your left. Pull the flap open, and lay it flat (Fig. 11-22, *B*, p. 224).

  f Repeat step 7e for the other side flap (Fig. 11-22, *C*, p. 224).

  g Grasp the outside of the fourth flap. Stand back and away from the package, and pull the flap back (Fig. 11-22, *D*, p. 224). Let the flap lay flat. Do not let the flap touch your uniform or any contaminated surface.

  h Remember that the 1-inch (2.5 cm) margin on the inside of the wrapper is contaminated. The rest of the inside wrapper is sterile. Do not let any contaminated item touch this area.

8 Opening a wrapped sterile package while holding it (Fig. 11-23, p. 225):

  a Hold the package in your left hand if you are right-handed. Hold it in your right hand if you are left-handed.

  b Hold the package so that the top flap points toward you.

  c Reach behind the top flap, and open it away from you.

  d Open each side flap away from the package.

  e Open the fourth flap toward you.

  f Do not touch the inside wrapper or the package contents.

  g Hold the package so the RN can grasp the contents. The RN wears sterile gloves.

  h Do the following to transfer the package contents to a sterile field:

    • Hold the package wrapper back and away from the sterile field (Fig. 11-24, *A*, p. 225).

    • Drop the contents onto the sterile field (Fig. 11-24, *B*, p. 225).

9 Opening a peel-back package:

  a Read the package instructions.

  b Two flaps: grasp the two flaps, and gently peel the flaps back (Fig. 11-25, p. 225).

  c One flap: hold the package, and pull back the flap (Fig. 11-26, p. 225).

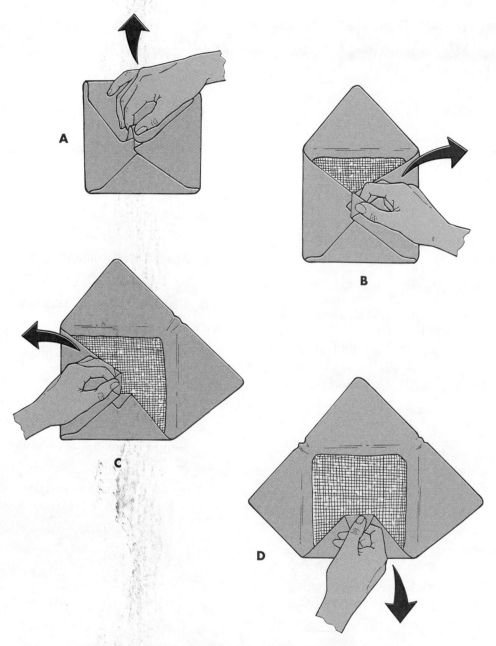

Fig. 11-22 *Opening a sterile package on a flat surface.*

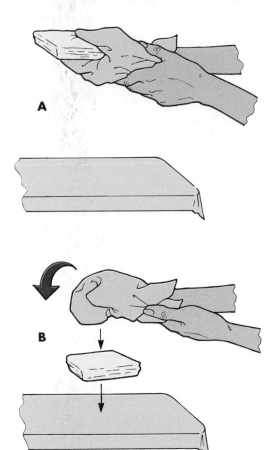

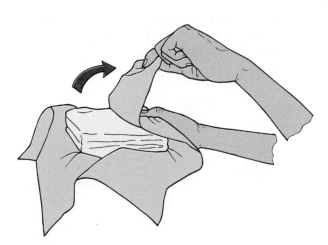

Fig. 11-23 *Opening a sterile package while holding it. Note that package is held away from the person so that the wrapper is not contaminated.*

Fig. 11-24 *Transferring package contents to a sterile field.* **A,** *Hold the wrapper back after opening the package.* **B,** *Drop the contents onto the sterile field.*

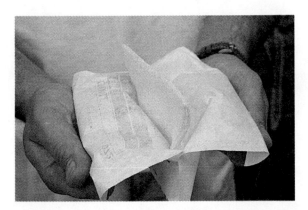

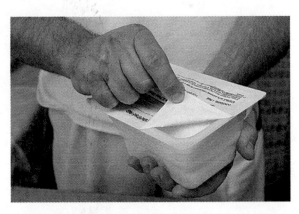

Fig. 11-25 *The flaps of a peel-back package are carefully peeled back.*

Fig. 11-26 *The flap of a one-flap package is pulled back.*

✦ Opening and pouring sterile solutions

Sterile solutions are usually obtained from the supply area. The container is sealed. The outside of the container and the cap is unsterile. The inside of the cap and container is sterile.

Inspect the container when collecting your supplies. Make sure it is not cracked or broken. Check that the seal is intact. Return the bottle to the supply department if it is cracked or broken or if the seal is broken.

Some sterile packages contain sterile solutions. If so, the container is sterile. The container is opened while wearing sterile gloves.

Sterile solutions are poured into sterile containers. Do not pour a sterile solution into a clean container. This contaminates the sterile solution.

✧ OPENING AND POURING A STERILE SOLUTION

PROCEDURE ALERT

- Does your state allow assistive personnel to perform the procedure?
- Is the procedure in your job description?
- Do you have the necessary training and education?
- Is an RN available to answer questions and to supervise you?

PRE-PROCEDURE

1 Obtain the correct solution.

2 Inspect the container for cracks and breaks.

3 Check the seal. It must be intact.

PROCEDURE

4 Hold the container so the label is in your palm. This protects the label from becoming wet from dripping solution.

5 Twist off the cap to break the seal.

6 Place the cap, inside up, on a clean surface.

7 Hold the container 4 to 6 inches over the sterile bowl (Fig. 11-27). Do not let the container touch the sterile bowl.

8 Pour the solution into the sterile bowl. Pour slowly to avoid splashing.

POST-PROCEDURE

9 Recap the container. Discard the container if it is empty or remaining solution will not be used.

10 Do the following if remaining solution will be used:

    a Make sure the remaining solution was not contaminated.

    b Label the container with the person's name, the date, and the time.

    c Store the container. Follow agency policy.

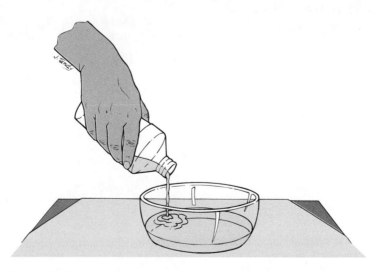

Fig. 11-27 Sterile solution is poured into a sterile bowl. Care is taken to avoid spills or splashing.

Setting Up a Sterile Field

The sterile field is your sterile work area. Once the sterile field is set up, you can add other sterile items to the field. You can use the inside wrapper of a sterile package or a sterile drape for your sterile field. Drapes often provide larger sterile fields than the inside of the sterile package.

A sterile drape is inside sterile packaging. You open the package as described earlier. Remember, the inside 1-inch margin (2.5 cm) of the drape is contaminated.

SETTING UP A STERILE FIELD

PROCEDURE ALERT

- Does your state allow assistive personnel to perform the procedure?

- Is the procedure in your job description?

- Do you have the necessary training and education?

- Is an RN available to answer questions and to supervise you?

PROCEDURE

1 Follow Pre-Procedure steps listed in *Opening a Sterile Package.*

2 Open the sterile package (see *Opening a Sterile Package*).

3 Pick up the folded top edge of the drape with your thumb and index finger.

4 Remove the drape from the package. Lift it away from you and let it unfold (Fig. 11-28, *A*). Discard the packaging.

5 Do not let the drape touch your uniform, the outer packaging, or any other surface.

6 Pick up the other corner of the drape. Hold the drape away from you and other contaminated surfaces.

7 Lay the drape on your work surface (Fig. 11-28, *B*). Start with the bottom half (the side away from you).

8 Add other sterile items to the sterile field:

   a Open each sterile package.

   b Hold the package wrapper back and away from the sterile field.

   c Drop the contents onto the sterile field, or use a transfer forceps.

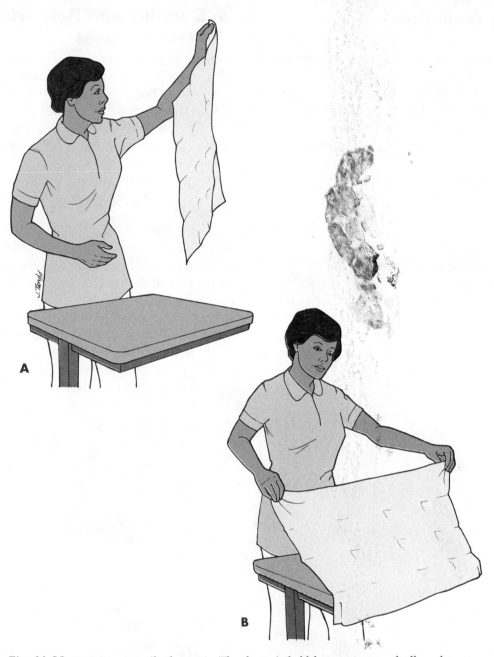

Fig. 11-28 *Opening a sterile drape.* **A,** *The drape is held by a corner and allowed to open freely.* **B,** *The drape is placed over a work surface. Note that it is held at two corners.*

Using a transfer forceps

Forceps are instruments used to pick up, hold, and transfer items (see Fig. 11-20). You use sterile forceps to transfer sterile items to or within a sterile field. You also use them to handle sterile items during a procedure. Remember the following when using sterile forceps:

- Hold sterile forceps above your waist.
- Hold wet forceps so the tips are lower than your wrist.
- Keep sterile forceps within your sight.
- Make sure the forceps do not touch the outside of any packaging.
- Make sure the forceps do not touch the 1-inch margin (2.5 cm) around the drape.
- Lay the forceps down carefully within the sterile field.
  - Not wearing sterile gloves: lay the tips within the sterile field and the handles outside the sterile field.
  - Wearing sterile gloves: lay the entire forceps within the sterile field.

✦ Donning and Removing Sterile Gloves

Sterile gloves are put on after setting up the sterile field. After putting on sterile gloves, you can handle sterile items within the sterile field. You cannot touch anything outside the sterile field.

In operating rooms and delivery areas, the closed method of sterile gloving is followed. A sterile gown is donned and then sterile gloves. You will learn sterile gowning and closed gloving if you work in those areas. The open gloving method is used for sterile procedures at the bedside.

Sterile gloves are disposable. They come in peel-back packaging. A variety of sizes let them fit each person snugly. The insides are powdered for ease in donning the gloves. Also, the right glove and left glove are marked on the package.

Always keep sterile gloved hands above your waist and within your vision. You can touch items only within the sterile field. If your gloves become contaminated, you must remove the gloves and put on a new pair. Also replace gloves that are torn, cut, or punctured.

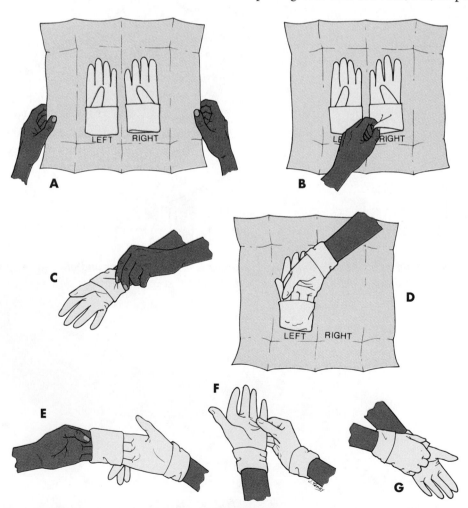

Fig. 11-29 *Donning sterile gloves.* **A,** *Open the inner wrapper to expose the gloves.* **B,** *Pick up the glove at the cuff with your thumb, index finger and middle finger.* **C,** *Slide your fingers and hand into the glove.* **D,** *Reach under the cuff of the other glove with your fingers.* **E,** *Pull on the glove.* **F,** *Adjust each glove for comfort.* **G,** *Slide your fingers under the cuffs to pull them up.*

◈ DONNING AND REMOVING STERILE GLOVES

PROCEDURE ALERT

- Does your state allow assistive personnel to perform the procedure?

- Is the procedure in your job description?

- Do you have the necessary training and education?

- Is an RN available to answer questions and to supervise you?

PROCEDURE

1 Follow Pre-Procedure steps listed in *Opening a Sterile Package*.

2 Use the peel-back method to open the package of sterile gloves.

3 Remove the inner package. Place it on a clean work surface. Have your work surface at waist height.

4 Read any manufacturer's instructions or information on the inner package. The package may be labeled with left, right, up, and down.

5 Arrange the inner package for left, right, up, and down. Have the left glove on your left and the right glove on your right. Have the cuffs near you with the fingers pointing away.

6 Use the thumb and index finger of each hand to grasp the folded edges of the inner package.

7 Fold back the inner package to expose the gloves (Fig. 11-29, *A*). Do not touch or otherwise contaminate the inside of the package or the gloves. The inside of the inner package is a sterile field.

8 Note that each glove has a cuff about 2 to 3 inches wide. The cuffs and insides of the gloves are not sterile.

9 Put on the right glove if you are right-handed. Put on the left glove if you are left-handed.

 a Pick up the glove with your other hand. Use your thumb and index and middle fingers (Fig. 11-29, *B*).

 b Touch only the cuff and the inside of the glove.

 c Turn the hand to be gloved palm side up.

 d Lift the cuff up. Slide your fingers and hand into the glove (Fig. 11-29, *C*).

 e Pull the glove up over your hand. If some fingers get stuck, leave them that way until the other glove is on. *Do not use your ungloved hand to straighten the glove. Do not let the outside of the glove touch any nonsterile surface.*

 f Leave the cuff turned down.

10 Put on the other glove with your gloved hand.

 a Reach under the cuff of the second glove with the four fingers of your gloved hand (Fig. 11-29, *D*). Keep your gloved thumb close to your gloved palm.

 b Pull on the second glove (Fig. 11-29, *E*). Your gloved hand cannot touch the cuff or any other surface. Hold the thumb of your first gloved hand away from your gloved palm.

11 Adjust each glove with the other hand. The gloves should be smooth and comfortable (Fig. 11-29, *F*).

12 Slide your fingers under the cuffs to pull them up (Fig. 11-29, *G*).

13 Touch only sterile items.

14 Remove the gloves as in Figure 11-14, p. 212.

REVIEW QUESTIONS

Circle T *if the statement is true or* F *if the statement is false.*

1 T F Microbes are pathogens in their natural environments.

2 T F An infection results from the invasion and growth of microbes in the body.

3 T F An item is sterile if nonpathogens are present.

4 T F You hold your hands and forearms up during the handwashing procedure.

5 T F Unused items in a person's room are used for another person.

6 T F A person has immunity against hepatitis B. The person will develop the disease.

7 T F The 1-inch edge around a sterile field is contaminated.

8 T F A sterile package has a watermark. The package is contaminated.

9 T F You wear sterile gloves to set up a sterile field.

10 T F The inside and cuffs of sterile gloves are contaminated.

Circle the best *answer.*

11 Pathogens need the following to grow *except*
  a Water
  b Light
  c Oxygen
  d Nourishment

12 The person with an infection may have
  a Fever, nausea, vomiting, rash, and/or sores
  b Pain or tenderness, redness, and/or swelling
  c Fatigue, loss of appetite, and/or a discharge
  d All of the above

13 Microbes enter and leave the body through the
  a Respiratory tract and/or breaks in the skin
  b Gastrointestinal system and/or the blood
  c Reproductive system and/or urinary system
  d All of the above

14 Which does not prevent nosocomial infections?
  a Handwashing before and after giving care
  b Sterilizing all items used for care
  c Surgical asepsis
  d Standard Precautions

15 When cleaning equipment, do the following *except*
  a Rinse the item in cold water before cleaning
  b Wash the item with soap and hot water
  c Use a brush if necessary
  d Clean from the dirtiest area to the cleanest

16 Isolation precautions
  a Prevent infection
  b Destroy pathogens
  c Keep pathogens within a certain area
  d Destroy pathogens and nonpathogens

17 Standard Precautions
  a Are used for all patients
  b Prevent the spread of pathogens through the air
  c Require gowns, masks, gloves, and protective eyewear
  d All of the above

18 Gloves are worn when in contact with
  a Blood
  b Body fluids
  c Secretions and excretions
  d All of the above

19 A mask
  a Can be reused
  b Is clean on the inside
  c Is contaminated when moist
  d Should fit loosely for breathing

REVIEW QUESTIONS—cont'd

20 Proper use of personal protective equipment involves the following *except*

a Washing disposable gloves for reuse

b Removing protective equipment before leaving the work area

c Discarding cracked or torn utility gloves

d Wearing gloves when touching contaminated items or surfaces

21 When are contaminated work surfaces cleaned?

a After completing a task

b Immediately when there is obvious contamination

c After blood or other potentially infectious material is spilled

d All of the above

22 These statements are about surgical asepsis. Which is *false?*

a A sterile item can touch only another sterile item.

b Wet items are held up.

c If you cannot see an item, it is contaminated.

d Sterile items are kept above your waist.

23 You opened a container of sterile solution. The cap is

a Dropped in the sterile field

b Held in your hand

c Discarded

d Placed so the inside is up

24 You are using sterile transfer forceps. Which is *incorrect?*

a Hold forceps above your waist and within your sight.

b Hold forceps so the tips are lower than your wrist.

c Always hold forceps with sterile gloved hands.

d Do not let forceps touch the outside of any packaging.

Answers to these questions are on p. 851.

12 Body Mechanics

- Define the key terms in this chapter
- Explain the purpose and rules of using good body mechanics
- Identify comfort and safety measures for lifting, turning, and moving persons in bed
- Know the basic bed positions
- Explain the purpose of a transfer belt
- Explain why good body alignment and position changes are important
- Identify the comfort and safety measures for positioning persons in bed
- Position persons in the basic bed positions and in a chair
- Perform the procedures described in this chapter

KEY TERMS

base of support The area on which an object rests

body alignment The way in which body parts are aligned with one another; posture

body mechanics Using the body in an efficient and careful way

dorsal recumbent position The back-lying or supine position

Fowler's position A semisitting position; the head of the bed is elevated 45 to 60 degrees

friction The rubbing of one surface against another

gait belt A transfer or safety belt

lateral position The side-lying position

logrolling Turning the person as a unit, in alignment, with one motion

posture The way in which body parts are aligned with one another; body alignment

prone position Lying on the abdomen with the head turned to one side

reverse Trendelenburg's position The head of the bed is raised, and the foot of the bed is lowered

safety belt A transfer belt

semi-Fowler's position The head of the bed is raised 45 degrees, and the knee portion is raised 15 degrees; or the head of the bed is raised 30 degrees

shearing When skin sticks to a surface and muscles slide in the direction the body is moving

side-lying position The lateral position

Sims' position A side-lying position in which the upper leg is sharply flexed so that it is not on the lower leg and the lower arm is behind the person

supine position The back-lying or dorsal recumbent position

transfer belt A belt used to hold onto a person during a transfer or when walking with the person; a gait belt or safety belt

Trendelenburg's position The head of the bed is lowered, and the foot of the bed is raised

Y ou will turn and reposition patients in bed. You also transfer patients to and from chairs, wheelchairs, and stretchers. During these and other activities, you must use your body correctly. This protects you and patients from injury.

BODY MECHANICS

Body mechanics means using the body in an efficient and careful way. It involves good posture and balance and using the strongest and largest muscles for work. You must focus on the person's and your own body mechanics. Good body mechanics reduce the risk of injury.

Posture (body alignment) is the way body parts (head, trunk, arms, legs) are aligned with one another. Good body alignment (posture) lets the body move and function with strength and efficiency. Standing, sitting, and lying down require good alignment.

Base of support is the area on which an object rests. A good base of support is needed for balance (Fig. 12-1). When standing, your feet are your base of support. Stand with your feet apart for a wider base of support and more balance.

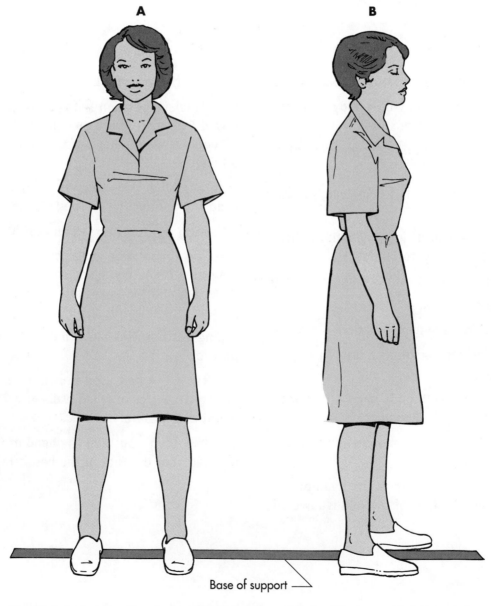

A   **B**

Base of support

Fig. 12-1 A, *Anterior (front) view of an adult in good body alignment with feet apart for a wide base of support.* **B,** *Lateral (side) view of an adult with good posture and alignment.*

The strongest and largest muscles are in the shoulders, upper arms, hips, and thighs. Use these muscles to lift and move heavy objects. Otherwise, you place strain and exertion on smaller and weaker muscles. This causes fatigue and injury. Back injuries are risks. Good body mechanics involve:

- Bending your knees and squatting to lift a heavy object (Fig. 12-2). Do not bend from your waist. Bending from the waist places strain on small back muscles.
- Holding items close to your body and base of support (see Fig. 12-2). This involves upper arm and shoulder muscles. Holding objects away from your body places strain on small muscles in your lower arms.

All activities require good body mechanics. Follow the rules in Box 12-1 to safely and efficiently lift and move persons and heavy objects.

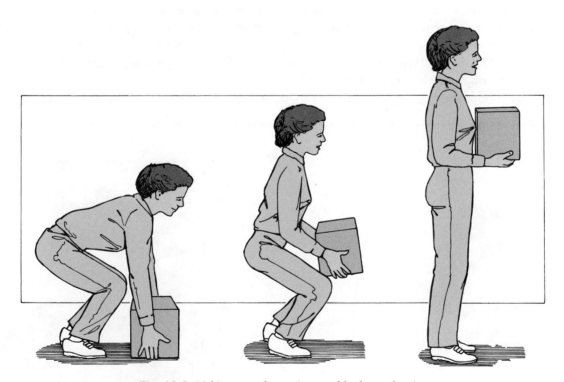

Fig. 12-2 *Picking up a box using good body mechanics.*

BOX 12-1

RULES FOR BODY MECHANICS

- Keep your body in good alignment with a wide base of support.
- Use the stronger and larger muscles in your shoulders, upper arms, thighs, and hips.
- Keep objects close to your body when you lift, move, or carry them (see Fig. 12-2).
- Avoid unnecessary bending and reaching. Raise the bed so it is close to your waist. Adjust the overbed table so it is at your waist level.
- Face your work area. This prevents unnecessary twisting.
- Push, slide, or pull heavy objects whenever you can rather than lifting them.
- Widen your base of support when pushing or pulling. Move your front leg forward when pushing. Move your rear leg back when pulling (Fig. 12-3).
- Use both hands and arms to lift, move, or carry heavy objects.
- Turn your whole body when changing the direction of your movement. Move your feet in the direction of the turn.
- Work with smooth and even movements. Avoid sudden or jerky motions.
- Get help from a co-worker if the patient cannot assist with turning or moving.
- Get help from a co-worker to move heavy objects or persons. Avoid lifting or moving patients by yourself.
- Bend your hips and knees to lift heavy objects from the floor (see Fig. 12-2). Straighten your back as the object reaches thigh level. Your leg and thigh muscles work to raise the item off the floor and to waist level.
- Do not lift objects higher than chest level. Do not lift above your shoulders. Use a step stool to reach an object higher than chest level.
- Wear a body support (Fig. 12-4) to help you use good body mechanics.

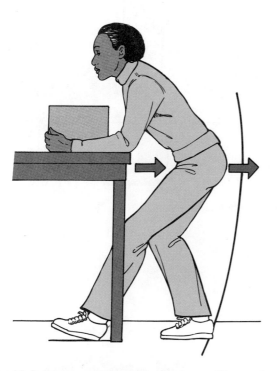

Fig. 12-3 *Move your rear leg back when pulling an item.*

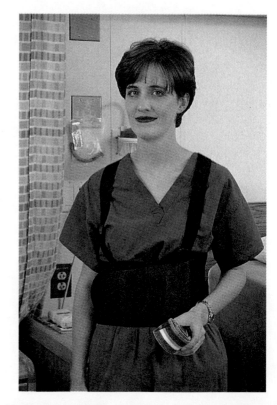

Fig. 12-4 *A body support helps in using good body mechanics.*

LIFTING AND MOVING PERSONS IN BED

Some persons need help moving and turning in bed. You must use the bed correctly, follow the rules of body mechanics, and keep the person in good body alignment. Also, position the person in good body alignment after moving or turning (pp. 264-266).

The Bed

Beds are raised horizontally to give care. This reduces bending or reaching. The lowest horizontal position lets the person get out of bed with ease. The head of the bed is kept flat or raised to varying degrees. Most beds are electric. Controls are on a side panel, a bed rail, or the footboard (Fig. 12-5). The person is taught how to safely use the controls and is told about position restrictions. (See Focus on Home Care.)

HOME CARE

Some home care patients have hospital beds. Electric beds are common. Some are operated manually. Manually operated beds have cranks at the foot of the bed (Fig. 12-6). The left crank raises or lowers the head of the bed. The right crank adjusts the knee portion. The center crank raises or lowers the entire bed. The cranks are pulled up for use. They are kept down at all other times. Cranks in the up position are safety hazards. Anyone walking past may bump into them.

Other home care patients use their regular beds. You cannot raise regular beds to give care. Therefore you will bend more when giving care. You must use good body mechanics to avoid injuring yourself.

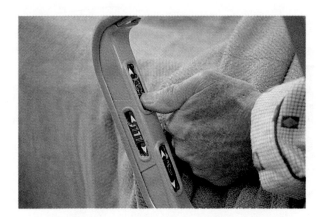

Fig. 12-5 *Controls for an electric bed.*

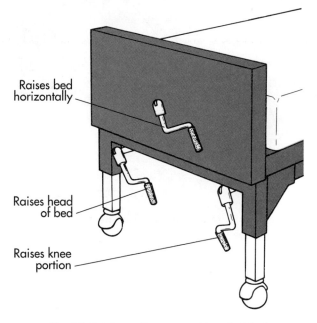

Raises bed horizontally

Raises head of bed

Raises knee portion

Fig. 12-6 *Manually operated hospital bed.*

Bed positions

The five basic bed positions are:

- **Flat**—this is the usual sleeping position. The position is needed after spinal cord surgery or injury and cervical traction (see Chapter 30).
- **Fowler's position**—a semisitting position. The head of the bed is elevated 45 to 60 degrees (Fig. 12-7). Persons with heart and respiratory disorders usually breathe more easily in this position. Eating, watching television, visiting, and reading are easier in Fowler's position.
- **Semi-Fowler's position**—the head of the bed is raised 45 degrees, and the knee portion is raised 15 degrees (Fig. 12-8). This position is comfortable and allows for easier breathing. However, raising the knee portion can interfere with circulation. Check with the RN before positioning a person in semi-Fowler's position. Many agencies define semi-Fowler's position as when the head of the bed is raised 30 degrees and the knee portion is *not* raised.

- **Trendelenburg's position**—the head of the bed is lowered, and the foot of the bed is raised (Fig. 12-9). The position promotes venous blood flow from the lower extremities to the heart. It is also used to drain secretions from the lungs (see p. 506). A doctor's order is required. Blocks are placed under the legs at the foot of the bed or the bedframe is tilted.
- **Reverse Trendelenburg's position**—the head of the bed is raised, and the foot of the bed is lowered (Fig. 12-10). The position promotes stomach emptying. Blocks are put under the legs at the head of the bed, or the bedframe is tilted. A doctor's order is required. (See Focus on Home Care.)

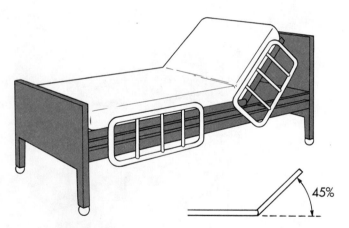

Fig. 12-7 *Fowler's position.*

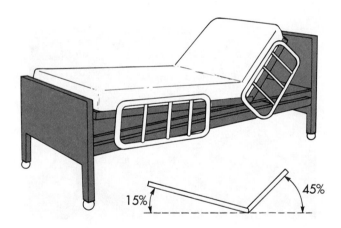

Fig. 12-8 *Semi-Fowler's position.*

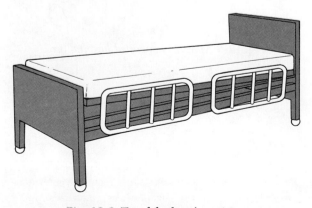

Fig. 12-9 *Trendelenburg's position.*

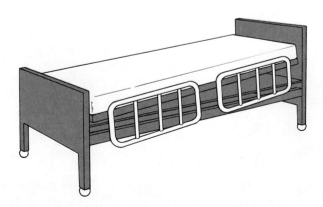

Fig. 12-10 *Reverse Trendelenburg's position.*

HOME CARE

focus on

Backrests are used with regular beds for Fowler's and semi-Fowler's position (Fig. 12-11). Check the head board to make sure it is sturdy. It needs to provide support when the patient leans against the backrest. Large, sturdy sofa pillows are useful if a backrest is not available.

OLDER PERSONS

focus on

Older persons are at great risk for shearing. Their skin is fragile and easily torn. Use a lift or turning sheet when lifting and moving older persons.

Other comfort and safety measures for moving persons in bed include the following:

- Ask the RN about limits or restrictions in positioning or moving the person.
- Decide how to move the person and how much help you need.
- Ask co-workers to help *before* starting the procedure.
- Cover and screen the person to protect the right to privacy.
- Protect tubes or drainage containers connected to the person.

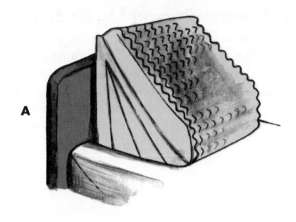
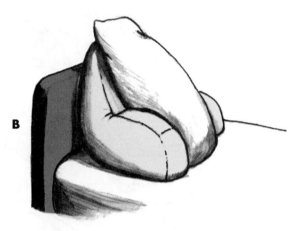

Fig. 12-11 *Backrests for regular beds.* **A,** *A wedge pillow.* **B,** *A study pillow with armrests.* (From Birchenall J, Streight M: Mosby's textbook for the home care aide, *St Louis, 1997, Mosby.*)

Comfort and Safety

The person's skin is protected during lifting and moving. Friction and shearing injure the skin. Both cause infection and pressure ulcers (see Chapter 14). **Friction** is the rubbing of one surface against another. When moved in bed, the person's skin rubs against the sheet. **Shearing** is when the skin sticks to a surface and muscles slide in the direction the body is moving (Fig. 12-12). Shearing occurs when the person slides down in bed or is moved in bed. Reduce friction and shearing by rolling or lifting the person. A cotton drawsheet (see Chapter 13) serves as a *lift sheet (turning or pull sheet)* to move the person in bed and reduce friction. (See Focus on Older Persons.)

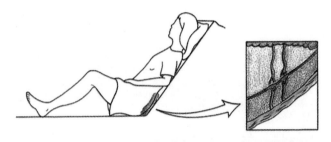

Fig. 12-12 *When the head of the bed is raised to a sitting position, skin on the buttocks stays in place. However, internal structures move forward as the person slides down in bed. Skin is pinched between the mattress and hip bones.*

✦ Moving the Person Up in Bed

Patients often slide down toward the middle and foot of the bed. They are moved up in bed for good body alignment and comfort. You can usually move children up in bed alone. Depending on your size and strength, you may be able to move lightweight adults alone. However, it is best to have help. This protects you and the person from injury.

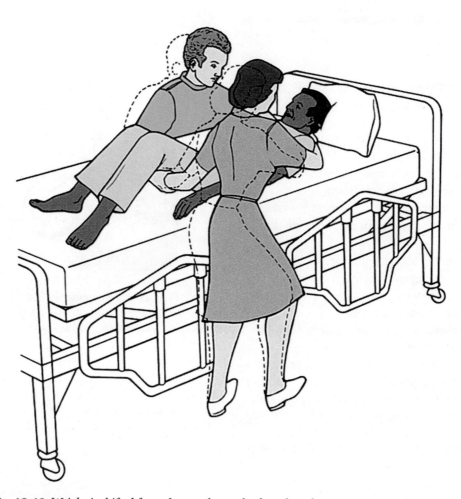

Fig. 12-13 *Weight is shifted from the rear leg to the front leg when moving a person up in bed.*

✦ MOVING THE PERSON UP IN BED WITH ASSISTANCE

PRE-PROCEDURE

1 Ask a co-worker to help you.

2 Wash your hands.

3 Identify the person. Check the ID bracelet, and call the person by name.

4 Explain the procedure to the person.

5 Provide for privacy.

6 Lock the bed wheels.

7 Raise the bed to the best level for body mechanics.

PROCEDURE

8 Lower the head of the bed to a level appropriate for the person. The bed should be as flat as possible.

9 Place the pillow against the headboard if the person can be without it. This prevents the person's head from hitting the headboard when being moved up.

10 Stand on one side of the bed. Your co-worker stands on the other side.

11 Lower the bed rails.

12 Stand with a wide base of support. Point the foot near the head of the bed toward the head of the bed. Face that direction.

13 Bend your hips and knees.

14 Place one arm under the person's shoulder and one arm under the buttocks. Your co-worker does the same. Grasp each other's forearms.

15 Have the person flex both knees.

16 Explain that you will move on the count of "3." The person should push against the bed with the feet if able.

17 Move the person to the head of the bed on the count of "3." Shift your weight from your rear leg to your front leg (Fig. 12-13).

18 Repeat steps 12 through 17 if necessary.

POST-PROCEDURE

19 Put the pillow under the person's head and shoulders. Straighten linens. Make sure the person is comfortable and in good body alignment (see p. 264).

20 Place the call bell within reach.

21 Raise or lower bed rails as instructed by the RN.

22 Raise the head of the bed to a level appropriate for the person.

23 Lower the bed to its lowest position.

24 Unscreen the person.

25 Wash your hands.

✦ Moving the Person Up in Bed With a Lift Sheet

With a co-worker's help, you can easily move a person up in bed with a lift sheet (turning sheet). Friction and shearing are reduced, and the person is lifted more evenly. A flat sheet folded in half or a drawsheet is used for the lift sheet. Place the lift sheet under the person from the head to above the knees. Use lift sheets to move persons who are unconscious, paralyzed, or recovering from spinal surgery or who have spinal cord injuries. Also use them for older persons.

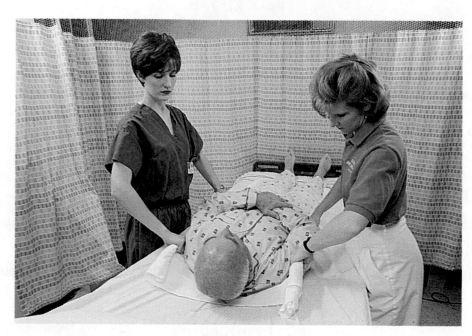

Fig. 12-14 *A lift sheet is used to move the person up in bed. The lift sheet extends from the person's head to above the knees. The lift sheet is rolled close to the person and held near the shoulders and buttocks.*

MOVING THE PERSON UP IN BED WITH A LIFT SHEET

PRE-PROCEDURE

1 Ask a co-worker to help you.

2 Wash your hands.

3 Identify the person. Check the ID bracelet, and call the person by name.

4 Explain the procedure to the person.

5 Provide for privacy.

6 Lock the bed wheels.

7 Raise the bed to the best level for body mechanics.

PROCEDURE

8 Lower the head of the bed to a level appropriate for the person. It should be as flat as possible.

9 Place the pillow against the headboard if the person can be without it.

10 Stand on one side of the bed. Your helper stands on the other side.

11 Lower the bed rails.

12 Stand with a broad base of support. Point the foot near the head of the bed toward the head of the bed. Face that direction.

13 Roll the sides of the lift sheet up close to the person.

14 Grasp the rolled up lift sheet firmly near the person's shoulders and buttocks (Fig. 12-14). Make sure you support the person's head.

15 Bend your hips and knees.

16 Slide the person up in bed on the count of "3." Shift your weight from your rear leg to your front leg.

17 Unroll the lift sheet.

POST-PROCEDURE

18 Put the pillow under the person's head and shoulders. Straighten linens. Make sure the person is comfortable and in good body alignment (see p. 264).

19 Place the call bell within reach.

20 Raise or lower bed rails as instructed by the RN.

21 Raise the head of the bed to a level appropriate for the person.

22 Lower the bed to its lowest position.

23 Unscreen the person.

24 Wash your hands.

✦ Moving the Person to the Side of the Bed

Repositioning and care procedures require moving the person to the side of the bed. The person is moved to the side of the bed before turning. Otherwise, after turning, the person lies on the side of the bed, not in the middle.

One method involves moving the person in segments. One person can sometimes do this. The lift sheet method is used for persons with spinal cord injuries or those recovering from spinal surgery. It is also safer for older persons and those with arthritis. When using a lift sheet, you need a co-worker to help you.

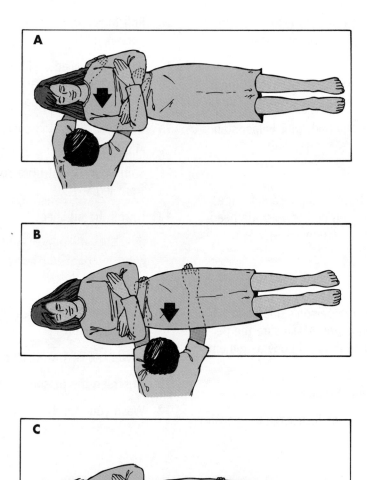

Fig. 12-15 *Moving the person to the side of the bed in segments.*

✦ MOVING THE PERSON TO THE SIDE OF THE BED

PRE-PROCEDURE

1 Ask a co-worker to help if you will use a lift sheet.

2 Wash your hands.

3 Identify the person. Check the ID bracelet, and call the person by name.

4 Explain the procedure to the person.

5 Provide for privacy.

6 Lock the bed wheels.

7 Raise the bed to the best level for body mechanics.

PROCEDURE

8 Lower the head of the bed to a level appropriate for the person. The bed should be as flat as possible.

9 Stand on the side of the bed to which you will move the person.

10 Make sure the far bed rail is raised. Lower the one near you. (Both bed rails are lowered for Step 14).

11 Stand with your feet about 12 inches apart and with one foot in front of the other. Flex your knees.

12 Cross the person's arms over the person's chest.

13 *Method 1:* Moving the person in segments:

  a Place your arm under the person's neck and shoulders. Grasp the far shoulder.

  b Place your other arm under the midback.

  c Move the upper part of the person's body toward you. Rock backward, and shift your weight to your rear leg (Fig. 12-15, *A*).

  d Place one arm under the person's waist and one under the thighs.

  e Rock backward to move the lower part of the person toward you (Fig. 12-15, *B*).

  f Repeat the procedure for the legs and feet (Fig. 12-15, *C*). Your arms should be under the person's thighs and calves.

14 *Method 2:* Moving the person with a lift sheet:

  a Roll the lift sheet up close to the person (see Fig. 12-14).

  b Grasp the rolled up lift sheet near the person's shoulders and buttocks. Make sure you support the head.

  c Rock backward on the count of "3," moving the person toward you. Your co-worker rocks backward slightly and then forward toward you while keeping the arms straight.

  d Unroll the lift sheet.

POST-PROCEDURE

15 Make sure the person is comfortable, in good body alignment (see p. 264), and positioned as directed by the RN. Reposition the pillow under his or her head and shoulders.

16 Place the call bell within reach.

17 Raise or lower bed rails as instructed by the RN.

18 Lower the bed to its lowest position.

19 Unscreen the person.

20 Wash your hands.

✦ Turning Persons

Turning persons onto their sides helps prevent complications from bedrest. Certain medical and nursing procedures require the side-lying position. Persons are turned toward or away from you. The direction depends on the person's condition and the situation.

✦ TURNING A PERSON

PRE-PROCEDURE

1 Wash your hands.

2 Identify the person. Check the ID bracelet, and call the person by name.

3 Explain the procedure to the person.

4 Provide for privacy.

5 Lock the bed wheels.

6 Raise the bed to the best level for body mechanics.

PROCEDURE

7 Lower the head of the bed to a level appropriate for the person. The bed should be as flat as possible.

8 Stand on the side of the bed opposite to where you will turn the person. The far bed rail must be up.

9 Lower the bed rail near you.

10 Move the person to the side near you.

11 Cross the person's arms over the person's chest. Cross the leg near you over the far leg.

12 *Method 1:* Moving the person away from you:

   a Stand with a wide base of support. Flex your knees.

   b Place one hand on the person's shoulder and the other on the buttock near you.

   c Push the person gently toward the other side of the bed (Fig. 12-16). Shift your weight from your rear leg to your front leg.

13 *Method 2:* Moving the person toward you:

   a Raise the bed rail.

   b Go to the other side. Lower the bed rail.

   c Stand with a wide base of support. Flex your knees.

   d Place one hand on the person's far shoulder and the other on the far hip.

   e Roll the person toward you gently (Fig. 12-17).

POST-PROCEDURE

14 Make sure the person is comfortable and in good body alignment (see p. 264).

15 Place the call bell within reach.

16 Raise or lower bed rails as instructed by the RN.

17 Lower the bed to its lowest position.

18 Unscreen the person.

19 Wash your hands.

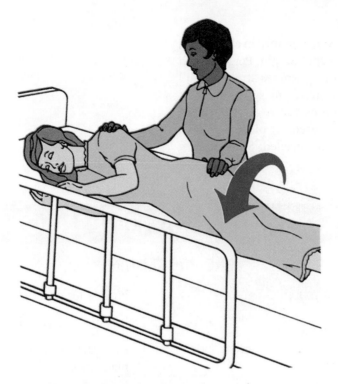

Fig. 12-16 *Turning the person away from you.*

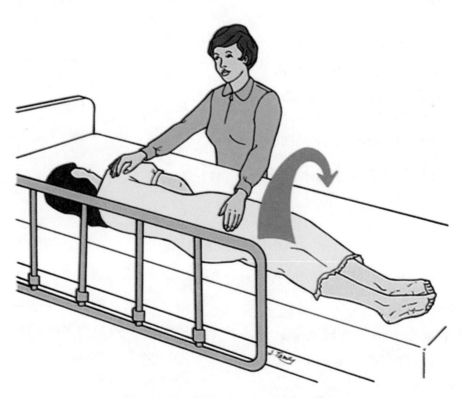

Fig. 12-17 *Turning the person toward you.*

Logrolling

Logrolling is turning the person as a unit, in alignment, with one motion. The spine is kept straight. Persons with spinal cord injuries must keep their spines straight at all times. So must persons recovering from spinal surgery. Rolling over in one motion keeps the back in straight alignment. This method is often used for older persons.

Two or three staff members are needed. Sometimes a turning sheet is used.

LOGROLLING THE PERSON

PRE-PROCEDURE

1 Ask a co-worker to help you.

2 Wash your hands.

3 Identify the person. Check the ID bracelet, and call the person by name.

4 Explain the procedure to the person.

5 Provide for privacy.

6 Lock the bed wheels.

7 Raise the bed to the best level for body mechanics.

PROCEDURE

8 Make sure the bed is flat.

9 Raise the bed rail on the side to which the person will be turned.

10 Stand on the other side. Lower the bed rail.

11 Move the person as a unit to the side of the bed near you. Use the turning sheet.

12 Place the person's arms across the chest. Place a pillow between the knees (Fig. 12-18, *A*). Raise the bed rail. Go to the other side, and lower the bed rail.

13 Position yourself near the shoulders and chest. Your co-worker stands near the buttocks and thighs.

14 Stand with a broad base of support. One foot is in front of the other.

15 Ask the person to hold his or her body rigid.

16 Roll the person toward you as in Fig. 12-18, *A*, or use a turn sheet as in Fig. 12-18, *B*.

17 Turn the person as a unit.

POST-PROCEDURE

18 Make sure the person is comfortable and in good body alignment (see p. 264). Use pillows as directed by the RN:

   a One pillow against the back for support.

   b One pillow under the head and neck if allowed.

   c One pillow or folded bath blanket between the legs.

   d A small pillow under the arm and hand.

19 Place the call bell within reach.

20 Raise or lower bed rails as instructed by the RN.

21 Lower the bed to its lowest position.

22 Unscreen the person.

23 Wash your hands.

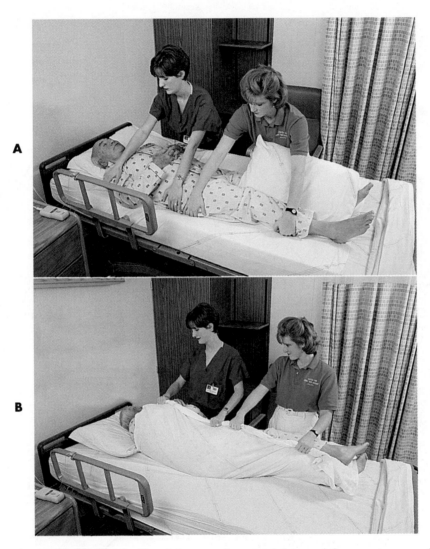

Fig. 12-18 *Logrolling.* **A,** *A pillow is between the person's legs, and the arms are crossed on the chest. The person is on the far side of the bed.* **B,** *A turning sheet is used to logroll a person.*

✦ SITTING ON THE SIDE OF THE BED

Persons sit on the side of the bed *(dangle)* for many reasons. Some increase activity in stages. They progress from bedrest to sitting on the side of the bed and then to sitting in a chair. Walking is the next step. Surgical patients sit on the side of the bed some time after surgery. While dangling their legs, they cough and deep breathe. They also move their legs back and forth and in circles to stimulate circulation. The procedure is also part of preparing a person to walk or for transfer to a chair or wheelchair.

Two staff members may be needed. Support the person if he or she has problems with balance or coordination.

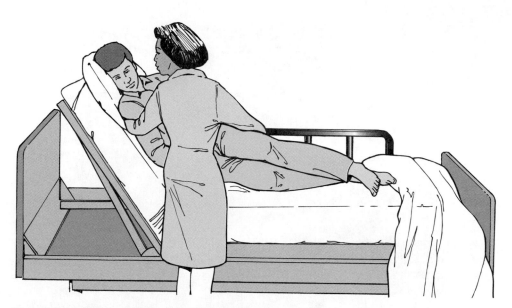

Fig. 12-19 *Helping the person sit on the side of the bed. The person is supported under the shoulders and under the thighs.*

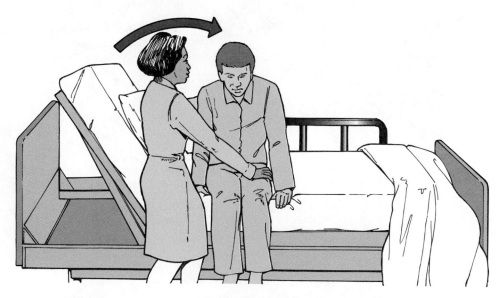

Fig. 12-20 *The person sits upright as the legs and feet are pulled over the edge of the bed.*

HELPING THE PERSON SIT ON THE SIDE OF THE BED (DANGLE)

PRE-PROCEDURE

1 Explain the procedure to the person.

2 Wash your hands.

3 Identify the person. Check the ID bracelet, and call the person by name.

4 Decide what side of the bed to use.

5 Move furniture to provide moving space.

6 Provide for privacy.

7 Position the person in a side-lying position facing you.

8 Lock the bed wheels.

9 Raise the bed to the best level for body mechanics.

PROCEDURE

10 Stand near the person's waist. This protects the person from falling out of bed.

11 Raise the head of the bed so the person is in a sitting position.

12 Lower the bed rail.

13 Stand by the person's hips. Turn so you face the far corner of the foot of the bed.

14 Slide one arm under the person's neck and shoulders. Grasp the far shoulder. Place your other hand under the thighs near the knees (Fig. 12-19).

15 Pivot toward the foot of the bed while pulling the person's feet and legs over the edge of the

bed. As the legs go over the edge of the mattress, the trunk is upright (Fig. 12-20).

16 Ask the person to hold onto the edge of the mattress. This supports the person in the sitting position.

17 Do not leave the person alone. Provide support if necessary.

18 Ask how the person feels. Check pulse and respirations. Help the person lie down if necessary.

19 Reverse the procedure to return the person to bed.

20 Lower the head of the bed after the person lies down. Help him or her move to the center of the bed.

POST-PROCEDURE

21 Make sure the person is comfortable and in good body alignment (see p. 264). Cover the person.

22 Place the call bell within reach.

23 Lower the bed to its lowest position.

24 Return furniture to its proper location.

25 Unscreen the person.

26 Wash your hands.

27 Report the following to the RN:

- How well the activity was tolerated

- The length of time the person dangled

- Pulse and respiratory rates

- The amount of assistance needed

- Other observations or patient complaints

TRANSFERRING PERSONS

Persons are often moved from beds to chairs, wheelchairs, or stretchers. Some need little help in transferring. Sometimes 2 or 3 people are needed. The rules of body mechanics apply to transfers. So do the safety and comfort measures for lifting and moving persons.

✦ Applying Transfer Belts

A **transfer belt** (**gait belt** or **safety belt**) is used to transfer unsteady and disabled persons. The belt goes around the person's waist. You grasp the belt to support the person during the transfer. The belt is called a **gait belt** when used for walking with a person. Many agencies require staff to use these belts when transferring or walking patients. (See Focus on Long-Term Care.)

✦ APPLYING A TRANSFER BELT

PROCEDURE

1 Wash your hands.

2 Identify the person. Check the ID bracelet, and call the person by name.

3 Explain the procedure to the person.

4 Provide for privacy.

5 Assist the person to a sitting position.

6 Apply the belt around the person's waist over clothing. Do not apply it over bare skin.

7 Tighten the belt so it is snug. It should not cause discomfort or impair breathing.

8 Make sure that a woman's breasts are not caught under the belt.

9 Place the buckle off center in the front or in the back for the person's comfort (Fig. 12-21).

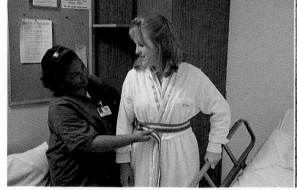
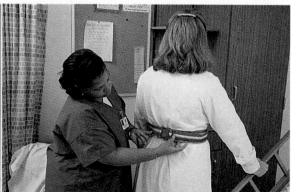

Fig. 12-21 *Transfer belt (gait or safety belt).* **A,** *The belt is positioned off center in the front.* **B,** *The belt buckle is positioned at the back.*

✤ Transferring the Person to a Chair or Wheelchair

Safety is important for chair and wheelchair transfers. You must prevent falls. The person wears shoes or slippers with nonskid soles to prevent sliding or slipping on the floor. The chair or wheelchair must support the person's weight. The number of staff members needed for a transfer depends on the person's physical capabilities, condition, and size.

The person is helped out of bed on his or her strong side. If the left side is weak, get the person out of bed on the right side. When transferring, the strong side moves first and pulls the weaker side along. Transfers from the weak side are awkward and unsafe.

Text continued on p. 260

TRANSFERRING THE PERSON TO A CHAIR OR WHEELCHAIR

PRE-PROCEDURE

1 Explain the procedure to the person.

2 Collect:

- Wheelchair or arm chair
- One or two bath blankets
- Robe and shoes
- Paper or sheet
- Transfer belt if needed

3 Wash your hands.

4 Identify the person. Check the ID bracelet, and call the person by name.

5 Provide for privacy.

6 Decide which side of the bed to use. Move furniture to provide moving space.

PROCEDURE

7 Place the chair at the head of the bed. The chair back is even with the headboard (Fig. 12-22, p. 257).

8 Place a folded bath blanket on the seat. Lock wheelchair wheels, and raise the footrests.

9 Lower the bed to its lowest position. Lock the bed wheels.

10 Fanfold top linens to the foot of the bed.

11 Place the paper or sheet under the person's feet. Put shoes on the person.

12 Help the person dangle. Make sure his or her feet touch the floor.

13 Help the person put on a robe.

14 Apply the transfer belt if it will be used.

15 Help the person stand. Use this method if using a transfer belt:

a Stand in front of the person.

b Have the person hold onto the mattress. Or ask the person to place his or her fists on the bed by the thighs.

c Make sure the person's feet are flat on the floor.

d Have the person lean forward.

e Grasp the transfer belt at each side.

f Brace your knees against the person's knees. Block his or her feet with your feet (Fig. 12-23, p. 257).

g Ask the person to push down on the mattress and to stand on the count of "3." Pull the person into a standing position as you straighten your knees (Fig. 12-24, p. 257).

Continued

TRANSFERRING THE PERSON TO A CHAIR OR WHEELCHAIR—cont'd

PROCEDURE—cont'd

16 Use this method if a transfer belt is not used:

   a Follow Step 15 a-c.

   b Place your hands under the person's arms. Your hands are around the person's shoulder blades (Fig. 12-25).

   c Have the person lean forward.

   d Brace your knees against the person's knees. Block his or her feet with your feet.

   e Ask the person to push down on the mattress and to stand on the count of "3." Pull the person up into a standing position as you straighten your knees.

17 Support the person in the standing position. Hold the transfer belt or keep your hands around the person's shoulder blades. Continue to block the person's feet and knees with your feet and knees. This helps prevent falling.

18 Turn the person so he or she can grasp the far arm of the chair. The legs will touch the edge of the chair as in Figure 12-26 on p. 258.

19 Continue to turn the person until the other armrest is grasped.

20 Lower him or her into the chair as you bend your hips and knees. The person assists by leaning forward and bending the elbows and knees (Fig. 12-27, p. 258).

21 Make sure the buttocks are to the back of the seat. Position the person in good alignment.

22 Position the person's feet on the wheelchair footrests.

23 Cover the person's lap and legs with a bath blanket. Keep the blanket off the floor and the wheels.

24 Remove the transfer belt if used.

25 Position the chair as the person prefers.

POST-PROCEDURE

26 Make sure the call bell and other necessary items are within reach.

27 Unscreen the person.

28 Wash your hands.

29 Report the following to the RN:

- The pulse rate if taken

- How well the activity was tolerated

- Complaints of lightheadedness, pain, discomfort, difficulty breathing, weakness, or fatigue

- The amount of assistance required to transfer the person

30 Reverse the procedure to return the person to bed.

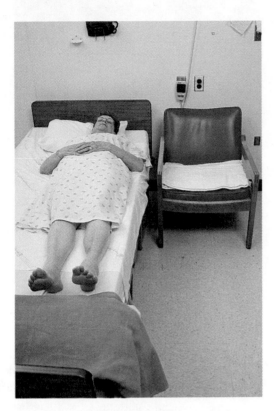

Fig. 12-22 *The chair is positioned next to and even with the headboard.*

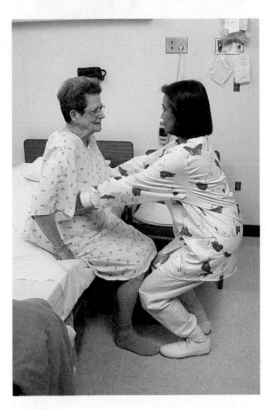

Fig. 12-23 *Prevent the person from sliding or falling by bracing the person's knees and feet with your own knees and feet.*

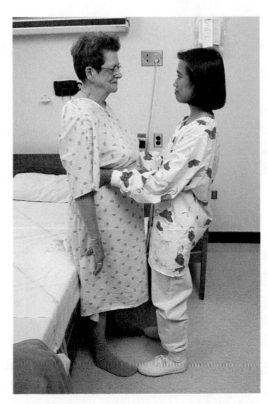

Fig. 12-24 *The person is pulled up to a standing position and supported by holding the transfer belt and blocking the person's knees and feet.*

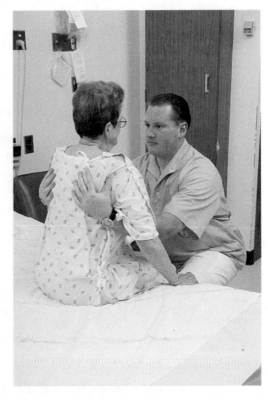

Fig. 12-25 *A person being prepared to stand. The hands are placed under the person's arms and around the shoulder blades.*

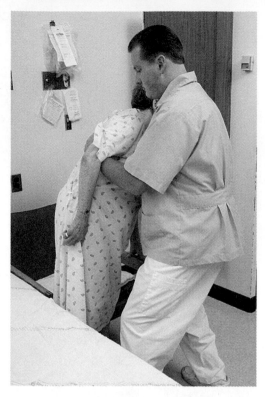 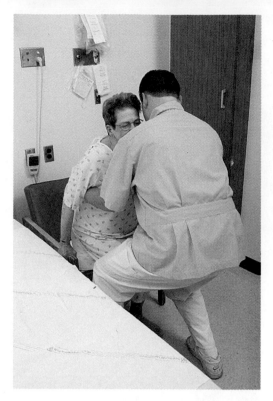

Fig. 12-26 *The person is supported as she grasps the far arm of the chair. The legs are against the chair.*

Fig. 12-27 *The person holds the arm rests, leans forward, and bends the elbows and knees while being lowered into the chair.*

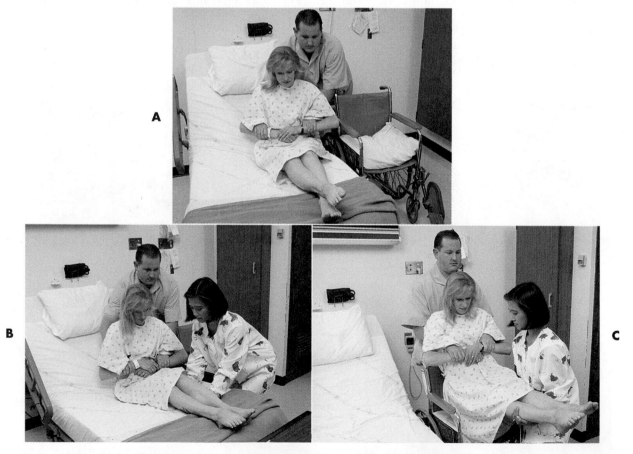

Fig. 12-28 *Transferring the person to a wheelchair.* **A,** *The person's forearms are held.* **B,** *The thighs and calves are held to support the lower extremities during a transfer.* **C,** *The person is lowered into the chair.*

TRANSFERRING THE PERSON TO A WHEELCHAIR WITH ASSISTANCE

PRE-PROCEDURE

1 Ask a co-worker to help you.

2 Explain the procedure to the person.

3 Collect:

- Wheelchair with removable armrests
- Bath blankets
- Shoes
- Cushion if used

4 Wash your hands.

5 Identify the person. Check the ID bracelet, and call the person by name.

6 Provide for privacy.

7 Decide which side of the bed to use. Move furniture to provide moving space.

PROCEDURE

8 Fanfold top linens to the foot of the bed.

9 Assist the person to the side of the bed near you. Help him or her to a sitting position by raising the head of the bed.

10 Place the wheelchair at the side of the bed, even with the person's hips.

11 Remove the armrest near the bed. Put the cushion or a folded bath blanket on the seat.

12 Lock wheelchair and bed wheels.

13 Stand behind the wheelchair. Put your arms under the person's arms, and grasp the person's forearms (Fig. 12-28, *A*).

14 Have your co-worker grasp the person's thighs and calves (Fig. 12-28, *B*).

15 Bring the person toward the chair on the count of "3." Lower him or her into the chair as in Figure 12-28, *C*.

16 Make sure the person's buttocks are to the back of the seat. Position the person in good alignment.

17 Put the armrest back on the wheelchair.

18 Put the shoes on the person. Position the person's feet on the footrests.

19 Cover the person's lap and legs with a blanket. Keep the blanket off the floor and wheels.

20 Position the chair as the person prefers.

POST-PROCEDURE

21 Make sure the call bell and other necessary items are within reach.

22 Unscreen the person.

23 Wash your hands.

24 Report the following to the RN:

- The pulse rate if taken
- Complaints of lightheadedness, pain, discomfort, difficulty breathing, weakness, or fatigue
- How well the activity was tolerated

25 Reverse the procedure to return the person to bed.

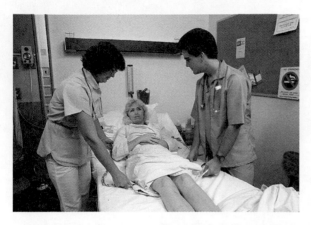

Fig. 12-29 *The sling of the mechanical lift is positioned under the person. The lower edge of the sling is behind the person's knees.*

⊕ Using a Mechanical Lift

Disabled persons are transferred with mechanical lifts. Lifts are used for transfers to chairs, stretchers, tubs, shower chairs, toilets, whirlpools, or cars. Before using a lift, make sure it works. Also, compare the person's weight and the lift's weight limit. Do not use the lift if a person's weight exceeds the lift's capacity.

At least two staff members are needed. The manufacturer's instructions are followed for a safe transfer. The following procedure is used as a guide.

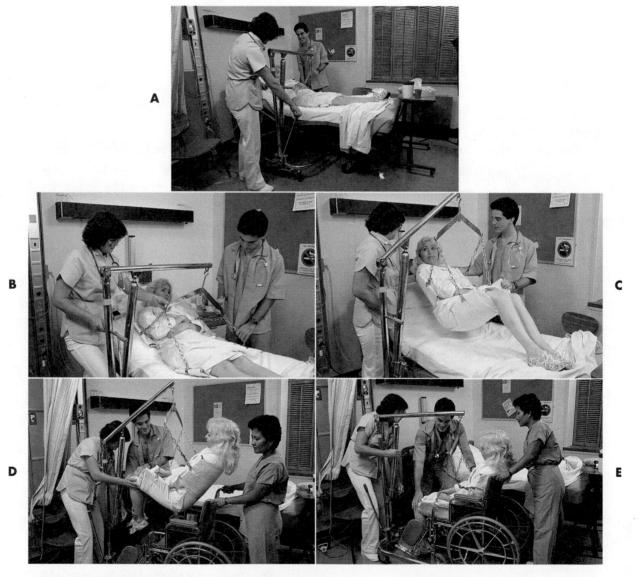

Fig. 12-30 **A,** *The lift is over the person. The lift's legs are spread to widen the base of support.* **B,** *The sling is attached to a swivel bar.* **C,** *The lift is raised until the sling and person are off of the bed.* **D,** *The person's legs are supported as the person and lift are moved away from the bed.* **E,** *The person is guided into a chair.*

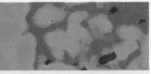
PRE-PROCEDURE

1 Ask a co-worker to help you.

2 Explain the procedure to the person.

3 Collect:

- Mechanical lift

- Arm chair or wheelchair

- Slippers

- Bath blanket

4 Wash your hands.

5 Identify the person. Check the ID bracelet, and call the person by name.

6 Provide for privacy.

PROCEDURE

7 Center the sling under the person (Fig. 12-29). Turn the person from side to side as if making an occupied bed to position the sling (see Chapter 13). Position the sling according to the manufacturer's instructions.

8 Place the chair at the head of the bed. It should be even with the headboard and about 1 foot away from the bed. Place a folded bath blanket in the chair.

9 Lock the bed wheels, and lower the bed to its lowest position.

10 Raise the lift so it can be positioned over the person.

11 Position the lift over the person (Fig. 12-30, A).

12 Lock the lift wheels in position.

13 Attach the sling to the swivel bar (Fig. 12-30, B)

14 Raise the head of the bed to a sitting position.

15 Cross the person's arms over the chest. Let him or her hold onto the straps or chains but not the swivel bar.

16 Pump the lift high enough until the person and sling are free of the bed (Fig. 12-30, C).

17 Ask your co-worker to support the person's legs as you move the lift and person away from the bed (Fig. 12-30, D).

18 Position the lift so that the person's back is toward the chair.

19 Lower the person into the chair. (Follow the manufacturer's instructions for lowering the lift.) Guide the person into the chair as in Figure 12-30, E.

20 Lower the swivel bar to unhook the sling. Leave the sling under the person unless otherwise indicated.

21 Put the slippers on the person. Position the person's feet on wheelchair footrests.

22 Cover the person's lap and legs with a blanket. Keep the blanket off the floor and wheels.

23 Position the chair as the person prefers.

POST-PROCEDURE

24 Make sure the call bell and other necessary items are within reach.

25 Wash your hands.

26 Report the following to the RN:

- The pulse rate if taken

- Complaints of lightheadedness, pain, discomfort, difficulty breathing, weakness, or fatigue

- How well the activity was tolerated

27 Reverse the procedure to return the person to bed.

✦ Moving the Person to a Stretcher

Stretchers are used to transport persons to other areas. They are used for persons who cannot sit up, for those who must stay in a lying position, and for those who are seriously ill. The stretcher is covered with a folded flat sheet or bath blanket. A pillow and extra blankets are available. With the RN's permission, raise the head of the stretcher to Fowler's or semi-Fowler's position. This increases the person's comfort.

Safety straps are used when the person is on the stretcher. The stretcher's rails are kept up during the transport. Move the person feet first so the co-worker at the head of the stretcher can watch the person's breathing and color during the transport. Never leave a person on a stretcher unattended.

At least three staff members are needed for a safe transfer. Remember, keep the person in good body alignment and use good body mechanics.

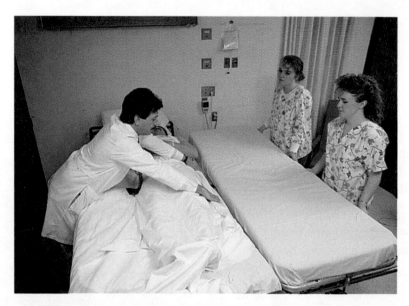

Fig. 12-31 *The stretcher is against the bed and is held in place.*

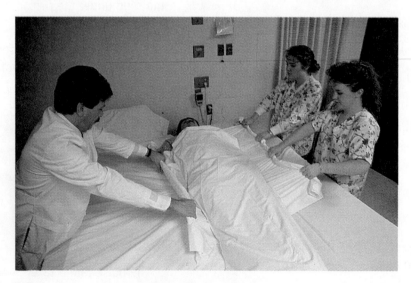

Fig. 12-32 *A drawsheet is used to transfer the person from the bed to a stretcher.*

✦ TRANSFERRING A PERSON TO A STRETCHER

PRE-PROCEDURE

1 Ask two co-workers to help you.

2 Explain the procedure to the person.

3 Collect:

- Stretcher covered with a sheet or bath blanket
- Bath blanket
- Pillow(s) if needed

4 Wash your hands.

5 Identify the person. Check the ID bracelet, and call the person by name.

6 Provide for privacy.

7 Raise the bed to its highest level.

PROCEDURE

8 Cover the person with a bath blanket. Fanfold top linens to the foot of the bed.

9 Loosen the cotton drawsheet on each side.

10 Lower the head of the bed so it is as flat as possible.

11 Lower the bed rail on the side to which you will move the person.

12 Ask your co-workers to help move the person to the side of the bed. Use the drawsheet.

13 Go to the other side of the bed. Lower the bed rail. Protect the person from falling by holding the far arm and leg.

14 Have your co-workers position the stretcher next to the bed, and stand behind the stretcher (Fig. 12-31).

15 Lock the wheels of the bed and stretcher.

16 Roll up and grasp the drawsheet at the hip and mid-chest levels.

17 Ask your co-workers to roll up and grasp the drawsheet. This supports the entire length of the person's body.

18 Transfer the person to the stretcher on the count of "3" by lifting and pulling him or her (Fig. 12-32). Make sure the person is centered on the stretcher.

19 Place a pillow or pillows under the person's head and shoulders if allowed.

20 Make sure the person is covered and comfortable.

21 Fasten safety straps. Raise the rails.

22 Unlock the stretcher's wheels. Transport the person.

POST-PROCEDURE

23 Wash your hands.

24 Report the following to the RN:

- The time of the transport
- Where the person was transported
- Who accompanied him or her
- How the transfer was tolerated

25 Reverse the procedure to return the person to bed.

POSITIONING

The person must be properly positioned at all times. Regular position changes and good alignment promote comfort and well-being. Breathing is easier, and circulation is promoted. Proper positioning also helps prevent many complications. These include pressure ulcers (see Chapter 14) and contractures (see Chapter 22). Some persons are repositioned every hour or every 2 hours.

The doctor may order certain positions or position restrictions. Follow these guidelines to safely position patients:

- Ask the RN about position changes for a person.
- Know how often to turn a person and to what positions.
- Use good body mechanics.
- Ask a co-worker to help you if indicated.
- Explain the procedure to the person.
- Be gentle when moving the person.
- Provide for privacy.
- Place the call bell within the person's reach after positioning.
- Use pillows as directed for support and alignment.

Fowler's Position

Fowler's position involves raising the head of the bed 45 to 60 degrees. Good alignment involves keeping the spine straight, supporting the head with a small pillow, and supporting the arms with pillows (Fig. 12-33). The RN may have you place a small pillow under the lower back, thighs, and ankles.

Supine Position

The **supine (dorsal recumbent) position** is the back-lying position. The bed is flat, the head and shoulders are supported on a pillow, and arms and hands are at the person's sides. The hands may be supported on small pillows with the palms down (Fig. 12-34). A rolled towel is placed under the lower back. Often a small pillow is under the ankles.

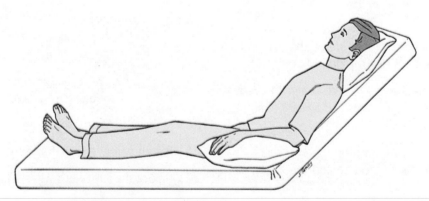

Fig. 12-33 *Fowler's position. Pillows are used to maintain alignment.*

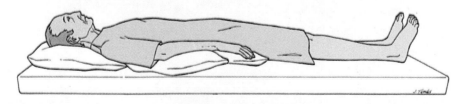

Fig. 12-34 *Person in supine position.*

Prone Position

Persons in the **prone position** lie on their abdomen with their head turned to one side. Small pillows are placed under the head, abdomen, and lower legs (Fig. 12-35). Arms are flexed at the elbows with the hands near the head.

Lateral Position

A person in the **lateral (side-lying) position** lies on one side or the other (Fig. 12-36). A pillow is under the head and neck. The upper leg and thigh are supported with pillows. A small pillow is under the upper hand and arm, and a pillow is positioned against the person's back.

Sims' Position

The **Sims' position** is a side-lying position. The upper leg is sharply flexed so it is not on the lower leg, and the lower arm is behind the person (Fig. 12-37). Good alignment involves placing a pillow under the person's head and neck, supporting the upper leg with a pillow, and placing a pillow under the upper arm and hand.

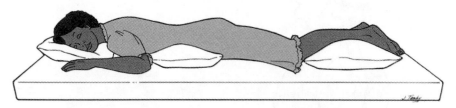

Fig. 12-35 *Person in prone position.*

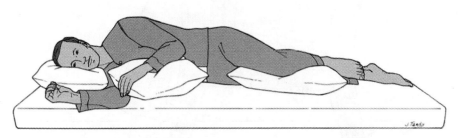

Fig. 12-36 *Person in lateral position with pillows used for support.*

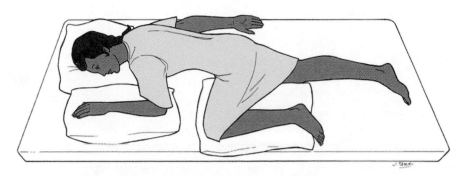

Fig. 12-37 *Person supported with pillows in Sims' position.*

Chair Position

Persons who sit in a chair must hold their upper body and head erect. The person's back and buttocks are against the back of the chair. Feet are flat on the floor or on wheelchair footrests. Backs of the knees and calves are slightly away from the edge of the seat (Fig. 12-38). The RN may ask you to put a small pillow between the person's lower back and the chair. (*Remember,* a pillow is not used behind the back if restraints are used. See p. 171.)

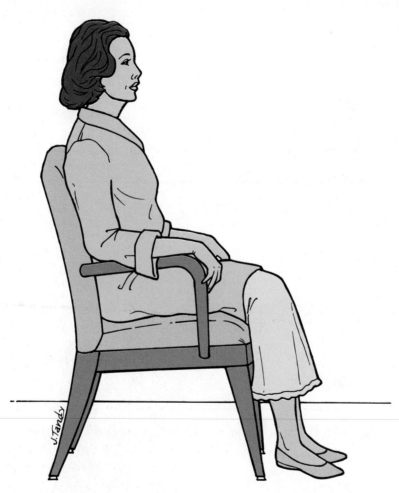

Fig. 12-38 *Person positioned in a chair. The person's feet are flat on the floor, the calves do not touch the chair, and the back is straight and against the back of the chair.*

REVIEW QUESTIONS

Circle T *if the statement is true or* F *if the statement is false.*

1 T F Body mechanics means the way body segments are aligned with one another.

2 T F Good body mechanics help protect you and your patients from injury.

3 T F Base of support is the area on which an object rests.

4 T F Objects are kept away from the body when lifting, moving, or carrying them.

5 T F Face the direction you are working to prevent unnecessary twisting.

6 T F Push, slide, or pull heavy objects rather than lift them.

7 T F Ask the RN about limitations or restrictions in positioning or moving a person.

8 T F The right to privacy is protected when moving, lifting, or transferring persons.

9 T F A lift sheet should extend from the shoulders to above the knees.

10 T F A person is moved to the side of the bed before being turned to the side-lying position.

11 T F Logrolling is rolling the person in segments.

12 T F Persons with spinal cord injuries are logrolled.

13 T F A transfer belt is part of a mechanical lift.

14 T F You are going to transfer Mrs. Lund from the bed to a chair. Move her from the direction of the weak side of her body.

15 T F Repositioning prevents deformities and pressure on body parts.

16 T F The head of the bed is elevated 45 to 60 degrees for the supine position.

17 T F The Sims' position is a side-lying position.

18 T F Sliding the person reduces friction and shearing.

19 T F Body mechanics involve using small muscles.

20 T F Mr. Smith is being transferred from the bed to a chair. He should wear nonskid shoes.

Answers to these questions are on p. 851.

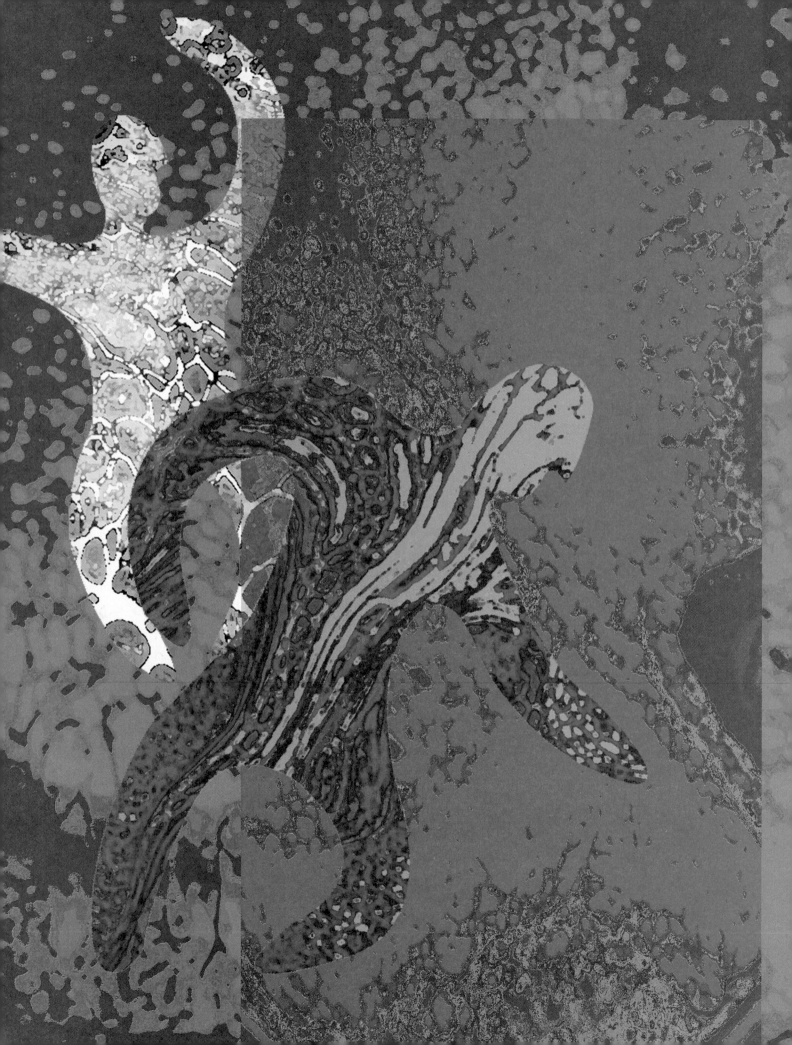

Unit IV
Assisting With Comfort Needs

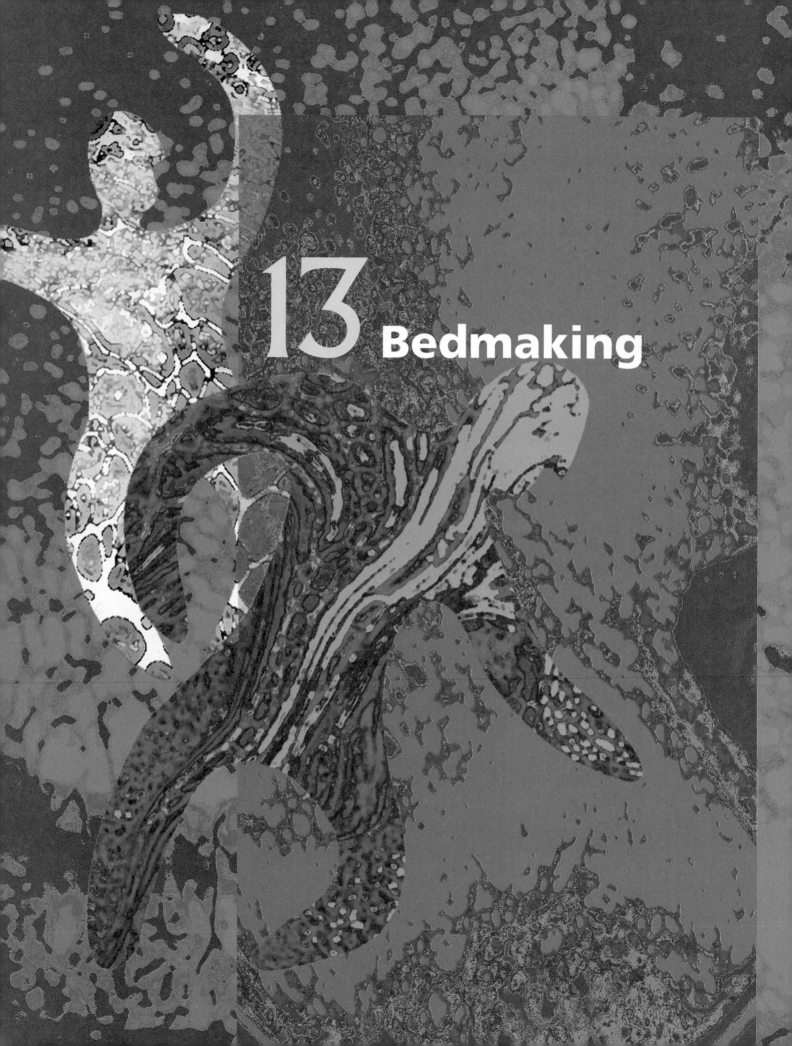

13 Bedmaking

- Define the key terms in this chapter
- Describe the differences between open, closed, occupied, and surgical beds
- Explain the purposes of plastic drawsheets and cotton drawsheets
- Handle linens according to the rules of medical asepsis
- Perform the procedures described in this chapter

KEY TERMS

drawsheet A small sheet placed over the middle of the bottom sheet; it helps keep the mattress and bottom linens clean and dry; can be used to turn and move the person in bed; the cotton drawsheet

plastic drawsheet A drawsheet placed between the bottom sheet and the cotton drawsheet to keep the mattress and bottom linens clean and dry

Bedmaking is an important function. A clean, neat bed helps the person's comfort. Beds are usually made in the morning after baths. They are also made while patients are taking showers or when out of the room. People like their beds made and rooms clean before visitors arrive.

Linens are straightened whenever they are loose or wrinkled. Check linens for crumbs after meals and properly remove them. Also straighten linens at bedtime. Linens are changed whenever they become wet, soiled, or damp. Follow Standard Precautions and the Bloodborne Pathogen Standard for contact with the person's blood, body fluids, secretions, or excretions.

Beds are made in the following ways:

- A *closed bed* is not in use. Top linens are not folded back, and the bed is ready for a new patient (Fig. 13-1, p. 272).
- An *open bed* is in use. Top linens are folded back so the patient can get into bed. A closed bed becomes an open bed when the top linens are folded back (Fig. 13-2, p. 272).
- An *occupied bed* is made with the patient in it (Fig. 13-3, p. 272).
- A *surgical bed* is made to move a patient from a stretcher to the bed. It also is called a *postoperative bed, recovery bed,* or *anesthesia bed* (Fig. 13-4, p. 272).

LINENS

When handling linens and making beds, follow the rules of medical asepsis. Your uniform is considered dirty. Therefore always hold linens away from your body and

uniform. Never shake linens in the air. Shaking them spreads microbes. Clean linens are placed on a clean surface. Never put clean or dirty linens on the floor.

Collect clean linens in the order of use. Be sure to collect enough linens. If the person has two pillows, get two pillowcases. The person may need extra blankets for warmth. Do not bring unneeded linens to a person's room. Extra linen is considered contaminated and is not used for another person.

Collect linens in the following order:

- Mattress pad
- Bottom sheet (flat sheet or contour sheet)
- Plastic drawsheet (optional)
- Cotton drawsheet
- Top sheet (flat sheet)
- Blanket
- Bedspread
- Pillowcase(s)
- Bath towel(s)
- Hand towel
- Washcloth
- Hospital gown
- Bath blanket

Use one arm to hold the linens and the other hand to pick them up. The item you will use first is at the bottom of your stack. (You picked up the mattress pad first, so it is at the bottom. The bath blanket is on top.) You need the mattress pad first. To get it on top, simply place your arm over the bath blanket. Then turn the stack over onto the arm on the bath blanket (Fig. 13-5, p. 273). The arm that held the linens is now free. Place the clean linens on a clean surface.

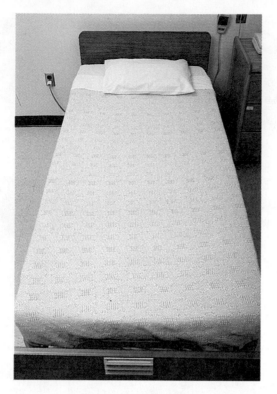

Fig. 13-1 *Closed bed.*

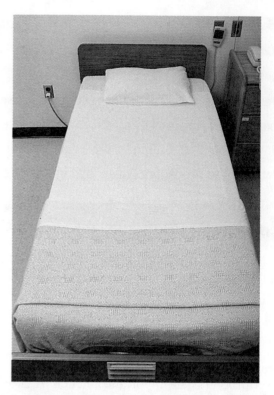

Fig. 13-2 *Open bed. Top linens are folded to the foot of the bed.*

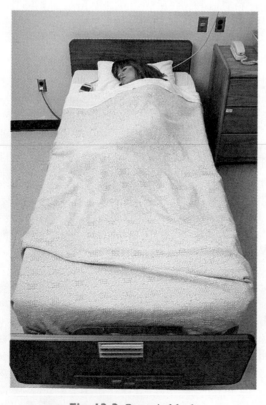

Fig. 13-3 *Occupied bed.*

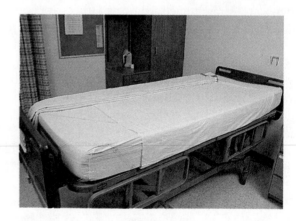

Fig. 13-4 *Surgical bed.*

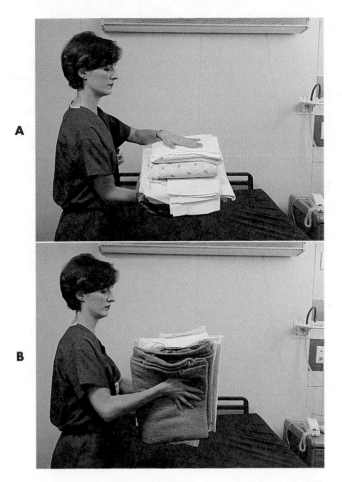

Fig. 13-5 **A,** *The arm is placed over the top of the stack of linens.* **B,** *The stack of linens is turned over onto the arm. Note that linens are held away from the body.*

LONG-TERM CARE

focus on

Policies about linen changes vary among nursing centers. Generally, linens are not changed every day. Remember, the center is the person's home. People do not change linens every day in their homes. A complete linen change is usually done weekly. Pillowcases, top and bottom sheets, and drawsheets (if used) may be changed twice a week. However, linens are changed if wet, soiled, or very wrinkled.

HOME CARE

focus on

Linen changes in the home are usually done weekly. However, follow the patient's routine. Change linens more often if the patient asks you to do so. Always change linens that are wet, soiled, or very wrinkled. Contact the RN if the person refuses to have linens changed.

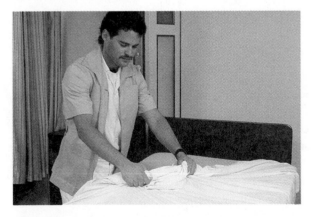

Fig. 13-6 *Roll linens away from you when removing them from the bed.*

When removing dirty linens, roll the linens away from you. The side that touched the person is inside the roll. The side that has not touched the person is outside (Fig. 13-6).

Top and bottom sheets, drawsheets, and pillowcases are changed daily in hospitals. The mattress pad, plastic drawsheet, blanket, and bedspread are reused for the same person. They are reused if not soiled, wet, or very wrinkled. If a person was discharged, remove all linens and make a closed bed. *Remember, wet, damp, or soiled linens are changed right away.* (See Focus on Long-Term Care and Focus on Home Care.)

A **drawsheet** is a small sheet placed over the middle of the bottom sheet. It helps keep the mattress and bottom linens clean and dry. A **plastic drawsheet** is waterproof. It protects the mattress and bottom linens from dampness and soiling. It is placed between the bottom sheet and cotton drawsheet. The cotton drawsheet protects the person from contact with the plastic and absorbs moisture. However, discomfort and skin breakdown may occur. The plastic retains heat, and plastic drawsheets are hard to keep tight and wrinkle free.

Many agencies use waterproof pads instead of plastic drawsheets. Plastic drawsheets are usually used only for persons with bowel or bladder control problems or those with excessive wound drainage.

Cotton drawsheets are often used without plastic drawsheets. Plastic-covered mattresses cause some persons to

HOME CARE

A flat sheet folded in half can serve as a cotton drawsheet. Usually a twin size sheet is easier to use for this purpose. The RN tells you what to use.

Medical supply stores sell plastic draw-sheets and waterproof pads. The RN discusses the need for these items with the patient and family. Some patients place plastic mattress protectors on their beds. These do not protect the bottom linens (cotton drawsheet, bottom sheet, and mattress pad). Some place a piece of plastic under the drawsheet. Again, the RN tells you what is safe to use for the person. Do not use plastic trash bags or dry-cleaning bags. These are not strong enough to protect the linens and mattress. They slide easily and can move out of place. The danger of suffocation is great if the bag covers the person's nose and mouth.

perspire heavily. This increases discomfort. A cotton drawsheet reduces heat retention and absorbs moisture. Cotton drawsheets are often used as lift or turning sheets (see Chapter 12). When used for this purpose, they are not tucked in at the sides.

The bedmaking procedures that follow include plastic and cotton drawsheets so you learn how to use them. Ask the RN about their use. (See Focus on Home Care at left.)

GENERAL RULES

Your job description will include making beds. No matter what type of bed you make, safety and medical asepsis are important. Box 13-1 lists the rules for bed-making. (See Focus on Home Care and Focus on Children on p. 275.)

RULES FOR BEDMAKING

- Use good body mechanics at all times.
- Follow the rules of medical asepsis.
- Practice Standard Precautions.
- Follow the Bloodborne Pathogen Standard.
- Wash your hands before handling clean linen and after handling dirty linen.
- Bring enough linen to the person's room.
- Never shake linens. Shaking linens spreads microorganisms.
- Extra linen in a person's room is considered contaminated. Do not use it for other patients. Put it with the dirty laundry.
- Hold linens away from your uniform. Dirty and clean linen must not touch your uniform.
- Never put dirty linens on the floor or on clean linens. Follow agency policy about dirty linen.
- Keep bottom linens tucked in and wrinkle free.
- Cover a plastic drawsheet with a cotton drawsheet. A plastic drawsheet must not touch the person's body.
- Straighten and tighten loose sheets, blankets, and bedspreads whenever necessary.
- Make as much of one side of the bed as possible before going to the other side. This saves time and energy.

focus on

HOME CARE

Many home care patients do not have hospital beds. You will see twin, regular, queen, and king size beds. Water beds, sofa sleepers, cots, and recliners also are common. Remember, you are in the person's home. Make the bed according to the person's wishes. No matter the type of bed, follow the rules in Box 13-1. If the person's wishes are unsafe, contact the RN.

focus on

CHILDREN

Cribs and crib linens present safety hazards. Mattresses, linens, and bumper pads pose many dangers. They can lead to strangulation and suffocation. Report any safety hazard to the RN. Always follow these safety rules:

- The crib mattress must be firm. A soft mattress can cover the baby's nose and mouth. This prevents breathing.
- The mattress must fit snugly in the crib frame. Otherwise the baby's head can get caught between the mattress and the frame. The baby can strangulate.
- The space between the mattress and crib sides should be no more than 2 inches. Only two adult fingers should fit in the space. If more than two fingers fit, the mattress does not fit.
- The mattress must be at least 26 inches lower than the top of the crib rails. This protects the baby from falling out of the crib. The mattress is lowered when the baby can stand in the crib.
- Plastic trash bags and dry-cleaning bags are not used to protect the mattress.

- Bumper pads must fit snugly against the slats. Otherwise the baby's head can get caught between the bumper pads and the slats. Strangulation can occur.
- Bumper pads are secured in place with at least six ties.
- Bumper pad ties must be away from the baby. Avoid long ties. The baby can get entangled in the ties and strangulate.
- Bumper pads are removed when the baby can stand in the crib.
- Do not tuck blankets and top sheets under the crib. A baby can get caught in them.
- Pillows are not used for babies. The pillow can cover the baby's nose and mouth. The baby can suffocate in the pillow.
- Blankets, comforters, and other linens are checked for loose threads and loose trim. Loose threads and trim can cause strangulation.
- Comforters are checked for loose stitching. Stuffing can come out if not stitched properly. The child can inhale the stuffing and suffocate.

✦ THE CLOSED BED

A closed bed is made after a person is discharged. It is made ready for a new patient. The bed is made after the bed frame and mattress are cleaned and disinfected.

Text continued on p. 281

LONG-TERM CARE

focus on

In long-term care, a closed bed also means that the linens are not folded back as in the open bed. Closed beds are made for residents who are up for most or all of the day. Clean linens are used as needed.

HOME CARE

focus on

In home care, a closed bed also means that linens are not folded back. Closed beds are made for patients who are up for most or all of the day. Clean linens are used as needed.

✦ MAKING A CLOSED BED

PRE-PROCEDURE

1 Wash your hands.

2 Collect clean linen:

- Mattress pad
- Bottom sheet
- Plastic drawsheet (optional)
- Cotton drawsheet
- Top sheet
- Blanket
- Bedspread
- Two pillowcases
- Bath towel(s)
- Hand towel
- Washcloth
- Hospital gown
- Bath blanket

3 Place linen on a clean surface.

4 Raise the bed for good body mechanics.

5 Move the mattress to the head of the bed.

6 Put the mattress pad on the mattress. It is even with the top of the mattress.

7 Place the bottom sheet on the mattress pad (Fig. 13-7, p. 278):

  a Unfold it lengthwise.

  b Place the center crease in the middle of the bed.

  c Position the lower edge even with the bottom of the mattress.

  d Place the large hem at the top and the small hem at the bottom.

  e Face hem-stitching downward.

8 Pick the sheet up from the side to open it. Fanfold it toward the other side of the bed (Fig. 13-8, p. 278).

MAKING A CLOSED BED—cont'd

PROCEDURE

9   Go to the head of the bed. Tuck the top of the sheet under the mattress. Make sure the sheet is tight and smooth.

10   Make a mitered corner (Fig. 13-9, p. 279).

11   Place the plastic drawsheet on the bed about 14 inches from the top of the mattress.

12   Open the plastic drawsheet, and fanfold it toward the other side of the bed.

13   Place a cotton drawsheet over the plastic drawsheet. It must cover the entire plastic drawsheet (Fig. 13-10, p. 279).

14   Open the cotton drawsheet, and fanfold it toward the other side of the bed.

15   Tuck both drawsheets under the mattress. Or tuck each in separately.

16   Go to the other side of the bed.

17   Miter the top corner of the bottom sheet.

18   Pull the bottom sheet tight so there are no wrinkles. Tuck in the sheet.

19   Pull the drawsheets tight so there are no wrinkles. Tuck both in together, or pull each tight and tuck them in separately (Fig. 13-11, p. 280).

20   Go to the other side of the bed.

21   Put the top sheet on the bed:

   a   Unfold it lengthwise.

   b   Place the center crease in the middle.

   c   Place the large hem at the top, even with the top of the mattress.

   d   Open the sheet and fanfold the extra part toward the other side.

   e   Face hem-stitching outward.

   f   Do not tuck the bottom in yet.

   g   Never tuck top linens in on the sides.

22   Place the blanket on the bed:

   a   Unfold it so the center crease is in the middle.

   b   Put the upper hem about 6 to 8 inches from the top of the mattress.

   c   Open the blanket, and fanfold the extra part toward the other side.

   d   If steps 28 and 29 are not done, turn the top sheet down over the blanket. Hem-stitching is down.

23   Place the bedspread on the bed:

   a   Unfold it so the center crease is in the middle.

   b   Place the upper hem even with the top of the mattress.

   c   Open the bedspread, and fanfold the extra part toward the other side.

   d   Make sure the bedspread facing the door is even and covers all the top linens.

24   Tuck in top linens together at the foot of the bed. They should be smooth and tight. Make a mitered corner.

25   Go to the other side.

26   Straighten all top linen, working from the head of the bed to the foot.

27   Tuck in the top linens together. Make a mitered corner.

28   Turn the top hem of the bedspread under the blanket to make a cuff (Fig. 13-12, p. 280).

29   Turn the top sheet down over the spread. Hem-stitching is down. (Steps 28 and 29 are not done in some agencies. The bedspread covers the pillow. Be sure to tuck the spread under the pillow.)

Continued

MAKING A CLOSED BED—cont'd

PROCEDURE—cont'd

30 Place the pillow on the bed.

31 Open the pillowcase so it is flat on the bed.

32 Put the pillowcase on the pillow as in Figure 13-13 on p. 280. Fold extra pillowcase material under the pillow at the seam end of the pillowcase.

33 Place the pillow on the bed so the open end is away from the door. The seam of the pillowcase is toward the head of the bed.

POST-PROCEDURE

34 Attach the call bell to the bed.

35 Lower the bed to its lowest position.

36 Put towels, washcloth, gown, and bath blanket in the bedside stand.

37 Wash your hands.

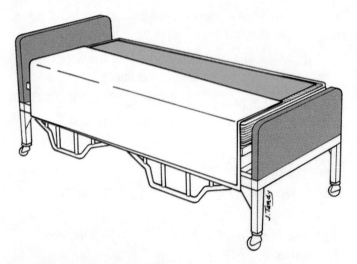

Fig. 13-7 *The bottom sheet is on the bed with the center crease in the middle. The lower edge of the sheet is even with the bottom of the mattress.*

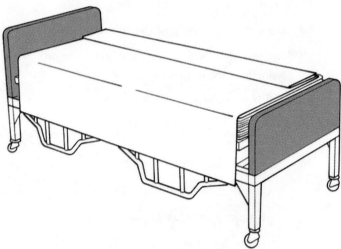

Fig. 13-8 *The bottom sheet is fanfolded to the other side of the bed.*

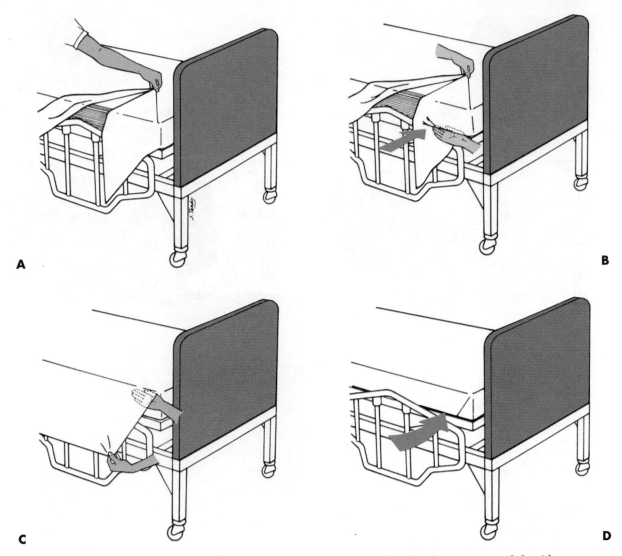

A
B
C
D

Fig. 13-9 *Making a mitered corner.* **A,** *Bottom sheet is tucked under the mattress and the side of the sheet is raised onto the mattress.* **B,** *The remaining portion of the sheet is tucked under the mattress.* **C,** *The raised portion of the sheet is brought off the mattress.* **D,** *The entire side of the sheet is tucked under the mattress.*

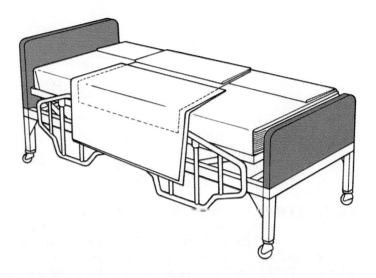

Fig. 13-10 *The cotton drawsheet completely covers the plastic drawsheet.*

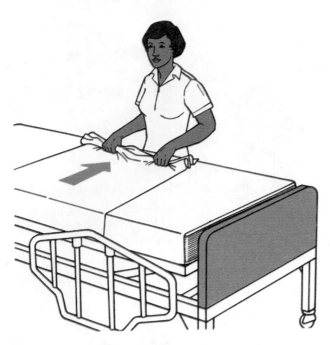

Fig. 13-11 *The drawsheet is pulled tight to remove wrinkles.*

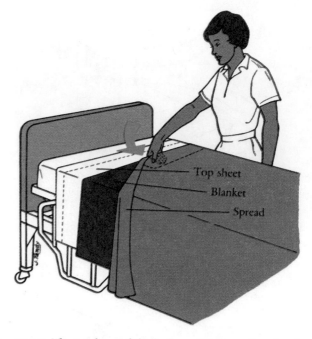

Fig. 13-12 *The top hem of the bedspread is turned under the top hem of the blanket to make a cuff.*

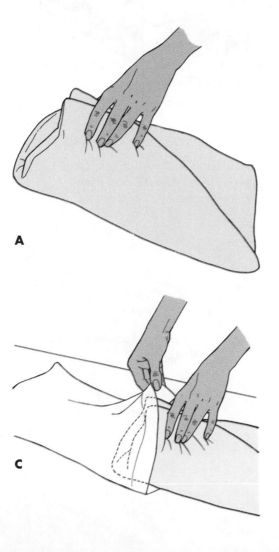

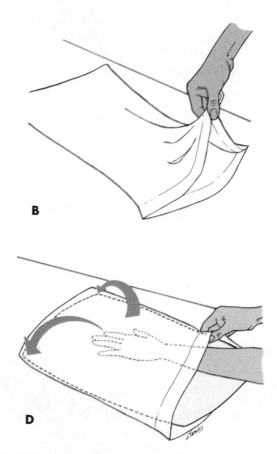

Fig. 13-13 *Putting a pillowcase on a pillow.* **A,** *Grasp the corners of the pillow at the seam end and form a V with the pillow.* **B,** *The pillowcase is flat on the bed; the pillowcase is opened with the free hand.* **C,** *The V end of the pillow is guided into the pillowcase.* **D,** *The V end of the pillow falls into the corners of the pillowcase.*

THE OPEN BED

A closed bed becomes an open bed by folding the top linens back. Open beds are made for newly admitted persons arriving by wheelchair. They are also made for persons who are out of bed when their beds are being made.

MAKING AN OPEN BED

PROCEDURE

1 Wash your hands.

2 Collect linen for a closed bed.

3 Make a closed bed.

4 Fanfold top linens to the foot of the bed (see Fig. 13-2).

5 Attach the call bell to the bed.

6 Lower the bed to its lowest position.

7 Put towels, washcloth, gown, and bath blanket in the bedside stand.

8 Follow agency policy for dirty linen.

9 Wash your hands.

◆ THE OCCUPIED BED

An occupied bed is made when a person cannot get out of bed because of illness or injury. You must keep the person in good body alignment. You must know about restrictions or limitations in the person's movement or positioning. Explain each step of the procedure to the person before it is done.

Text continued on p. 287

MAKING AN OCCUPIED BED

PRE-PROCEDURE

1 Explain the procedure to the person.

2 Wash your hands.

3 Collect the following:

- Gloves
- Linen bag
- Clean linen (see *Making a Closed Bed,* p. 276).

4 Place linen on a clean surface.

5 Provide for privacy.

6 Remove the call bell.

7 Raise the bed for good body mechanics.

8 Lower the head of the bed to a level appropriate for the person. It should be as flat as possible.

9 Lower the bed rail near you. Make sure the far one is up and secure.

10 Put on gloves if linens are soiled with blood, body fluids, secretions, or excretions.

11 Loosen top linens at the foot of the bed.

12 Remove the bedspread and blanket separately. Fold them as in Figure 13-14 on p. 284 if you will reuse them.

13 Cover the person with a bath blanket for warmth and privacy:

a Unfold a bath blanket over the top sheet.

b Ask the person to hold onto the bath blanket. If he or she cannot, tuck the top part under the person's shoulders.

c Grasp the top sheet under the bath blanket at the shoulders. Bring the sheet down to the foot of the bed. Remove the sheet from under the blanket (Fig. 13-15, p. 285).

14 Move the mattress to the head of the bed.

15 Position the person on the side of the bed away from you. Adjust the pillow for the person's comfort. It should be on the far side of the bed.

16 Loosen bottom linens from the head to the foot of the bed.

17 Fanfold bottom linens one at a time toward the person: cotton drawsheet, plastic drawsheet, bottom sheet, and mattress pad (Fig. 13-16, p. 285). Do not fanfold the mattress pad if it will be reused.

18 Place a clean mattress pad on the bed. Unfold it lengthwise so the center crease is in the middle. Fanfold the top part toward the person. If reusing the mattress pad, straighten and smooth any wrinkles.

MAKING AN OCCUPIED BED—cont'd

PRE-PROCEDURE—cont'd

19 Place the bottom sheet on the mattress pad so hem-stitching is away from the person. Unfold the sheet so the crease is in the middle. The small hem should be even with the bottom of the mattress. Fanfold the top part toward the person.

20 Make a mitered corner at the head of the bed. Tuck the sheet under the mattress from the head to the foot.

21 Pull the fanfolded plastic drawsheet toward you over the bottom sheet. Tuck excess material under the mattress. Do the following if you are using a clean plastic drawsheet (Fig. 13-17, p. 286):

  a Place the plastic drawsheet on the bed about 14 inches from the mattress top.

  b Fanfold the top part toward the person.

  c Tuck in the excess material.

22 Place the cotton drawsheet over the plastic drawsheet. It must cover the entire plastic drawsheet. Fanfold the top part toward the person. Tuck in excess material.

23 Raise the bed rail. Go to the other side, and lower the bed rail.

24 Position the person on the side of the bed away from you. Adjust the pillow for the person's comfort.

25 Loosen bottom linens. Remove soiled linen one piece at a time. Remove and discard the gloves.

26 Straighten and smooth the mattress pad.

27 Pull the clean bottom sheet toward you. Make a mitered corner at the top. Tuck the sheet under the mattress from the head to the foot of the bed.

28 Pull the drawsheets tightly toward you. Tuck both under together or tuck each in separately.

29 Position the person supine in the center of the bed. Adjust the pillow for comfort.

30 Put the top sheet on the bed. Unfold it lengthwise. Make sure the crease is in the middle, the large hem is even with the top of the mattress, and hem-stitching is on the outside.

31 Ask the person to hold onto the top sheet so you can remove the bath blanket. You may have to tuck the top sheet under the person's shoulders. Remove the bath blanket.

32 Place the blanket on the bed. Unfold it so the crease is in the middle. Unfold the blanket so it covers the person. The upper hem should be 6 to 8 inches from the top of the mattress.

33 Place the bedspread on the bed. Unfold it so the center crease is in the middle and it covers the person. The top hem is even with the mattress top.

34 Turn the top hem of the bedspread under the blanket to make a cuff.

35 Bring the top sheet down over the bedspread to form a cuff.

36 Go to the foot of the bed.

37 Lift the mattress corner with one arm. Tuck all top linens under the mattress together. Be sure the linens are loose enough to allow movement of the person's feet. Make a mitered corner.

38 Raise the bed rail. Go to the other side, and lower the bed rail.

39 Straighten and smooth top linens.

40 Tuck the top linens under the mattress as in step 37. Make a mitered corner.

41 Change the pillowcase(s).

42 Place the call bell within reach.

43 Raise or lower bed rails as instructed by the RN.

Continued

✦ MAKING AN OCCUPIED BED—cont'd

POST-PROCEDURE

44 Raise the head of the bed to a level appropriate for the person. Make sure the person is comfortable.

45 Lower the bed to its lowest position.

46 Put towels, washcloth, gown, and bath blanket in the bedside stand.

47 Unscreen the person. Thank him or her for cooperating.

48 Follow agency policy for dirty linen.

49 Wash your hands.

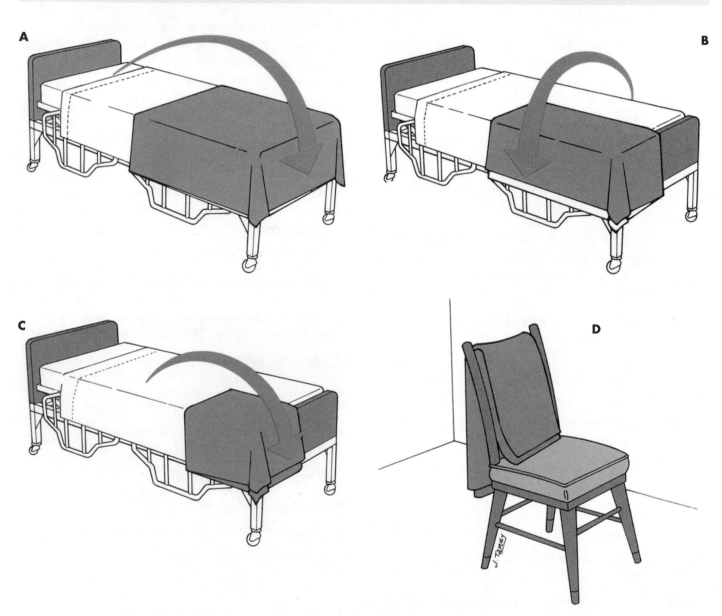

Fig. 13-14 *Folding linen for reuse.* **A,** *The top edge of the blanket is folded down to the bottom edge.* **B,** *The blanket is folded from the far side of the bed to the near side.* **C,** *The top edge of the blanket is folded down to the bottom edge again.* **D,** *The folded blanket is placed over the back of a straight chair.*

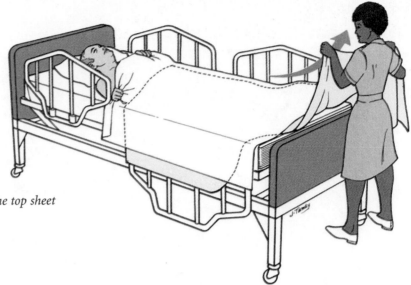

Fig. 13-15 *The person holds onto the bath blanket. The top sheet is removed from under the bath blanket.*

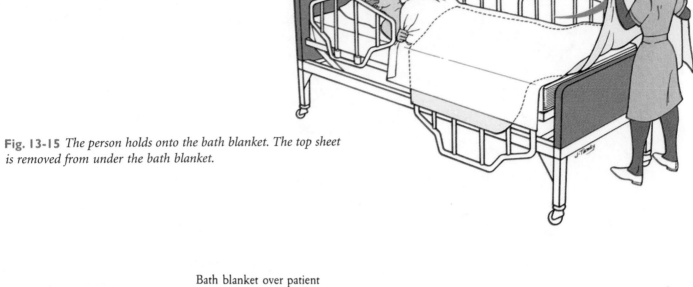

Bath blanket over patient

Old cotton drawsheet

A

Old plastic drawsheet

Old bottom sheet

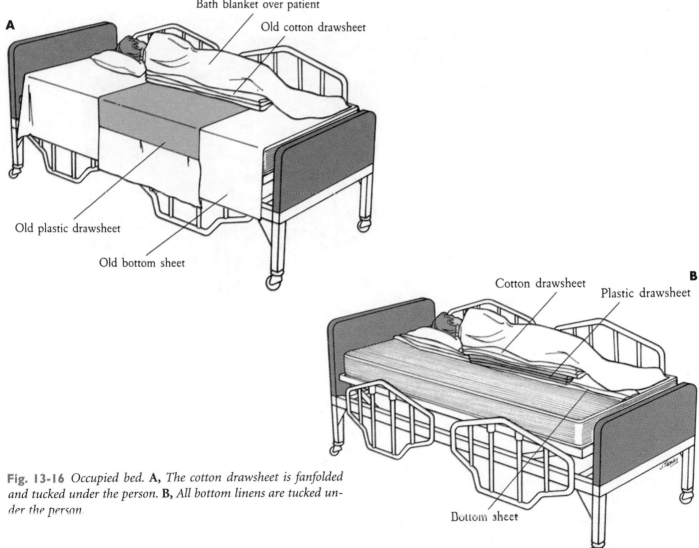

Cotton drawsheet

Plastic drawsheet

B

Bottom sheet

Fig. 13-16 *Occupied bed.* **A,** *The cotton drawsheet is fanfolded and tucked under the person.* **B,** *All bottom linens are tucked under the person.*

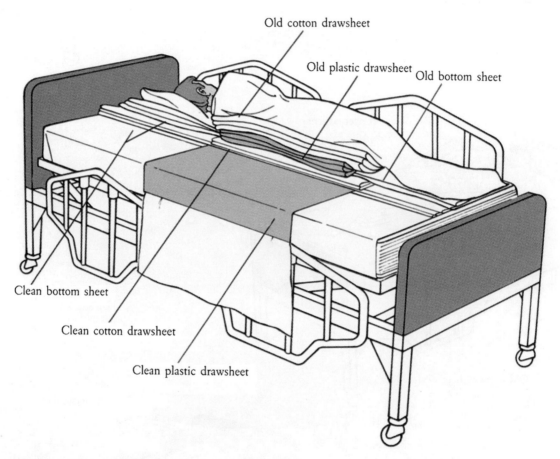

Old cotton drawsheet

Old plastic drawsheet

Old bottom sheet

Clean bottom sheet

Clean cotton drawsheet

Clean plastic drawsheet

Fig. 13-17 *A clean bottom sheet and plastic drawsheet are on the bed with both fanfolded and tucked under the person. The clean cotton drawsheet is put in place in step 22.*

THE SURGICAL BED

The surgical bed (recovery bed, postoperative bed, or anesthesia bed) is a form of the open bed. Top linens are folded for transferring the person from a stretcher to the bed. The term *surgical bed* and its other names imply that the person had surgery. However, this bed is used for persons who arrive on a stretcher. If the bed is made for a postoperative (surgical) patient, a complete linen change is done.

MAKING A SURGICAL BED

PROCEDURE

1 Wash your hands.

2 Collect the following:

- Clean linen (see *Making a Closed Bed*, p. 276)
- IV pole
- Tissues
- Kidney basin
- Gloves
- Laundry bag
- Other equipment as requested by the RN

3 Place linen on a clean surface.

4 Remove the call bell.

5 Raise the bed for good body mechanics.

6 Remove all linen from the bed. Wear gloves for contact with the person's blood, body fluids, secretions, or excretions.

7 Make a closed bed (See *Making a Closed Bed*, p. 276). Do not tuck the top linens under the mattress.

8 Fold all top linens at the foot of the bed back onto the bed. The fold is even with the edge of the mattress (Fig. 13-18, p. 288).

9 Fanfold linen lengthwise to the side of the bed farthest from the door (Fig. 13-19, p. 288).

10 Put the pillowcase(s) on the pillow(s).

11 Place the pillow(s) on a clean surface.

12 Leave the bed in its highest position.

13 Make sure both bed rails are down.

14 Put the towels, washcloth, gown, and bath blanket in the bedside stand.

15 Place the tissues and kidney basin on the bedside stand. Place the IV pole near the head of the bed.

16 Move all furniture away from the bed. Allow enough room for the stretcher and for the staff to move about.

17 Do not attach the call bell to the bed.

18 Follow agency policy for soiled linen.

19 Wash your hands.

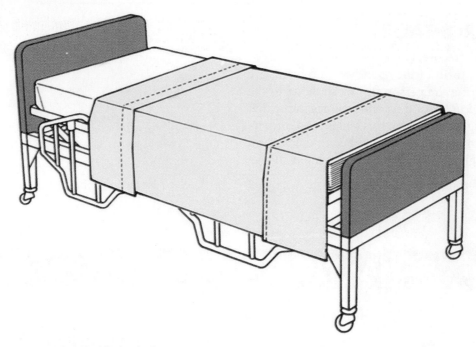

Fig. 13-18 *Surgical bed. The bottom of the top linens is folded back onto the bed. The fold is even with the edge of the mattress.*

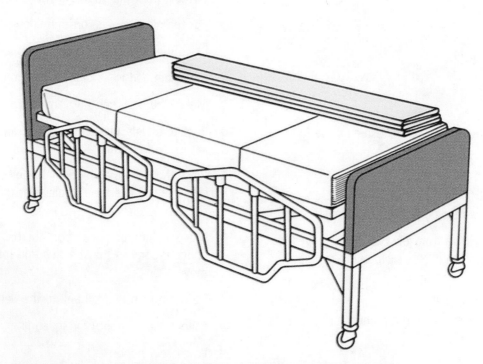

Fig. 13-19 *A surgical bed with the top linens fanfolded lengthwise to the opposite side of the bed.*

REVIEW QUESTIONS

Circle T *if the statement is true or* F *if the statement is false.*

1 T F Linens are changed whenever soiled, wet, or damp.

2 T F A surgical bed is only for persons who had surgery.

3 T F Linens are held away from your body and uniform.

4 T F Dirty linens are put on the floor.

5 T F Extra linen in a person's room is used for another person.

6 T F Complete linen changes are required for closed beds and surgical beds.

7 T F A cotton drawsheet is always used when a plastic drawsheet is used.

8 T F The hem-stitching of the bottom sheet is placed downward away from the person.

9 T F A cotton drawsheet must completely cover the plastic drawsheet.

10 T F The upper hem of the bedspread is even with the top of the mattress.

11 T F Top linens are fanfolded to the foot of the bed for an open bed.

12 T F A person is screened when an occupied bed is made.

13 T F When making an occupied bed, the far bed rail is up at all times.

14 T F After a surgical bed is made, it is left in its lowest position.

15 T F A cotton drawsheet is used only with a plastic drawsheet.

Answers to these questions are on p. 851.

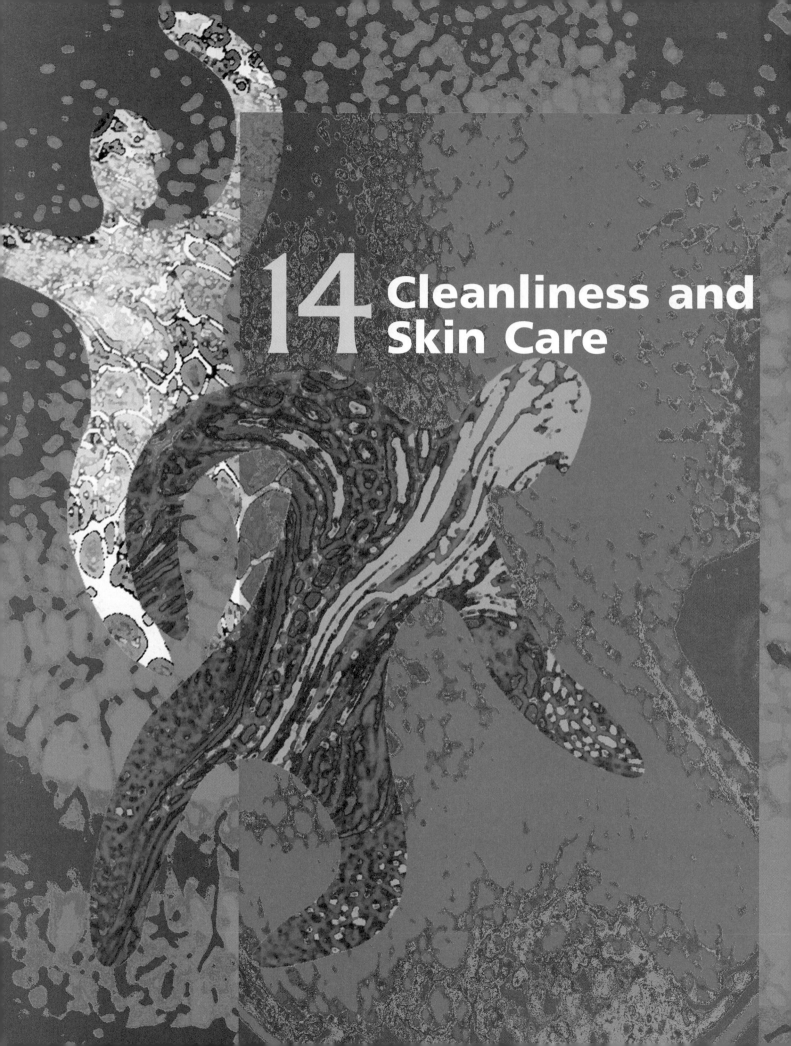

14 Cleanliness and Skin Care

- Define the key terms in this chapter
- Explain the importance of cleanliness and skin care
- Describe the routine care given before and after breakfast, after lunch, and in the evening
- Describe the importance of oral hygiene and the observations to report
- Describe the rules for bathing and the observations to make
- Identify the safety precautions for persons taking tub baths or showers
- Explain the purposes of a back massage
- Identify the purposes of perineal care
- Describe the signs, symptoms, and causes of pressure ulcers
- Locate the pressure points of the body in the prone, supine, lateral, Fowler's, and sitting positions
- Describe how to prevent pressure ulcers
- Perform the procedures described in this chapter

KEY TERMS

AM care Routine care performed before breakfast; early morning care

aspiration Breathing fluid or an object into the lungs

bedsore A decubitus ulcer, a pressure sore, a pressure ulcer

decubitus ulcer A bedsore, pressure sore, or pressure ulcer

early morning care AM care

epidermal stripping Removing the epidermis (outer skin layer) with tape

evening care HS care or PM care

HS care Care given in the evening at bedtime (hour of sleep [HS]); evening care or PM care

morning care Care given after breakfast; cleanliness and skin care measures are more thorough at this time

oral hygiene Measures performed to keep the mouth and teeth clean; mouth care

pericare Perineal care

perineal care Cleansing the genital and anal areas

plaque A thin film that sticks to the teeth; it contains saliva, microorganisms, and other substances

PM care HS care or evening care

pressure sore A bed sore, decubitus ulcer, or pressure ulcer

pressure ulcer Any injury caused by unrelieved pressure; a decubitus ulcer, bedsore, or pressure sore

tartar Hardened plaque on teeth

Cleanliness and skin care promote comfort, safety, and health. The skin is the body's first line of defense against disease. Intact skin prevents microbes from entering the body and causing an infection. Likewise, mucous membranes of the mouth, genital area, and anus must be clean and intact. Besides cleansing, good hygiene prevents body and breath odors. It also promotes relaxation and increases circulation.

Culture and personal choice affect hygiene. Some people take showers. Others take tub baths. Some bathe at bedtime. Others bathe in the morning. Bathing frequency also varies. Some bathe daily or twice a day—such as before work and after work or exercise. Some people do not have water for bathing. Others cannot afford soap, deodorant, shampoo, toothpaste, or other hygiene products.

Patients usually need some help with personal hygiene. Illness, age, and the changes of aging affect the ability to practice hygiene. Perspiration, vomiting, urinary and bowel elimination, drainage from wounds or body openings, bed rest, and activity all affect cleanliness and skin care needs. The RN uses the nursing process to meet the person's hygiene needs. The RN and the nursing care plan tell you how to meet the person's hygiene needs.

DAILY CARE OF THE PERSON

People usually have hygiene routines and habits. For example, teeth are brushed and the face and hands washed on awakening. These and other hygiene measures may be done routinely before and after meals and at bedtime.

Infants, young children, and some weak or disabled adults need help with hygiene. Routine care is given at certain times. However, you assist with personal hygiene whenever necessary.

Before Breakfast

Routine care before breakfast is **early morning care** or AM **care**. Night shift or day shift staff give AM care. They get patients ready for breakfast or morning tests. Personal hygiene measures at this time include:

- Assisting persons to the bathroom or offering the commode, bedpan, or urinal
- Helping persons wash their face and hands
- Assisting with oral hygiene
- Positioning persons in Fowler's position or in a chair for breakfast
- Straightening bed linens
- Straightening patient units

After Breakfast

Morning care is given after breakfast. Cleanliness and skin care measures are more thorough. Routine morning care usually involves:

- Assisting persons to the bathroom or offering the commode, bedpan, or urinal
- Helping persons wash their face and hands
- Assisting with oral hygiene
- Shaving patients
- Providing showers, tub baths, or bed baths
- Giving perineal care
- Giving back massages
- Changing gowns or pajamas
- Brushing and combing hair
- Changing bed linens
- Straightening patient units

Afternoon Care

Routine hygiene is performed after lunch and the evening meal. If done before visiting hours, patients feel more refreshed. They also can visit with family and friends without interruption. Afternoon care involves:

- Assisting persons to the bathroom or offering the commode, bedpan, or urinal
- Helping patients wash their face and hands
- Assisting with oral hygiene
- Changing gowns or pajamas
- Brushing or combing hair if needed
- Changing damp or soiled bed linens
- Straightening patient units

Evening Care

Care given at bedtime is **HS care**, **evening care**, or PM **care**. (HS stands for *hour of sleep*.) Hygiene measures are performed before the person is ready for sleep. HS care promotes comfort and relaxation. It involves:

- Assisting persons to the bathroom or offering the commode, bedpan, or urinal
- Helping patients wash their face and hands
- Assisting with oral hygiene
- Changing damp or soiled linens and straightening all other linens
- Changing gowns or pajamas if needed
- Giving back massages
- Straightening patient units

ORAL HYGIENE

Oral hygiene (mouth care) keeps the mouth and teeth clean. This prevents mouth odors and infections. It also increases comfort and makes food taste better. *Cavities (dental caries)* are prevented. So is periodontal disease *(gum disease, pyorrhea)*. Periodontal disease is an inflammation of the tissues around the teeth. Poor oral hygiene allows the buildup of plaque and tartar. **Plaque** is a thin film that sticks to teeth. It contains saliva, bacteria, and other substances. Plaque leads to tooth decay or cavities. When plaque hardens, it is called **tartar.** Tartar builds up at the gum line near the neck of the tooth. Tartar buildup leads to periodontal disease. The gums are red, swollen, and bleed easily. As the disease progresses, bone is destroyed and teeth loosen. Tooth loss is common.

Illness and disease often cause a bad taste in the mouth. Some drugs and diseases cause a whitish coating on the mouth and tongue. Others cause redness and swelling of the mouth and tongue. Dry mouth is common from oxygen, smoking, decreased fluid intake, and anxiety. Some drugs cause dry mouth.

The RN assesses the person's need for mouth care. Then the RN decides the type of mouth care and assistance needed. Oral hygiene is given on awakening, after each meal, and at bedtime. Many people also practice oral hygiene before meals.

Equipment

A toothbrush, toothpaste, dental floss, and mouthwash are needed. The toothbrush should have soft bristles. Persons with dentures need a denture cleaner, denture cup, and denture brush or regular toothbrush. Sponge swabs are used for persons with sore, tender mouths and for unconscious patients.

Follow Standard Precautions and the Bloodborne Pathogen Standard when giving oral hygiene. You have contact with the person's mucous membranes. Gums may bleed during oral care. Also, the mouth contains many microbes. Pathogens spread through sexual contact may be in the mouths of some persons.

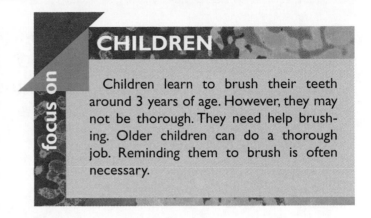

CHILDREN

focus on

Children learn to brush their teeth around 3 years of age. However, they may not be thorough. They need help brushing. Older children can do a thorough job. Reminding them to brush is often necessary.

✧ Brushing Teeth

Many people perform oral hygiene themselves. Others need help gathering and setting up equipment. You may have to brush the teeth of persons who are very weak or who cannot use or move their arms. Report the following observations to the RN:

- Dry, cracked, swollen, or blistered lips
- Redness, swelling, irritation, sores, or white patches in the mouth or on the tongue
- Bleeding, swelling, or redness of the gums

(See Focus on Children.)

Text continued on p. 297

ASSISTING THE PERSON TO BRUSH THE TEETH

PRE-PROCEDURE

1 Explain the procedure to the person.

2 Wash your hands.

3 Collect the following:

- Toothbrush
- Toothpaste or dentifrice
- Mouthwash
- Dental floss
- Water glass with cool water
- Straw
- Kidney basin
- Face towel
- Paper towels

4 Place the paper towels on the overbed table. Arrange items on top of them.

5 Identify the person. Check the ID bracelet, and call the person by name.

6 Provide for privacy.

7 Raise the head so the person can brush with ease.

PROCEDURE

8 Place the towel over the person's chest. This protects the gown and linens from spills.

9 Lower the bed rail if up.

10 Place the overbed table in front of the person. Adjust table height for the person.

11 Allow the person to brush the teeth.

12 Remove the towel when the person is done.

13 Move the overbed table next to the bed. Lower it to a level appropriate for the person.

POST-PROCEDURE

14 Make sure the person is comfortable.

15 Place the call bell within reach.

16 Raise or lower bed rails as instructed.

17 Clean and return items to their proper place.

18 Wipe off the overbed table with the paper towels and discard them.

19 Unscreen the person.

20 Follow agency policy for dirty linen.

21 Wash your hands.

22 Report your observations to the RN.

BRUSHING THE PERSON'S TEETH

PRE-PROCEDURE

1 Explain the procedure to the person.

2 Wash your hands.

3 Collect gloves and items listed in *Assisting the Person to Brush the Teeth.*

4 Place the paper towels on the overbed table. Arrange items on top of them.

5 Identify the person. Check the ID bracelet, and call the person by name.

6 Provide for privacy.

7 Raise the bed to the best level for good body mechanics.

PROCEDURE

8 Raise the head of the bed so the person can sit comfortably. Position the person in a side-lying position on the side near you if he or she cannot sit up.

9 Lower the bed rail near you. Make sure the far bed rail is up.

10 Place the towel over the person's chest. This protects the gown and linens from spills.

11 Position the overbed table so you can reach it with ease. Adjust the height as needed.

12 Put on the gloves.

13 Apply toothpaste to the toothbrush.

14 Hold the toothbrush over the kidney basin. Pour some water over the brush.

15 Brush the person's teeth gently as shown in Figure 14-1 on p. 296.

16 Let the person rinse the mouth with water. Hold the kidney basin under the person's chin (Fig. 14-2, p. 296). Repeat this step as necessary.

17 Floss the person's teeth (see *Flossing the Person's Teeth,* p. 297).

18 Let the person use mouthwash. Hold the kidney basin under the chin.

19 Remove the towel when done.

20 Remove and discard the gloves.

POST-PROCEDURE

21 Make sure the person is comfortable.

22 Place the call bell within reach.

23 Lower the bed to its lowest position.

24 Raise or lower bed rails as instructed by the RN.

25 Clean and return equipment to its proper place.

26 Wipe off the overbed table with the paper towels and discard them.

27 Lower the overbed table to a level appropriate for the person.

28 Unscreen the person.

29 Follow agency policy for dirty linen.

30 Wash your hands.

31 Report your observations to the RN.

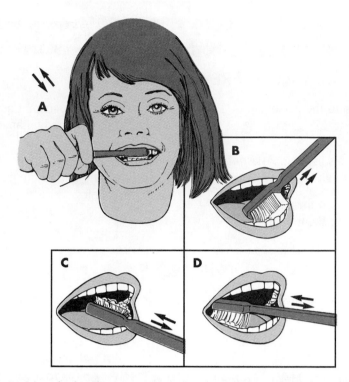

Fig. 14-1 A, *Position the brush at a 45-degree angle to the gums. Brush with short strokes.* **B,** *Position the brush at a 45-degree angle against the inside of the front teeth. Brush from the gum to the crown of the tooth with short strokes.* **C,** *Hold the brush horizontally against the inner surfaces of the teeth. Brush back and forth.* **D,** *Position the brush on the biting surfaces of the teeth. Brush back and forth.*

Fig. 14-2 *The kidney basin is held under the person's chin.*

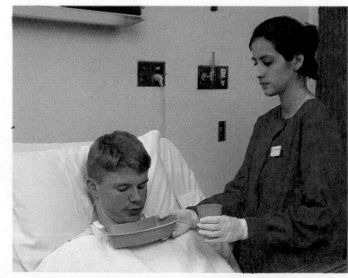

✤ Flossing

Flossing is a preventive measure. It removes plaque and tartar from the teeth. These substances cause serious gum disease that leads to loosening and loss of teeth. Flossing also removes food from between the teeth. It is usually done after brushing but can be done at other times. Some people floss after meals. If done only once a day, bedtime is the best time to floss.

You need to floss for persons who cannot tend to oral hygiene. (See Focus on Children.)

focus on CHILDREN

Preschoolers and older children need to floss. You need to floss for preschoolers. Older children can floss themselves. However, they need reminding and some supervision.

✦ FLOSSING THE PERSON'S TEETH

PRE-PROCEDURE

1. Explain to the person what you are going to do.

2. Wash your hands.

3. Collect the following:
   - Kidney basin
   - Water glass with cool water
   - Dental floss
   - Face towel
   - Paper towels
   - Gloves

4. Place the paper towels on the overbed table. Arrange items on top of them.

5. Identify the person. Check the ID bracelet, and call the person by name.

6. Provide for privacy.

7. Raise the bed to the best level for good body mechanics.

PROCEDURE

8. Raise the head of the bed so the person can sit comfortably. Position the person in a side-lying position near you if he or she cannot sit up.

9. Place the towel over the person's chest.

10. Position the overbed table so you can reach it with ease. Adjust the height as needed.

11. Lower the bed rail near you. Make sure the far bed rail is up.

12. Put on the gloves.

13. Break off an 18-inch piece of floss from the dispenser.

14. Hold the floss between the middle fingers of each hand (Fig. 14-3, *A*, p. 298).

15. Stretch the floss with your thumbs.

16. Start at the upper back tooth on the right side, and work around to the left side.

17. Move the floss gently up and down between the teeth (Fig. 14-3, *B*, p. 298). Move floss up and down from the top of the crown to the gum line.

18. Move to a new section of floss after every second tooth.

19. Floss the lower teeth. Hold the floss with your index fingers (Fig. 14-3, *C*, p. 298). Use up and down motions, and go under the gums as for the upper teeth. Start on the right side, and work around to the left side.

20. Let the person rinse his or her mouth. Hold the kidney basin under the chin. Repeat rinsing as necessary.

21. Remove the towel when done.

22. Remove and discard the gloves.

Continued

FLOSSING THE PERSON'S TEETH—cont'd

POST-PROCEDURE

23 Follow steps 21 through 30 for *Brushing the Person's Teeth,* p. 295.

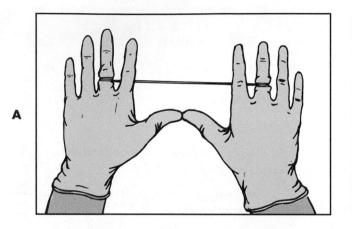

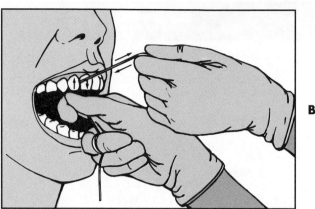

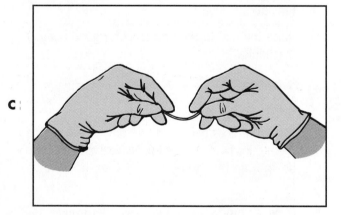

Fig. 14-3 A, *Dental floss is held between the middle fingers to floss the upper teeth.* **B,** *Floss is moved in up-and-down motions between the teeth. Floss is moved up and down from the crown to the gum line.* **C,** *Floss is held with the index fingers to floss the lower teeth.*

Mouth Care for the Unconscious Person

Unconscious persons need special mouth care. They cannot eat and drink, they breathe with their mouths open, and they usually receive oxygen (see Chapter 21). These factors cause mouth dryness. They also cause crusting on the tongue and mucous membranes. Good mouth care helps keep the mouth clean and moist. It also prevents infection.

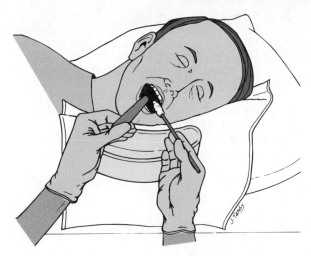

Fig. 14-4 *The head of the unconscious person is turned well to the side to prevent aspiration. A padded tongue blade is used to keep the mouth open while cleaning the mouth with swabs.*

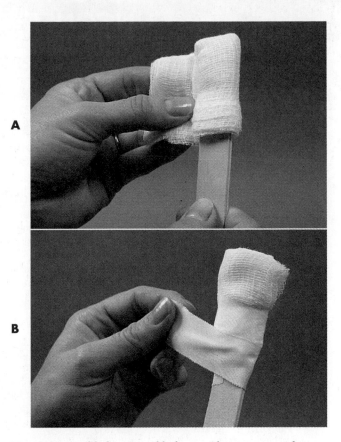

Fig. 14-5 *Padded tongue blade.* **A,** *Place two wooden tongue blades together, and wrap gauze around the top half.* **B,** *Tape the gauze in place.*

The RN tells you what cleaning agent to use. Use sponge swabs to apply the cleaning agent. Apply petroleum jelly to the lips after cleaning to prevent cracking.

Unconscious persons usually cannot swallow. Protect them from choking and aspiration. **Aspiration** is the breathing of fluid or an object into the lungs. To prevent aspiration, position the person on one side with the head turned well to the side (Fig. 14-4). In this position, excess fluid runs out of the mouth. This reduces the risk of aspiration. Using only a small amount of fluid also reduces the risk of aspiration. Sometimes oral suctioning (see Chapter 21) is part of the procedure.

The person's mouth is kept open with a padded tongue blade. (Figure 14-5 shows how to make a padded tongue blade.) Do not use your fingers to hold the mouth open. The person can bite down on them. The bite breaks the skin and creates a portal of entry for microbes. An infection could develop.

Unconscious persons cannot speak or respond to what is happening. However, some can hear. Always assume that unconscious persons can hear. Explain what you are doing step by step. Also tell the person when you are done and when you are leaving the room.

Mouth care is given at least every 2 hours. The RN assesses the person's needs and then writes a care plan. Check with the RN and the nursing care plan. They tell you how often to do oral hygiene and what to use. Unconscious persons are also repositioned at least every 2 hours. Combining mouth care, skin care, and other comfort measures increases their comfort and safety.

✦ Denture Care

Dentures are cleaned for persons who cannot do so themselves. Mouth care is given, and dentures are cleaned as often as natural teeth. Remember, dentures are the person's property. They are costly. Losing or damaging dentures is negligent conduct.

Dentures are slippery when wet. They easily break or chip if dropped onto a hard surface such as floors or sinks. You must hold them firmly. During cleaning, firmly hold them over a basin of water lined with a towel. Hot water causes them to warp. Do not use hot water to clean or store dentures. If not worn, store dentures in a container of cool water. Otherwise, dentures can dry out and warp.

Dentures are generally removed at bedtime. Some people choose not to wear their dentures. Others wear dentures for eating and remove them after meals. Remind patients not to wrap dentures in tissues or napkins. Otherwise they are easily discarded.

Many patients clean their own dentures. However, they may need help collecting and cleaning items. They may also need help getting to the bathroom.

Text continued on p. 303

PROVIDING MOUTH CARE FOR AN UNCONSCIOUS PERSON

PRE-PROCEDURE

1   Wash your hands.

2   Collect the following:

  • Cleaning agent as directed by the RN

  • Sponge swabs

  • Padded tongue blade

  • Water glass with cool water

  • Face towel

  • Kidney basin

  • Petroleum jelly

  • Paper towels

  • Gloves

3   Place the paper towels on the overbed table. Arrange items on top of them.

4   Identify the person. Check the ID bracelet, and call the person by name.

5   Explain the procedure to the person.

6   Provide for privacy.

7   Raise the bed to the best level for good body mechanics.

PROCEDURE

8   Lower the bed rail near you. Make sure the far bed rail is up.

9   Put on the gloves.

10 Position the person in a side-lying position on the side toward you. Turn his or her head well to the side.

11 Place the towel under the person's face.

12 Place the kidney basin under the chin.

13 Position the overbed table so you can reach it. Adjust the height as needed.

14 Separate the upper and lower teeth with the padded tongue blade.

15 Clean the mouth using the sponge swabs moistened with the cleaning agent (see Fig. 14-4).

  a   Clean the chewing and inner surfaces of the teeth.

  b   Clean the outer surfaces of the teeth.

  c   Swab the roof of the mouth, inside of the cheeks, and the lips.

  d   Swab the tongue.

  e   Moisten a clean swab with water, and swab the mouth to rinse.

  f   Place used swabs in the kidney basin.

16 Apply petroleum jelly to the person's lips.

17 Remove the towel.

18 Remove and discard the gloves.

19 Explain that the procedure is done and that you will reposition him or her.

20 Reposition the person.

21 Raise the bed rail. Make sure both bed rails are up.

POST-PROCEDURE

22 Make sure the call bell is within reach.

23 Lower the bed to its lowest position.

24 Clean and return equipment to its proper place. Discard disposable items.

25 Unscreen the person.

26 Tell the person that you are leaving the room.

27 Follow agency policy for dirty linen.

28 Wash your hands.

29 Report your observations to the RN.

PRE-PROCEDURE

1 Explain the procedure to the person.

2 Wash your hands.

3 Collect the following:

- Denture brush or toothbrush

- Denture cup labeled with the person's name and room number

- Denture cleaner or toothpaste

- Water glass with cool water

- Straw

- Mouthwash

- Kidney basin

- Two face towels

- Gauze squares

- Gloves

4 Identify the person. Check the ID bracelet, and call the person by name.

5 Provide for privacy.

PROCEDURE

6 Lower the bed rail if up.

7 Place a towel over the person's chest.

8 Put on the gloves.

9 Ask the person to remove the dentures. Carefully place them in the kidney basin.

10 Remove the dentures using gauze if the person cannot do so. (The gauze lets you get a good grip on the slippery dentures.)

   a Grasp the upper denture with your thumb and index finger (Fig. 14-6, p. 302). Move the denture up and down slightly to break the seal. Gently remove the denture once the seal is broken. Place it in the kidney basin.

   b Remove the lower denture by grasping it with your thumb and index finger. Turn it slightly, and lift it out of the person's mouth. Place it in the kidney basin.

11 Raise the bed rail if instructed by the RN.

12 Take the kidney basin, denture cup, brush, and denture cleaner or toothpaste to the sink.

13 Line the sink with a towel, and fill it with water.

14 Rinse each denture under warm running water. Return them to the denture cup.

15 Apply denture cleaner or toothpaste to the brush.

16 Brush the dentures as in Figure 14-7 on p. 302.

17 Rinse dentures under cool running water. Handle them carefully; do not drop them.

18 Place them in the denture cup. Fill it with cool water until the dentures are covered.

19 Clean the kidney basin.

20 Bring the denture cup and kidney basin to the bedside table.

21 Lower the bed rail if up.

22 Position the person for oral hygiene.

23 Assist the person to rinse his or her mouth with mouthwash. Hold the kidney basin under the chin.

24 Ask the person to insert the dentures. Insert them if the person cannot.

   a Grasp the upper denture firmly with your thumb and index finger. Raise the upper lip with the other hand, and insert the denture. Use your index fingers to gently press on the denture to make sure it is securely in place.

   b Grasp the lower denture securely with your thumb and index finger. Pull down slightly on the lower lip, and insert the denture. Gently press down on it to make sure it is in place.

Continued

✦ PROVIDING DENTURE CARE—cont'd

PROCEDURE—cont'd

25 Put the denture cup in the top drawer of the bedside stand if the dentures are not reinserted.

26 Remove the towel.

27 Remove the gloves.

POST-PROCEDURE

28 Make sure the person is comfortable.

29 Make sure the call bell is within reach.

30 Raise or lower bed rails as instructed by the RN.

31 Unscreen the person.

32 Clean and return equipment to its proper place. Discard disposable items.

33 Follow agency policy for dirty linen.

34 Wash your hands.

35 Report your observations to the RN.

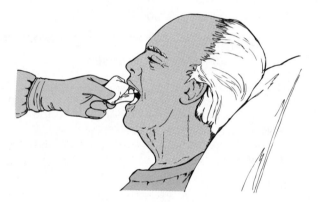

Fig. 14-6 *Remove the upper denture by grasping it with the thumb and index finger of one hand. Use a piece of gauze to grasp the slippery denture.*

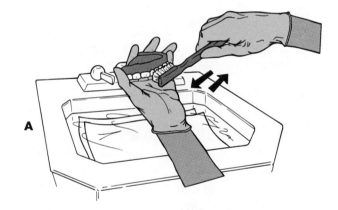

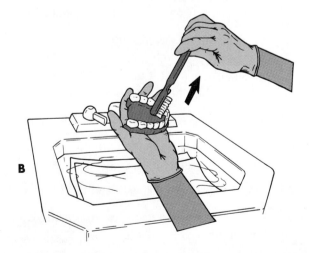

Fig. 14-7 **A,** *Outer surfaces of the upper denture are brushed with back-and-forth motions. Note that the denture is held over the sink, which is filled halfway with water and lined with a towel.* **B,** *Position the brush vertically to clean the inner surfaces of the denture. Use upward strokes.*

BOX 14-1

RULES FOR BATHING

- Ask the RN what type of bath a person is to have.
- Find out which skin care products to use. Allow personal choice when possible.
- Assist the person to the bathroom or offer the commode, bedpan, or urinal. Bathing usually stimulates the need to urinate. Comfort and relaxation increase if urination needs are met.
- Collect equipment before starting the procedure.
- Protect the person's privacy. Properly screen the person, and close doors.
- Cover the person for warmth and privacy.
- Reduce drafts by closing doors and windows.
- Protect the person from falling.
- Use good body mechanics at all times.
- Make sure water temperature is not too hot, particularly for older persons.
- Keep soap in the soap dish between latherings. This prevents soapy water. If a tub bath is taken, the person will not slip on the soap.
- Wash from the cleanest to the dirtiest areas.
- Encourage the person to help as much as is safely possible.
- Rinse the skin thoroughly to remove all soap.
- Pat the skin dry to avoid irritating or breaking the skin.
- Bathe the skin whenever feces or urine is on the skin.

BATHING

Bathing cleans the skin and mucous membranes of the genital and anal areas. Microbes, dead skin, perspiration, and excess oils are removed. A bath also is refreshing and relaxing. Circulation is stimulated and body parts exercised. You make observations during the bath. The bath also gives you time to get to know the person.

A person may get a complete or partial bed bath, a tub bath, or a shower. The method depends on the person's condition, self-care abilities, and personal choice. Bathing usually occurs after breakfast. However, a person who normally bathes at bedtime should continue the practice if possible.

Bathing frequency is a personal matter. Some people bathe daily. Others take a complete bath only once or twice a week. Personal choice, weather, physical activity, and illness affect how often a person bathes. Illness usually increases the need for bathing because of fever and increased perspiration. Other illnesses and dry skin may require bathing every 2 or 3 days.

The rules for bed baths, showers, and tub baths are listed in Box 14-1. Table 14-1 on p. 304 describes common skin care products. (See Focus on Children and Focus on Older Persons.)

focus on CHILDREN

Younger and school-age children may not bathe every day. The RN collects information about the child's bathing practices on admission. The child's nursing care plan reflects the child's normal practices and needs during illness.

focus on OLDER PERSONS

Age affects bathing frequency. Dry skin occurs with aging. Soap also dries the skin. Dry skin is easily damaged. Therefore older persons usually need a complete bath once a week. Partial baths are taken the other days. Some bathe daily but do not always use soap. Thorough rinsing is essential when using soap. Lotions and oils help keep the skin soft.

TABLE 14-1 COMMON SKIN CARE PRODUCTS

Type	Purpose	Nursing Care Considerations
Soaps	Clean the skin Remove dirt, dead skin, skin oil, some microbes, and perspiration	Tend to dry and irritate the skin Dry skin is easily injured and causes itching and discomfort Skin must be rinsed well to remove all soap Not needed for every bath; plain water can clean the skin Plain water is often used for older persons because of dry skin People with dry skin may prefer soaps containing bath oils Not used if a person has very dry skin
Bath oils	Keep the skin soft and prevent drying	Some soaps contain bath oil Liquid bath oil can be added to bath water Showers and tubs become slippery from bath oils; safety precautions are necessary to prevent falls
Creams and lotions	Protect the skin from the drying effect of air and evaporation	Do not feel greasy but leave an oily film on the skin Most are scented
Powders	Absorb moisture and prevent friction when two skin surfaces rub together	Usually applied under the breasts, under the arms, and in the groin area, and sometimes between the toes Applied to dry skin in a thin, even layer Excessive amounts cause caking and crusts that can irritate skin
Deodorants	Mask and control body odors	Applied to the axillae (under arms) Not applied to irritated skin Do not take the place of bathing
Antiperspirants	Reduce the amount of perspiration	Applied to the axillae (under arms) Not applied to irritated skin Do not take the place of bathing

Observations

Observe the skin during bathing procedures. Report the following observations to the RN:

- The color of the skin, lips, nail beds, and sclera (whites of the eyes)
- The location and description of rashes
- Dry skin
- Bruises or open skin areas
- Pale or reddened areas, particularly over bony parts
- Drainage or bleeding from wounds or body openings
- Skin temperature
- Complaints of pain or discomfort

✦ The Complete Bed Bath

The *complete bed bath* involves washing the person's entire body in bed. Persons who are unconscious, paralyzed, in a cast or traction, or weak from illness or surgery generally require bed baths. You give complete bed baths to persons who cannot bathe themselves.

Ask the RN about the person's ability to assist with the bath. Also ask about any activity or position limits. Remember to follow Standard Precautions and the Bloodborne Pathogen Standard.

A bed bath is often a new experience for patients. Some are embarrassed to have another person see their bodies. Some persons fear exposure. Every person must get an explanation about the bed bath procedure and how the body is covered to protect privacy.

The following bed bath procedure is for adults. (See Focus on Children and Focus on Older Persons.)

Text continued on p. 311

focus on CHILDREN

See Chapter 34 for bathing infants. Follow the adult procedure for bathing toddlers and older children. Infants and young children have fragile skin. Lower water temperatures are used. Ask the RN about what water temperature to use.

focus on OLDER PERSONS

Older persons also have fragile skin. Lower water temperatures are used. Ask the RN about what water temperature to use.

✦ GIVING A COMPLETE BED BATH

PRE-PROCEDURE

1 Identify the person. Check the ID bracelet, and call the person by name.

2 Explain the procedure to the person.

3 Offer the bedpan or urinal. Provide for privacy.

4 Wash your hands.

5 Collect clean linen for a closed bed. Place linen on a clean surface.

6 Collect the following:

- Wash basin

- Soap dish with soap

- Bath thermometer

- Orange stick or nail file

- Washcloth

- Two bath towels and two face towels

- Bath blanket

- Gown or pajamas

- Equipment for oral hygiene

- Body lotion

- Talcum powder

- Deodorant or antiperspirant

- Brush and comb

- Other toilet articles if requested

- Paper towels

- Gloves

Continued

GIVING A COMPLETE BED BATH—cont'd

PROCEDURE

7 Arrange items on the overbed table. Adjust the height as needed. Use the bedside stand if necessary.

8 Close doors and windows to prevent drafts.

9 Provide for privacy.

10 Raise the bed to the best level for good body mechanics.

11 Remove the call bell, and lower the bed rail near you.

12 Provide oral hygiene.

13 Remove top linens, and cover the person with a bath blanket (see *Making an Occupied Bed*, p. 282).

14 Lower the head of the bed to a level appropriate for the person. Keep it as flat as possible. Let the person have at least one pillow.

15 Place paper towels on the overbed table.

16 Raise the bed rail near you. Go fill the wash basin. (Both bed rails must be up.)

17 Fill the wash basin 2/3 full with water. Water temperature should be 110° to 115° F (43° to 46° C) for adults. These higher water temperatures are needed because the water cools rapidly.

18 Place the basin on the overbed table on top of the paper towels.

19 Lower the bed rail.

20 Place a face towel over the person's chest.

21 Make a mitt with the washcloth (Fig. 14-8, p. 308). Use a mitt throughout the procedure.

22 Wash around the person's eyes with water. Do not use soap. Gently wipe from the inner aspect with a corner of the mitt (Fig. 14-9, p. 308). Clean around the far eye first. Repeat this step for around the near eye.

23 Ask the person if you should use soap to wash the face.

24 Wash the face, ears, and neck. Rinse and dry the skin well using the towel on the chest.

25 Help the person move to the side of the bed near you.

26 Remove the gown. Do not expose the person.

27 Place a bath towel lengthwise under the far arm.

28 Support the arm with your palm under the person's elbow. His or her forearm rests on your forearm.

29 Wash the arm, shoulder, and underarm with long, firm strokes (Fig. 14-10, p. 308). Rinse and pat dry.

30 Place the basin on the towel. Put the person's hand into the water (Fig. 14-11, p. 309). Wash it well. Clean under fingernails with an orange stick or nail file.

31 Encourage the person to exercise the hand and fingers.

32 Remove the basin, and dry the hand well. Cover the arm with the bath blanket.

33 Repeat steps 27 to 32 for the near arm.

34 Place a bath towel over the chest crosswise. Hold the towel in place, and pull the bath blanket from under the towel to the waist.

35 Lift the towel slightly, and wash the chest (Fig. 14-12, p. 309). Do not expose the person. Rinse and pat dry, especially under breasts.

36 Move the towel lengthwise over the chest and abdomen. Do not expose the person. Pull the bath blanket down to the pubic area.

37 Lift the towel slightly, and wash the abdomen (Fig. 14-13, p. 310). Rinse and pat dry.

38 Pull the bath blanket up to the shoulders, covering both arms. Remove the towel.

39 Change the water if it is soapy or cool. Raise the bed rail before you leave the bedside. Lower it when you return.

40 Uncover the far leg. Do not expose the genital area. Place a towel lengthwise under the foot and leg.

GIVING A COMPLETE BED BATH—cont'd

PROCEDURE—cont'd

41 Bend the knee and support the leg with your arm. Wash it with long, firm strokes. Rinse and pat dry.

42 Place the basin on the towel near the foot.

43 Lift the leg slightly. Slide the basin under the foot.

44 Place the foot in the basin (Fig. 14-14, p. 310). Use an orange stick or nail file to clean under toenails if necessary.

45 Remove the basin, and dry the leg. Cover the leg with the bath blanket. Remove the towel.

46 Repeat steps 40 to 45 for the near leg.

47 Change the water. Raise the bed rail before leaving the bedside. Lower it when you return.

48 Turn the person onto the side away from you. Keep him or her covered with the bath blanket.

49 Uncover the back and buttocks. Do not expose the person. Place a towel lengthwise on the bed along the back.

50 Wash the back, working from the back of the neck to the lower end of the buttocks. Use long, firm, continuous strokes (Fig. 14-15, p. 310). Rinse and dry well.

51 Give a back massage. (The person may prefer to have the back massage after the bath.)

52 Turn the person onto his or her back.

53 Change the water for perineal care. Raise the bed rail before you leave the bedside. Lower it when you return.

54 Let the person wash the genital area. Adjust the overbed table so he or she can reach the wash basin, soap, and towels with ease. Place the call bell within reach. Ask the person to signal when finished. Make sure the person understands what to do. Answer the call bell promptly. Provide perineal care if the person cannot do so (see *Perineal Care,* p. 318).

55 Give a back massage if you have not already done so.

56 Apply deodorant or antiperspirant. Apply lotion and powder as directed by the RN or as requested by the person. Use only a thin layer of powder.

57 Put a clean gown or pajamas on the person.

58 Comb and brush the hair.

59 Make the bed. Attach the call bell.

POST-PROCEDURE

60 Make sure the person is comfortable.

61 Lower the bed to its lowest position.

62 Raise or lower bed rails as instructed by the RN.

63 Empty and clean the wash basin. Return it and other supplies to their proper place.

64 Wipe off the overbed table with the paper towels and discard them.

65 Unscreen the person.

66 Follow agency policy for dirty linen.

67 Wash your hands.

68 Report your observations to the RN (see p. 304).

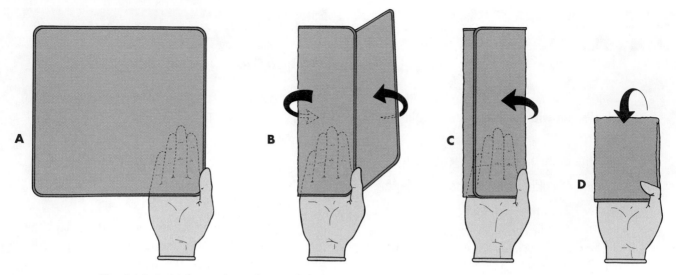

Fig. 14-8 A, *Make a mitt with a washcloth by grasping the near side of the washcloth with your thumb.* **B,** *Bring the washcloth around and behind your hand.* **C,** *Fold the side of the washcloth over your palm as you grasp it with your thumb.* **D,** *Fold the top of the washcloth down and tuck it under next to your palm.*

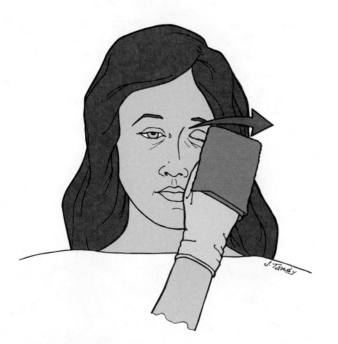

Fig. 14-9 *Wash around the person's eyes with a mitted washcloth. Wipe from the inner to the outer aspect of the eye.*

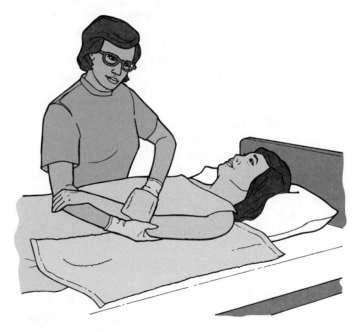

Fig. 14-10 *Wash the person's arm with firm, long strokes using a mitted washcloth.*

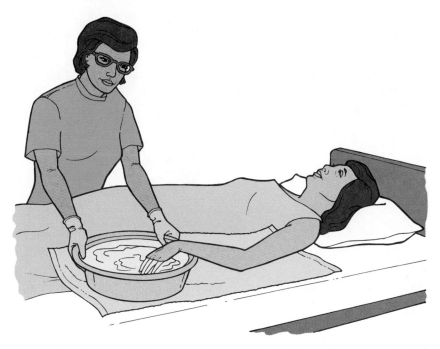

Fig. 14-11 *The person's hands are washed by placing the wash basin on the bed.*

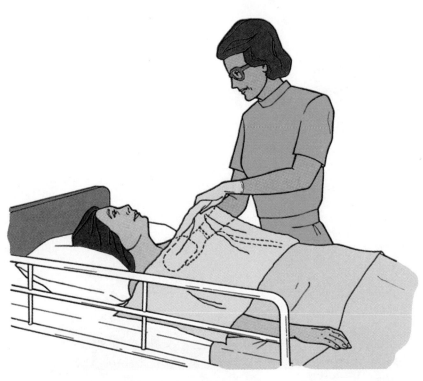

Fig. 14-12 *The person's breasts are not exposed during the bath. A bath towel is placed horizontally over the chest area. The towel is lifted slightly to reach under to wash the breasts and chest.*

Fig. 14-13 *The bath towel is turned so that it is vertical to cover the breasts and abdomen. The towel is lifted slightly to bathe the abdomen. The bath blanket covers the pubic area.*

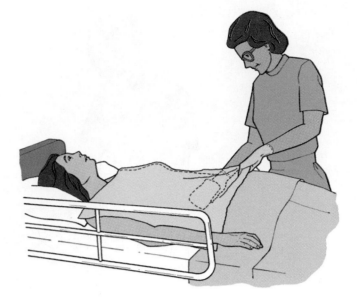

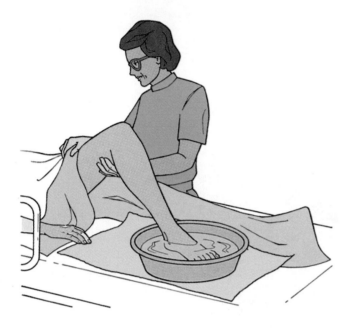

Fig. 14-14 *The foot is washed by placing it in the wash basin on the bed.*

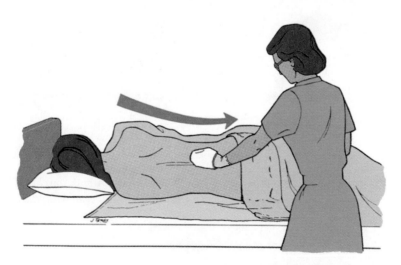

Fig. 14-15 *The back is washed with long, firm, continuous strokes. Note that the person is in a side-lying position. A towel is placed lengthwise on the bed to protect the linens from water.*

✦ The Partial Bath

The partial bath involves bathing the face, hands, axillae (underarms), genital and rectal areas, back, and buttocks. These areas develop odors or cause discomfort if not clean. You give partial bed baths to persons who cannot bathe themselves. Persons who are able bathe themselves in bed or at the bathroom sink. You assist as needed, especially with washing the back.

The general rules for bathing apply for partial bed baths. The considerations involved in giving a complete bed bath also apply.

GIVING A PARTIAL BATH

PRE-PROCEDURE

1 Follow steps 1 through 9 in *Giving a Complete Bed Bath,* p. 305.

PROCEDURE

2 Make sure the bed is in the lowest position.

3 Assist with oral hygiene. Adjust the height of the overbed table to an appropriate level.

4 Remove top linen. Cover the person with a bath blanket.

5 Place the paper towels on the overbed table.

6 Fill the wash basin with water. Water temperature should be 110° to 115° F (43° to 46° C) for adults.

7 Place the basin on the overbed table on top of the paper towels.

8 Raise the head of the bed so the person can bathe comfortably. Assist him or her to sit at the bedside if allowed this position.

9 Position the overbed table so the person can easily reach the basin and supplies.

10 Help the person remove the gown or pajamas.

11 Ask the person to wash easy-to-reach body parts (Fig. 14-16, p. 312). Explain that you will wash the back and those areas that cannot be reached.

12 Place the call bell within reach. Ask him or her to signal if help is needed or when bathing is complete.

13 Leave the room after washing your hands.

14 Return when the call light is on. Knock before entering.

15 Change the bath water.

16 Ask what was washed. Wash areas the person could not reach. The face, hands, axillae, genital and rectal areas, back, and buttocks are washed for the partial bath.

17 Give a back massage.

18 Apply lotion, powder, and deodorant or antiperspirant.

19 Help the person put on a clean gown or pajamas.

20 Assist with hair care.

21 Assist him or her to a chair. Otherwise, turn the person onto the side away from you.

22 Make the bed.

23 Lower the bed to its lowest position.

24 Assist the person to return to bed.

Continued

GIVING A PARTIAL BATH—cont'd

POST-PROCEDURE

25 Make sure the person is comfortable.

26 Place the call bell within reach.

27 Raise or lower bed rails as instructed by the RN.

28 Empty and clean the basin. Return the basin and supplies to their proper place.

29 Wipe off the overbed table with the paper towels and discard them.

30 Unscreen the person.

31 Follow agency policy for dirty linen.

32 Wash your hands.

33 Report your observations to the RN (see p. 304).

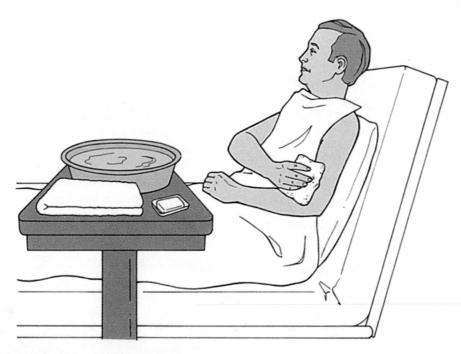

Fig. 14-16 *The person is bathing himself in bed. Necessary equipment is within his reach.*

⬥ Tub Baths and Showers

Many people prefer tub baths or showers. However, burns from hot water and falls are risks. A tub bath can cause a person to feel faint, weak, or tired. These are greater risks for persons who were on bed rest. A bath lasts no longer than 20 minutes. The RN's approval is needed for a person to take a tub bath.

Some patients use shower chairs. Shower chairs are made of plastic or metal and have wheels on the legs. The shower chair is wheeled into the shower stall. Water drains through a round open area in the seat. The wheels are locked during the shower so the chair does not move.

Some rooms have private baths or showers. If not, reserve the tub or shower room. Also clean the tub or shower before use. This prevents the spread of microbes and infection. The person is protected from falls and chilling. Practice these safety measures for tub baths and showers:

- Place a bath mat in the tub or on the shower floor, unless there are nonskid strips or a nonskid surface.
- Place needed items within the person's reach. This includes the call bell.
- Drain the tub before the person gets out of the tub. Keep the person covered to protect from exposure and chilling.
- Have the person use safety bars when getting into and out of the tub.

- Avoid using bath oils. They make tub and shower surfaces slippery.
- Do not leave weak or unsteady persons unattended.
- Stay within hearing distance of the shower or tub if the person can be left alone. Wait outside the shower curtain or door. You will be nearby if the person calls for you or has an accident.
- Have the person use safety bars for support when getting into or out of the tub or shower.

(See Focus on Children.)

Some agencies have portable tubs. The sides are lowered, and the person is transferred from the bed to the tub. Then the sides are raised. The person is transported to the tub room in the portable tub. The tub is filled and the person bathed in the usual manner. After the bath the tub is drained. The person is transported back to the room in the tub.

focus on CHILDREN

Many older children enjoy showers. The RN tells you how much help and supervision to give the child. Remember, independence is important to older children.

⬥ ASSISTING WITH A TUB BATH OR SHOWER

PRE-PROCEDURE

1 Reserve the bathtub or shower if necessary.

2 Identify the person. Check the ID bracelet, and call the person by name.

3 Explain the procedure to the person.

4 Wash your hands.

5 Collect the following:

- Washcloth and two bath towels

- Soap

- Bath thermometer (for a tub bath)

- Clean gown or pajamas

- Deodorant and other toilet articles as requested

- Robe and nonskid slippers or shoes

- Rubber bath mat if needed

- Disposable bath mat

Continued

ASSISTING WITH A TUB BATH OR SHOWER

PROCEDURE

6 Place items in the bathroom or shower room in the space provided or on a chair.

7 Clean the tub or shower if needed.

8 Place a rubber bath mat in the tub or on the shower floor. Do not block the drain.

9 Place a disposable bath mat on the floor in front of the tub or shower.

10 Put the *occupied* sign on the door.

11 Return to the person's room. Provide for privacy.

12 Help the person sit on the side of the bed.

13 Help the person put on a robe and slippers.

14 Assist the person to the bathroom or shower room. Use a wheelchair if necessary.

15 *For a tub bath:*

   a Have the person sit on the chair by the tub.

   b Fill the tub halfway with warm water (105° F; 41° C).

   For a shower:

   a Turn on the shower.

   b Adjust water temperature and pressure.

16 Help the person remove slippers, robe, and gown.

17 Assist the person into the tub or shower (Fig. 14-17). If using a shower chair, place it in position and lock the wheels.

18 Assist with washing if necessary.

19 Ask the person to use the call bell when done or when help is needed.

20 Remind the person not to stay in the tub longer than 20 minutes.

21 Place a towel across the chair.

22 Leave the room only if the person can be left unattended. Otherwise stay in the room or remain nearby. Wash your hands if you leave the room.

23 Check the person every 5 minutes.

24 Return when he or she signals for you. Knock before entering.

25 Turn off the shower.

26 Help the person out of the tub or shower and onto the chair.

27 Help the person dry off. Pat gently.

28 Assist with lotion, powder, and deodorant or antiperspirant as needed.

29 Help the person put on a clean gown or pajamas, a bathrobe, and slippers or shoes.

30 Help the person return to the room and to bed.

31 Provide a back massage.

32 Assist with hair care.

33 Make sure the person is comfortable.

34 Raise or lower side rails as instructed by the nurse.

35 Place the call bell within reach.

36 Clean the tub or shower. Remove soiled linen, and discard disposable items. Put the *unoccupied* sign on the door. Return supplies to their proper place.

37 Follow agency policy for dirty linen.

38 Wash your hands.

39 Report your observations to the nurse.

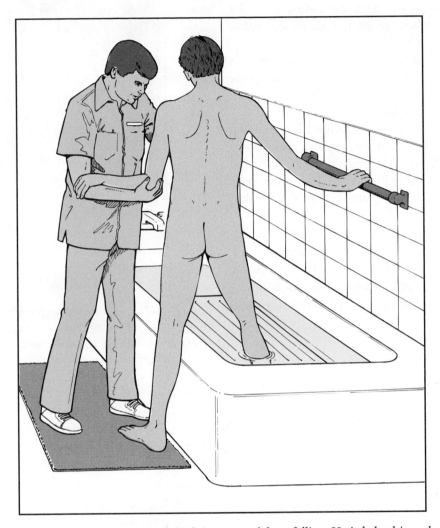

Fig. 14-17 *The person taking a tub bath is protected from falling. He is helped into the tub. A bath mat is in the tub, the tub is filled halfway with water, and a floor mat is in front of the tub.*

✦ THE BACK MASSAGE

The back massage (back rub) relaxes muscles and stimulates circulation. A massage is normally given after the bath and with HS care. It should last 3 to 5 minutes. Observe the skin before starting the procedure. Look for breaks in the skin, bruises, reddened areas, and other signs of skin breakdown.

Lotion reduces friction when giving the massage. It is warmed before being applied. Warm lotion by placing the bottle in the bath water or holding it under warm water. Or rub some between your hands.

The prone position is best for a massage. The side-lying position is often used. Use firm strokes, and always keep your hands in contact with the person's skin. After the massage, apply some lotion to the elbows, knees, and heels to keep the skin soft. These bony areas are at risk for skin breakdown.

Some persons should not have back massages as described in this procedure. They are dangerous for those with certain heart diseases, back injuries, back surgeries, skin diseases, and some lung disorders. Check with the RN before giving back massages to persons with these conditions.

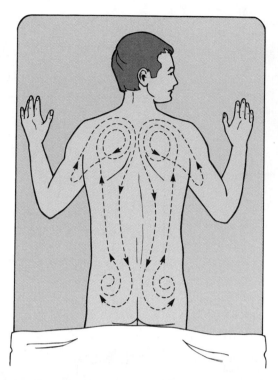

Fig. 14-18 *The person lies in the prone position for a back massage. Stroke upward from the buttocks to the shoulders, down over the upper arms, back up the upper arms, across the shoulders, and down the back to the buttocks.*

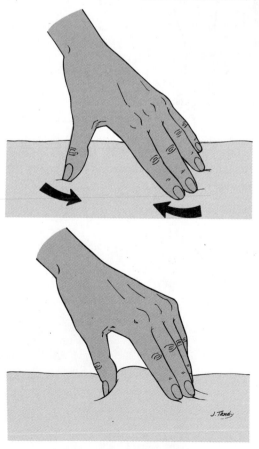

Fig. 14-19 *Kneading is done by picking up tissue between the thumb and fingers.*

GIVING A BACK MASSAGE

PRE-PROCEDURE

1 Identify the person. Check the ID bracelet, and call the person by name.

2 Explain the procedure to the person.

3 Wash your hands.

4 Collect the following:

- Bath blanket

- Bath towel

- Lotion

5 Provide for privacy.

6 Raise the bed to the best level for good body mechanics.

PROCEDURE

7 Lower the bed rail.

8 Position the person in the prone or side-lying position with the back toward you.

9 Expose the back, shoulders, upper arms, and buttocks. Cover the rest of the body with the bath blanket.

10 Lay the towel on the bed along the back.

11 Warm some lotion between your hands.

12 Explain that the lotion may feel cool and wet.

13 Apply lotion to the lower back area.

14 Stroke up from the buttocks to the shoulders. Then stroke down over the upper arms. Stroke up the upper arms, across the shoulders, and down the back to the buttocks (Fig. 14-18). Use firm strokes. Keep your hands in contact with the person's skin.

15 Repeat step 14 for at least 3 minutes.

16 Knead by grasping skin between your thumb and fingers (Fig. 14-19). Knead half of the back starting at the buttocks and moving up to the shoulder. Then knead down from the shoulder to the buttocks. Repeat on the other half of the back.

17 Massage bony areas. Use circular motions with the tips of your index and middle fingers.

18 Use fast movements to stimulate and slow movements to relax the person.

19 Stroke with long, firm movements to end the massage. Tell the person you are finishing.

20 Cover the person. Remove the towel and bath blanket.

POST-PROCEDURE

21 Make sure the person is comfortable.

22 Lower the bed to its lowest position.

23 Raise or lower bed rails as instructed by the RN.

24 Place the call bell within reach.

25 Return lotion to its proper place.

26 Unscreen the person.

27 Follow agency policy for dirty linen.

28 Wash your hands.

29 Report your observations to the RN.

✦ PERINEAL CARE

Perineal care (pericare) involves cleaning the genital and anal areas. These areas are warm, moist, and dark. They provide a place for microbes to grow. The genital and anal areas are cleaned to prevent infection and odors and to promote comfort.

Perineal care is done at least daily during the bath. The procedure is also done whenever the area is soiled with urine or feces. Persons with certain disorders need perineal care more often. It is given before and after some surgeries and after childbirth.

Patients do their own perineal care if able. Otherwise it is given by nursing staff. Many people and nursing staff find the procedure embarrassing, especially when given to the other sex. People may not know the terms *perineum* and *perineal*. Most understand *privates, private parts, crotch, genitals*, or the *area between your legs*. Use terms the person understands. The term must also be in good taste professionally.

Standard Precautions, medical asepsis, and the Bloodborne Pathogen Standard are followed. Work from the cleanest area to the dirtiest. The urethral area is the clean-

est, the anal area the dirtiest. Therefore clean from the urethra to the anal area. The perineal area is very delicate and easily injured. Use warm water, not hot. Washcloths are used if pericare is part of the bath. The RN may have you use cotton balls or swabs at other times. The area is rinsed thoroughly. Pat dry after rinsing to reduce moisture and promote comfort. (See Focus on Children.)

Text continued on p. 323

focus on CHILDREN

Children of all ages need perineal care. In children who wear diapers, the perineal area is often exposed to urine and feces. Inadequate wiping after urinating and bowel movements is a common problem in younger children. Older children may hesitate to clean the genital and anal areas.

✦ GIVING FEMALE PERINEAL CARE

PRE-PROCEDURE

1 Explain the procedure to the person.

2 Wash your hands.

3 Collect the following:

- Soap dish with soap

- At least four washcloths

- Bath towel

- Bath blanket

- Bath thermometer

- Waterproof pad

- Gloves

- Paper towels

4 Arrange items on the overbed table.

5 Identify the person. Check the ID bracelet, and call her by name.

6 Provide for privacy.

7 Raise the bed to the best level for good body mechanics.

PROCEDURE

8 Lower the bed rail.

9 Cover the person with a bath blanket. Move top linens to the foot of the bed.

10 Position the person on her back.

11 Position the waterproof pad under her buttocks.

12 Drape the person as in Figure 14-20 on p. 320.

13 Raise the bed rail.

GIVING FEMALE PERINEAL CARE—cont'd

PROCEDURE—cont'd

14 Fill the wash basin. Water temperature is about 105° to 109° F (41° to 43° C).

15 Place the basin on the overbed table on top of the paper towels.

16 Lower the bed rail.

17 Help the person flex her knees and spread her legs.

18 Put on the gloves.

19 Fold the corner of the bath blanket between the person's legs onto her abdomen.

20 Wet the washcloths. Squeeze out excess water from washcloths before using them.

21 Apply soap to a washcloth.

22 Separate the labia. Clean downward from front to back with one stroke (Fig. 14-21, p. 321).

23 Repeat steps 21 and 22 until the area is clean. Use a different part of the washcloth for each stroke.

24 Rinse the perineum with a clean washcloth. Separate the labia. Stroke downward from front to back. Repeat the step as necessary. Use a different part of the washcloth for each stroke.

25 Pat the area dry with the towel.

26 Fold the blanket back between her legs.

27 Help the person lower her legs and turn onto her side away from you.

28 Apply soap to a washcloth.

29 Clean the rectal area. Clean from the vagina to the anus with one stroke (Fig. 14-22, p. 321).

30 Repeat steps 28 and 29 until the area is clean. Use a different part of the washcloth for each stroke.

31 Rinse the rectal area with a washcloth. Stroke from the vagina to the anus. Repeat the step as necessary using a different part of the washcloth for each stroke.

32 Pat the area dry with the towel.

33 Remove and discard the gloves.

POST-PROCEDURE

34 Position the person so she is comfortable.

35 Return linens to their proper position, and remove the bath blanket.

36 Lower the bed to its lowest position.

37 Raise or lower bed rails as instructed by the RN.

38 Place the call bell within reach.

39 Empty and clean the wash basin.

40 Return the basin and supplies to their proper place.

41 Wipe off the overbed table with the paper towels and discard them.

42 Unscreen the person.

43 Follow agency policy for dirty linen.

44 Wash your hands.

45 Report your observations to the RN:
  • Any odors
  • Redness, swelling, discharge, or irritation
  • Complaints of pain, burning, or other discomfort

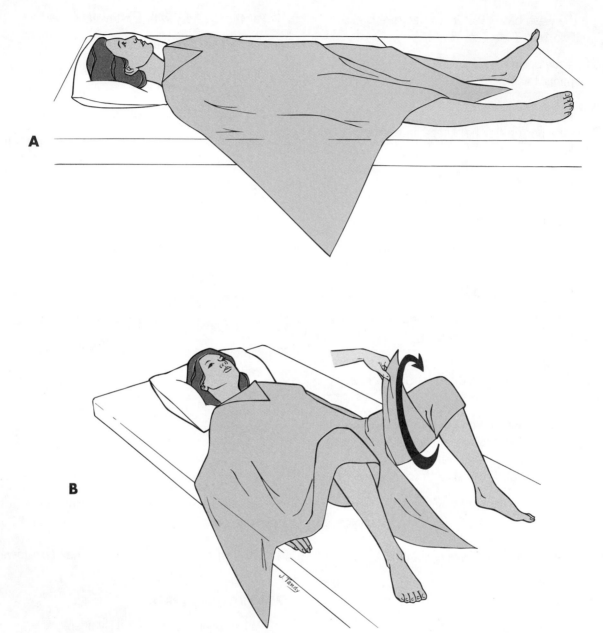

Fig. 14-20 **A,** *Drape the person for perineal care by positioning the bath blanket like a diamond: one corner is at the neck, there is a corner at each side, and one corner is between the person's legs.* **B,** *Wrap the blanket around the leg by bringing the corner around under the leg and over the top. Tuck the corner under the hip.*

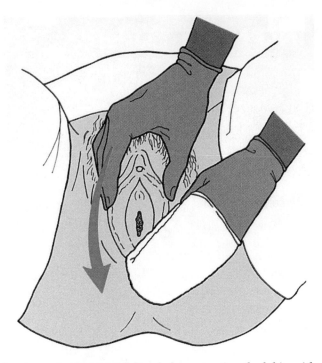

Fig. 14-21 *Perineal care is given to the female by separating the labia with one hand. Use a mitted washcloth to cleanse between the labia with downward strokes.*

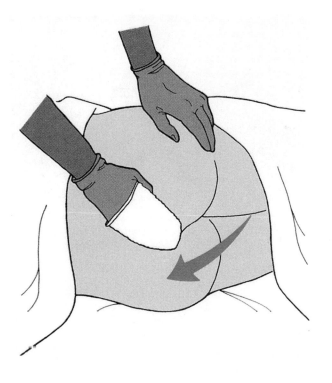

Fig. 14-22 *The rectal area is cleaned by wiping from the vagina to the anus. The side-lying position allows the anal area to be cleaned more thoroughly.*

GIVING MALE PERINEAL CARE

PRE-PROCEDURE

1   Follow steps 1 through 21 in *Female Perineal Care*, p 318.

PROCEDURE

2   Retract the foreskin if the person is uncircumcised (Fig. 14-23).

3   Grasp the penis.

4   Clean the tip using a circular motion. Start at the urethral opening and work outward (Fig. 14-24). Repeat this step as necessary. Use a different part of the washcloth each time.

5   Rinse the area with another washcloth.

6   Return the foreskin to its natural position.

7   Clean the shaft of the penis with firm downward strokes. Rinse the area.

8   Help the person flex his knees and spread his legs.

9   Clean the scrotum and rinse well.

10   Pat dry the penis and scrotum.

11   Fold the bath blanket back between his legs.

12   Help him lower his legs and turn onto his side away from you.

13   Clean the rectal area (see *Female Perineal Care*). Rinse and dry well.

14   Remove and discard the gloves.

POST-PROCEDURE

15   Follow steps 34 through 45 in *Female Perineal Care.*

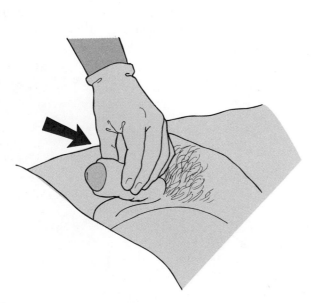

Fig. 14-23 *The foreskin of the uncircumcised male is pulled back for perineal care. It is returned to the normal position immediately after cleaning.*

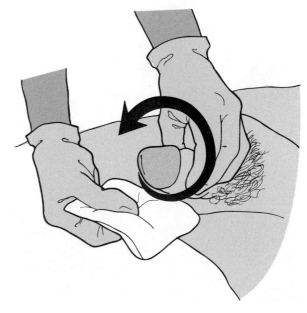

Fig. 14-24 *The penis is cleaned with circular motions starting at the urethra.*

PRESSURE ULCERS

A **pressure ulcer (decubitus ulcer, bedsore, pressure sore)** is any injury caused by unrelieved pressure. It usually occurs over a bony prominence. Prominence means to stick out. Therefore a bony prominence is an area where the bone sticks out or projects out from the flat surface of the body. The shoulder blades, elbows, hip bones, sacrum, knees, ankle bone, heels, and toes are bony prominences.

Causes

Pressure, friction, and shearing are common causes of skin breakdown and pressure ulcers. Other factors include breaks in the skin, poor circulation to an area, moisture, dry skin, and irritation by urine and feces.

Pressure occurs when the skin over a bony prominence is squeezed between hard surfaces. The bone itself is one hard surface. The other is usually the mattress. The squeezing or pressure prevents blood flow to the skin and underlying tissues. Lack of blood flow means oxygen and nutrients cannot get to the cells. Therefore the involved skin and tissues die (Fig. 14-25).

Friction scrapes the skin. An open area, the scrape is a portal of entry for microbes. The open area needs to heal. A good blood supply to the area is necessary. Infection is prevented so healing occurs. A poor blood supply or an infection can lead to a pressure ulcer.

Shearing is when the skin sticks to a surface (usually the bed or chair) and deeper tissues move downward (see Fig. 12-12, p. 241). This occurs when a person is sitting in a chair or in Fowler's position. Shearing occurs when the person slides down in the bed or chair. Blood vessels and tissues are damaged. Therefore blood flow to the area is reduced.

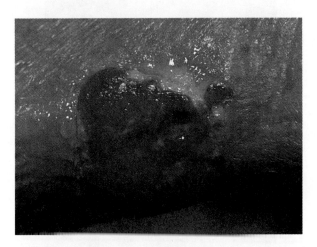

Fig. 14-25 *A pressure ulcer.*

Focus on

CHILDREN

Infants and children also are at risk for pressure ulcers. Pressure, friction, and shearing are causes. **Epidermal stripping** is another cause, especially in newborns. Epidermal stripping is removing the epidermis (outer skin layer) with tape. Remember, newborns have fragile skin. Risk factors for pressure ulcers in infants and children include poor mobility, lack of bowel and bladder control (incontinence), and poor nutrition. Infection is another risk factor.

Persons at Risk

Persons at risk for pressure ulcers are those who:
- Are confined to bed or chair
- Are unable to move
- Have loss of bowel or bladder control
- Have poor nutrition
- Have altered mental awareness
- Have problems sensing pain or pressure
- Have circulatory problems
- Are older, obese, very thin, or malnourished

(See Focus on Children.)

Signs of Pressure Ulcers

The first sign of a pressure ulcer is pale skin or a reddened area. The person may complain of pain, burning, or tingling in the area. Some do not feel anything unusual. Box 14-2 on p. 324 describes the four stages of pressure ulcer development.

Sites

Pressure ulcers usually occur over bony areas. The bony areas are called *pressure points* because they bear the weight of the body in a certain position. Pressure from body weight can reduce the blood supply to the area. Figure 14-27 on pp. 325-326 shows the pressure points for the bed positions and the sitting position. In obese people, pressure ulcers can develop in areas where skin is in contact with skin. Friction results when this occurs. Pressure ulcers can develop between abdominal folds, the legs, and the buttocks and underneath the breasts.

Text continued on p. 326

STAGES OF PRESSURE ULCERS

Stage 1 The skin is red. The color does not return to normal when the skin is relieved of pressure (Fig. 14-26, *A*).

Stage 2 The skin cracks, blisters, or peels (Fig. 14-26, *B*). There may be a shallow crater.

Stage 3 The skin is gone, and the underlying tissues are exposed (Fig. 14-26, *C*). The exposed tissue is damaged. There may be drainage from the area.

Stage 4 Muscle and bone are exposed and damaged (Fig. 14-26, *D*). Drainage is likely.

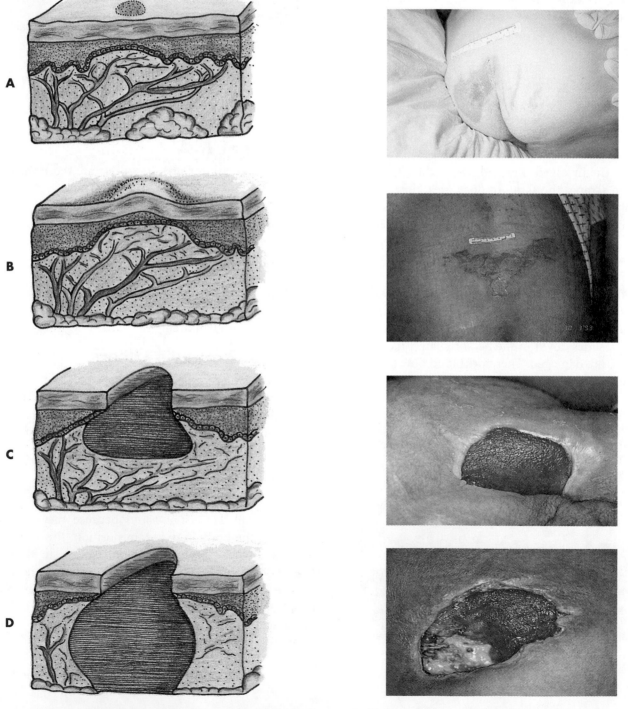

A

B

C

D

Fig. 14-26 *Stages of pressure ulcers.* **A,** *Stage 1.* **B,** *Stage 2.* **C,** *Stage 3.* **D,** *Stage 4. (From Potter PA, Perry AG:* Fundamentals of nursing: concepts, process, and practice, *ed 4, St Louis, 1997, Mosby.)*

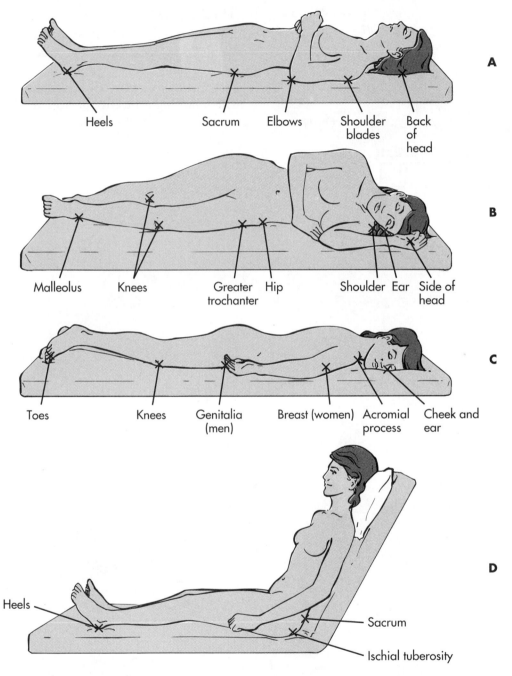

Fig. 14-27 *Pressure points.* **A,** *The supine position.* **B,** *The lateral position.* **C,** *The prone position.* **D,** *Fowler's position.*   *Continued*

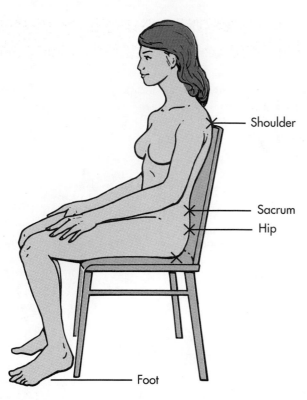

Fig. 14-27 E, *The sitting position.*

Prevention

Preventing pressure ulcers is much easier than trying to heal them. Good nursing care, cleanliness, and skin care are essential. The measures listed in Box 14-3 help prevent skin breakdown and pressure ulcers.

Treatment

Pressure ulcer treatment is directed by the doctor. Wound care (see Chapter 28), drugs, treatments, and special equipment are ordered to promote healing. The RN and nursing care plan tell you about a person's treatment. The following protective devices are often ordered.

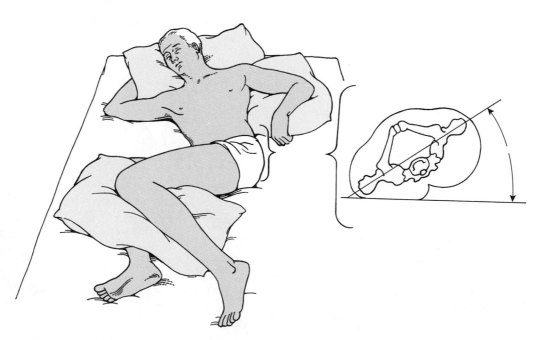

Fig. 14-28 *The 30-degree lateral position. Pillows are placed under the head, shoulder, and leg. This position inclines (lifts up) the hip to avoid pressure on the hip. The person does not lie on the hip as in the side-lying position.* (From Potter PA, Perry AG: Fundamentals of nursing: concepts, process, and practice, *ed 4, St Louis, 1997, Mosby.*)

BOX 14-3

MEASURES TO PREVENT PRESSURE ULCERS

- Reposition the person at least every 2 hours or as scheduled in the person's care plan. Some persons are repositioned every 15 minutes. Use pillows for support as instructed by the RN. The 30-degree lateral position is recommended (Fig. 14-28).
- Prevent shearing and friction during lifting and moving procedures.
- Prevent shearing by not raising the head of the bed more than 30 degrees or as instructed by the RN.
- Prevent friction by applying a thin layer of cornstarch to the bottom sheets.
- Provide good skin care. The skin must be clean and dry after bathing. Make sure the skin is free of moisture from urine, feces, perspiration, and wound drainage.
- Minimize skin exposure to moisture. Check incontinent persons (those without bowel or bladder control) often. Also check persons who perspire heavily and those with wound drainage. Change linens and clothing as needed, and provide good skin care.
- Check with the RN before using soap. Remember, soap can dry and irritate the skin.
- Apply a moisturizer to dry areas such as the hands, elbows, legs, ankles, and heels. The RN tells you what to use and the areas that need attention.
- Give a back massage when repositioning the person. Do not massage bony areas.
- Keep linens clean, dry, and free of wrinkles.
- Apply powder where skin touches skin.
- Do not irritate the skin. Avoid scrubbing or vigorous rubbing when bathing or drying the person.
- Avoid massaging over pressure points. *Never rub or massage reddened areas.*
- Use pillows and blankets to prevent skin from being in contact with skin and to reduce moisture and friction.
- Keep the heels off the bed. Use pillows or other devices as instructed by the RN. Place the pillows or devices under the lower legs from midcalf to the ankles.
- Use protective devices as instructed by the RN.
- Remind persons sitting in chairs to shift their position every 15 minutes. This decreases pressure on bony points.
- Report any signs of skin breakdown or pressure ulcers immediately to the RN.

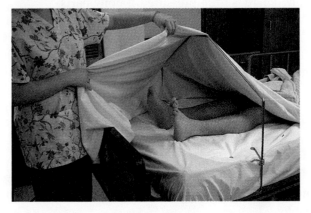

Fig. 14-29 *A bed cradle is placed on top of the bed. Linens are brought over the top of the cradle.*

Bed cradle

A bed cradle (Anderson frame) is a metal frame placed on the bed and over the patient. Top linens are brought over the cradle to prevent pressure on the legs and feet (Fig. 14-29). Top linens are tucked in at the bottom of the mattress and mitered. They are also tucked under both sides of the mattress to protect the person from air drafts and chilling. (See Focus on Home Care on p. 328.)

HOME CARE

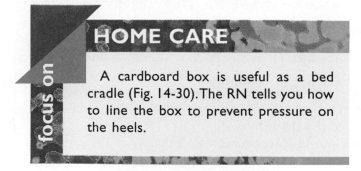

A cardboard box is useful as a bed cradle (Fig. 14-30). The RN tells you how to line the box to prevent pressure on the heels.

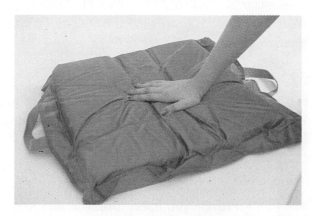

Fig. 14-31 *Flotation pad.*

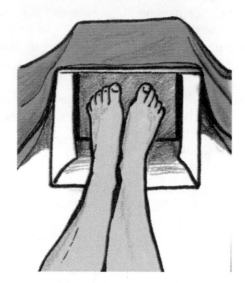

Fig. 14-30 *A box serves as a bed cradle. It keeps top linens off the person's feet.* (From Birchenall J, Streight M: Mosby's textbook for the home care aide, St Louis, 1997, Mosby.)

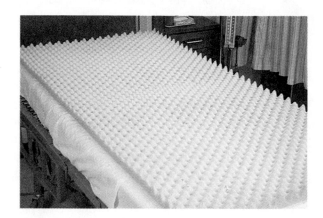

Fig. 14-32 *Eggcrate-type mattress on the bed.*

Flotation pads

Flotation pads or cushions (Fig. 14-31) are like water beds. They are made of a gel-like substance. The outer case is heavy plastic. They are used for chairs and wheelchairs. The pad is placed in a pillowcase so the plastic does not touch the skin.

Eggcrate-type mattress

The eggcrate-type mattress is a foam pad that looks like an egg carton (Fig. 14-32). Peaks in the mattress distribute the person's weight more evenly. The eggcrate-type mattress is placed on top of the regular mattress. Only a bottom sheet covers the eggcrate-type mattress. Before the bottom sheet is put on, the eggcrate-type mattress is put in a special cover. The cover protects against moisture and soiling.

Special beds

Some beds have air flowing through the mattresses. The *person floats* on the mattress. Body weight is distributed evenly. There is little pressure on bony parts.

Another type of bed allows repositioning without moving the person. Depending on the bed, the person is turned to the prone or supine position or tilted various degrees. Body alignment does not change. Pressure points change as the position changes. There is little friction.

Some beds constantly rotate from side to side. These beds are useful for persons with spinal cord injuries.

Other equipment

Trochanter rolls and footboards also are used to prevent and treat pressure ulcers. These are described in Chapter 22.

Circle T *if the statement is true or* F *if the statement is false.*

1 T F Cleanliness and skin care are needed for comfort, safety, and health.

2 T F Mrs. Boyd asks for a back massage as part of HS care. You can tell her that back massages are given during morning care.

3 T F Mrs. Boyd's toothbrush has hard bristles. They are good for oral hygiene.

4 T F Unconscious persons are supine for mouth care.

5 T F Your fingers are used to keep an unconscious person's mouth open for oral hygiene.

6 T F Mrs. Boyd has a lower denture. It is washed in warm water over a hard surface.

7 T F Bath oils cleanse and soften the skin.

8 T F Powders absorb moisture and prevent friction.

9 T F Deodorants reduce the amount of perspiration.

10 T F The RN says that Mrs. Boyd can have a tub bath. Mrs. Boyd says that she usually takes half-hour baths at home. You can let her take a 30-minute bath.

11 T F You can give permission for showers but not tub baths.

12 T F Weak persons can be left alone in the shower if they are sitting.

13 T F A back massage relaxes muscles and stimulates circulation.

14 T F Perineal care helps prevent infection.

15 T F A reddened area is the first sign of a pressure ulcer.

16 T F Bony areas are common sites for pressure ulcers.

17 T F Shearing and friction can cause pressure ulcers.

Circle the best *answer.*

18 You brush Mrs. Boyd's teeth and note the following. Which do you report to the RN?
 a Bleeding, swelling, or redness of the gums
 b Irritations, sores, or white patches in the mouth or on the tongue
 c Lips that are dry, cracked, swollen, or blistered
 d All of the above

19 Which is *not* a purpose of bathing?
 a Increasing circulation
 b Promoting drying of the skin
 c Exercising body parts
 d Refreshing and relaxing the person

20 Soaps do the following *except*
 a Remove dirt and dead skin
 b Remove pigment
 c Remove skin oil and perspiration
 d Dry the skin

21 Which action is *wrong* when bathing Mrs. Boyd?
 a Cover her for warmth and privacy.
 b Rinse her skin thoroughly to remove all soaps.
 c Wash from the dirtiest to cleanest area.
 d Pat her skin dry.

22 Water for Mrs. Boyd's complete bed bath should be at least
 a 100° F c 110° F
 b 105° F d 120° F

23 You are going to give Mrs. Boyd a back massage. Which is *incorrect*?
 a The massage should last about 5 minutes.
 b Lotion is warmed before being applied.
 c Your hands are always in contact with the skin.
 d The side-lying position is best.

24 Which will *not* prevent pressure ulcers?
 a Repositioning the person every 2 hours
 b Applying lotion to dry areas
 c Scrubbing and rubbing the skin vigorously
 d Keeping bed linens clean, dry, and free of wrinkles

Answers to these questions are on pp. 851-852.

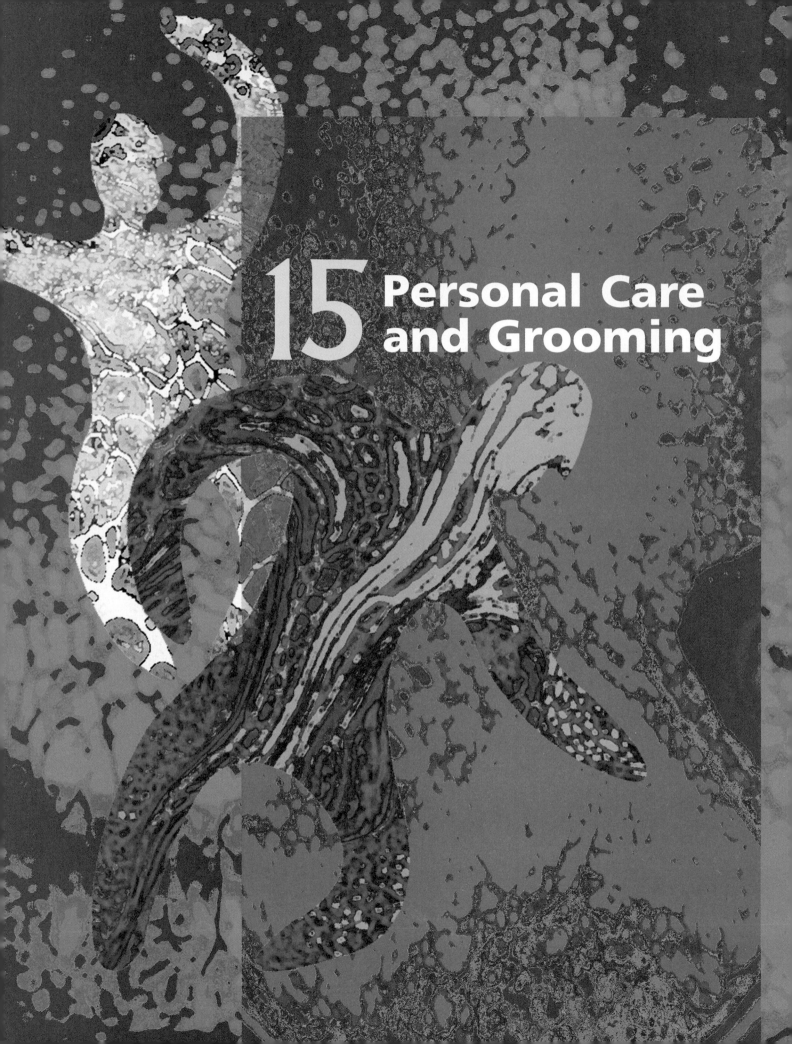

15 Personal Care and Grooming

- Define the key terms in this chapter
- Explain the importance of hair care
- Identify the factors that affect hair care
- Explain how to care for matted and tangled hair
- Describe ways to shampoo a person's hair
- Explain why shaving is important
- Identify the measures that are practiced when shaving a person
- Explain why nail and foot care are important
- Describe the rules for changing hospital gowns and clothing
- Perform the procedures described in this chapter

KEY TERMS

alopecia Hair loss

dandruff The excessive amount of dry, white flakes from the scalp

hirsutism Excessive body hair in women and children

pediculosis (lice) The infestation with lice

pediculosis capitis The infestation of the scalp *(capitis)* with lice

pediculosis corporis The infestation of the body *(corporis)* with lice

pediculosis pubis The infestation of the pubic *(pubis)* hair with lice

Cleanliness and skin care meet basic physical and safety and security needs. Clean and intact skin protects against infection. Bathing and back massage promote circulation, exercise, comfort, and relaxation. For many people, being clean is necessary for love and belonging and self-esteem needs.

Hair care, shaving, and nail care also are important to many people. People vary in how much attention they give to such matters. Some want only clean hair. Others want hair styled in a certain way. Clean hands are enough for some people. Others want nails clean, manicured, and polished. Shaving and beard grooming are important to many men. Likewise, many women shave their legs and underarms.

A simple bath often takes much energy. Acutely ill persons usually are concerned with the basic physical needs necessary for survival. Interest in other personal care and grooming measures usually increases as the person gains strength.

HAIR CARE

How the hair looks and feels affects mental well-being. Illness and disability can interfere with hair care. Patients are assisted with hair care whenever necessary.

The RN uses the nursing process to meet the person's hair care needs. Culture, personal choice, skin and scalp condition, health history, and self-care ability are considered by the RN. These terms are common in nursing care plans.

- **Alopecia** means hair loss. Hair loss may be complete or partial. Male pattern baldness occurs with aging and is the result of heredity. Hair also thins in some women with aging. Cancer treatments (radiation therapy to the head and chemotherapy) often cause alopecia in both men and women. Skin disease is another cause. Other causes include stress, poor nutrition, pregnancy, some drugs, and hormone changes. Except for hair loss from aging, the hair grows back in many cases.

- **Hirsutism** is excessive body hair in women and children. It is the result of heredity and abnormal amounts of male hormones.
- **Dandruff** is the excessive amount of dry, white flakes from the scalp. Itching often occurs. Sometimes the eyebrows and ear canals are involved. Medicated shampoos correct the problem.
- **Pediculosis (lice)** is the infestation with lice. Lice are parasites. Lice bites cause severe itching in the affected body area. **Pediculosis capitis** is the infestation of the scalp *(capitis)* with lice. **Pediculosis pubis** is the infestation of the pubic *(pubis)* hair with lice. Both head and pubic lice attach their eggs to hair shafts. **Pediculosis corporis** is the infestation of the body *(corporis)* with lice. Lice eggs attach to clothing and furniture. Lice easily spread to other persons through clothing, furniture, bed linen, and sexual contact. Medicated shampoos, lotions, and creams are used to treat lice. Thorough bathing is necessary. So is washing clothing and linen in hot water.

✵ Brushing and Combing Hair

Brushing and combing hair are part of morning care. They also are done as needed during the day. Many people want their hair styled before visitors arrive. Encourage patients to do their own hair care. Assist as needed. Perform hair care for those who cannot do so. Let the person choose how to brush, comb, and style hair.

Long hair easily matts and tangles. Daily brushing and combing prevent the problem. So does braiding. Do not braid hair unless the person gives consent. *Never cut hair to remove matted or tangled hair.*

Brushing brings scalp oils along the hair shaft. Scalp oils help keep hair soft and shiny. Brushing and combing keep hair from tangling and matting. When brushing and combing hair, start at the scalp. Then brush or comb to the hair ends.

Talk to the RN if the person has matted or tangled hair. The RN may have you comb or brush through the matting and tangling. To do this, take a small section of hair near the ends. Then comb or brush through to the hair ends. Working up to the scalp, add small sections of hair. Comb or brush through each longer section to the hair ends. Finally, brush or comb from the scalp to the hair ends. *Never cut matted or tangled hair.*

Special measures are needed for curly, coarse, and dry hair. Use a wide-toothed comb for curly hair. Start at the neckline. Work upward, lifting and fluffing hair outward. Continue until you reach the forehead. Wetting the hair or applying a conditioner or petroleum jelly makes combing easier. The person may have certain practices or use special hair care products. The RN asks the patient about personal preferences and routine hair care measures. These become part of the person's care plan. The person can guide you when giving hair care.

When giving hair care, place a towel across the shoulders to protect the person's gown. If the person is in bed, give hair care before changing the pillowcase. If done after a linen change, place a towel across the pillow to collect falling hair. (See Focus on Children on p. 333.)

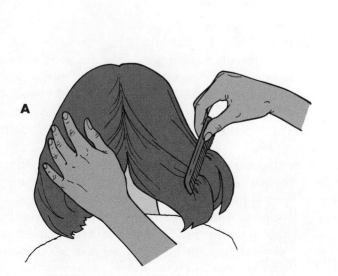
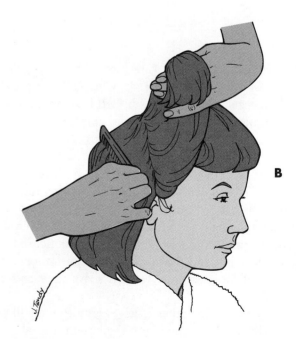

Fig. 15-1 **A,** *Part hair down the middle, and divide it into two main sections.* **B,** *Then part the main section into two smaller sections.*

✦ BRUSHING AND COMBING A PERSON'S HAIR

PRE-PROCEDURE

1 Identify the person. Check the ID bracelet, and call the person by name.

2 Explain the procedure to the person.

3 Collect the following:

  • Comb and brush

  • Bath towel

  • Hair care items as requested by the person

4 Arrange items on the bedside stand.

5 Wash your hands.

6 Provide for privacy.

PROCEDURE

7 Lower the bed rail.

8 Help the person to a chair or to Fowler's position if possible. The person puts on a robe and nonskid slippers when up.

9 Place a towel across the shoulders or across the pillow.

10 Ask the person to remove eyeglasses. Put them in the glass case. Put the case inside the bedside stand.

11 Part hair into two sections (Fig. 15-1, *A*). Divide one side into two sections (Fig. 15-1, *B*).

12 Brush the hair. Start at the scalp, and brush toward the hair ends (Fig. 15-2).

13 Style the hair as the person prefers.

14 Remove the towel.

15 Let the person put on the eyeglasses.

POST-PROCEDURE

16 Assist the person to a comfortable position.

17 Raise or lower bed rails as instructed by the RN.

18 Place the call bell within reach.

19 Unscreen the person.

20 Clean and return items to their proper place.

21 Follow agency policy for dirty linen.

22 Wash your hands.

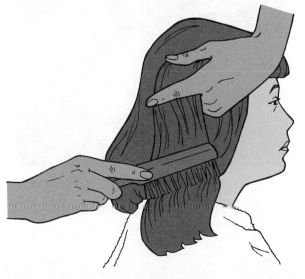

Fig. 15-2 *Brush hair by starting at the scalp and brushing down to the hair ends.*

focus on

CHILDREN

Hairstyles are important to adolescents. Many school-age children also are concerned about hairstyles. Do not make judgments about the child's hairstyle. Style hair in a manner that pleases the child and parents. Remember not to style hair according to your standards or customs.

✦ Shampooing

Most people shampoo at least once a week. Some shampoo two or three times a week. Others shampoo every day. Many factors affect frequency. These include the condition of the hair and scalp, hairstyle, and personal choice. Shampoo and hair conditioner also involve personal choice.

Patients often need help shampooing. Personal choice is followed whenever possible. However, safety is important and the RN's approval is needed. Tell the RN if a shampoo is requested. Do not wash a person's hair unless a RN asks you to do so.

The shampooing method depends on the person's condition, safety factors, and personal choice if possible. The RN decides which method to use. Dry and style hair as quickly as possible after shampooing. Women may want hair curled or rolled up before drying. Consult with the RN before curling or rolling up a person's hair.

Shampooing during the shower or tub bath

Persons who shower can usually shampoo at the same time. A hand-held nozzle is used for those using shower chairs or taking tub baths. A spray of water is directed to the hair. Place an extra towel, shampoo, and hair conditioner within the person's reach. Assist as necessary.

Shampooing at the sink

The chair is placed so the person faces away from the sink. The person's head is tilted back over the edge of the sink. A folded towel is placed over the sink edge to protect the neck. A water pitcher or hand-held nozzle is used to wet and rinse the hair.

Shampooing a person on a stretcher

The stretcher is positioned in front of a sink. A pillow is placed under the head and neck, and the head is tilted over the edge of the sink (Fig. 15-3). A water pitcher or hand-held nozzle is used to wet and rinse the hair. Safety measures include locking the stretcher wheels, using the safety straps, and raising the far rail.

Shampooing a person in bed

This method is for those who cannot be out of bed. The person's head and shoulders are moved to the edge of the bed if the position is allowed. A rubber or plastic trough is placed under the head to protect the linens and mattress from water. The trough also drains water into a basin placed on a chair by the bed (Fig. 15-4). A water pitcher is used to wet and rinse the hair. (See Focus on Older Persons and Focus on Home Care on p. 335.)

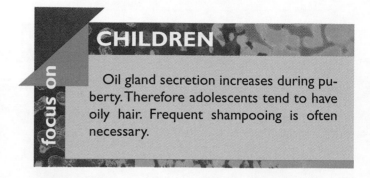

CHILDREN

focus on

Oil gland secretion increases during puberty. Therefore adolescents tend to have oily hair. Frequent shampooing is often necessary.

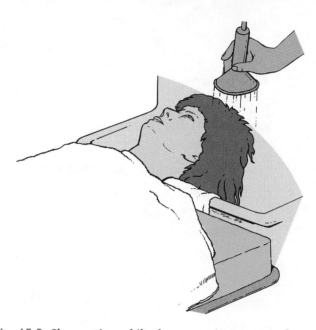

Fig. 15-3 *Shampooing while the person is on a stretcher. The stretcher is in front of the sink.*

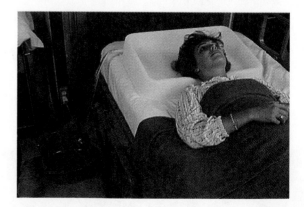

Fig. 15-4 *A trough is used when shampooing a person in bed. The trough is directed to the side of the bed so water drains into a collecting basin.*

OLDER PERSONS

focus on

Oil gland secretion decreases with aging. Older persons may shampoo less often than younger adults.

HOME CARE

focus on

You can make a trough from a plastic shower curtain or tablecloth. A plastic drop cloth for painting also is useful. Avoid plastic trash bags. They slip and slide easily and are not sturdy. To make a trough, place the plastic under the patient's head. Make a raised edge around the plastic to prevent water from spilling over the sides. Direct the ends of the plastic into the basin. This directs water into the basin.

✦ SHAMPOOING THE PERSON'S HAIR

PRE-PROCEDURE

1 Explain the procedure to the person.

2 Wash your hands.

3 Collect the following:

- Two bath towels
- Face towel or washcloth folded lengthwise
- Shampoo
- Hair conditioner if requested
- Bath thermometer
- Pitcher or hand-held nozzle
- Gloves (optional)

- Equipment for the shampoo in bed (if needed):
  - Trough
  - Basin or pail
  - Bath blanket
  - Waterproof pad
- Comb and brush
- Hair dryer

4 Arrange items nearby.

5 Identify the person. Check the ID bracelet, and call the person by name.

6 Provide for privacy.

PROCEDURE

7 Position the person for the method you are going to use.

8 Place a bath towel across the shoulders or across the pillow under the person's head.

9 Brush and comb the hair to remove snarls and tangles.

10 Obtain water. Water temperature should be about 105° F (40.5° C).

11 Ask the person to hold the face towel or washcloth over the eyes.

12 Apply water until the hair is completely wet. Use the pitcher or nozzle.

13 Apply a small amount of shampoo.

14 Work up a lather with both hands. Start at the hairline, and work toward the back.

Continued

SHAMPOOING THE PERSON'S HAIR—cont'd

PROCEDURE—cont'd

15 Massage the scalp with your fingertips.

16 Rinse the hair.

17 Repeat steps 13 through 15.

18 Rinse the hair thoroughly.

19 Apply conditioner and rinse as directed on the container.

20 Wrap the person's head with a bath towel.

21 Dry his or her face with the towel or washcloth used to protect the eyes.

22 Help the person raise the head if appropriate.

23 Rub the hair and scalp with the towel. Use the second towel if the first is wet.

24 Comb the hair to remove snarls and tangles. A woman may want hair curled or rolled up.

25 Dry the hair as quickly as possible.

POST-PROCEDURE

26 Make sure the person is comfortable.

27 Place the call bell within reach.

28 Raise or lower bed rails as instructed by the RN.

29 Clean and return equipment to its proper place. Discard disposable items.

30 Follow agency policy for dirty linen.

31 Wash your hands.

BOX 15-1

RULES FOR SHAVING

- Follow Standard Precautions and the Bloodborne Pathogen Standard.
- Protect the bed linens by placing a towel under the part being shaved.
- Soften the skin before shaving.
- Encourage the person to do as much for himself or herself as safely possible.
- Hold the skin taut as necessary.
- Shave in the direction of hair growth when shaving the male face and female underarms.
- Shave upward, starting at the ankle, when shaving legs.
- Rinse the body part thoroughly.
- Apply direct pressure to any nicks or cuts.
- Report nicks and cuts to the RN immediately.

SHAVING

A clean-shaven face is important for the comfort and well-being of many men. Likewise, many women shave their legs and underarms. Persons may prefer electric shavers or razor blades. With electric shavers, practice safety precautions for using electrical equipment. Razor blades can cause nicks or cuts. Follow Standard Precautions and the Bloodborne Pathogen Standard to prevent contact with the person's blood. Also follow the rules listed in Box 15-1 when shaving men or the legs and underarms of women.

◆ Shaving Men

The beard and skin are softened before shaving with a razor blade. Soften the skin by applying a warm washcloth or face towel to the face for a few minutes. Then lather the face with soap and water or a shaving cream. Be careful not to cut or irritate the skin while shaving.

SHAVING A MAN

PRE-PROCEDURE

1 Explain the procedure to the person.

2 Wash your hands.

3 Collect the following:

- Wash basin
- Bath towel
- Face towel
- Washcloth
- Bath thermometer
- Razor or shaver
- Mirror
- Shaving cream or soap
- Shaving brush
- After-shave lotion
- Tissues
- Paper towel
- Gloves

4 Arrange items on the overbed table.

5 Identify the person. Check the ID bracelet, and call the person by name.

6 Provide for privacy.

7 Raise the bed to the best level for good body mechanics. Raise the bed rails.

PROCEDURE

8 Fill the wash basin. Water temperature should be about 115° F (46° C).

9 Place the basin on the overbed table on top of the paper towels.

10 Lower the bed rail.

11 Position the person in semi-Fowler's position if allowed or on his back.

12 Adjust lighting to clearly see the person's face.

13 Place the bath towel over his chest.

14 Position the overbed table within easy reach and at a comfortable working height.

15 Put on the gloves.

16 Wash the person's face. Do not dry.

17 Place a washcloth or face towel in the water and wet it thoroughly. Wring it out.

18 Apply the washcloth or towel to the face to soften the beard. Remove it after 3 to 5 minutes.

19 Apply shaving cream to the face with your hands. Use a shaving brush if using soap for lather.

20 Tighten the razor blade to the razor.

21 Hold the skin taut with one hand.

22 Shave in the direction of hair growth. Use shorter strokes around the chin and lips (Fig. 15-5, p. 338).

23 Rinse the razor often and wipe with tissues.

24 Apply direct pressure to any bleeding areas.

25 Wash off any remaining shaving cream or soap. Dry with a towel.

26 Apply after-shave lotion if requested.

27 Remove the towel.

28 Remove the gloves.

29 Move the overbed table to the side of the bed.

Continued

✦ SHAVING A MAN—cont'd

POST-PROCEDURE

30 Make sure the person is comfortable.

31 Place the call bell within reach.

32 Lower the bed to its lowest position.

33 Raise or lower bed rails as instructed by the RN.

34 Clean and return equipment and supplies to their proper place. Discard disposable items.

35 Wipe off the overbed table with the paper towels. Discard the paper towels.

36 Position the table as appropriate for the person.

37 Unscreen the person.

38 Follow agency policy for dirty linen.

39 Wash your hands.

40 Report any nicks or bleeding to the RN.

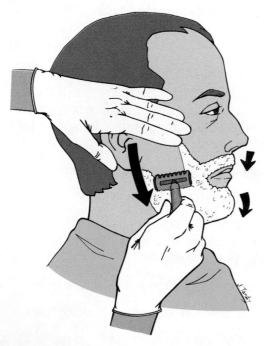

Fig. 15-5 *Shave in the direction of hair growth. Use longer strokes on the larger areas of the face. Use short strokes around the chin and lips.*

Caring for Mustaches and Beards

Beards and mustaches need daily care. Food can collect in hair. So can mouth and nose drainage. Daily washing and combing usually is enough. Ask the person how to groom his beard or mustache. *Never trim or shave a beard or mustache without the person's consent.*

Shaving Female Legs and Underarms

Many women shave their legs and underarms. This practice varies among cultures. Some women shave only the lower legs. Others shave to mid-thigh and others shave the entire leg.

Women's legs and underarms are shaved after bathing when the skin is soft. Soap and water or a shaving cream is used for lather. Needed shaving items are collected with the bath items. Use the kidney basin to rinse the razor rather than using the bath water.

Shaving underarms and legs is similar to shaving the male face. Practice the measures in Box 15-1.

✦ CARE OF NAILS AND FEET

Nails and feet need special attention to prevent infection, injury, and odors. Hangnails, ingrown nails (nails that grow in at the side), and nails torn away from the skin cause skin breaks. These breaks are portals of entry for microbes. Long or broken nails can scratch skin or snag clothing.

The feet are easily infected and injured. Dirty feet, socks, or stockings harbor microbes and cause odors. Shoes and socks provide a warm, moist environment for the growth of microbes. Injuries occur from stubbing toes, stepping on sharp objects, or being stepped on. Shoes that fit poorly cause blisters. Healing is prolonged in persons with poor circulation to the feet. Diabetes mellitus and vascular disease are common causes of poor circulation. Infections or foot injuries are particularly serious for older persons and persons with circulatory disorders. Gangrene and amputation are serious complications (see Chapter 30). Trimming and clipping toenails can easily result in injuries. *Therefore assistive personnel do not cut or trim toenails.*

Cleaning and trimming fingernails are easier after soaking. Use nail clippers to cut fingernails. *Never use scissors.* Be very careful when clipping and trimming fingernails. You must not damage surrounding tissues. Also, check with the RN about the water temperature. The feet are easily burned. Persons with decreased sensation or circulatory problems may not feel hot temperatures. (See Focus on Home Care.)

focus on HOME CARE

Tub baths are a good time for soaking toes. If soaking is done at other times, the person can sit on the side of the tub and soak the feet. Make sure the person can step into and out of the tub. Otherwise, soak the feet in a basin.

If the position is comfortable for the person, fingers can soak in the sink. Or a bowl is useful if a small basin is not available.

✦ GIVING NAIL AND FOOT CARE

PRE-PROCEDURE

1 Explain the procedure to the person.

2 Wash your hands.

3 Collect the following:

- Wash basin
- Bath thermometer
- Bath towel
- Face towel
- Washcloth
- Kidney basin
- Nail clippers

- Orange stick
- Emery board or nail file
- Lotion or petroleum jelly
- Paper towels
- Disposable bath mat
- Gloves (optional)

4 Arrange items on the overbed table.

5 Identify the person. Check the ID bracelet, and call the person by name.

6 Provide for privacy.

PROCEDURE

7 Help the person to a bedside chair. Place the call bell within reach.

8 Place the bath mat under the feet.

9 Fill the wash basin. Water temperature should be 105° F (40.5° C) unless otherwise instructed by the RN.

10 Place the basin on the bath mat. Help the person put the feet into the basin.

11 Position the overbed table in front of the person. It should be low and close to the person.

12 Fill the kidney basin. Water temperature should be 105° to 110° F (40.5° to 43.3° C).

Continued

GIVING NAIL AND FOOT CARE—cont'd

PROCEDURE—cont'd

13 Place the basin on the overbed table on top of the paper towels.

14 Place the person's fingers into the basin. Position the arms so he or she is comfortable (Fig. 15-6).

15 Let the feet and fingernails soak for 10 to 20 minutes. Rewarm the water as needed.

16 Clean under the fingernails with the orange stick.

17 Remove the kidney basin, and dry the fingers thoroughly.

18 Clip fingernails straight across with the nail clippers (Fig. 15-7).

19 Shape nails with an emery board or nail file.

20 Push cuticles back with the orange stick or a washcloth (Fig. 15-8).

21 Move the overbed table to the side.

22 Scrub calloused areas of the feet with a washcloth.

23 Remove the feet from the basin. Dry thoroughly.

24 Apply lotion or petroleum jelly to the feet.

POST-PROCEDURE

25 Assist the person back to bed and to a comfortable position. Place the call bell within reach.

26 Raise or lower bed rails as instructed by the RN.

27 Clean and return equipment and supplies to their proper place. Discard disposable items.

28 Unscreen the person.

29 Follow agency policy for dirty linen.

30 Wash your hands.

31 Report your observations to the RN:

- Reddened, irritated, or calloused areas
- Breaks in the skin

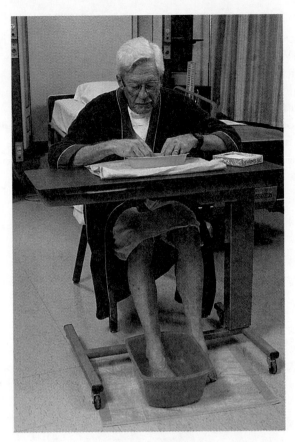

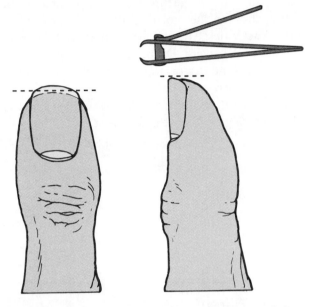

Fig. 15-7 *Clip fingernails straight across. Use a nail clipper.*

Fig. 15-6 *Nail and foot care. The feet soak in a foot basin, and the fingers soak in a kidney basin.*

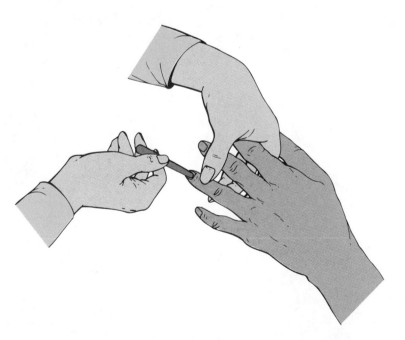

Fig. 15-8 *Push the cuticle back with an orange stick.*

CHANGING HOSPITAL GOWNS AND CLOTHING

Hospital gowns or pajamas are changed after the bath and when wet or soiled. Persons who wear regular clothing during the day change into a gown or pajamas for bed. Then they dress in the morning. Patients may need help with these activities. The following rules are followed:

- Provide for privacy. Do not expose the person.
- Encourage the person to do as much as possible.
- Allow the person to choose what to wear.
- Remove clothing from the strong or *good* side first.
- Put clothing on the weak side first.

✦ Changing Hospital Gowns

Special measures are needed for arm injuries, paralysis, or IV infusions. If there is injury or paralysis, the gown is removed from the good arm first. Support the weak arm while removing the gown. Put the clean gown on the weak arm first and then on the good arm.

Some agencies have special gowns for persons receiving IV infusions. The gowns open along the entire sleeve and close with ties, snaps, or velcro. Standard hospital gowns may be used for persons with IV infusions.

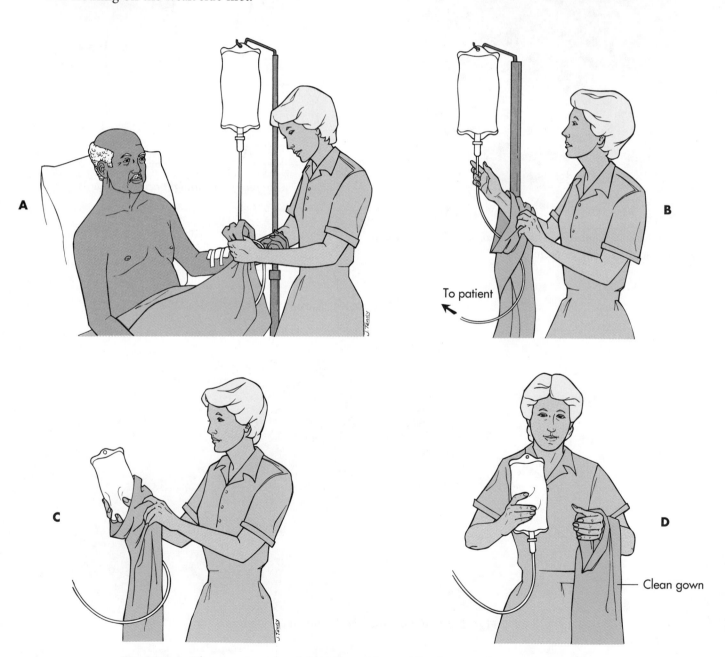

To patient

Clean gown

Fig. 15-9 A, *The gown is removed from the good arm. The sleeve on the arm with the IV is gathered up, slipped over the IV site and tubing, and removed from the arm and hand.* **B,** *The gathered sleeve is slipped along the IV tubing to the bag.* **C,** *The IV bag is removed from the pole and passed through the sleeve.* **D,** *The gathered sleeve of the clean gown is slipped over the IV bag at the shoulder part of the gown.*

CHANGING THE GOWN OF A PERSON WITH AN IV

PRE-PROCEDURE

1 Explain the procedure to the person.

2 Wash your hands.

3 Get a clean gown.

4 Identify the person. Check the ID bracelet, and call the person by name.

5 Provide for privacy.

PROCEDURE

6 Untie the back of the gown. Free parts of the gown that the person is lying on.

7 Remove the gown from the arm with no IV.

8 Gather up the sleeve of the arm with the IV. Slide it over the IV site and tubing. Remove the arm and hand from the sleeve (Fig. 15-9, *A*).

9 Keep the sleeve gathered. Slide your arm along the tubing to the bag (Fig. 15-9, *B*).

10 Remove the bag from the pole. Slide the bag and tubing through the sleeve (Fig. 15-9, *C*). Do not pull on the tubing. Keep the bag above the person's arm.

11 Hang the IV bag on the pole.

12 Gather the sleeve of the clean gown that will go on the arm with the IV infusion.

13 Remove the bag from the pole. Quickly slip the gathered sleeve over the bag at the shoulder part of the gown (Fig. 15-9, *D*). Hang the bag on the pole.

14 Slide the gathered sleeve over the tubing, hand, arm, and IV site. Then slide the sleeve onto the person's shoulder.

15 Put the other side of the gown on the person.

16 Fasten the back of the gown.

POST-PROCEDURE

17 Make sure the person is comfortable.

18 Place the call bell within reach.

19 Lower the bed to its lowest position.

20 Raise or lower bed rails as instructed by the RN.

21 Unscreen the person.

22 Follow agency policy for dirty linen.

23 Wash your hands.

24 Ask the RN to check the IV flow rate.

✦ Dressing and Undressing

Clothing changes are usually necessary on admission and discharge. Some people enter and leave the agency in a gown or pajamas. Most wear street clothes. The rules listed on p. 342 are followed when dressing or undressing individuals. (See Focus on Long-Term Care and Focus on Home Care.)

LONG-TERM CARE

focus on

Most residents wear street clothes during the day. Some dress and undress themselves. Others need help. Remember, personal choice is a resident right. Allow the person to choose what to wear.

HOME CARE

focus on

Patients often wear street clothes during the day. Some wear nightgowns and pajamas and robes. The procedures that follow apply to nightgowns, pajamas, and robes as well as street clothes.

✦ UNDRESSING A PERSON

PRE-PROCEDURE

1 Explain the procedure to the person.

2 Wash your hands.

3 Get a bath blanket.

4 Identify the person. Check the ID bracelet, and call the person by name.

5 Provide for privacy.

6 Raise the bed to the best level for good body mechanics.

PROCEDURE

7 Lower the bed rail on the person's weak side.

8 Position him or her supine.

9 Cover the person with the bath blanket. Fanfold linens to the foot of the bed. Do not expose the person during the procedure.

10 Remove garments that open in the back:

    a Raise the person's head and shoulders. Or turn him or her onto the side away from you.

    b Undo buttons, zippers, ties, or snaps.

    c Bring the sides of the garment to the sides of the person (Fig. 15-10, p. 346). Do the following if he or she is in a side-lying position:

      • Tuck the far side under the person.

      • Fold the near side onto the chest (Fig. 15-11, p. 346).

    d Position the person supine.

UNDRESSING A PERSON—cont'd

PROCEDURE—cont'd

e Slide the garment off the shoulder on the strong side. Remove it from the arm (Fig. 15-12, p. 346).

f Repeat step 10e for the weak side.

11 Remove garments that open in the front:

a Undo buttons, zippers, snaps, or ties.

b Slide the garment off the shoulder and arm on the strong side.

c Raise the head and shoulders. Bring the garment over to the weak side (Fig. 15-13, p. 346). Lower the head and shoulders.

d Remove the garment from the weak side.

e Do the following if you cannot raise the person's head and shoulders:

- Turn the person toward you. Tuck the removed part under the person.

- Turn him or her onto the side away from you.

- Pull the side of the garment out from under the person. Make sure he or she will not lie on it when supine.

- Return the person to the supine position.

- Remove the garment from the weak side.

12 Remove pullover garments:

a Undo any buttons, zippers, ties, or snaps.

b Remove the garment from the strong side.

c Raise the head and shoulders. You may need to turn the person onto the side away from you. Bring the garment up to the person's neck (Fig. 15-14, p. 347).

d Remove the garment from the weak side.

e Bring the garment over the person's head.

f Position him or her in the supine position.

13 Remove pants or slacks:

a Remove shoes or slippers.

b Position the person supine.

c Undo buttons, zippers, ties, snaps, or buckles.

d Remove the belt if one is worn.

e Ask the person to lift the buttocks off the bed. Slide the pants down over the hips and buttocks (Fig. 15-15, p. 347). Have the person lower the hips and buttocks.

f Do the following if the person cannot raise the hips off the bed:

- Turn the person toward you.

- Slide the pants off the hip and buttock on the strong side (Fig. 15-16, p. 347).

- Turn the person away from you.

- Slide the pants off the hip and buttock on the weak side (Fig. 15-17, p. 347).

g Slide the pants down the legs and over the feet.

14 Dress or put a clean gown or pajamas on the person.

15 Help the person get out of bed if he or she is to be up. Cover the person and remove the bath blanket if the person will not be up.

16 Lower the bed.

POST-PROCEDURE

17 Raise or lower bed rails as instructed by the RN.

18 Place the call bell within reach.

19 Unscreen the person.

20 Follow agency policy for soiled clothing.

21 Report your observations to the RN.

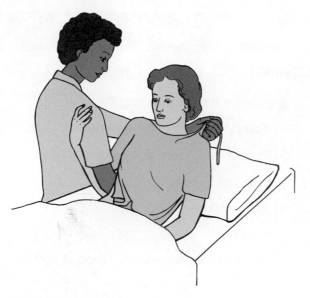

Fig. 15-10 *The sides of the garment are brought from the back to the sides of the person.*

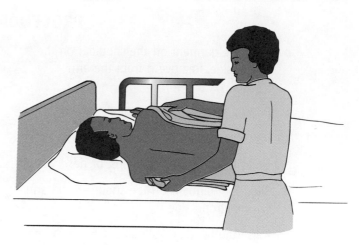

Fig. 15-11 *A garment that opens in back is removed from the person in the side-lying position. The far side of the garment is tucked under the person. The near side is folded onto the person's chest.*

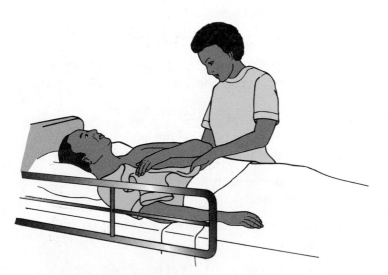

Fig. 15-12 *The garment is removed from the strong side first.*

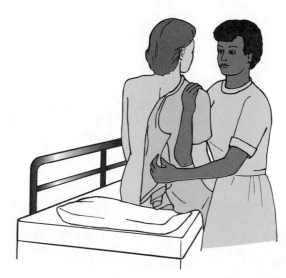

Fig. 15-13 *A front-opening garment is removed with the person's head and shoulders raised. The garment is removed from the strong side first. Then it is brought around the back to the weak side.*

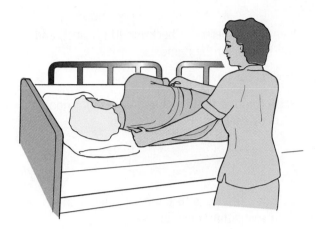

Fig. 15-14 *A pullover garment is removed from the strong side first. Then the garment is brought up to the person's neck so that it can be removed from the weak side.*

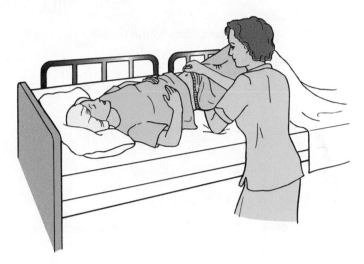

Fig. 15-15 *The person lifts the hips and buttocks for removing the pants. The pants are slid down over the hips and buttocks.*

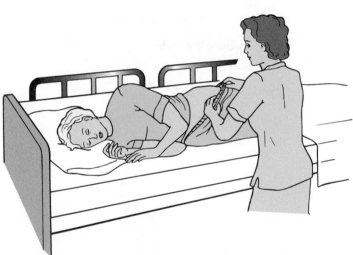

Fig. 15-16 *Pants are removed in the side-lying position. They are removed from the strong side first. They are slid over the hips and buttocks.*

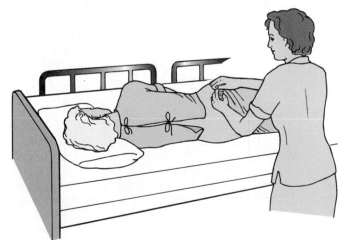

Fig. 15-17 *The person is turned onto the other side. The pants are removed from the weak side.*

✦ DRESSING THE PERSON

PRE-PROCEDURE

1 Explain the procedure to the person.

2 Wash your hands.

3 Get a bath blanket and necessary clothing.

4 Identify the person. Check the ID bracelet, and call the person by name.

5 Provide for privacy.

6 Raise the bed to a level appropriate for good body mechanics.

PROCEDURE

7 Undress the person if indicated.

8 Lower the bed rail on the person's strong side.

9 Position the person supine.

10 Cover the person with the bath blanket. Fanfold linens to the foot of the bed. Do not expose the person during the procedure.

11 Put on garments that open in the back.

   a Slide the garment onto the arm and shoulder of the weak side.

   b Slide the garment onto the arm and shoulder of the strong side.

   c Raise the person's head and shoulders.

   d Bring the sides to the back if he or she is in a semisitting position.

   e Do the following if the person is in a side-lying position:

     • Turn the person toward you.

     • Bring one side of the garment to the person's back (Fig. 15-18, *A*).

     • Turn the person away from you.

     • Bring the other side to the person's back (Fig. 15-18, *B*).

   f Fasten buttons, snaps, ties, or zippers.

   g Position the person in the supine position.

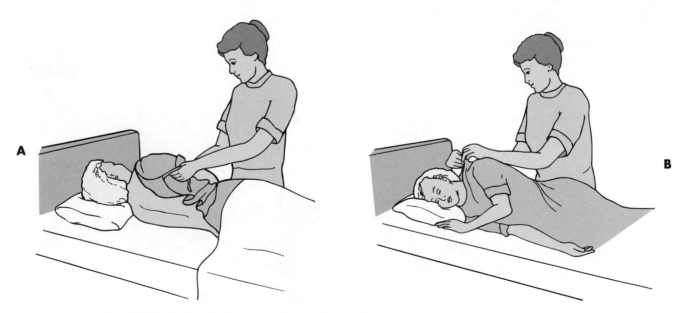

Fig. 15-18 A, *The side-lying position can be used to put on garments that open in the back. Turn the person toward you after the garment is put on the arms. The side of the garment is brought to the person's back.* **B,** *Then turn the person away from you. The other side of the garment is brought to the back and fastened.*

DRESSING THE PERSON—cont'd

PROCEDURE—cont'd

12 Put on garments that open in the front:

  a Slide the garment onto the arm and shoulder on the weak side.

  b Raise the person's head and shoulders. Bring the other side of the garment around to the back. Lower the person to the supine position. Slide the garment onto the arm and shoulder of the strong arm.

  c Do the following if the person cannot raise the head and shoulders:

    • Turn the person toward you.

    • Tuck the garment under him or her.

    • Turn the person away from you.

    • Pull the garment out from under him or her.

    • Turn the person back to the supine position.

    • Slide the garment over the arm and shoulder of the strong arm.

  d Fasten buttons, snaps, ties, or zippers.

13 Put on pullover garments:

  a Position the person supine.

  b Bring the neck of the garment over the head.

  c Slide the arm and shoulder of the garment onto the person's weak side.

  d Raise the person's head and shoulders.

  e Bring the garment down.

  f Slide the arm and shoulder of the garment onto the person's strong side.

  g Do the following if the person cannot assume a semisitting position:

    • Turn the person toward you.

    • Tuck the garment under him or her.

    • Turn the person away from you.

    • Pull the garment out from under him or her.

    • Return the person to the supine position.

    • Slide the arm and shoulder of the garment onto the strong side.

  h Fasten buttons, snaps, ties, or zippers.

14 Put on pants or slacks:

  a Slide the pants over the feet and up the legs.

  b Ask him or her to raise the hips and buttocks off the bed.

  c Bring the pants up over the buttocks and hips.

  d Ask the person to lower the hips and buttocks.

  e Do the following if the person cannot raise the hips and buttocks:

    • Turn person onto strong side.

    • Pull the pants over the buttock and hip on the weak side.

    • Turn the person onto the weak side.

    • Pull the pants over the buttock and hip on the strong side.

    • Return the person to the supine position.

  f Fasten buttons, ties, snaps, the zipper, and the belt buckle.

15 Put socks and shoes or slippers on the person.

16 Help the person to the chair if he or she can be up. Otherwise, help the person assume a comfortable position in bed.

17 Cover the person, and remove the bath blanket.

18 Lower the bed to its lowest position.

POST-PROCEDURE

19 Raise or lower bed rails as instructed by the RN.

20 Make sure the call bell is within reach.

21 Unscreen the person.

22 Follow agency policy for soiled clothing.

23 Report your observations to the RN.

REVIEW QUESTIONS

Circle the best *answer.*

1 You read the word *alopecia* in Mr. Lee's medical record. The term means
   a Excessive body hair
   b Dry, white flakes from the scalp
   c An infestation of lice
   d Hair loss

2 You are going to brush a woman's hair. The hair is not matted or tangled. When brushing the hair, start at
   a The forehead
   b The hair ends
   c The scalp
   d The back of the neck

3 Brushing is important to keep the hair
   a Soft and shiny
   b Clean
   c Free from pediculosis
   d All of the above

4 Mr. Lee wants his hair washed. You should
   a Wash his hair during his shower
   b Wash his hair at the sink
   c Shampoo him in bed
   d Follow the RN's instructions

5 When shaving Mr. Lee, you need to do the following *except*
   a Practice Standard Precautions
   b Follow the Bloodborne Pathogen Standard
   c Shave in the opposite direction of hair growth
   d Make sure the skin is soft before shaving

6 Mr. Lee is nicked during shaving. Your first action is to
   a Wash your hands
   b Apply direct pressure
   c Report the nick to the RN immediately
   d Switch to an electric razor

7 Mr. Lee has a mustache and beard. You think he would be more comfortable without facial hair. You can shave his beard and mustache.
   a True
   b False

8 You are going to cut a person's fingernails. You should use
   a Toenail clippers
   b Scissors
   c An emery board
   d Nail clippers

9 You can cut and trim toenails.
   a True
   b False

REVIEW QUESTIONS—cont'd

10 Fingernails are trimmed
  a Before they are soaked
  b After they are soaked
  c Before the toenails are trimmed
  d After the toenails are trimmed

11 Clothing is removed from the strong side first.
  a True
  b False

12 The person is allowed to choose what to wear.
  a True
  b False

Answers to these questions are on p. 850.

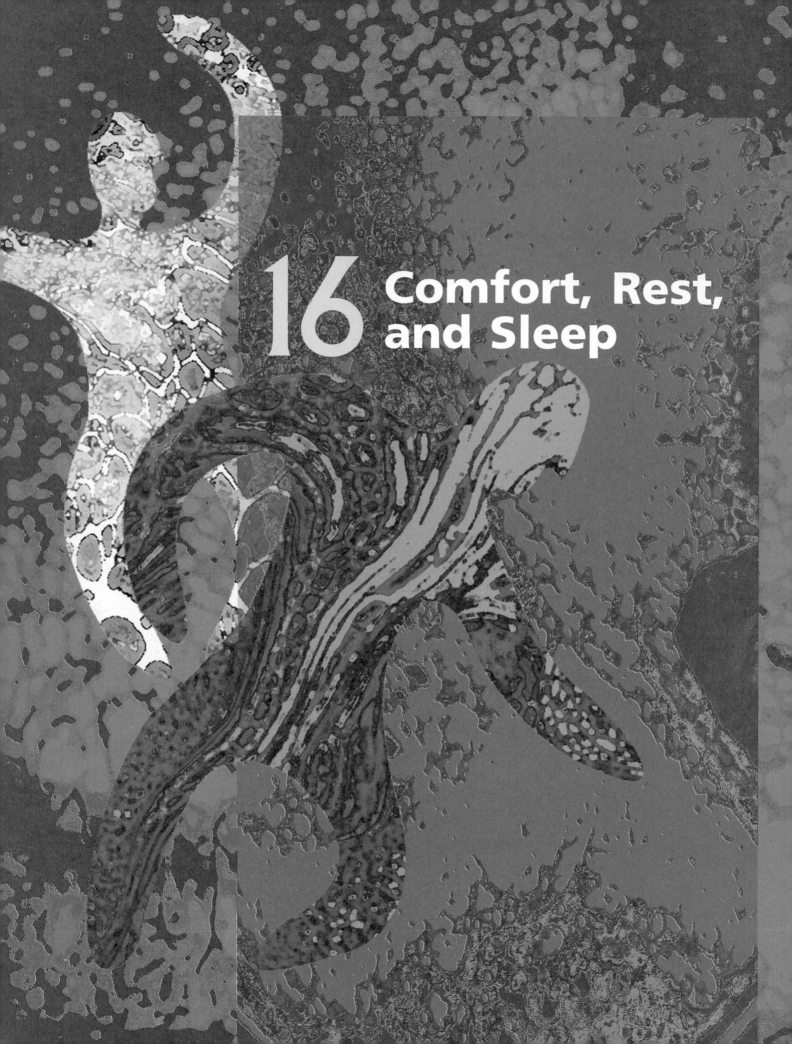

16 Comfort, Rest, and Sleep

OBJECTIVES

- Define the key terms in this chapter
- Explain why comfort, rest, and sleep are important
- Describe four types of pain
- Explain why pain is a personal experience
- Describe the factors that affect pain
- List the signs and symptoms of pain
- List the nursing measures that relieve pain
- Explain why meeting basic needs is important for rest
- Describe the nursing measures that promote rest
- Identify when rest is needed
- Describe the factors that affect sleep
- Describe the common sleep disorders
- Explain circadian rhythm and how it affects sleep
- Describe the stages of sleep
- Know the sleep requirements for each age-group
- List the nursing measures that promote sleep
- List the OBRA requirements for comfort, rest, and sleep

KEY TERMS

acute pain Pain that is felt suddenly from injury, disease, trauma, or surgery; it generally lasts less than 6 months

chronic pain Pain that lasts longer than 6 months; it may be constant or occur off and on

circadian rhythm Daily rhythm based on 24-hour cycle

comfort A state of well-being; the person has no physical or emotional pain and is calm and at peace

discomfort To ache, hurt, or be sore; pain

distraction To change the person's center of attention

enuresis Urinary incontinence in bed at night

guided imagery Creating and focusing on an image

insomnia A chronic condition in which the person cannot sleep or stay asleep throughout the night

nonREM sleep NREM sleep

NREM sleep The stage of sleep when there is *no rapid eye movement;* nonREM sleep

pain Discomfort

phantom pain Pain felt in a body part that is no longer there

radiating pain Pain felt at the site of tissue damage and in nearby areas

relaxation To be free from mental or physical stress

REM sleep The stage of sleep when there is *rapid eye movement*

rest To be calm, at ease, and relaxed; to be free of anxiety and stress

sleep A state of unconsciousness, reduced voluntary muscle activity, and lowered metabolism

Comfort, rest, and sleep are needed for well-being. The total person—the physical, emotional, social, and spiritual—is affected by comfort, rest, and sleep problems. People need to be comfortable and free of pain. Discomfort and pain can be physical or emotional. Whatever the cause, discomfort and pain affect rest and sleep.

Rest and sleep restore energy and well-being. Illness and injury increase the need for rest and sleep. The body needs more energy for healing and repair. When a person is ill or injured, more energy than normal is needed to perform daily activities.

COMFORT

Comfort is a state of well-being. There is no physical or emotional pain. The person is calm and at peace. Age, illness, and activity affect comfort. So do factors like temperature, ventilation, noise, odors, and lighting. Those factors are controlled to meet the person's needs.

Temperature and Ventilation

Heating, air conditioning, and ventilation systems maintain comfortable temperatures and provide fresh air. A temperature range of 68° to 74° F is usually comfortable for most healthy people. A comfortable temperature for one person may be too hot or too cold for another.

Stale room air and lingering odors affect comfort and rest. A good ventilation system provides fresh air and moves room air. Drafts can occur as air moves. Some persons are sensitive to drafts. Adequate clothing is necessary. Move patients away from drafty areas when possible. (See Focus on Children, Focus on Older Persons, and Focus on Home Care.)

Odors

Many odors are pleasant, like food aromas and flower scents. Others are unpleasant. Draining wounds, vomitus, and bowel movements have unpleasant smells. These odors can embarrass the person. Body, breath, and smoking odors may offend patients, visitors, and staff. Ill and older persons often have a reduced sense of smell. They may not notice odors. Good nursing care, good ventilation, and good housekeeping practices help eliminate odors. Odors are reduced by:

- Emptying and washing bedpans and kidney basins promptly
- Changing soiled linens promptly
- Cleaning incontinent persons promptly
- Providing good personal hygiene to prevent body and breath odors
- Using room deodorizers when necessary and if allowed by the agency

focus on CHILDREN

Infants generally need higher room temperatures for comfort. They also are sensitive to drafts. Adequate clothing and blankets are needed for warmth.

focus on OLDER PERSONS

Aging results in the loss of the fatty tissue layer. This increases the older person's sensitivity to cold. Higher room temperatures are often necessary. Sweaters, lap blankets, socks, and extra blankets are often needed for warmth. Older persons need protection from drafts and extreme cold.

focus on HOME CARE

Some homes do not have air conditioning. Some have inadequate heating systems. Extremely high or low temperatures can threaten the person's health and safety. Report extremely high or low temperatures to the RN immediately, especially in very warm and very cold weather. See Chapter 10 if space heaters are used in the home.

Smoke odors cause special problems. Most agencies ban smoking. Patients, staff, and visitors cannot smoke anywhere in the building. If you smoke, follow the employer's policy. Wash your hands after handling smoking materials and before giving care. Smoke odors cling to your uniform, hair, and breath. Your own personal hygiene is important. (See Focus on Long-Term Care at top left on p. 355.)

Noise

Ill people are sensitive to noises and sounds around them. They are often disturbed by common health care sounds. The clanging of metal bedpans, urinals, and wash basins is annoying. So is the clatter of dishes and trays. Loud talking and laughing in hallways and at the nurses' station, loud televisions and radios, ringing telephones, and buzzing intercoms are often irritating. So is noise from equipment needing repair or oil.

When in a strange place, people want to know the cause and meaning of new sounds. This is part of the basic need for safety and security. Patients may find some sounds dangerous, frightening, or irritating. They may become upset, anxious, and uncomfortable. Remember, noise to one person may not be noise to another. For example, loud stereo music may please a teenager but irritate parents.

Health care agencies are designed to reduce noise. Drapes, carpeting, and acoustical tiles help absorb noise. Plastic items make less noise than metal equipment. Reduce noise by controlling the loudness of your voice. Also, handle equipment carefully. Keeping equipment working properly and promptly answering telephones and intercoms also decrease noise.

Lighting

Good lighting is needed for the safety and comfort of patients and staff. Glares, shadows, and dull lighting can cause falls, headaches, and eyestrain. People usually relax and rest better in dim light. However, a bright room is more cheerful and stimulating.

Adjust lighting to meet the person's changing needs. Pull shades or draw drapes to control natural light. Adjust the overbed light to provide soft, medium, and bright lighting. Some agencies have ceiling lights over beds. These provide low to very bright light. Bright lighting is helpful when giving care. Light controls should be within the person's reach. (See Focus on Long-Term Care above right.)

PAIN

Discomfort or **pain** means to ache, hurt, or be sore. Discomfort is unpleasant. Comfort and discomfort are subjective (see p. 63). That is, you cannot see, hear, touch, or smell the person's comfort or discomfort. You must rely on what the person tells you. You must report

complaints to the RN. The information is used for the nursing process.

Pain is personal. It differs for each person. What *hurts* to one person may *ache* to another. What one person calls *sore*, another may call *aching*. Pain is subjective. If a person complains of pain or discomfort, the person *has* pain or discomfort. You must believe the person. Remember, you cannot see, hear, feel, or smell the pain.

Pain is a warning from the body. It means there is damage to body tissues. Pain often causes the person to seek health care.

Types of Pain

There are different types of pain. The doctor uses the type of pain when diagnosing. The type of pain also is used in the nursing process:

- **Acute pain** is felt suddenly from injury, disease, trauma, or surgery. There is tissue damage. Acute pain lasts a short time, usually less than 6 months. It decreases with healing.
- **Chronic pain** lasts longer than 6 months. Pain is constant or occurs off and on. There is no longer tissue damage. Chronic pain remains long after healing. Arthritis and cancer are common causes of chronic pain.
- **Radiating pain** is felt at the site of tissue damage and in nearby areas. Pain from a heart attack is often felt in the left side of the chest, left jaw, left shoulder, and left arm. A diseased gallbladder can cause pain in the right upper abdomen, the back, and the right shoulder (Fig. 16-1, p. 356).
- **Phantom pain** is felt in a body part that is no longer there. A person with an amputated leg may still sense leg pain (see Chapter 30).

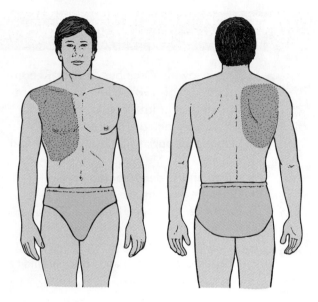

Fig. 16-1 *Gallbladder pain radiates to the right upper abdomen, the back, and the right shoulder.*

Factors Affecting Pain

A person may handle pain well one time and poorly the next time. Many factors affect reactions to pain.

Past experience

We learn from past experiences. They help us know what to do or what to expect. Whether it is going to school, driving a car, taking a test, shopping, having a baby, or caring for children, the past prepares us for similar events at another time. We also learn from the past experiences shared by family and friends.

A person may have had pain before. The severity of pain, its cause, how long it lasted, and if relief occurred all affect the person's current response to pain. Knowing what to expect can help or hinder how the person handles pain.

Some people have not had pain. When pain is felt, the person may be very afraid and anxious. Fear and anxiety affect pain.

Anxiety

Anxiety relates to feelings of fear, dread, worry, and concern. The person feels uneasy and tense. The person may feel troubled or threatened or sense danger. Something is wrong but the person does not know what or why.

Pain and anxiety are related. Pain can cause anxiety. Anxiety increases how much pain the person feels. Lessening anxiety helps reduce pain. For example, the nurse explains to Mr. Smith that he will have pain after surgery. The nurse also explains that medication will be given for the pain. Mr. Smith knows the cause of the pain and what

to expect. This helps reduce his anxiety and therefore the amount of pain felt.

Rest and sleep

Rest and sleep restore energy. They reduce body demands, and the body repairs itself. Lack of needed rest and sleep affects how a person thinks and copes with daily life. Ill and injured persons need more sleep than usual. Many also have pain. Lack of rest and sleep affect how the person deals with pain. Pain seems worse when the person is tired or restless. Also, the person usually pays more attention to pain when tired and unable to rest or sleep.

Attention

The more a person thinks about the pain, the worse it can seem. Sometimes pain is so severe that it is all the person thinks about. However, even mild pain can seem worse if the person thinks about it all the time. Pain often seems worse at night. Activity is less, it is quiet, there are no visitors, the radio or television is off, and others are asleep. When unable to sleep, the person has time to think about the pain.

Personal and family duties

How a person deals with pain often relates to personal and family obligations. Often pain is ignored if children must be cared for. Some people go to work when having pain. Others deny pain because they fear a serious illness. The illness can interfere with earning money, going to school, or caring for children, a partner, or ill parents.

The value or meaning of pain

Some people view pain as a sign of weakness. It also may mean a serious illness and the need for painful tests and treatments. Therefore pain is ignored or denied. Sometimes pain results in pleasure. The pain of childbirth is one example.

For some persons, pain means not having to work or assume daily routines. Pain is used to avoid certain people or things. Pain is useful for the person. Some people like doting and pampering by others. The person values and wants such attention.

Support from others

Pain is often easier to deal with when family and friends offer comfort and support. The pain of childbirth is easier when a loving father gives support and encouragement. A child bears pain much better when comforted by a caring mother, father, or family member. The use of touch by a valued person is very comforting. Just being nearby also helps.

Some people do not have caring family or friends. They must deal with pain alone. Being alone can increase anx-

TOP TEN COUNTRIES OF ORIGIN OF IMMIGRANTS TO THE UNITED STATES*: PAIN REACTIONS

Country	Pain Reactions
Mexico	Emotional self-restraint and stoic inhibition of strong feelings and emotional expression are seen. Expression of pain may be a self-help relief mechanism. Pain relief might be refused as a means for atonement.
	During labor the loud verbal repetition of "Aye, yie, yie" requires long, slow breaths, thus becoming a culturally and medically appropriate method of pain relief.
Vietnam	Pain may be severe before relief is requested.
Philippines	People may appear stoic, believing that pain is the will of God and that God will give them the strength to bear it.
Former Soviet Union	People are communicative about pain. Some prefer injections for pain relief.
Dominican Republic	None reported.
Mainland China	Strong negative feelings, such as anger and pain, are often suppressed.
	A display of emotion is considered a weakness of character. Because it is considered impolite to accept something the first time it is offered, pain relief interventions must be offered more than once.
India	The person has a quiet acceptance of pain and will accept some relief measures.
El Salvador	None reported.
Poland	Tolerance of pain is valued. Pain may be expressed by facial grimaces or by crying out.
United Kingdom	None reported.

From Geissler EM: *Pocket guide to cultural assessment*, St Louis, 1994, Mosby.
*Information based on data gathered through 1992 by the U.S. Department of Immigration and Naturalization Services.

iety. It also gives the person more time to think about the pain. Facing pain alone is hard for everyone, especially children and older persons.

Culture

Culture affects how a person responds to pain (Box 16-1). In some cultures the person in pain is stoic. To be stoic means to show no reaction to joy, sorrow, pleasure, or pain. Strong verbal and nonverbal reactions to pain are seen in other cultures. (See Focus on Children and Focus on Older Persons on p. 358.)

Signs and Symptoms

You cannot see, hear, feel, or smell the person's pain. You must rely on what the person tells you. Promptly report to the RN any information you collect about pain. Use the person's exact words when you report and record. The RN needs the following information when assessing the person's pain:

- *Location.* Where is the pain? Ask the person to point to the area of pain (Fig. 16-2, p. 358). Remember, pain can radiate. Ask the person if the pain is anywhere else and to point to those areas.

- *Onset and duration.* When did the pain start? How long has the pain lasted?
- *Intensity.* Does the person complain of mild, moderate, or severe pain? Ask the person to rate the pain on a scale of 1 to 10, with 10 being the most severe.
- *Description.* Ask the person to describe the pain. Box 16-2 on p. 358 lists some words used to describe pain. Write down what the person says. Use the person's words when reporting to the RN.
- *Factors causing pain.* These are called *precipitating* factors. To precipitate means to cause. Such factors include moving or turning in bed, coughing or deep breathing, and exercising. Ask what the person was doing before the pain started and when it started.
- *Vital signs.* What are the person's pulse, respirations, and blood pressure? Increases in these vital signs often occur with pain.
- *Other signs and symptoms.* Does the person have other symptoms: dizziness, nausea, vomiting, weakness, numbness or tingling, or others? Box 16-3 on p. 359 lists the signs and symptoms that often occur with pain.

CHILDREN

Children may not understand pain. They know it feels bad. Their pain experiences are fewer. They do not know what to expect. They also have fewer ways of dealing with the pain. Adults can take some pain drugs bought in stores. They also know that heat or cold applications help to relieve pain. They can distract their attention away from the pain. Music, working, reading, and hobbies are distracting for some adults. Children do not know how to relieve their own pain. They rely on adults for help.

Infants, toddlers, and preschool children have difficulty alerting adults to pain. Infants cry, fuss, and are restless. Such behaviors also mean hunger and the need for a diaper change. Toddlers and preschool children may not have the words to express pain. Adults must be alert for behaviors and situations that signal pain.

OLDER PERSONS

Older persons may have decreased pain sensations. They do not feel pain, or it may not feel severe. This places them at greater risk for undetected disease or injury. Remember, pain occurs with tissue damage. Therefore pain alerts the person to illness or injury. If pain is not felt, the person does not know to seek health care.

Some older persons have many health problems that cause pain. Chronic pain may mask new pain. Older persons may also ignore or deny new pain. They may think it is related to an existing health problem. Like other adults, older persons often deny or ignore pain because of what it may mean.

Thinking and reasoning are affected in some older persons. Some cannot verbally communicate pain. Nursing staff must be alert for the signs of pain.

BOX 16-2

WORDS USED TO DESCRIBE PAIN

- Aching
- Burning
- Cramping
- Crushing
- Dull
- Gnawing
- Knifelike
- Piercing
- Pressure
- Sharp
- Sore
- Squeezing
- Stabbing
- Throbbing
- Viselike

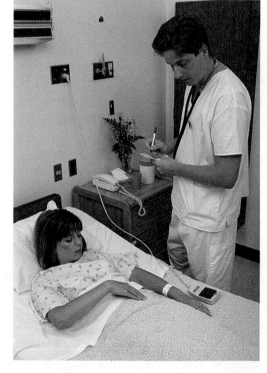

Fig. 16-2 *The person points to the area of pain.*

BOX 16-3 SIGNS AND SYMPTOMS OF PAIN

Body Responses
- Increased pulse, respirations, and blood pressure
- Sweating (diaphoresis)
- Nausea
- Vomiting
- Pale skin (pallor)

Behaviors
- Changes in speech: slow or rapid; loud or quiet
- Crying
- Gasping

Behaviors—cont'd
- Grimacing
- Groaning
- Grunting
- Holding the affected body part (splinting)
- Irritability
- Maintaining one position; refusing to move
- Moaning
- Quietness
- Restlessness
- Rubbing
- Screaming

BOX 16-4 NURSING MEASURES TO PROMOTE COMFORT AND RELIEVE PAIN

- Position the person in good body alignment; use pillows for support.
- Keep bed linens tight and wrinkle-free.
- Make sure the person is not lying on drainage tubes.
- Offer the bedpan or urinal, or assist the person to the bathroom or commode.
- Provide blankets for warmth and to prevent chilling.
- Use correct lifting, moving, and turning procedures.
- Wait one-half hour after pain medication was given before performing procedures.
- Give a back massage.
- Provide soft music to distract the person.
- Use touch to provide comfort.
- Allow family members and friends at the bedside as requested by the person.
- Avoid sudden or jarring movements of the bed.
- Handle the person gently.
- Practice safety measures if the person is receiving strong pain medication or sedatives:
  - Keep the bed in the low position.
  - Raise bed rails as directed.
  - Check on the person every 10 to 15 minutes.
  - Provide assistance when the person is up.
  - Apply warm or cold applications as directed by the RN.
  - Provide a calm, quiet, darkened environment.

Nursing Measures

The RN uses the nursing process to promote comfort and relieve pain. Box 16-4 lists the nursing measures that are often part of care plans. You learned how to perform most of the measures in earlier chapters (Fig. 16-3, p. 360).

You also learned why they are important for comfort.

Other measures are often needed to control pain. These include distraction, relaxation, and guided imagery. The RN may ask you to assist with these measures. The RN instructs you on how to properly perform them.

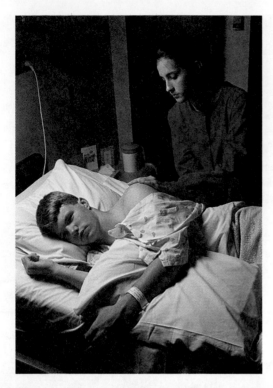

Fig. 16-3 *Measures are implemented to relieve pain. The person is positioned in good body alignment with pillows used for support. The room is darkened. Blankets provide warmth. A back massage provides touch and promotes relaxation.*

Distraction means to change the person's center of attention. The person's attention is moved away from the pain. Listening to music, playing games, singing, praying, watching television, and needlework are some ways to distract attention.

Relaxation means to be free from mental or physical stress. This state reduces pain and anxiety. The RN teaches the person relaxation techniques. The person is taught to breathe deeply and slowly and to contract and relax muscle groups. A comfortable position and a quiet room are important.

Guided imagery is creating and focusing on an image. The person is asked to create a pleasant scene. The RN notes this on the care plan so the staff uses the same image with the person. The RN uses a calm, soft voice when helping the person focus on the image. Soft music, a blanket for warmth, and a darkened room may help. The RN coaches the person to focus on the image and then to practice relaxation exercises.

Doctors often order medications to control or relieve pain. Nurses give these medications. Such medications can cause drowsiness, dizziness, and coordination problems. Therefore the person is protected from injury. The RN alerts you to any needed safety measures. (See Focus on Children.)

REST

Rest means being calm, at ease, and relaxed. The person is free of anxiety and stress. Rest may involve physical inactivity. Or the person may do things that he or she finds calming and relaxing. Examples include reading, music, television, needlework, prayer, gardening, baking, golf, walking, and carpentry (Fig. 16-4).

Basic needs must be met for a person to rest. Thirst, hunger, elimination needs, and pain or discomfort can affect rest. You can promote rest by meeting physical needs. A comfortable position and good body alignment also are important. A quiet environment promotes rest. So does a clean, dry, and wrinkle-free bed. Some people rest easier in a clean, neat, and uncluttered room.

Safety and security needs must be met. The person must feel safe from falling or other injuries. The person is secure with the call bell within reach. Understanding the reasons for treatments also helps the person feel safe. So does knowing how procedures are done. That is why you always explain the procedure before it is performed.

Many persons have rituals or routines before resting. These may include going to the bathroom, brushing teeth, washing the face and hands, praying, having a snack or beverage, locking doors, or making sure children or loved ones are safe at home. The person may want a favorite blanket or afghan. Follow routines and rituals whenever possible.

Love and belonging are important for rest. Visits or telephone calls from family and friends may help the person relax. The person knows that others care and are concerned. Reading cards and letters may also help the person relax and rest.

Esteem needs relate to feeling good about oneself. A person may find hospital gowns embarrassing. Others fear exposure. Many persons rest better wearing their own gowns or pajamas. Personal appearance also affects esteem. Hair care, being clean and free of body odors, and other hygiene and grooming measures all help people feel

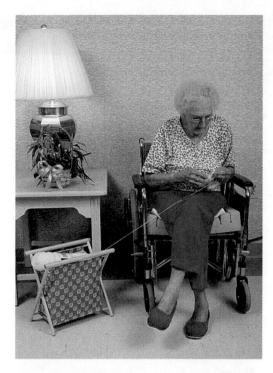

Fig. 16-4 *Needlework is relaxing for this lady.*

good about themselves. If esteem needs are met, the person may rest easier.

Some people are refreshed after resting for 15 or 20 minutes. Others need more time. Health care routines usually allow time for afternoon rest.

Ill or injured persons need to rest more often. Some need to rest during or after a procedure. For example, a bath tires Mr. Smith. So does getting dressed. You need to let him rest before making the bed. Some people need a few hours to complete oral hygiene, bathing, grooming, and dressing. Others need to rest after meals. Do not push the person beyond his or her limits. Allow rest periods as they are needed. Do not rush the person.

Distraction, relaxation, and guided imagery also promote rest. So does a back massage. You must plan and organize care so that the person can rest without interruptions.

The doctor may order bed rest for a person. Bed rest, its complications, and how to prevent complications are presented in Chapter 22.

SLEEP

Sleep is a state of unconsciousness, reduced voluntary muscle activity, and lowered metabolism. An unconscious person is unaware of the environment and cannot respond to people and things in the environment. The unconsciousness is temporary. People awake from sleep. Alarm clocks, voices, and crying babies easily awaken sleeping persons. Voluntary muscles are skeletal muscles. During

sleep, there are no voluntary arm or leg movements. Metabolism is the burning of food and energy for use by the body. Less energy is needed during sleep. Thus metabolism is reduced during sleep.

Sleep is a basic need. It lets the mind and body rest. The body saves energy. Body functions slow. Vital signs fall. That is, blood pressure, temperature, pulse, and respirations are less than when awake. Tissue healing and repair occur during sleep. Sleep lowers stress, tension, and anxiety. It refreshes and renews the person. That is, the person regains energy and mental alertness. The person thinks and functions better after needed sleep.

Circadian Rhythm

Sleep occurs regularly. It is part of circadian rhythm. Circadian comes from the Latin words *circa* meaning *about* and *dies* meaning *day*. **Circadian rhythm** is a pattern based on a 24-hour cycle. It is a daily rhythm called the *day-night cycle* or *body rhythm*. Functioning is affected by circadian rhythm. Some people function better in the morning. They are more alert and active; they think and react better. Others do better in the evening.

Circadian rhythm includes a sleep-wake cycle. The person's *biological clock* signals the time for sleep and the time to wake up. You have usual times for going to sleep and waking up. You may awaken before the alarm clock goes off. That is all part of your biological clock. Health care agencies often interfere with a person's circadian rhythm and the sleep-wake cycle. Sleep problems easily occur.

Many people work evening and night shifts. They include health care workers, police officers, fire fighters, fast-food workers, and factory workers. Their bodies must adjust to changes in the sleep-wake cycle.

Sleep Cycle

There are two phases of sleep. *Nonrapid eye movement* is **NREM sleep** or **nonREM sleep**. NREM sleep has four stages. Sleep goes from light to deep as the person moves through the four stages.

The *rapid eye movement* phase is called **REM sleep**. The person is hard to arouse. Mental restoration occurs during REM sleep. Events and problems of the previous day are thought to be reviewed during REM sleep. The person prepares for the next day.

Box 16-5 on p. 362 shows the stages of NREM and REM sleep. There are usually 4 to 6 cycles of NREM and REM sleep during the 7 to 8 hours of sleep each night. Stage 1 of NREM is usually not repeated.

Sleep Requirements

Sleep needs vary for each age-group. The amount needed decreases with age (Table 16-1, p. 362). Infants

BOX 16-5

SLEEP CYCLE

Stage 1: NREM Sleep
- Lightest sleep level
- Lasts a few minutes
- Gradual fall in vital signs
- Gradual lowering of metabolism
- Person feels drowsy and relaxed
- Person easily aroused
- Daydreaming feeling after being aroused

Stage 2: NREM Sleep
- Sound sleep
- Relaxation increases
- Still easy to arouse
- Lasts 10 to 20 minutes
- Body functions continue to slow

Stage 3: NREM Sleep
- First stages of deep sleep
- Hard to arouse the person
- Person rarely moves
- Muscles relax completely
- Vital signs fall
- Lasts 15 to 30 minutes

Stage 4: NREM Sleep
- Deepest stage of sleep
- Hard to arouse the person
- Body rests and is restored
- Vital signs much lower than when awake
- Lasts about 15 to 30 minutes
- Sleepwalking and **enuresis** (urinary incontinence in bed at night) may occur

REM Sleep
- Vivid, full-color dreaming
- Usually starts 50 to 90 minutes after sleep has begun
- Rapid eye movements
- Blood pressure, pulse, and respirations may fluctuate
- Voluntary muscles are relaxed
- Mental restoration occurs
- Hard to arouse the person
- Lasts about 20 minutes

Modified from Potter PA, Perry AG: *Fundamentals of nursing: concepts, process and practice*, ed 4, St Louis, 1997, Mosby.

TABLE 16-1

AVERAGE SLEEP REQUIREMENTS

Age-Group	Hours Per Day
Newborns (birth to 4 weeks)	14 to 18
Infants (4 weeks to 1 year)	12 to 14
Toddlers (1 to 3 years)	11 to 12
Preschoolers (3 to 6 years)	11 to 12
Middle and late childhood (6 to 12 years)	10 to 11
Adolescents (12 to 18 years)	8 to 9
Young adults (18 to 40 years)	7 to 8
Middle-age adults (40 to 65 years)	7
Older adults (65 years and older)	5 to 7

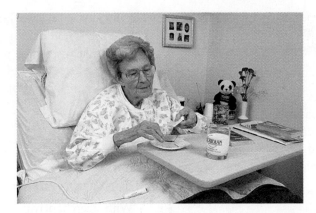

Fig. 16-5 *A bedtime snack of milk, cheese, and crackers helps to promote sleep.*

need more sleep than toddlers. Toddlers need more than preschool children. School-age children need more than teenagers. Older persons need less sleep than middle-age adults.

Factors Affecting Sleep

Several factors affect the amount and quality of sleep. Quality relates to how well the person slept and if needed amounts of NREM and REM sleep were obtained.

- *Illness.* Illness increases the need for sleep. However, the signs and symptoms of illness can interfere with sleep. They include pain, nausea, vomiting, coughing, difficulty breathing, diarrhea, frequent voiding, and itching. Treatments and therapies can also interfere with sleep. Often patients are awakened for treatments or medications. Traction or a cast can cause uncomfortable positions. The emotional effects of illness can affect sleep. These include fear, anxiety, and worry.
- *Nutrition.* Weight loss or gain affects sleep. The need for sleep increases with weight gain. It decreases with weight loss. Some foods affect sleep. Those with caffeine (chocolate, coffee, tea, colas) prevent sleep. The protein L-tryptophan tends to help sleep. It is found in milk, cheese, and beef (Fig. 16-5).
- *Exercise.* Exercise is good for the body. It improves health and fitness. Exercise requires energy. The person usually feels good after exercising. Eventually the person tires. Being tired helps the person sleep well at night. Exercising right before bedtime interferes with sleep. Exercise causes the release of substances into the bloodstream that stimulate the body. Therefore there should be at least 2 hours between exercise and bedtime.
- *Environment.* People adjust to their usual sleeping environments. They get used to such things as the bed, pillows, noises in the home or neighborhood, lighting, and a sleeping partner. Any change in the usual environment can affect the amount and quality of sleep.
- *Drugs and other substances.* Some drugs promote sleep. These are commonly called *sleeping pills.* Drugs given for anxiety, depression, and pain may cause the person to sleep. However, these drugs and sleeping pills reduce the length of REM sleep. Remember, mental restoration occurs during REM sleep. Behavior problems and sleep deprivation can occur. Alcohol is a drug. Alcohol tends to cause drowsiness and sleep. However, it interferes with REM sleep. Those under the influence of alcohol may awaken during sleep. Difficulty returning to sleep is common. Some drugs contain caffeine. As stated earlier, caffeine is a stimulant and prevents sleep. Besides in drugs, it is found in coffee, tea, chocolate, and colas. The side effects of some drugs can disrupt sleep. These include frequent voiding and nightmares.
- *Life-style changes.* Life-style relates to a person's daily routines and way of living. Work, school, play, and social events are all part of life-style. Life-style changes can affect sleep. Travel, vacation, and social events often affect usual bedtimes and when the person awakens. Children usually stay up later during school holidays. They may sleep later, too. If work hours change, the person needs to change sleep hours. Such changes affect normal sleep-wake cycles and the circadian rhythm.
- *Emotional problems.* Fear, worry, and anxiety affect sleep. These may be caused by work, personal, or family problems. Loss of a close family member or friend is another cause. Money problems are stressful. People may have difficulty falling asleep, or they awaken often. Difficulty getting back to sleep may occur.

BOX 16-6

SIGNS AND SYMPTOMS OF SLEEP DISORDERS

- Hand tremors
- Slowed responses to questions, conversations, or situations
- Reduced word memory; difficulty finding the right word
- Decreased reasoning and judgment
- Irregular pulse
- Red, puffy eyes
- Dark circles under the eyes
- Moodiness; mood swings
- Disorientation
- Irritability
- Fatigue
- Sleepiness
- Agitation
- Restlessness
- Decreased attention
- Hallucinations (see Chapter 31)
- Coordination problems
- Slurred speech

Sleep Disorders

Sleep disorders involve repeated sleep problems. The amount and quality of sleep are affected. Sleep disorders affect life-style. Box 16-6 lists the signs and symptoms that occur.

Insomnia

Insomnia is a chronic condition in which the person cannot sleep or stay asleep throughout the night. There are three forms of insomnia:
- Unable to fall asleep
- Unable to stay asleep
- Early awakening and unable to fall back asleep

Emotional problems are common causes of insomnia.

The fear of dying during sleep is another cause. Some people are afraid of not waking up. This may occur after recent heart disease or after being told of a terminal illness. The fear of not being able to sleep is another cause. The physical and emotional discomforts of illness can also cause insomnia.

The RN plans measures to promote sleep. However, the emotional or physical problems causing the insomnia also are treated.

Sleep deprivation

With sleep deprivation, the amount and quality of sleep are decreased. Sleep is interrupted. NREM and REM sleep stages are not completed. Illness and hospital care are common causes of sleep deprivation. Patients in intensive care units (ICUs) are at great risk. ICU lights are on much of the time. The many care measures and sounds from equipment interfere with sleep. Factors that affect sleep can also lead to sleep deprivation. Sleep deprivation results in many of the signs and symptoms listed in Box 16-6.

Sleepwalking

The person who sleepwalks leaves the bed and walks about. The person is not aware of sleepwalking and has no memory of the event on awakening. Children sleepwalk more than adults. The event may last 3 to 4 minutes or longer.

Stress, fatigue, and some medications can cause sleepwalking. The person needs protection from injury. The risk of falling is great. Intravenous infusions, catheters, nasogastric tubes, and other tubes are also sources of injury. The tubes or catheters can be pulled out of the body when the person gets out of bed. Guide sleepwalkers back to bed. They startle easily. Awaken them gently.

Promoting Sleep

The RN assesses the person's sleep patterns. Your observations are important. Report any of the signs and symptoms listed in Box 16-6. The RN plans measures to promote sleep (Box 16-7). Check the care plan so that you give the correct care. Also, report your observations so the RN can evaluate if the goal of a regular sleep pattern was met. (See Focus on Older Persons and Focus on Long-Term Care.)

BOX 16-7

NURSING MEASURES TO PROMOTE SLEEP

- Organize care to allow for uninterrupted rest.
- Avoid physical activity before bedtime.
- Encourage the person to avoid tending to business or family matters before bedtime.
- Let bedtime be flexible: bedtime should be when the person is tired and fatigued, not because it is a certain time.
- Provide a comfortable room temperature.
- Allow the person to take a warm bath or shower.
- Provide a bedtime snack (milk).
- Avoid caffeine (coffee, tea, colas, chocolate).
- Avoid alcoholic beverages.
- Have the person void before going to bed; change diapers.
- Follow bedtime rituals.
- Make sure the person wears loose-fitting nightwear.
- Provide adequate warmth (blankets, socks) for those who tend to be cold.
- Reduce noise.
- Darken the room by closing shades, blinds, and the privacy curtain. Shut off or dim lights.
- Dim lights in hallways and the nursing unit.
- Make sure linens are clean, dry, and wrinkle-free.
- Position the person in good alignment.
- Support body parts as ordered.
- Make sure the person is in a comfortable position.
- Give a back massage.
- Implement measures to relieve pain.
- Allow the person to read. Read to children.
- Allow the person to listen to music.
- Allow the person to watch television.
- Assist with relaxation exercises as ordered.
- Sit and talk with patients.

focus on OLDER PERSONS

Older persons have less energy than younger people. Many older persons take naps during the day. You need to let the person sleep. Organize the person's care to allow for uninterrupted naps.

focus on LONG-TERM CARE

Many residents have specific rituals and routines before bedtime. They are allowed if safe. The person may perform personal hygiene measures in a certain order. Some residents like to check on friends in the center before going to bed. Some are given the responsibility of turning off lights at bedtime. A bedtime snack may be important. Watching certain television shows in bed may be a bedtime routine. Others may read the Bible, pray, or say a rosary before going to sleep. Whatever the routine or ritual, it is important to the resident.

The resident is involved in planning care. The person is allowed to choose when to take a nap or go to sleep. The person also has the right to choose what measures are helpful in promoting comfort, rest, and sleep. You must follow the care plan and the resident's wishes.

REVIEW QUESTIONS

Circle the best *answer.*

1 These statements are about pain. Which is *false?*

  a Pain is objective. It can be seen, heard, smelled, or felt.

  b Pain is a warning from the body. It means there is damage to tissues.

  c Pain is personal. It is different for each person.

  d Pain is used to make diagnoses.

2 A person complains of pain in the left side of the chest, up into the left jaw, and down to the left shoulder and left arm. This is

  a Acute pain

  b Chronic pain

  c Radiating pain

  d Phantom pain

3 Mr. Smith complains of pain. You should do the following *except*

  a Ask him to point to where he feels the pain

  b Ask him when the pain started

  c Ask him to describe the pain

  d Ask to look at the pain

4 The RN gives Mr. Smith medication for pain. A procedure is scheduled for this time. You should

  a Perform the procedure before the medication is given

  b Perform the procedure right after the medication is given

  c Wait one-half hour to let the medication take effect

  d Omit the procedure for the day

5 Mr. Smith is protected from injury after receiving pain medication. You should do the following *except*

  a Keep the bed in the high position

  b Raise bed rails as directed

  c Check on him every 10 to 15 minutes

  d Provide assistance if he needs to get up

6 Which measure will not help relieve pain?

  a Provide blankets as needed.

  b Keep the room well lighted.

  c Provide soft music.

  d Give a back massage.

7 Mr. Smith's care plan has the following nursing measures. Which will *not* help him rest or sleep?

  a Have patient urinate before rest or sleep.

  b Assist patient to assume a comfortable position.

  c Assist patient to ambulate before rest or sleep.

  d Allow him to choose sleep attire.

8 Mr. Smith tires very easily. His morning care includes a bath, hair care, and getting dressed. His bed is made after he is dressed. When should he rest?

  a After morning care is completed.

  b After his bath and before hair care.

  c After you make the bed.

  d Whenever he needs to.

9 These statements are about sleep. Which is *false?*

  a Tissue healing and repair occur during sleep.

  b Voluntary muscle activity increases during sleep.

  c Sleep refreshes and renews the person.

  d All of the above

10 Mr. Smith was awake several nights when he first entered the hospital. Which is *true?*

  a His circadian rhythm may be affected.

  b NREM and REM sleep are affected.

  c His biological clock will still tell him when to sleep and wake up.

  d His functioning will not be affected.

11 Mr. Smith is 35 years old. When healthy, he probably needs about

  a 12 to 14 hours of sleep per day

  b 8 to 9 hours of sleep per day

  c 7 to 8 hours of sleep per day

  d About 6 hours of sleep per day

REVIEW QUESTIONS—cont'd

12 Mr. Smith asks for a snack. He said a friend brought him a chocolate chip cheesecake and some beef summer sausage. He asks for milk with his snack. Which foods will prevent sleep?

a Chocolate

b Cheese

c Milk

d Beef

13 Mr. Smith has difficulty sleeping, and he awakens several times during the night. He has difficulty answering your questions and seems moody. His pulse is irregular, and his eyes are red and puffy. He is showing signs of

a Insomnia

b Sleep deprivation

c Enuresis

d Distraction

14 These measures are part of Mr. Smith's care plan. Which should you question?

a Let Mr. Smith choose his bedtime.

b Provide a bedtime snack of hot tea and a cheese sandwich.

c Make sure his cast is properly supported.

d Follow his bedtime rituals.

Answers to these questions are on p. 850.

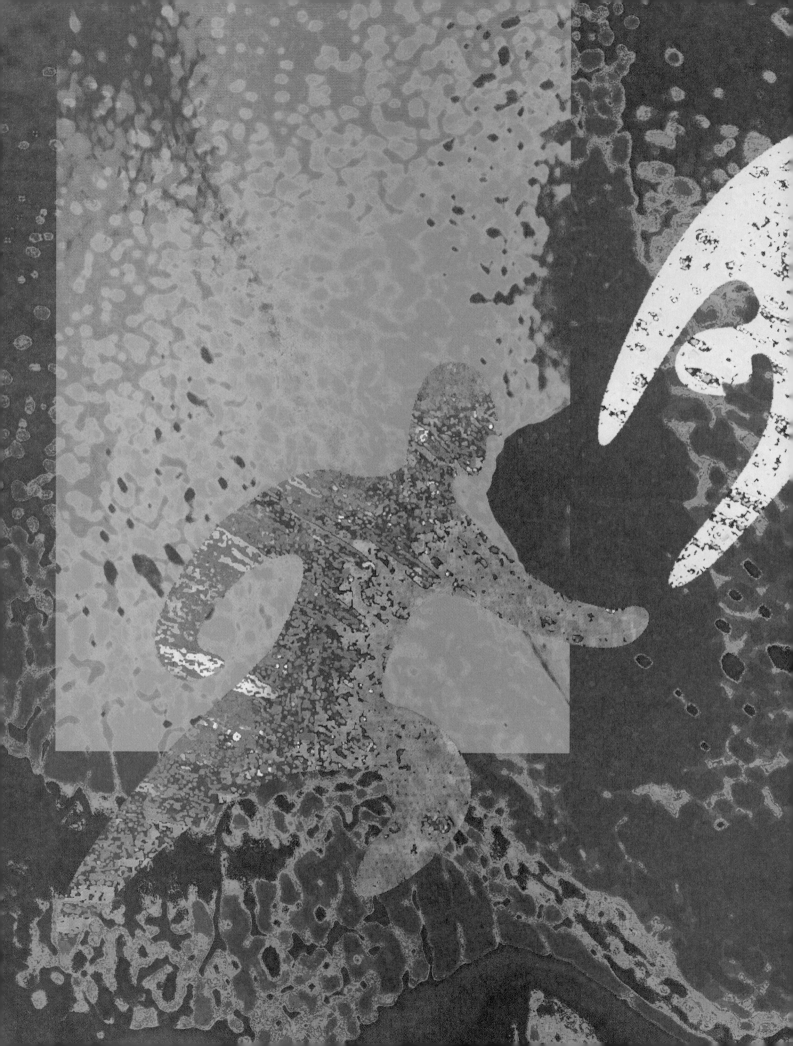

Unit V
Assisting With Physical Needs

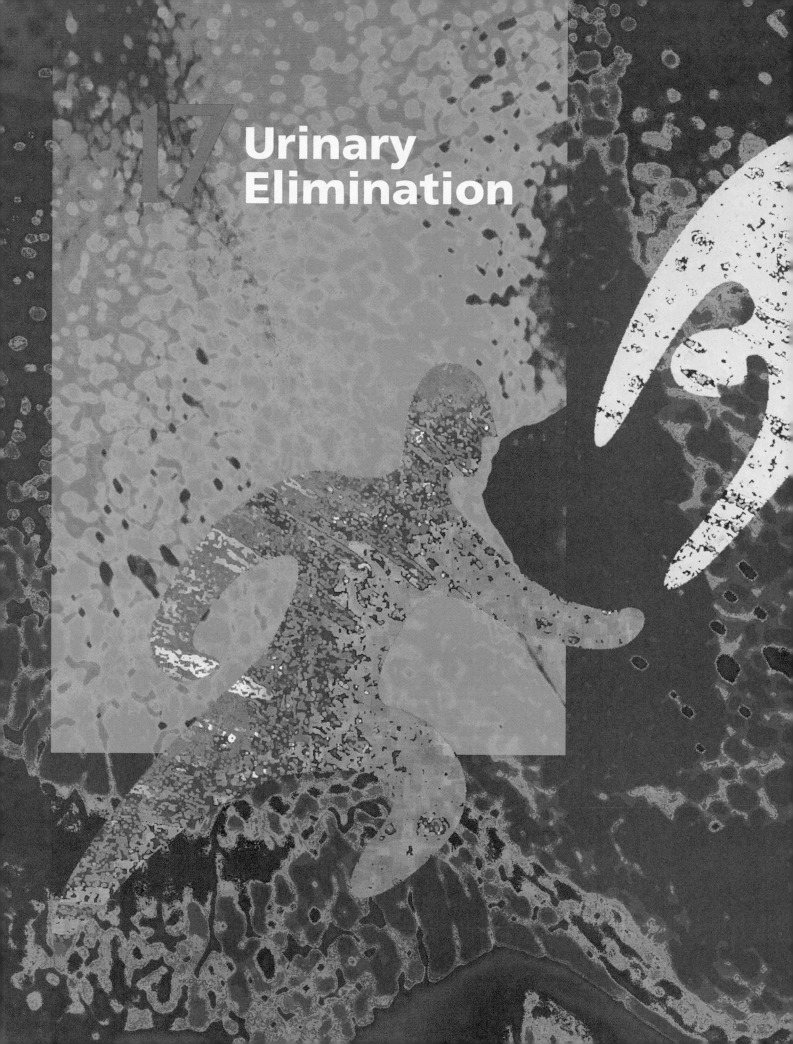

17 Urinary Elimination

- Define the key terms in this chapter
- Identify the characteristics of normal urine
- Describe the rules for maintaining normal urinary elimination
- List the observations to be made about urine
- Describe urinary incontinence and the care required
- Explain why catheters are used
- Describe the rules for caring for persons with catheters
- Explain the differences between straight, indwelling, and condom catheters
- Explain the purpose of bladder irrigations
- Describe two methods of bladder training
- Describe the rules for collecting urine specimens
- Perform the procedures described in this chapter

KEY TERMS

acetone Ketone bodies that appear in the urine because of the rapid breakdown of fat for energy

catheter A tube used to drain or inject fluid through a body opening

catheterization The process of inserting a catheter

dysuria Painful or difficult *(dys)* urination *(uria)*

functional incontinence The involuntary, unpredicted loss of urine from the bladder

glucosuria Sugar *(glucos)* in the urine *(uria)*; glycosuria

glycosuria Sugar *(glycos)* in the urine *(uria)*; glucosuria

hematuria Blood *(hemat)* in the urine *(uria)*

irrigation The process of washing out, flushing out, clearing, or cleaning a tube or body cavity

ketone body Acetone

meniscus The curved surface of a column of liquid

micturition The process of emptying urine from the bladder; urination or voiding

mixed incontinence A combination of urge and stress incontinence

nocturia Frequent urination *(uria)* at night *(noct)*

oliguria Scant amount *(olig)* of urine *(uria)*; usually less than 500 ml in 24 hours

overflow incontinence The loss of urine when the bladder is too full

polyuria The production of abnormally large amounts *(poly)* of urine *(uria)*

reflex incontinence The loss of urine at predictable intervals; unconscious incontinence

residual urine The amount of urine left in the bladder after voiding

stress incontinence The loss of small amounts of urine with exercise and certain movements

unconscious incontinence Reflex incontinence

urge incontinence The involuntary loss of urine after feeling a strong need to void

urinary frequency Voiding at frequent intervals

urinary incontinence The inability to control the loss of urine from the bladder

urinary urgency The need to void immediately

urination The process of emptying urine from the bladder; micturition or voiding

voiding Urination or micturition

Eliminating waste is a physical need. The respiratory, digestive, integumentary, and urinary systems all remove body wastes. The digestive system rids the body of solid wastes. The lungs rid the body of carbon dioxide. Sweat contains water and other substances. Blood contains waste products from body cells burning food for energy. The urinary system removes waste products from the blood and maintains the body's water balance (see Chapter 7).

NORMAL URINATION

The healthy adult excretes about 1500 ml (milliliters) (3 pints) of urine a day. Many factors affect urine production. They include age, disease, the amount and kinds of fluid ingested, dietary salt, and drugs. Some substances increase urine production. Examples are coffee, tea, alcohol, and some drugs. A diet high in salt causes the body to retain water. When water is retained, less urine is produced.

Urination, micturition, and **voiding** mean the process of emptying urine from the bladder. Urination patterns depend on many factors. The amount of fluid ingested, personal habits, and available toilet facilities affect frequency. So do activity, work, and illness. People usually urinate at bedtime, after getting up, and before meals. Some people urinate every 2 to 3 hours. The need to urinate at night disturbs sleep.

MAINTAINING NORMAL URINATION

Some persons need help getting to the bathroom. Others use bedpans, urinals, or commodes. Follow the rules listed in Box 17-1 to help maintain normal elimination.

What to Report to the RN

Urine is normally pale yellow, straw colored, or amber. It is clear with no particles. A faint odor is normal. Observe urine for color, clarity, odor, amount, and particles. Some foods normally affect urine color. Red food dyes, beets, blackberries, and rhubarb cause red-colored urine. Carrots and sweet potatoes cause bright yellow urine. Certain drugs cause changes in urine color. Asparagus causes a urine odor.

Ask the RN to observe any urine that looks or smells abnormal. Report complaints of urgency, burning on urination, or dysuria. **Dysuria** means painful or difficult *(dys)* urination *(uria)*. Also report the problems described in Table 17-1. The RN uses the information for the nursing process.

BOX 17-1

RULES FOR MAINTAINING NORMAL ELIMINATION

- Practice medical asepsis and Standard Precautions. Also follow the Bloodborne Pathogen Standard.
- Provide fluids as instructed by the RN.
- Follow the person's normal voiding routines and habits. Check with the RN and the nursing care plan.
- Help the person to the bathroom when the request is made. Or provide the commode, bedpan, or urinal. The need to void may be urgent.
- Help the person assume a normal position for voiding if possible. Women sit or squat; men stand.
- Warm the bedpan or urinal.
- Cover the person for warmth and privacy.
- Provide for privacy. Pull the curtain around the bed, close room and bathroom doors, and pull drapes or window shades. Leave the room if the person can be alone.
- Tell the person that running water, flushing the toilet, or playing music can mask urination sounds. Some persons are embarrassed about voiding with others close by.
- Remain nearby if the person is weak or unsteady.
- Place the call bell and toilet tissue within reach.
- Allow the person enough time to void. Do not rush the person.
- Promote relaxation. Some people like to read when eliminating.
- Run water in a nearby sink if the person has difficulty starting the stream. Or place the person's fingers in some water.
- Provide perineal care as needed.
- Have the person wash his or her hands after voiding. Provide a wash basin, soap, washcloth, and towel. Assist as necessary.
- Offer the bedpan or urinal at regular times. Some people are embarrassed or are too weak to ask.

TABLE 17-1 COMMON URINARY ELIMINATION PROBLEMS

	Definition	Causes
dysuria	Painful or difficult *(dys)* urination *(uria)*	Urinary tract infection, trauma, urinary tract obstruction
hematuria	Blood *(hemat)* in the urine *(uria)*	Kidney disease, urinary tract infection, trauma
nocturia	Frequent urination *(uria)* at night *(noct)*	Excessive fluid intake, kidney disease, disease of the prostate
oliguria	Scant amount *(olig)* of urine *(uria)*, usually less than 500 ml in 24 hours	Inadequate fluid intake, shock, burns, kidney disease, heart failure
polyuria	The production of abnormally large amounts *(poly)* of urine *(uria)*	Drugs, excessive fluid intake, diabetes mellitus, hormone imbalance
urinary frequency	Voiding at frequent intervals	Excessive fluid intake, bladder infections, pressure on the bladder, drugs
urinary incontinence	Inability to control the loss of urine from the bladder	Trauma, disease, urinary tract infections, reproductive or urinary tract surgeries, aging, fecal impaction, constipation, not getting to the bathroom
urinary urgency	The need to void immediately	Urinary tract infection, fear of incontinence (see p. 380), full bladder, stress

✦ Bedpans

Bedpans are used when persons cannot be out of bed. Women use bedpans for voiding and bowel movements. Men use them only for bowel movements. Bedpans are made of plastic or stainless steel. Stainless steel bedpans are often cold. They are warmed with water and dried before use.

A *fracture pan* has a thinner rim and is only about ½-inch deep at one end (Fig. 17-1). The smaller end is placed under the buttocks (Fig. 17-2, p. 374). Fracture pans are used for persons with casts or those in traction.

Follow medical asepsis, Standard Precautions, and the Bloodborne Pathogen Standard when handling bedpans and their contents.

Text continued on p. 377

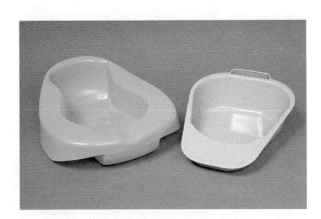

Fig. 17-1 *The regular bedpan and the fracture pan.*

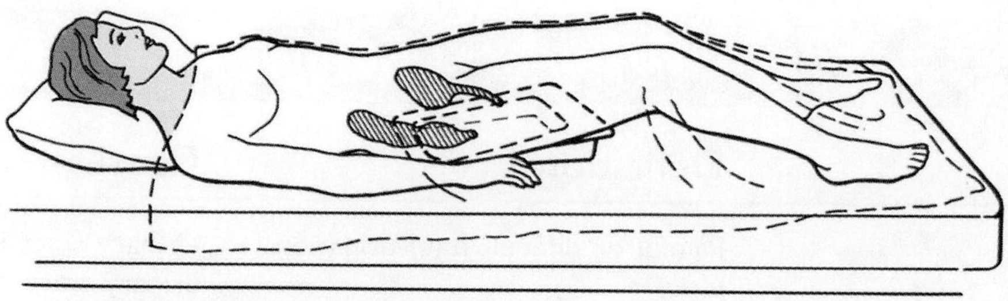

Fig. 17-2 *A person positioned on a fracture pan. The smaller end is placed under the buttocks.*

GIVING THE BEDPAN

PRE-PROCEDURE

1   Provide for privacy.

2   Put on gloves.

3   Collect the following:

  • Bedpan

  • Bedpan cover

  • Toilet tissue

4   Arrange equipment on the chair or bed.

5   Explain the procedure to the person.

6   Raise the bed to the best level for good body mechanics.

PROCEDURE

7   Make sure the bed rails are up.

8   Warm and dry the bedpan if necessary.

9   Lower the bed rail.

10 Position the person supine. Raise the head of the bed slightly.

11 Fold the top linens and gown out of the way. Keep the lower body covered.

12 Ask the person to flex the knees and raise the buttocks by pushing against the mattress with his or her feet.

13 Slide your hand under the lower back, and help him or her raise the buttocks.

14 Slide the bedpan under the person (Fig. 17-3, p. 376).

15 Do the following if the person cannot assist in getting on the bedpan:

  a   Turn the person onto the side away from you.

  b   Place the bedpan firmly against the buttocks (Fig. 17-4, *A*, p. 376).

  c   Push the bedpan down and toward the person (Fig. 17-4, *B*, p. 376).

  d   Hold the bedpan securely. Turn the person onto the back. Make sure the bedpan is centered under the person.

16 Return top linens to their proper position.

17 Raise the head of the bed so the person is in a sitting position.

GIVING THE BEDPAN—cont'd

PROCEDURE—cont'd

18 Make sure the person is correctly positioned on the bedpan (Fig. 17-5, p. 376).

19 Raise the bed rail.

20 Place the toilet tissue and call bell within reach.

21 Ask the person to signal when done or when help is needed.

22 Remove the gloves.

23 Leave the room, and close the door. Wash your hands.

24 Return when the person signals. Knock before entering.

25 Lower the bed rail and the head of the bed.

26 Put on gloves.

27 Ask the person to raise the buttocks. Remove the bedpan. Or hold the bedpan securely and turn him or her onto the side away from you.

28 Clean the genital area if the person cannot do so. Clean from front to back with toilet tissue. Use fresh tissue for each wipe. Provide perineal care if necessary.

29 Cover the bedpan. Take it to the bathroom or dirty utility room. Raise the bed rail before leaving the bedside.

30 Note the color, amount, and character of urine or feces.

31 Empty and rinse the bedpan. Clean it with a disinfectant.

32 Return the bedpan and clean cover to the bedside stand.

33 Remove soiled gloves. Put on clean gloves.

34 Help the person wash the hands.

35 Remove the gloves.

POST-PROCEDURE

36 Make sure the person is comfortable.

37 Place the call bell within reach.

38 Raise or lower bed rails as instructed by the RN.

39 Lower the bed to its lowest position.

40 Unscreen the person.

41 Follow agency policy for soiled linen.

42 Wash your hands.

43 Report your observations to the RN.

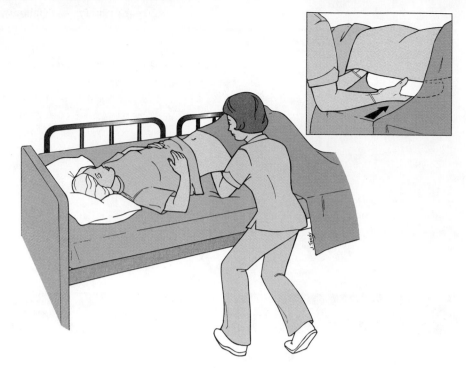

Fig. 17-3 *The person raises the buttocks off the bed with help. The bedpan is slid under the person.*

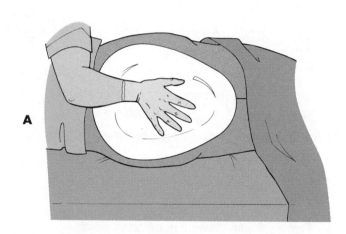

A

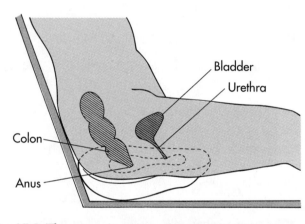

Fig. 17-5 *The person is positioned on the bedpan so the urethra and anus are directly over the opening.*

Bladder
Urethra
Colon
Anus

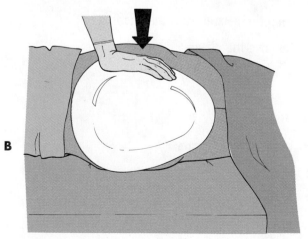

B

Fig. 17-4 **A,** *Position the person on one side, and place the bedpan firmly against the buttocks.* **B,** *Push downward on the bedpan and toward the person.*

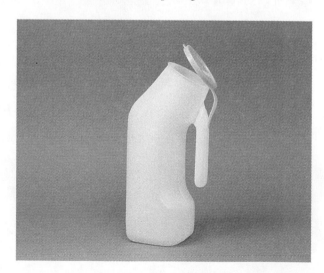

Fig. 17-6 *A urinal.*

✦ Urinals

Men use urinals to void (Fig. 17-6). Plastic urinals have caps at the top and hook-type handles. The urinal hooks to the bed rail within the man's reach. The man stands to use the urinal if possible. Otherwise he sits on the side of the bed or lies in bed. Some men stand with the support of 1 or 2 people. You may have to place and hold the urinal for some men.

Remind men to hang urinals on bed rails and to signal when urinals need emptying. Discourage men from placing urinals on overbed tables and bedside stands. The overbed table is used for eating and as a work surface. Bedside stands are used for supplies. For these reasons, table surfaces must not be contaminated with urine.

Follow medical asepsis, Standard Precautions, and the Bloodborne Pathogen Standard when handling urinals and their contents. Empty urinals promptly to prevent odors and the spread of microbes. A filled urinal spills easily, causing safety hazards. Also, it is an unpleasant sight and a source of odor. Urinals are cleaned like bedpans.

GIVING THE URINAL

PROCEDURE

1 Provide for privacy.

2 Determine if the man will stand or stay in bed.

3 Put on gloves.

4 Give him the urinal if he is in bed. Remind him to tilt the bottom down to prevent spills.

5 Do the following if he is going to stand:

   a Help him sit on the side of the bed.

   b Put nonskid slippers on him.

   c Assist him to a standing position.

   d Provide support if he is unsteady.

   e Give him the urinal.

6 Position the urinal between his legs if necessary. Position his penis in the urinal if he cannot hold the urinal.

7 Cover him to provide for privacy.

8 Place the call bell within reach. Ask him to signal when done or when he needs help.

9 Remove the gloves, and wash your hands.

10 Leave the room, and close the door.

11 Return when he signals for you. Knock before entering.

12 Put on gloves.

13 Cover the urinal. Take it to the bathroom or dirty utility room.

14 Note the color, amount, and character of the urine.

15 Empty the urinal, and rinse it with cold water. Clean it with a disinfectant.

16 Return the urinal to the bedside stand.

17 Remove soiled gloves. Put on clean gloves.

18 Help the person wash his hands.

19 Remove the gloves.

POST-PROCEDURE

20 Make sure he is comfortable.

21 Place the call bell within reach.

22 Raise or lower bed rails as instructed by the RN.

23 Unscreen him.

24 Follow agency policy for soiled linen.

25 Wash your hands.

26 Report your observations to the RN.

✦ Commodes

A bedside commode is a portable chair or wheelchair with an opening for a bedpan or container (Fig. 17-7). Persons unable to walk to the bathroom often use commodes. The commode allows a normal position for elimination. The bedpan or container is cleaned after use like the regular bedpan.

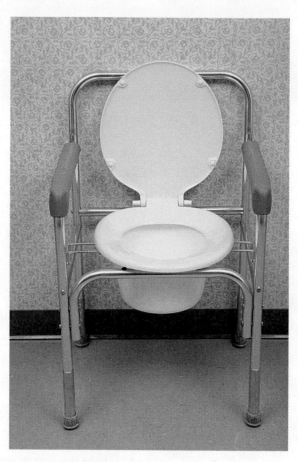

Fig. 17-7 *The bedside commode has a toilet seat with a container. The container slides out from under the toilet seat for emptying.*

✦ HELPING THE PERSON TO THE COMMODE

PRE-PROCEDURE

1 Explain the procedure to the person.

2 Provide for privacy.

3 Put on gloves.

4 Collect the following:
- Commode
- Toilet tissue
- Bath blanket

PROCEDURE

5 Bring the commode next to the bed. Remove the chair seat and lid from the container.

6 Help the person sit on the side of the bed.

7 Help him or her put on a robe and nonskid slippers.

8 Assist the person to the commode.

9 Place a bath blanket over his or her lap for warmth.

10 Place the toilet tissue and call bell within reach.

11 Ask him or her to signal when done or when help is needed.

12 Remove the gloves, and wash your hands.

13 Leave the room, and close the door.

14 Return when the person signals. Knock before entering.

15 Put on the gloves.

16 Help the person clean the genital area if indicated. Remove the gloves.

17 Help the person back to bed. Remove the robe and slippers. Raise the bed rail if instructed by the RN.

18 Put on clean gloves. Cover and remove the container from the commode. Clean the commode if necessary.

19 Take the container to the bathroom or dirty utility room.

20 Check urine and feces for color, amount, and character. Collect a specimen if one is needed.

21 Clean and disinfect the container.

22 Return the container to the commode. Return other supplies to their proper place.

23 Return the commode to its proper place.

24 Remove soiled gloves. Put on clean gloves.

25 Help the person wash the hands.

26 Remove the gloves.

POST-PROCEDURE

27 Make sure he or she is comfortable and the call bell is within reach.

28 Raise or lower bed rails as instructed by the RN.

29 Unscreen the person.

30 Follow agency policy for soiled linen.

31 Wash your hands.

32 Report your observations to the RN.

NURSING MEASURES FOR PERSONS WITH URINARY INCONTINENCE

- Keep records of the person's voidings. This includes incontinent episodes and successful use of the toilet, commode, bedpan, or urinal.
- Answer call bells promptly. The person may have an urgent need to void.
- Promote normal urinary elimination (see Box 17-1).
- Promote normal bowel elimination (see Chapter 18).
- Encourage urination at scheduled intervals.
- Follow the person's bladder training program (see p. 399).
- Encourage the person to wear clothing that is easy to remove. Incontinence can occur as the person is trying to deal with buttons, zippers, and undergarments.
- Encourage the person to do pelvic muscle exercises as instructed by the RN.
- Encourage fluid intake as directed by the RN.
- Decrease fluid intake before bedtime.
- Provide good skin care.
- Provide dry gowns and linens.
- Observe the skin for signs of breakdown.
- Use incontinence products as directed by the RN.

URINARY INCONTINENCE

Urinary incontinence is the involuntary loss of urine from the bladder. It may be temporary or permanent. There are different types of incontinence:

- **Urge incontinence** is the involuntary loss of urine after feeling a strong need to void. The person cannot stop urinating and cannot get to the bathroom in time. Urinary frequency, urinary urgency, and night-time voidings are common. Urinary tract infections, decreased bladder capacity, alcohol and caffeine intake, and increased fluid intake are causes.
- **Stress incontinence** is the loss of small amounts of urine with exercise and certain movements. Urine loss is usually small (less than 50 ml). Often called *dribbling*, stress incontinence occurs with laughing, sneezing, coughing, lifting, or other activities. Late pregnancy and obesity are other causes. The problem is common in women. Pelvic muscles weaken after multiple pregnancies and with aging.
- **Mixed incontinence** is a combination of urge and stress incontinence. This type is more common in older women.
- **Overflow incontinence** is the loss of urine when the bladder is too full. The person feels like the bladder is never completely empty. Much time is spent trying to void. However, the person only dribbles or has a weak stream of urine. Small amounts of urine are lost during the day and night. Nocturia is common. Fecal impaction, diabetes, and spinal cord injury are causes. Prostate enlargement is a common cause in men.

- **Functional incontinence** is the involuntary, unpredictable loss of urine. The person does not have nervous system or urinary system injuries. The person cannot use the bathroom, bedpan, urinal, or commode in time. Immobility, restraints, unanswered call bells, not having a call bell within reach, and not knowing where to find the bathroom also are causes. So is difficulty removing clothes. Confusion and disorientation are other causes.
- **Unconscious or reflex incontinence** is the loss of urine at predictable intervals. Urine is lost when the bladder is full. The person does not know the bladder is full and has no urge to void. Central nervous system disorders and injuries are common causes.

Incontinence is embarrassing. Clothing gets wet, odors develop, and the person is uncomfortable. Irritation, infection, and pressure ulcers can occur. Falling is a risk as the person tries to get to the bathroom quickly.

The RN uses the nursing process to meet the person's needs. Follow the RN's instructions and the nursing care plan. Nursing measures depend on the type of incontinence. The person's care plan may include some of the nursing measures listed in Box 17-2. *Good skin care and dry clothing and linens are always essential.* Following the rules for maintaining normal urinary elimination prevents incontinence in some people. Others need bladder training programs (see p. 399). Sometimes catheters are ordered. Some people wear garment protectors or incontinence pads (Fig. 17-8). Incontinence drawsheets help keep the person dry. The drawsheet has two layers and a

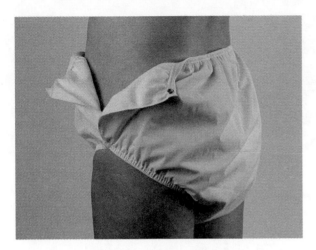

Fig. 17-8 *Garment protector (incontinence pad).*

waterproof back. Fluid passes through the first layer and is absorbed by the lower layer. A variety of incontinent products are available. The nurse selects products best suited to the person's needs.

Incontinence is linked to abuse, mistreatment, and neglect. Caring for these persons is stressful. They need frequent care and may wet again just after you gave skin care and changed wet gowns and linens. Do not lose patience. Their needs are great, and your role is to meet their needs. If you find yourself short-tempered and impatient, discuss the problem with the RN immediately. Remember, the person has the right to be free from abuse, mistreatment, or neglect. The incontinence is beyond the person's control. It is not something he or she chooses to let happen. Kindness, empathy, understanding, and patience are very important. (See Focus on Older Persons and Focus on Home Care.)

✦ CATHETERS

A **catheter** is a rubber or plastic tube used to drain or inject fluid through a body opening. Inserted through the urethra into the bladder, a urinary catheter drains urine. A *straight catheter* drains the bladder and is removed. An *indwelling catheter* (*retention* or *Foley catheter*) is left in the bladder so urine drains constantly into a drainage bag. A balloon near the tip of the catheter is inflated after the catheter is inserted. The balloon prevents the catheter from slipping out of the bladder (Fig. 17-9, p. 382). Tubing connects the catheter to the collection bag.

Catheter insertion (**catheterization**) is done by a nurse or doctor. Some states and agencies allow assistive personnel to perform catheterizations (see p. 386).

Catheters often are used before, during, and after surgery to keep the bladder empty. This reduces the risk of accidental bladder injury during surgery. After surgery, a full bladder causes pressure on nearby organs.

Catheters also allow hourly urinary output measurements in critically ill persons. They are a last resort for incontinence. Catheters do not treat the cause of incontinence, and the risk of infection is high. However, some persons have wounds and pressure ulcers that need protection from urine. Catheters can protect the wounds and pressure ulcers from contamination with urine.

Some patients are too weak or disabled to use the bedpan, commode, or toilet. Dying patients are an example. For these patients, catheters can promote comfort. Also, the person is protected from incontinence.

Catheters are inserted for diagnostic purposes. They are used to collect sterile urine specimens (see p. 405). Another test involves inserting a catheter to see how much urine is left in the bladder (**residual urine**). The catheter is inserted after the person voids.

You will care for persons with indwelling catheters. The rules listed in Box 17-3 on p. 382 promote their comfort and safety.

Text continued on p. 386

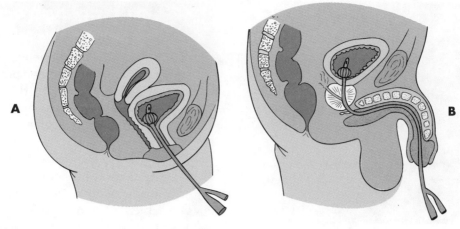

Fig. 17-9 A, *Indwelling catheter in the female bladder. The inflated balloon at the top prevents the catheter from slipping out through the urethra.* **B,** *Indwelling catheter with the balloon inflated in the male bladder.*

BOX 17-3

CARING FOR PERSONS WITH INDWELLING CATHETERS

- Follow the rules of medical asepsis, Standard Precautions, and the Bloodborne Pathogen Standard.
- Make sure urine flows freely through the catheter or tubing. Tubing should not have kinks. The person should not lie on the tubing.
- Keep the drainage bag below the bladder. This prevents urine from flowing backward into the bladder. Attach the drainage bag to the bed frame. *Never attach the drainage bag to the bed rail.* Otherwise the drainage bag is higher than the bladder when the bed rail is raised.
- Coil the drainage tubing on the bed, and pin it to the bottom linen (Fig. 17-10).
- Secure the catheter to the inner thigh as in Figure 17-10. Or secure it to the man's abdomen. This prevents excessive movement of the catheter and reduces friction at the insertion site. Secure the catheter with tape or other devices as ordered by the RN.
- Check for leaks. Check the site where the catheter connects to the drainage bag. Report any leaks to the RN immediately.
- Provide catheter care if ordered. Catheter care is done daily or twice a day (see *Catheter Care,* p. 384). Some agencies consider perineal care to be sufficient. Catheter care is sometimes needed after bowel movements and when vaginal drainage is present.
- Provide perineal care daily and after bowel movements.
- Empty the drainage bag at the end of the shift or at time intervals as directed by the RN. Measure and record the amount of urine (see *Emptying a Urinary Drainage Bag,* p. 386). Report increases or decreases in the amount of urine.
- Use a separate measuring container for each person. This prevents the spread of microbes from one person to another.
- Do not the let the drain on the drainage bag touch any surface.
- Report complaints to the RN immediately. These include complaints of pain, burning, the need to urinate, or irritation. Also report the color, clarity, and odor of urine and the presence of particles.
- Encourage fluid intake as instructed by the RN.

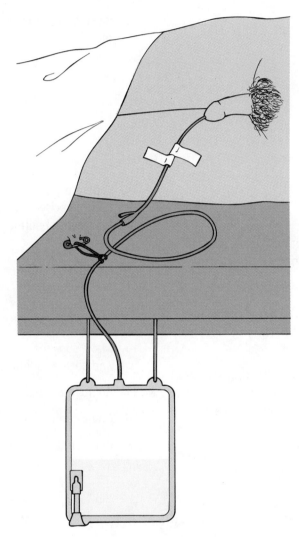

Fig. 17-10 *The drainage tubing is coiled on the bed and pinned to the bottom linens so urine flows freely. A rubber band is placed around the tubing with a clove hitch. The safety pin is passed through the loops and pinned to the linens. The catheter is taped to the inner thigh. Enough slack is left on the catheter to prevent friction at the urethra.*

GIVING CATHETER CARE

PRE-PROCEDURE

1 Explain the procedure to the person.

2 Wash your hands.

3 Collect the following:

   • Equipment for perineal care (see p. 318)

   • Gloves

   • Bed protector

   • Bath blanket

4 Identify the person. Check the ID bracelet against the assignment sheet.

5 Provide for privacy.

6 Raise the bed to the best level for good body mechanics.

PROCEDURE

7 Lower the bed rail.

8 Put on the gloves.

9 Cover the person with a bath blanket. Fanfold top linens to the foot of the bed.

10 Drape the person for perineal care (see Fig. 14-20, p. 320).

11 Fold back the bath blanket between the legs to expose the genital area.

12 Place the bed protector under the buttocks. Ask the person to flex the knees and raise the buttocks off the bed by pushing against the mattress with the feet.

13 Perform perineal care (see *Female Perineal Care, p. 318* or *Male Perineal Care*, p. 322).

14 Separate the labia (female) or retract the foreskin (uncircumcised male) as in Figure 17-11. Check for crusts, abnormal drainage, or secretions.

15 Clean the catheter from the meatus down the catheter about 4 inches (Fig. 17-12). Use soap and water and a clean washcloth. Avoid tugging or pulling on the catheter. Repeat if necessary with a clean washcloth.

16 Make sure the catheter is secured properly. Coil and secure tubing (see Fig. 17-10).

17 Remove the bed protector.

18 Cover the person, and remove the bath blanket.

19 Remove the gloves.

POST-PROCEDURE

20 Make sure the person is comfortable and the call bell is within reach.

21 Raise or lower bed rails as instructed by the RN.

22 Lower the bed to its lowest position.

23 Clean and return equipment to its proper place. Discard disposable items. (Wear gloves for this step.)

24 Unscreen the person.

25 Follow agency policy for soiled linen.

26 Wash your hands.

27 Report your observations to the RN.

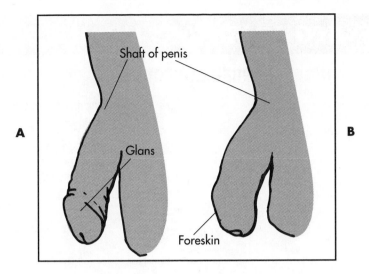

Fig. 17-11 A, *Circumcised male.* **B,** *Uncircumcised male.*

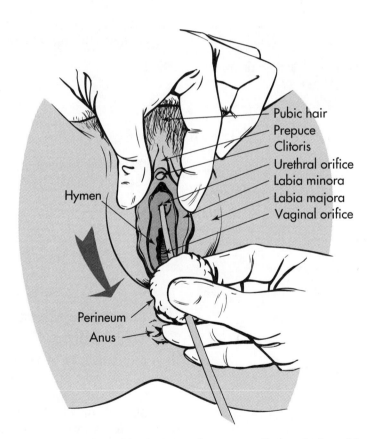

Fig. 17-12 *The catheter is cleaned beginning at the meatus. About 4 inches of the catheter is cleaned.*

◆ EMPTYING A URINARY DRAINAGE BAG

PRE-PROCEDURE

1 Collect equipment:
 • Graduate (measuring container)
 • Gloves
2 Wash your hands.

3 Explain the procedure to the person.
4 Identify the person. Check the ID bracelet against the assignment sheet.
5 Provide for privacy.

PROCEDURE

6 Put on the gloves.
7 Place the measuring container (graduate) so urine is collected when you open the drain.
8 Open the clamp on the bottom of the drainage bag.
9 Let all urine drain into the graduate. Do not let the drain touch the graduate (Fig. 17-13).
10 Close the clamp. Replace the clamped drain in the holder on the bag (see Fig. 17-10).

11 Measure urine.
12 Rinse the graduate, and return it to its proper place.
13 Remove the gloves, and wash your hands.
14 Record the time and amount on the intake and output (I&O) record (see Chapter 20).

POST-PROCEDURE

15 Unscreen the person.

16 Report the amount of urine and other observations to the RN.

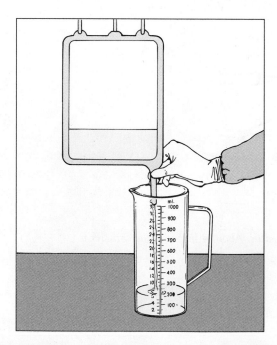

Fig. 17-13 *The clamp on the drainage bag is opened, and the drain is directed into the measuring container. The drain must not touch the inside of the container.*

◆ Inserting Straight and Indwelling Catheters

A catheterization requires a doctor's order. The doctor orders a straight catheter or an indwelling catheter (see p. 387). The straight catheter is removed after draining the bladder or obtaining a specimen. An indwelling catheter is left in place and attached to a closed drainage system. A closed drainage system means that nothing can enter the system from the catheter to the drainage bag.

Catheterizations require sterile technique. The urinary system is sterile. Catheterizations increase the risk of urinary tract infections (UTIs). These infections prolong the person's health care and recovery. Some cause life-threatening complications. See Chapter 11 to review surgical asepsis.

Before doing a catheterization, make sure:

- Your state allows assistive personnel to perform the procedure
- The procedure is in your job description
- You know the urinary tract structures (see Chapter 7)
- You receive the necessary education and training
- You feel comfortable with the procedure
- You are familiar with the agency's supplies and equipment
- You review the procedure with the RN
- An RN is available for questions and to supervise you

Equipment and supplies

The RN tells you what size catheter to use, what kind of catheter to use (straight or indwelling), and if a closed drainage system is needed. With this information, you select a straight or indwelling catheterization kit from the supply area. The kit has supplies for the procedure. All items in the kit are sterile. The kit contains:

- Catheter
- Sterile gloves
- Sterile drape for under the buttocks (female) or across the thighs (male)
- Fenestrated drape (*fenestrated* means with an opening or window) for the perineal area
- Forceps
- Basin for urine
- Lubricant
- Antiseptic solution
- Cotton balls
- Syringe with sterile water (see p. 405)
- Drainage bag and tubing (indwelling catheter kit)

Catheters are sized in the French scale. (The abbreviation "Fr" means French.) Either *Fr* follows the number or the # sign is before the number. The RN tells you what size to use. The following are guidelines:

- Children—8 or 10 Fr (#8 or #10)
- Women—14 or 16 Fr (#14 or #16)
- Men—14, 16, or 18 Fr (#14, #16, or #18)

You need good lighting for the procedure. A flashlight or gooseneck lamp helps you see the urinary meatus. Place the light source at the foot of the bed, and direct it at the perineal area.

Types of catheters

A straight catheter (Fig. 17-14, *A*) has one lumen (passageway). An indwelling catheter is double-lumen (Fig. 17-14, *B*). Sterile water is injected through one lumen to inflate the balloon. Urine drains from the bladder through the other lumen. Some indwelling catheters are triple-lumen (Fig. 17-14, *C*). The third lumen is for bladder treatments ordered by the doctor.

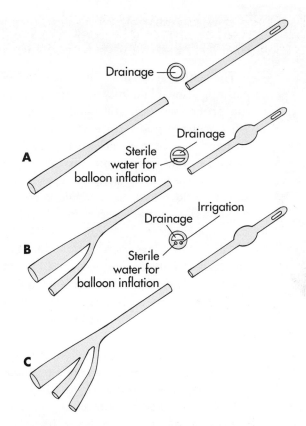

Fig. 17-14 *Types of catheters.* **A,** *Straight catheter (single lumen).* **B,** *Indwelling catheter (double-lumen) with balloon inflated.* **C,** *Indwelling catheter with a triple-lumen catheter. The balloon is inflated.*

Preparing the person

The RN explains the procedure and its need to the person. The RN also explains the care required while the catheter is in place. This helps the person understand what is happening and why. You also explain the procedure before beginning. During the procedure, explain to the person what you are doing step by step. This information helps meet the person's need for safety and security. The informed person is more relaxed and cooperative.

The procedure embarrasses some people. It involves exposing and touching the genitals. The person needs to know how privacy is protected during the procedure. Explain that you will draw the privacy curtain, close window shades or drapes, and close room doors. Also explain how draping is done and that the perineal area is exposed only for a short time. If the procedure embarrasses you, share your feelings with the RN. (See Focus on Children, Focus on Older Persons, and Focus on Home Care on p. 388.)

Text continued on p. 394

focus on CHILDREN

The child may not be cooperative. Although the child may not understand the procedure, you still need to explain what you are going to do. You are likely to need a parent or co-worker to help keep the child in position. Restricting the child's movement is likely to further upset the child. However, the child needs to be kept still so that the sterile field is not contaminated.

Adolescents are concerned about genital development. Having someone look at and touch the perineal area is embarrassing. You need to thoroughly explain what you are going to do. A professional manner is important.

Adolescent boys may have an erection when the genitals are touched. If this happens, cover the area and tell the boy you will give him some time alone. Tell him when you will return, and leave the room. Close the door as you leave the room, and knock on the door when you return. (This applies to adolescent boys and adult men of all ages.)

focus on OLDER PERSONS

When catheterizing women, they are positioned for perineal care. Older women may not be able to hold the position. You need a co-worker to help the patient maintain the position. Work as quickly as you can to complete the procedure.

If possible, catheterizations are avoided in older persons because of the risk of urinary tract infections (UTIs). Changes in the urinary system from aging increase the older person's risk for UTIs. These infections are especially serious for older persons. They can lead to serious health problems and death.

Enlargement of the prostate gland is a common problem in older men. The gland lies just below the bladder. When the gland enlarges, it can obstruct the urethra. Urine does not flow out of the bladder normally. The urine stream is less forceful. The bladder does not empty completely. Dribbling, frequent urination, and nocturia (urination at night) are common problems. Catheterization is sometimes necessary. A Coudé catheter is often used. It has a curved tip and is easier to pass around the obstruction. Because of the obstruction, a doctor or RN inserts a Coudé catheter.

focus on HOME CARE

Make sure an RN is available by phone in case problems arise. Remember that you cannot pick up the phone and dial with sterile gloves. Nor can you answer the phone. When you review the procedure with the RN, ask what you should do if problems occur.

INSERTING A STRAIGHT CATHETER

PROCEDURE ALERT

- Does your state allow assistive personnel to perform the procedure?

- Is the procedure in your job description?

- Do you have the necessary training and education?

- Is an RN available to answer questions and to supervise you?

PRE-PROCEDURE

1 Explain the procedure to the person.

2 Collect the following:

- Catheterization kit as directed by the RN (see p. 387)

- Sterile gloves (if not part of the kit)

- Flashlight or gooseneck lamp

- Bath blanket

- Soap

- Bath basin with warm water

- Washcloth

- Towel

- Disposable gloves

- Specimen container and laboratory requisition (if ordered)

- Trash bag

3 Identify the person. Check the ID bracelet against the assignment sheet.

4 Provide for privacy.

5 Raise the bed to the best level for good body mechanics. Make sure the far bed rail is raised.

PROCEDURE

6 Position the person supine. Cover the person with a bath blanket.

7 Position and drape the person as for perineal care (see Fig. 14-20, p. 320).

8 Put on the disposable gloves.

9 Provide perineal care (see *Giving Female Perineal Care*, p. 318 and *Giving Male Perineal Care*, p. 322).

10 Remove equipment and supplies used for perineal care. Also remove the gloves and wash your hands. (Make sure both bed rails are up when you leave the bedside. Lower the near bed rail when you return.)

11 Position the flashlight or gooseneck lamp at the foot of the bed. Direct the light source at the perineal area.

12 Arrange the overbed table and catheterization kit so you can create a sterile field.

13 Place the trash bag in a convenient location.

14 Open the catheterization kit. Follow directions on the package.

15 Put on the sterile gloves.

16 Organize the sterile field:

  a Open sterile packages and containers (cotton balls, antiseptic solution, specimen container, and lubricant).

  b Pour the antiseptic solution over the cotton balls.

17 Pick up the first sterile drape. Stand back and let it unfold.

18 Drape the person:

  a Draping a female:

- Hold the drape with both hands.

- Do not touch her or the bed with your gloves. Your gloves must touch only the sterile drape.

- Ask the woman to raise her buttocks off the bed.

- Slide the drape under her buttocks.

- Pick up the fenestrated drape and let it unfold.

- Drape it over the perineum. Expose only the labia.

Continued

PROCEDURE—cont'd

b Draping a male:

- Lift the penis with your nondominant hand. (This hand is now contaminated. It cannot touch any part of the sterile field.)

- Lay the drape over the thighs.

- Pick up the fenestrated drape with your sterile hand. Let it unfold.

- Position the drape over the penis.

- Lift the penis through the opening in the drape with your contaminated hand. Lay the penis on the drape.

19 Place the catheterization tray and its contents on the drape between the person's legs.

20 Lubricate the catheter:

a Female: lubricate about 1 to 2 inches (2.5 to 5 cm) of the catheter tip.

b Male: lubricate about 3 to 5 inches (7.5 to 12.5 cm) of the catheter tip.

21 Clean the meatus. Use a sterile cotton ball for each stroke. (Discard used cotton balls into the trash bag. Do not let the forceps touch the bag.)

a Female (Fig. 17-15, p. 392):

- Separate the labia majora with the thumb and index finger of your nondominant hand. (This hand is now contaminated and cannot touch any part of the sterile field.)

- Keep the labia separated until you insert the catheter.

- Use your sterile hand to pick up the forceps.

- Pick up a cotton ball with the forceps.

- Clean the labia minora on the side away from you. Wipe from the clitoris to the anus with one stroke.

- Clean the labia minora on the side near you. Wipe from clitoris to the anus with one stroke.

- Clean the meatus. Clean each side and down the middle. Wipe from the top to the meatus.

b Male (Fig. 17-16, p. 392):

- Pick up the penis with your contaminated hand.

- Retract the foreskin if the man is not circumcised.

- Hold the penis firmly behind the glans as in Figure 17-16. Maintain this position until you insert the catheter.

- Pick up a cotton ball using the sterile forceps.

- Clean the penis starting at the meatus. Use a circular motion.

- Wipe around the meatus using a circular motion.

- Clean to where your fingers are holding the penis.

22 Place the drainage end of the catheter into the collecting basin.

23 Pick up the catheter about 2 inches from the tip. Make sure the drainage end stays in the collecting basin.

24 Insert the catheter (Fig. 17-17, p. 392).

a Female:

- Make sure you can see the meatus. Also locate the vaginal opening.

- Ask the person to take a deep breath.

- Insert the catheter into the meatus until urine flows (about 3 inches). Insert gently and slowly. (Do not push the catheter if you feel resistance. Stop the procedure, and call for the RN.)

- Hold the catheter in place with your contaminated hand.

- If no urine flows, the catheter could be in the vagina. Leave the catheter in place, and get a new catheterization kit. Begin at step 14. If a co-worker is with you, ask that person to get you another catheter. Keep the labia retracted. Have the person peel back the packaging so that you can grasp the catheter. Lubricate the catheter and insert it. Remove the catheter from the vagina when urine flows.

PROCEDURE—cont'd

b Male:

- Hold the penis so it is upright as in Figure 17-16.

- Ask the person to bear down as if voiding.

- Insert the catheter into the meatus.

- Advance the catheter until urine flows (about 8 inches).

- Lay the penis on the drape. Hold the catheter in place with your contaminated hand.

- Do not force the catheter if you feel resistance. Stop the procedure and call for the RN.

25 Collect a urine specimen if ordered. Continue to hold the catheter in place with your contaminated hand.

a Hold the end of the catheter over the specimen container with your sterile hand. Collect about 30 ml of urine.

b Pinch the catheter to stop urine flow.

c Cover the specimen container, and set it aside.

26 Place the end of the catheter into the collecting basin.

27 Let the bladder empty according to the RN's instructions. Agency policy may require you to stop urine flow for 20 minutes after draining 750 ml or 1000 ml.

28 Note the amount of urine collected.

29 Remove the catheter slowly.

30 Return foreskin to its natural position.

31 Remove and discard the gloves. Gather equipment and supplies for disposal.

32 Cover the person, and remove the bath blanket.

33 Thank the person for cooperating.

POST-PROCEDURE

34 Make sure the person is comfortable.

35 Raise or lower bed rails as instructed by the RN.

36 Lower the bed to its lowest position.

37 Place the call bell within reach.

38 Clean the wash basin. Return reusable supplies to their proper place.

39 Wipe off the overbed table.

40 Unscreen the person.

41 Follow agency policy for dirty linen.

42 Wash your hands.

43 Report your observations to the RN:

a The amount of urine obtained

b Color, clarity, and odor of urine

c Any particles in the urine

d How the person tolerated the procedure

e Any other observations

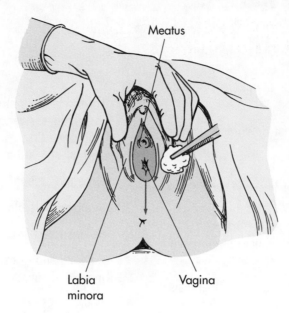

Fig. 17-15 *Cleaning the female meatus. Clean from top to bottom using a clean cotton ball for each stroke.* (*From Potter PA, Perry AG:* Fundamentals of nursing: concepts, process, and practice, *ed 4, St Louis, 1997, Mosby.*)

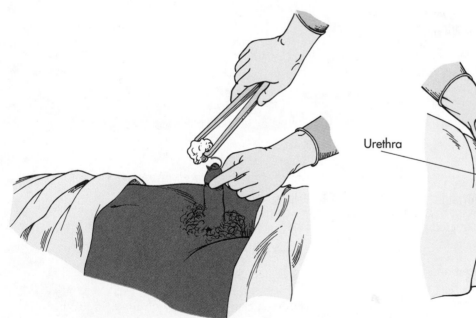

Fig. 17-16 *Cleaning the male meatus. Start at the meatus using circular motions. Clean downward to your fingers. Use a clean cotton ball for each stroke.* (*From Potter PA, Perry AG:* Fundamentals of nursing: concepts, process, and practice, *ed 4, St Louis, 1997, Mosby.*)

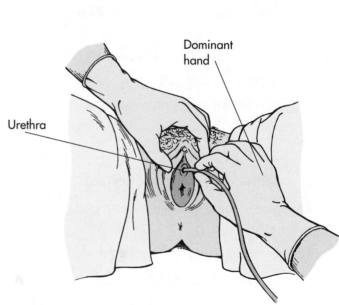

Fig. 17-17 *Inserting the catheter.* (*From Potter PA, Perry AG:* Fundamentals of nursing: concepts, process, and practice, *ed 4, St Louis, 1997, Mosby.*)

INSERTING AN INDWELLING CATHETER

PROCEDURE ALERT

- Does your state allow assistive personnel to perform the procedure?

- Is the procedure in your job description?

- Do you have the necessary training and education?

- Is an RN available to answer questions and to supervise you?

PRE-PROCEDURE

1 Explain the procedure to the person.

2 Collect equipment:

- Catheterization kit as directed by the RN (see p. 387).

- Flashlight or gooseneck lamp

- Bath blanket

- Soap

- Bath basin with warm water

- Washcloth

- Towel

- Disposable gloves

- Trash bag

- Nonallergenic tape

- Safety pin

3 Identify the person. Check the ID bracelet against the assignment sheet.

4 Provide for privacy.

5 Raise the bed to the best level for good body mechanics. Make sure the far bed rail is raised.

PROCEDURE

6 Follow steps 6–16 in *Inserting a Straight Catheter*, p. 389.

7 Make sure the catheter is attached to the collecting tubing and the drainage container. Make sure the drain is closed.

8 Test the balloon on the indwelling catheter (Fig. 17-18, p. 394). It must inflate and not leak:

   a Attach the prefilled syringe to the balloon valve.

   b Inject the water. The balloon should inflate.

   c Pull back on the syringe to withdraw the fluid.

   d Leave the syringe attached to the balloon port.

9 Drape the person as in *Inserting a Straight Catheter* (see steps 17 and 18).

10 Place the sterile catheterization tray and its contents on the drape between the person's legs.

11 Lubricate the catheter.

12 Clean the meatus.

13 Insert the catheter until urine appears.

14 Advance the catheter:

   a Female: advance the catheter another 2 inches after urine appears.

   b Male: advance the catheter another 2 or 3 inches after urine appears. (Check agency policy. Some agencies require advancing the catheter farther. This is done to make sure the balloon is inflated in the bladder not in the urethra [see step 16]).

15 Hold the catheter in place with your nondominant hand.

Continued

⬥ INSERTING AN INDWELLING CATHETER—cont'd

PROCEDURE—cont'd

16 Inflate the balloon. Inject the contents of the syringe. (Pull back on the syringe to withdraw the water if the person complains of pain or discomfort. Insert the catheter farther. Inject fluid again.)

17 Remove the syringe.

18 Let go of the catheter with your nondominant hand. Return foreskin to its natural position.

19 Pull on the catheter gently. You should feel resistance. Resistance means that the balloon is holding the catheter in place (see Fig. 17-9).

20 Secure the catheter in place. Allow enough slack so there is no pull on the catheter:

   a Female: tape the catheter to the inner thigh.

   b Male: tape the catheter to the top of the thigh or lower abdomen.

21 Secure the drainage container to the bed frame.

22 Coil tubing on the bed as in Fig. 17-10.

23 Remove and discard the gloves. Gather equipment and supplies for disposal.

24 Cover the person, and remove the bath blanket.

25 Thank the person for cooperating.

POST-PROCEDURE

26 Follow steps 34-43 in *Inserting a Straight Catheter.*

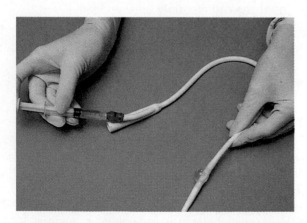

Fig. 17-18 *Testing the balloon. It should inflate and not leak.* (From Potter PA, Perry AG: Fundamentals of nursing: concepts, process, and practice, *ed 4, St Louis, 1997, Mosby.)*

⬥ Removing Indwelling Catheters

The doctor gives the order to remove the catheter. Some persons need bladder training before the catheter is removed (see p. 399). Dysuria and frequency are common problems after removing catheters.

Removing an indwelling catheter involves deflating the balloon. You need a syringe large enough to hold the balloon's contents. Check the label at the end of the catheter for balloon size. The RN also tells you what size syringe to use.

The RN tells you when to remove a catheter. Make sure you review the procedure with the RN. Make sure that your state allows assistive personnel to perform the procedure. The procedure must be in your job description.

REMOVING AN INDWELLING CATHETER

PROCEDURE ALERT

- Does your state allow assistive personnel to perform the procedure?

- Is the procedure in your job description?

- Do you have the necessary training and education?

- Is an RN available to answer questions and to supervise you?

PRE-PROCEDURE

1 Explain the procedure to the person.

2 Wash your hands.

3 Collect the following:

- Disposable towel

- Syringe as directed by the RN

- Trash receptacle

- Gloves

- Bath blanket

4 Identify the person. Check the ID bracelet against the assignment sheet.

5 Provide for privacy.

6 Raise the bed to the best level for body mechanics. Make sure the far bed rail is raised.

PROCEDURE

7 Position the person as for a catheterization.

8 Drape the person with a bath blanket.

9 Put on the gloves.

10 Remove the tape securing the catheter to the person.

11 Place the towel:

a Female: between her legs.

b Male: over his thighs.

12 Attach the syringe to the balloon port.

13 Pull back on the syringe slowly to withdraw all the water from the balloon. (Call for the RN if you cannot remove all the water.)

14 Withdraw the catheter gently. Do not withdraw the catheter while water is in the balloon.

15 Place the catheter in the trash receptacle.

16 Dry the perineal area with the towel.

17 Remove the gloves.

18 Cover the person, and remove the bath blanket. Make sure the person is comfortable.

19 Raise bed rails as instructed by the RN.

20 Lower the bed to its lowest position.

21 Place the call bell within reach.

POST-PROCEDURE

22 Put on gloves.

23 Take the drainage container to the bathroom.

24 Measure the amount of urine in the drainage bag. Note the amount.

25 Discard the urine.

26 Place the drainage bag in the trash container.

27 Remove and discard the gloves.

28 Wash your hands.

29 Report your observations to the RN (see p. 391).

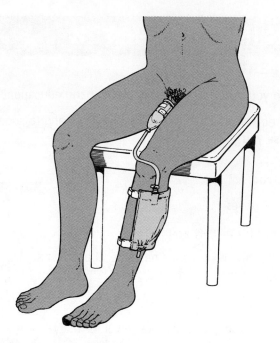

Fig. 17-19 *A condom catheter attached to a leg bag.*

◈ The Condom Catheter

Condom catheters (external catheter, urinary sheath) are often used for incontinent men. A condom catheter is a soft, rubber sheath that slides over the penis. Tubing connects the condom catheter and the drainage bag. Many men prefer leg bags (Fig. 17-19).

A new condom catheter is applied daily. The manufacturer's instructions are followed. The penis is thoroughly washed with soap and water and dried before applying a new catheter. Elastic tape secures the catheter in place. Elastic tape expands when the penis changes size. This allows blood flow to the penis. *Never use adhesive tape to secure catheters. It does not expand. Blood flow to the penis is cut off, injuring the penis.* Follow medical asepsis, Standard Precautions, and the Bloodborne Pathogen Standard when removing or applying condom catheters.

✦ APPLYING A CONDOM CATHETER

PRE-PROCEDURE

1 Explain the procedure to the man.

2 Wash your hands.

3 Collect the following:

- Condom catheter
- Elastic tape
- Drainage bag or leg bag
- Basin of warm water
- Soap
- Towel and washcloths
- Bath blanket

- Gloves

- Bed protector

- Paper towels

4 Arrange paper towels and equipment on the overbed table.

5 Identify the man. Check the ID bracelet against the assignment sheet.

6 Provide for privacy.

7 Raise the bed to the best level for good body mechanics. Make sure the far bed rail is up.

APPLYING A CONDOM CATHETER—cont'd

PROCEDURE

8   Lower the bed rail.

9   Cover the person with a bath blanket. Bring top linens to the foot of the bed.

10 Ask the person to raise his buttocks off the bed. Or turn him onto his side away from you.

11 Slide the bed protector under his buttocks.

12 Have the person lower his buttocks, or turn him onto his back.

13 Bring top linens up to cover his knees and lower legs.

14 Secure the drainage bag to the bed frame or have a leg bag ready. Close the drain.

15 Raise the bath blanket to expose the genital area.

16 Put on the gloves.

17 Remove the condom catheter:

   a   Remove the tape, and roll the sheath off the penis.

   b   Disconnect the drainage tubing from the condom.

   c   Discard the tape and condom.

18 Provide perineal care (see *Male Perineal Care,* p. 322). Observe the penis for skin breakdown or irritation.

19 Remove the protective backing from the condom. This exposes the adhesive strip.

20 Hold the penis firmly. Roll the condom onto the penis. Leave a 1-inch space between the penis and the end of the catheter (Fig. 17-20, p. 398).

21 Secure the condom with elastic tape. Apply tape in a spiral (Fig. 17-21, p. 398). Do not apply tape completely around the penis.

22 Connect the condom to the drainage tubing. Coil excess tubing on the bed as shown in Figure 17-10, or attach a leg bag.

23 Remove the bed protector.

24 Remove the gloves.

25 Return top linens, and remove the bath blanket.

POST-PROCEDURE

26 Make sure the person is comfortable.

27 Place the call bell within reach.

28 Raise or lower bed rails as instructed by the RN.

29 Lower the bed to its lowest position.

30 Put on clean gloves.

31 Clean and return the wash basin and other equipment. Return items to their proper place.

32 Unscreen the person.

33 Measure and record the amount of urine in the bag. Discard the collection bag and disposable items.

34 Remove the gloves and wash your hands.

35 Report your observations to the RN.

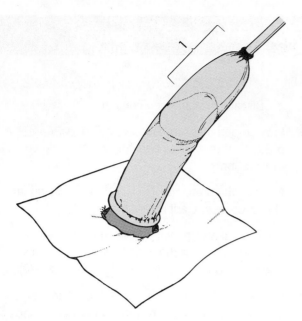

Fig. 17-20 *A condom catheter applied to the penis. There is a 1-inch space between the penis and the end of the catheter.*

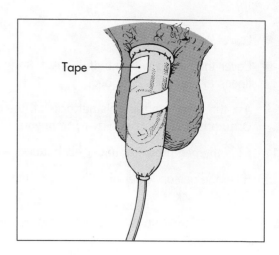

Fig. 17-21 *Tape is applied in spiral fashion to secure the condom catheter to the penis.*

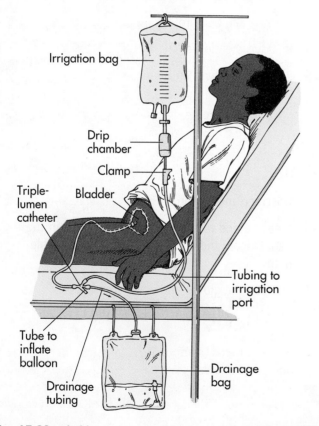

Fig. 17-22 *Bladder irrigation. The bag of irrigating solution hangs from an IV pole. The irrigating solution flows into the bladder through the irrigation port in the catheter. The solution and urine drain out of the bladder through the catheter's drainage port. The solution and urine collect in the drainage bag.* (From Potter PA, Perry AG: Fundamentals of nursing: concepts, process, and practice, ed 4, St Louis, 1997, Mosby.)

BLADDER IRRIGATIONS

An **irrigation** is the process of washing out, flushing out, clearing, or cleaning a tube or body cavity. Water, saline, or medicated solutions are used depending on the purpose and site of the irrigation. *Bladder irrigations* are done to wash out the bladder or to treat bladder infections. The doctor orders the procedure, the required solution, and the amount of solution. Sterile technique is required.

Bladder irrigations usually involve sterile saline or a medicated solution. A common irrigation procedure involves a triple-lumen catheter (Fig. 17-22). The irrigation bag is attached to one lumen and the drainage bag to another. The third lumen is for inflating the catheter balloon. The irrigation bag hangs from an IV pole. Solution flows into the bladder through the irrigation lumen in the catheter. It drains, along with urine, from the bladder through the drainage lumen in the catheter. The solution and urine collect in the drainage bag.

To measure urine output, the RN notes the amount of irrigating solution used. This amount is subtracted from the amount of fluid in the collection bag. The remaining amount is urine. For example, 1000 ml of irrigation solution was used. The drainage bag contained 1450 ml of fluid. Subtracting 1000 ml from 1450 ml leaves 450 ml of urine.

$$
\begin{array}{r}
1450 \text{ ml (solution and urine)} \\
- \underline{1000 \text{ ml (solution)}} \\
450 \text{ ml (urine)}
\end{array}
$$

RULES FOR COLLECTING URINE SPECIMENS

- Follow the rules of medical asepsis, Standard Precautions, and the Bloodborne Pathogen Standard.
- Use a clean container for each specimen.
- Use a container appropriate for the specimen.
- Label the container accurately. Write the person's full name, room and bed number, date, and time the specimen was collected.
- Do not touch the inside of the container or lid.
- Collect the specimen at the time specified.
- Ask the person not to have a bowel movement during specimen collection. The specimen must not contain fecal material.
- Ask the person to put toilet tissue in the toilet or wastebasket. The specimen must not contain tissue.
- Take the specimen and requisition slip to the laboratory or storage place. The specimen container should be in a plastic bag.

A bladder irrigation is done by RNs and LPNs. You may be asked to assist. Some states and agencies let assistive personnel perform the procedure. If assistive personnel are allowed to do the procedure, the agency will provide the necessary education and training.

BLADDER TRAINING

Bladder training programs are developed for persons with urinary incontinence. Some persons need bladder training after indwelling catheter removal. Voluntary control of urination is the goal. The bladder training program is part of the nursing care plan. You assist with bladder training as directed by the RN.

There are two basic methods for bladder training. With one, the person uses the toilet, commode, bedpan, or urinal at scheduled times. The person is given 15 to 20 minutes to start voiding. The rules for maintaining normal urination are followed. The normal position for urination is assumed if possible. Privacy is important.

The second method is used with catheters. Clamping the catheter prevents urine from draining out of the bladder. Usually the catheter is clamped for 1 hour at first. Eventually it is clamped for 3 to 4 hours at a time. Urine drains from the bladder when the catheter is unclamped. When the catheter is removed, urination is encouraged every 3 to 4 hours.

focus on CHILDREN

For infants and toddlers who are not toilet trained, a collection bag is applied to the genital area (see p. 408). Toilet-trained toddlers and young children have difficulty urinating into a collecting receptacle. Potty chairs and specimen pans are useful (see p. 438).

Urine specimens may embarrass older children and adolescents. They do not like clear specimen containers that show urine. Placing the urine specimen in a paper bag often is helpful.

COLLECTING URINE SPECIMENS

Urine specimens (samples) are collected for urine tests. Doctors use test results to make a diagnosis or evaluate treatment. Each specimen sent to the laboratory needs a requisition slip. The slip has the person's identifying information and the required test. Box 17-4 lists the rules to follow when collecting specimens. (See Focus on Children.)

The Random Urine Specimen

The random urine specimen is collected for a urinalysis. No special measures are needed. It is collected at any time. Many persons can collect the specimen themselves. Weak and very ill persons need assistance.

✦ COLLECTING A RANDOM URINE SPECIMEN

PRE-PROCEDURE

1 Explain the procedure to the person.

2 Wash your hands.

3 Collect the following:

   • Bedpan and cover, urinal, or specimen pan

   • Specimen container and lid

   • Label

   • Gloves

   • Plastic bag

PROCEDURE

4 Fill out the label. Put it on the container.

5 Put the container and lid in the bathroom.

6 Identify the person. Check the ID bracelet against the requisition slip.

7 Provide for privacy.

8 Put on the gloves.

9 Ask the person to urinate in the receptacle. Remind him or her to put toilet tissue into the wastebasket or toilet, not in the bedpan or specimen pan.

10 Take the receptacle to the bathroom.

11 Measure urine if I&O is ordered.

12 Pour about 120 ml (4 oz) of urine into the specimen container. Dispose of excess urine.

13 Place the lid on the specimen container. Put the container in the plastic bag.

14 Clean and return the receptacle to its proper place.

15 Help the person wash the hands.

16 Remove the gloves.

POST-PROCEDURE

17 Make sure the person is comfortable.

18 Place the call bell within reach.

19 Raise or lower bed rails as instructed by the RN.

20 Unscreen the person.

21 Wash your hands.

22 Report your observations to the RN.

23 Take the specimen and the requisition slip to the storage area or laboratory.

✦ The Midstream Specimen

The midstream specimen is also called a *clean-voided specimen* or a *clean-catch specimen*. The perineal area is cleaned before collecting the specimen. This reduces the number of microbes in the urethral area during specimen collection. The person starts to void into the toilet, bedpan, urinal, or commode. Then the stream is stopped and a sterile specimen container is positioned. The person voids into the container until the specimen is obtained.

Stopping the stream of urine is hard for many people. You may need to position and hold the specimen container in place after the person starts to void.

✦ COLLECTING A MIDSTREAM SPECIMEN

PRE-PROCEDURE

1 Explain the procedure to the person.

2 Wash your hands.

3 Collect the following:

- Clean-voided specimen kit with sterile specimen container
- Label
- Antiseptic solution
- Disposable gloves
- Sterile gloves (if not part of the kit)
- Bedpan, urinal, or commode if the person cannot use the bathroom
- Plastic bag
- Supplies for perineal care

4 Label the container with the requested information.

5 Identify the person. Check the ID bracelet against the requisition slip.

6 Provide for privacy.

PROCEDURE

7 Let the person complete perineal care if able. Place the call bell within reach.

8 Provide perineal care if the person cannot.

9 Open the sterile kit using sterile technique (see pp. 222–225).

10 Put on the sterile gloves.

11 Pour the antiseptic solution over the cotton balls.

12 Open the sterile specimen container. Do not touch the inside of the container or lid. Set the lid down so the inside is up.

13 Clean the perineum with cotton balls if the person cannot:

a Female:

- Spread the labia with your thumb and index finger. Use your nondominant hand. (This hand is now contaminated and must not touch anything sterile.)
- Clean down the urethral area from front to back. Use a clean cotton ball for each stroke.
- Keep the labia separated to collect the urine specimen (steps 15 and 16).

Continued

COLLECTING A MIDSTREAM SPECIMEN—cont'd

PROCEDURE—cont'd

b Male:

- Hold the penis with your nondominant hand.
- Clean the penis starting at the meatus. Use a cotton ball, and clean in a circular motion.
- Keep holding the penis until the specimen is collected (steps 15 and 16).

14 Ask the person to start urinating into the toilet, bedpan, commode, or urinal.

15 Pass the specimen container into the stream of urine. Keep the labia separated (Fig. 17-23).

16 Collect about 30 to 60 ml of urine (1 to 2 oz).

17 Remove the specimen container before the person stops urinating.

18 Release the labia or penis.

19 Let the person finish urinating into the toilet, bedpan, commode, or urinal.

20 Put the lid on the specimen container. Touch only the outside of the container or lid.

21 Wipe the outside of the container.

22 Place the container in a plastic bag.

23 Provide toilet tissue after the person finishes urinating.

24 Remove and empty the bedpan, commode container, or urinal.

25 Clean the bedpan, urinal, or commode container and other equipment. Return equipment to its proper place.

26 Remove soiled gloves. Put on clean gloves.

27 Let the person wash his or her hands.

28 Remove the gloves.

POST-PROCEDURE

29 Follow steps 17-23 in *Collecting a Random Urine Specimen.*

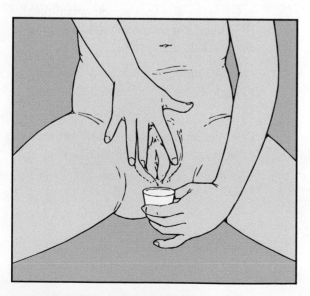

Fig. 17-23 *The labia are separated to collect a midstream specimen. (From Potter PA, Perry AG: Fundamentals of nursing: concepts, process, and practice, ed 4, St Louis, 1997, Mosby.)*

◆ The 24-Hour Urine Specimen

All urine voided during a 24-hour period is collected for a 24-hour urine specimen. Urine is chilled on ice or refrigerated during the collection period. This prevents the growth of microbes. A preservative is added to the collection container for some tests.

The person voids to begin the test; this voiding is discarded. *All* voidings during the next 24 hours are collected. The person and nursing staff must clearly understand the procedure and test period. The rules for collecting urine specimens are followed.

✦ COLLECTING A 24-HOUR URINE SPECIMEN

PRE-PROCEDURE

1 Review the procedure with the RN.

2 Explain the procedure to the person.

3 Wash your hands.

4 Collect the following:

- Urine container for a 24-hour collection

- Preservative from the laboratory if needed

- Bucket with ice if needed

- Two 24-hour urine specimen labels

- Funnel

- Bedpan, urinal, commode, or specimen pan

- Gloves

- Measuring containers

PROCEDURE

5 Label the specimen container.

6 Identify the person. Check the ID bracelet against the requisition slip.

7 Arrange equipment in the person's bathroom or dirty utility room.

8 Place one 24-hour specimen label in the bathroom or dirty utility room. Place the other near the bed.

9 Put on the gloves.

10 Offer the bedpan or urinal, or assist the person to the bathroom or bedside commode.

11 Ask the person to void.

12 Discard the specimen, and note the time. This starts the 24-hour collection period.

13 Clean the bedpan, urinal, commode, or specimen pan.

14 Remove the gloves.

15 Mark the time the test began and the time it ends on the room and bathroom labels. Also mark the specimen container.

16 Ask the person to use the bedpan, urinal, commode, or specimen pan when voiding during the next 24 hours. Tell the person to signal after voiding. Remind him or her not to have a bowel movement at the same time and not to put toilet tissue in the receptacle.

17 Put on the gloves.

18 Measure all urine if I&O is ordered.

19 Pour urine into the specimen container using the funnel. Do not spill any urine. Restart the test if you spill or discard urine.

20 Clean the bedpan, urinal, commode, or specimen pan. Remove the gloves.

21 Add ice to the bucket as necessary.

22 Ask the person to void at the end of the 24-hour period. Pour the urine into the specimen container.

23 Thank the person for cooperating.

POST-PROCEDURE

24 Make sure the person is comfortable.

25 Place the call bell within reach.

26 Raise or lower bed rails as instructed by the RN.

27 Remove the labels from the room and bathroom. Clean and return equipment to its proper place. Discard disposable items.

28 Wash your hands.

29 Report your observations to the RN.

30 Take the specimen and requisition slip to the laboratory.

✦ The Double-Voided Specimen

Fresh-fractional urine specimen is another term for a double-voided specimen. The person voids twice. The first time the bladder is emptied of "stale" urine. "Fresh" urine collects in the bladder after the first voiding. In 30 minutes the person voids again. The second voiding is usually a very small or "fractional" amount of urine.

Fresh-fractional specimens are used to test urine for glucose and ketones (see p. 410).

✦ COLLECTING A DOUBLE-VOIDED SPECIMEN

PRE-PROCEDURE

1 Explain the procedure to the person.

2 Wash your hands.

3 Collect the following:

- Bedpan, urinal, commode, or disposable specimen pan

- Two specimen containers

- Urine testing equipment

- Gloves

4 Identify the person. Check the ID bracelet against the assignment sheet.

5 Provide for privacy.

PROCEDURE

6 Put on the gloves.

7 Offer the bedpan or urinal, or assist the person to the bathroom or commode. A robe and nonskid slippers are worn when up.

8 Ask the person to urinate.

9 Take the receptacle to the bathroom.

10 Measure urine if I&O is ordered. Pour some urine into the specimen container.

11 Test the specimen in case you cannot obtain a second specimen. Discard the urine.

12 Clean the receptacle. Remove the gloves.

13 Return the receptacle to its proper place.

14 Help the person wash the hands.

15 Ask the person to drink an 8-ounce glass of water.

16 Make sure the person is comfortable, the bed rails are up if needed, and the call bell is within reach. Unscreen the person.

17 Wash your hands.

18 Return to the room in 20 to 30 minutes.

19 Repeat steps 5 through 17.

20 Report the results of the second test and any other observations to the RN.

✦ The Sterile Urine Specimen

With a closed drainage system, nothing can enter the system from the catheter to the drainage bag. You cannot disconnect the catheter from the drainage tubing to collect a specimen. Otherwise microbes enter the system. Nor can you collect a specimen from the drainage bag. The drainage bag is an environment for the growth of microbes. To collect a specimen, urine is withdrawn from the catheter under sterile conditions. A sterile needle and syringe are used. Microbes do not enter the system with sterile technique.

The catheter is self-sealing or has a collection port. Rubber catheters are self-sealing. Plastic, silicone, or silastic catheters are not. The RN tells you when to collect a sterile urine specimen and what type of catheter the person has. Before you perform this procedure make sure that:

- Your state allows assistive personnel to perform the procedure
- The procedure is in your job description
- You have the necessary education and training
- You know how to use the agency's supplies and equipment
- You are comfortable with the procedure
- You review the procedure with an RN
- An RN is available to answer questions and to supervise you

Handling syringes and needles

Syringes are made of plastic. A syringe has three parts (Fig. 17-24): the tip, barrel, and plunger. The needle attaches to the tip. The outside of the barrel is marked to show amounts. The inside of the barrel is for fluid. You use the plunger to inject or withdraw fluid. When you push the plunger in, fluid is injected. To withdraw fluid, pull the plunger back. The tip, inside of the barrel, and plunger shaft are sterile. You can touch only the outside of the barrel and the top of the plunger.

Needles are made of stainless steel. A needle has three parts (see Fig. 17-24): the hub, shaft, and bevel. The hub attaches to the syringe tip. The shaft varies in length ($\frac{1}{4}$ to 5 inches) and gauge (diameter). Needle gauges vary from #14 to #28. The smaller the gauge, the larger the needle diameter. The bevel (sharp part of the needle) is slanted. Bevels are short or long. Needles are sterile. You cannot touch any part of the needle. A needle cover caps the needle to prevent contamination or needle stick injuries.

Sterile syringes and needles are packaged together or separately in peel-back packaging (see p. 222). If separate, attach the capped needle to the syringe tip. To use the syringe and needle, pull the cap straight off the needle. *After use, discard the needle and syringe into a sharps disposable container. Do not remove the needle from the syringe. Do not recap the needle. Do not bend or break the needle. Follow Standard Precautions and the Bloodborne Pathogen Standard when using needles.*

The RN tells you what size syringe and needle to use. Depending on the test, a 3-ml or 30-ml syringe is used. Small-gauge needles (#23 or #25) are usually used. Large-gauge needles can leave holes in the catheter or collection port.

Text continued on p. 408

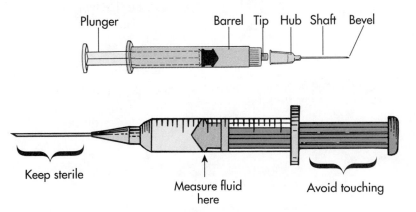

Plunger   Barrel Tip Hub Shaft Bevel

Keep sterile   Measure fluid here   Avoid touching

Fig. 17-24 *Parts of syringe and needle. Note that the needle, plunger shaft, and inside of the barrel are sterile.* (*From Potter PA, Perry AG:* Fundamentals of nursing: concepts, process, and practice, *ed 4, St Louis, 1997, Mosby.*)

COLLECTING A STERILE URINE SPECIMEN FROM AN INDWELLING CATHETER

PROCEDURE ALERT

- Does your state allow assistive personnel to perform the procedure?
- Is the procedure in your job description?
- Do you have the necessary training and education?
- Is an RN available to answer questions and to supervise you?

PRE-PROCEDURE

1. Explain the procedure to the person.

2. Wash your hands.

3. Put on gloves.

4. Clamp the drainage tube for 15 to 30 minutes as directed by the RN (Fig. 17-25). This lets urine collect in the catheter. (Provide privacy during this step.)

5. Remove the gloves, and wash your hands.

6. Collect the following:
   - Syringe and needle as directed by the RN
   - Antiseptic swabs
   - Sterile specimen container
   - Label
   - Plastic bag
   - Gloves

7. Provide for privacy.

PROCEDURE

8. Label the specimen container.

9. Identify the person. Check the ID bracelet against the requisition slip.

10. Put on gloves.

11. Open the specimen container. Set the container and lid in a convenient location. Set the lid down so the inside is up.

12. Expose the catheter site.

13. Clean the puncture site with an antiseptic swab. Use the collection port or end of a self-sealing catheter (just above where the catheter connects to the drainage tubing).

14. Unclamp the catheter.

15. Remove the needle cap. Pull the cap straight off the needle.

16. Insert the needle at a 90-degree angle into a collection port (Fig. 17-26). Insert the needle at a 30-degree angle into a self-sealing catheter (Fig. 17-27).

17. Pull back on the plunger to fill the syringe with urine.

18. Transfer syringe contents into the specimen container. Push down on the plunger to eject urine from the syringe. The needle must not touch the outside of the specimen container.

19. Put the lid on the specimen container. Place the container in a plastic bag.

20. Discard the syringe and needle into a sharps disposable container.

21. Unclamp the tubing. Make sure urine flows into the drainage bag.

22. Cover the person.

23. Remove the gloves.

POST-PROCEDURE

24 Make sure the person is comfortable.

25 Place the call bell within reach.

26 Unscreen the person.

27 Discard disposable supplies.

28 Wash your hands.

29 Report your observations to the RN.

30 Take the urine specimen and laboratory requisition slip to the laboratory.

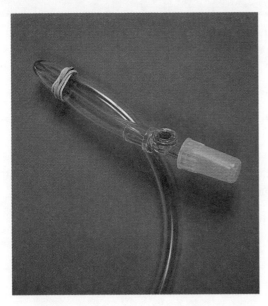

Fig. 17-25 *Catheter tubing is clamped with a rubber band.* (*From Elkin MK, Perry AG, Potter PA: Nursing interventions and clinical skills, St Louis, 1996, Mosby.*)

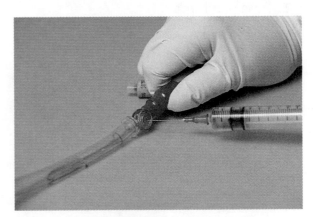

Fig. 17-26 *The needle is inserted at a 90-degree angle into the collection port.* (*From Elkin MK, Perry AG, Potter PA: Nursing interventions and clinical skills, St Louis, 1996, Mosby.*)

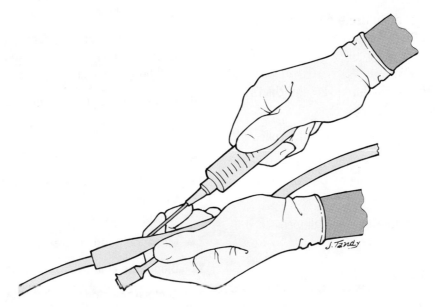

Fig. 17-27 *The needle is inserted at a 30-degree angle into a self-sealing catheter.*

Collecting a Specimen From an Infant or Child

Sometimes specimens are needed from infants and children who are not toilet trained. A collection bag is applied over the urethra. A parent or another staff member assists if the child is agitated.

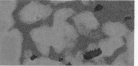

COLLECTING A URINE SPECIMEN FROM AN INFANT OR CHILD

PRE-PROCEDURE

1 Explain the procedure to the child and parents.

2 Wash your hands.

3 Collect the following:

- Collection bag

- Wash basin

- Cotton balls

- Bath towel

- Two diapers

- Specimen container

- Gloves

- Plastic bag

- Scissors

4 Identify the child. Check the ID bracelet against the requisition slip.

5 Provide for privacy.

PROCEDURE

6 Put on the gloves.

7 Remove and dispose of the diaper.

8 Clean the perineal area. Use a new cotton ball for each stroke. Rinse and dry the area.

9 Put on clean gloves.

10 Position the child on the back. Flex the child's knees, and separate the legs.

11 Remove the adhesive backing from the collection bag.

12 Apply the bag to the perineum. Do not cover the anus (Fig. 17-28).

13 Cut a slit in the bottom of a new diaper.

14 Diaper the child.

15 Pull the collection bag through the slit in the bottom of the diaper.

16 Remove the gloves.

17 Raise the head of the crib if allowed. This helps urine to collect in the bottom of the bag.

18 Unscreen the child.

19 Return to the room periodically. Check the bag to see if the child has urinated. (Wear gloves, and provide for privacy.)

20 Provide privacy if the child has urinated.

21 Remove the diaper.

22 Remove the collection bag gently.

23 Press the adhesive surfaces of the bag together. Or transfer urine to the specimen container through the drainage tab.

24 Clean the perineal area, rinse, and dry well.

25 Diaper the child.

26 Remove the gloves and wash your hands.

COLLECTING A URINE SPECIMEN FROM AN INFANT OR CHILD—cont'd

POST-PROCEDURE

27 Make sure the child is comfortable. Raise the bed rail.

28 Unscreen the child.

29 Write the requested information on the specimen container. Place the container in the plastic bag.

30 Clean and return equipment to its proper place. Discard disposable items. (Wear gloves for this step.)

31 Wash your hands.

32 Report your observations to the RN.

33 Take the requisition slip and the specimen to the storage area or laboratory.

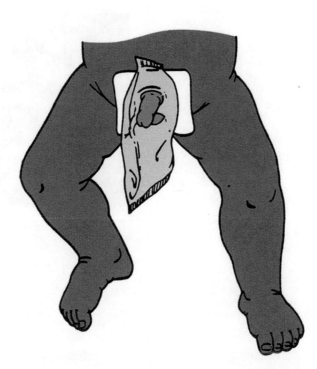

Fig. 17-28 *A disposable collection bag is applied to the perineal area of the infant. Urine collects in the bag for a specimen.*

TESTING URINE

The RN may ask you to do simple urine tests. You can test for ph, glucose, ketones, blood, and specific gravity using reagent strips. Some states allow assistive personnel to test specific gravity with urinometers. Straining urine for stones is another simple test.

Testing for pH

Urine pH measures if urine is acidic or alkaline. Changes in normal pH (4.6 to 8.0) occur from illness, foods, and medications. Use reagent strips to test for urine pH. A routine urine specimen is needed.

Testing for Glucose and Ketones

Diabetes mellitus is a chronic disease in which the pancreas fails to secrete enough insulin. The body needs insulin to use sugar for energy. Sugar builds up in the blood if it cannot be used. Some sugar appears in the urine. **Glucosuria** or **glycosuria** means sugar *(glucos, glycos)* in the urine *(uria)*.

The diabetic person may also have **acetone (ketone bodies, ketones)** in the urine. These appear in urine because of the rapid breakdown of fat for energy. The body uses fat for energy if it cannot use sugar. Urine is also tested for ketones.

The doctor orders the type and frequency of urine tests. They are usually done four times a day: 30 minutes before each meal (ac) and at bedtime (HS). The doctor uses the test results to regulate the person's medication and diet. You must be accurate when testing urine. Promptly report the results to the RN.

Double-voided specimens are best for testing urine for sugar and ketones. Reagent strips are used for testing.

Testing for Blood

Normal urine is free of blood. Injury and disease can cause blood *(hemat)* to appear in the urine *(uria)*. This is called **hematuria.** Sometimes blood is seen in the urine. At other times it is unseen *(occult).* You use reagent strips to test for occult blood. A routine urine specimen is needed.

Testing Specific Gravity

Urine contains particles and dissolved solids. Urine specific gravity measures the amount of these substances in comparison with water. When urine contains large amounts of particles and dissolved solids, urine is concentrated. The amount of water is less than normal, and the amount of substances is higher than normal. Urine is dark yellow. Specific gravity is high. Dilute urine contains large amounts of water and few substances. Urine is pale, and specific gravity is low.

A routine urine specimen is needed for the test.

◆ *Using reagent strips*

Reagent strips have different sections that change color when they react with urine. To use a reagent strip, dip the strip into urine. Then compare the strip with the color chart on the bottle (Fig. 17-29). The RN gives you specific instructions for the urine test ordered. You must read the manufacturer's instructions before you begin.

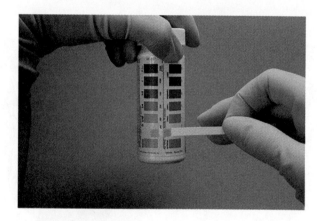

Fig. 17-29 *Reagent strip for sugar and ketones.*

TESTING URINE WITH REAGENT STRIPS

PRE-PROCEDURE

1 Explain the procedure to the person.

2 Wash your hands.

3 Identify the person. Check the ID bracelet against the assignment sheet.

PROCEDURE

4 Put on the gloves.

5 Collect the following:

- Urine specimen (routine specimen for ph, occult blood, and specific gravity; double-voided specimen for sugar and ketones)

- Reagent strip as ordered

- Gloves

6 Remove a strip from the bottle. Put the cap on the bottle immediately. Make sure it is tight.

7 Dip the strip test areas into the specimen.

8 Remove the strip after the correct amount of time (see the manufacturer's instructions).

9 Tap the strip gently against the container to remove excess urine.

10 Wait the required amount of time (see the manufacturer's instructions).

11 Compare the strip with the color chart on the bottle. Read the results.

12 Discard disposable items and the specimen.

POST-PROCEDURE

13 Clean and return equipment to its proper place.

14 Remove the gloves, and wash your hands.

15 Report the results and other observations to the RN.

✦ *Using a urinometer*

A *urinometer* measures *(meter)* the specific gravity of urine *(urino)*. This device has two parts (Fig. 17-30). The scale is calibrated in 0.001 units. The scale ranges from 1.000 to 1.060. The bottom part is a mercury-filled bulb. This part gives the urinometer weight. To measure specific gravity, the urinometer is placed in a cylinder of urine. The urinometer sinks into the urine and floats as in Figure 17-30.

Normal specific gravity is between 1.010 and 1.035. Place the urinometer at eye level to read the measurement. Read the measurement at the base of the *meniscus* of urine. (A meniscus is the curved surface of a column of liquid.)

Refractometers (Fig. 17-31, p. 412) are used by laboratory personnel to test urine for specific gravity. A drop of urine is placed on the prism. The refractometer is held toward light. Then the measurement is read.

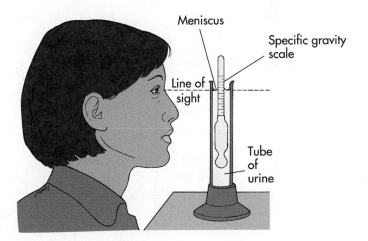

Meniscus
Specific gravity scale
Line of sight
Tube of urine

Fig. 17-30 *Urinometer for measuring specific gravity.*

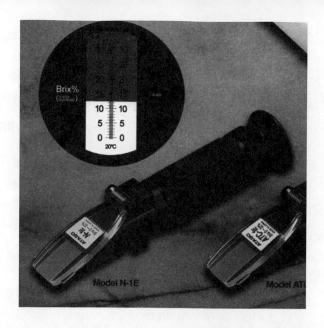

Fig. 17-31 *Refractometer. (From Perry AG, Potter PA:* Clinical Nursing Skills and Techniques, *ed 4, 1998, Mosby.)*

MEASURING SPECIFIC GRAVITY WITH A URINOMETER

PROCEDURE ALERT

- Does your state allow assistive personnel to perform the procedure?

- Is the procedure in your job description?

- Do you have the necessary training and education?

- Is an RN available to answer questions and to supervise you?

PRE-PROCEDURE

1 Explain the procedure to the person.

2 Wash your hands.

3 Collect a urinometer and gloves.

4 Identify the person. Check the ID bracelet against the assignment sheet.

5 Provide for privacy.

PROCEDURE

6 Put on the gloves.

7 Collect a urine specimen as directed by the RN.

8 Fill the glass cylinder about ¾ full (about 20 ml) with urine.

9 Place the urinometer into the cylinder.

10 Spin the urinometer between your thumb and index finger. Spin the urinometer again if it stops against the cylinder. The urinometer should float freely.

11 Place the urinometer at eye level.

12 Read the measurement at the base of the meniscus. Note the measurement.

13 Discard the urine, and clean the urinometer.

14 Clean the bedpan, urinal, or specimen pan.

15 Return equipment to its proper place.

16 Remove the gloves.

17 Help the person wash the hands.

POST-PROCEDURE

18 Make sure the person is comfortable.

19 Place the call bell within reach.

20 Raise or lower bed rails as instructed by the RN.

21 Unscreen the person.

22 Wash your hands.

23 Report your observations to the RN.

✦ Straining Urine

Stones (calculi) can develop in the kidneys, ureters, or bladder. Stones vary in size. Some are pinhead size; others are the size of an orange. Stones causing severe pain and damage to the urinary system may require surgical removal. Some stones exit the body through urine. Therefore all of the person's urine is strained. Passed stones are sent to the laboratory for examination.

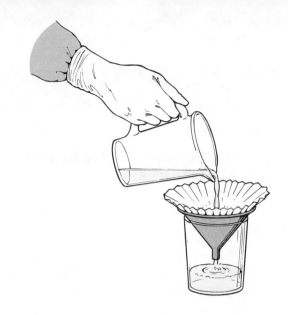

Fig. 17-32 *A disposable strainer is placed in a specimen container. Urine is poured through the strainer into the specimen container.*

✦ STRAINING URINE

PRE-PROCEDURE

1 Explain the procedure to the person. Also explain that the urinal, bedpan, commode, or specimen pan is used for voiding.

2 Wash your hands.

3 Collect the following:

 • Strainer or 4 × 4 gauze

 • Specimen container

 • Urinal, bedpan, commode, or specimen pan

 • Two labels stating that all urine is strained

 • Gloves

 • Plastic bag

4 Identify the person. Check the ID bracelet against the assignment sheet.

PROCEDURE

5 Arrange items in the person's bathroom.

6 Place one label in the bathroom. Place the other near the bed.

7 Put on the gloves.

8 Offer the bedpan or urinal. Or assist the person to the bedside commode or bathroom.

9 Provide for privacy, and remove the gloves.

10 Tell the person to signal after voiding.

11 Put on gloves.

12 Place the strainer or gauze into the specimen container.

13 Pour urine into the specimen container. Urine passes through the strainer or gauze (Fig. 17-32).

14 Place the strainer or gauze in the container if any crystals, stones, or particles appear.

15 Discard the urine.

16 Help the person clean the perineal area if necessary.

17 Clean and return equipment to its proper place.

18 Removed soiled gloves and put on clean gloves.

19 Help the person wash the hands.

20 Remove the gloves.

Continued

STRAINING URINE—cont'd

POST-PROCEDURE

21   Make sure the person is comfortable and the call bell is within reach.

22   Raise or lower bed rails as instructed by the RN.

23   Unscreen the person.

24   Label the specimen container with the requested information. Put the container in the plastic bag. (Wear gloves for this step.)

25   Wash your hands.

26   Report your observations to the RN.

27   Take the specimen and requisition slip to the laboratory.

REVIEW QUESTIONS

Circle the best answer.

1   Which is *false?*
   a   Urine is normally clear and yellow or amber in color.
   b   Urine normally has an ammonia odor.
   c   Micturition usually occurs before going to bed and on rising.
   d   A person normally voids about 1500 ml a day.

2   Which is *not* a rule for maintaining normal elimination?
   a   Help the person assume a normal position for urination.
   b   Provide for privacy.
   c   Help the person to the bathroom or commode, or provide the bedpan or urinal as soon as requested.
   d   Always stay with the person who is on a bedpan.

3   The best position for using a bedpan is
   a   Fowler's position
   b   The supine position
   c   The prone position
   d   The side-lying position

4   After a man uses the urinal, he should
   a   Put the urinal on the bedside stand
   b   Use the call bell
   c   Put the urinal on the overbed table
   d   Empty the urinal

5   Urinary incontinence
   a   Is always permanent
   b   Requires good skin care
   c   Is treated with an indwelling catheter
   d   Requires tests for sugar and ketones

6   A person has an indwelling catheter. Which is *incorrect?*
   a   Keep the drainage bag above the level of the bladder.
   b   Make sure the drainage tubing is free of kinks.
   c   Coil the drainage tubing on the bed.
   d   Tape the catheter to the inner thigh.

7   A person has an indwelling catheter. Which is *incorrect?*
   a   Tape any leaks at the connection site.
   b   Follow the rules of medical asepsis and Standard Precautions.
   c   Empty the drainage bag at the end of each shift.
   d   Report complaints of pain, burning, the need to urinate, or irritation immediately.

8   You are going to catheterize Mr. Clark. You need the following information from the RN *except*
   a   If a straight or indwelling catheter was ordered
   b   What size catheter to use
   c   What size needle to use
   d   If a urine specimen is needed

REVIEW QUESTIONS—cont'd

9 A catheterization requires

a Sterile technique
b Medical asepsis
c A closed drainage system
d Perineal care after the procedure

10 You are inserting a straight catheter. Which is part of the procedure?

a Attaching the catheter to a closed drainage system
b Testing the balloon before inserting the catheter
c Letting the bladder empty
d Tugging gently on the catheter to make sure it is in place

11 You are going to remove an indwelling catheter. You

a Attach a needle to a syringe
b Check the size of the balloon
c Tug on the catheter to make sure it is in place
d Use an alcohol swab to clean the site

12 You are going to remove a catheter with a 5 ml balloon. You withdraw only 3 ml. What should you do?

a Call for the RN.
b Inject the fluid.
c Pull out the catheter gently.
d Make sure the needle is attached to the syringe.

13 Mr. Powers has a condom catheter. You apply elastic tape

a Completely around the penis
b To the inner thigh
c To the abdomen
d In a spiral fashion

14 The goal of bladder training is to

a Remove the catheter
b Allow the person to walk to the bathroom
c Gain voluntary control of urination
d All of the above

15 When collecting a urine specimen, you should do the following *except*

a Label the container with the requested information
b Use the correct container
c Collect the specimen at the time specified
d Use sterile supplies

16 The perineum is cleaned immediately before collecting a

a Random specimen
b Midstream specimen
c 24-hour urine specimen
d Double-voided specimen

17 A 24-hour urine specimen involves

a Collecting all urine voided by a person during a 24-hour period
b Collecting a random specimen every hour for 24 hours
c A catheterization
d Testing the urine for sugar and acetone

18 Urine is tested for sugar and ketones

a At bedtime
b 30 minutes after meals and at bedtime
c 30 minutes before meals and at bedtime
d Before breakfast

19 Which specimen is best for sugar and ketone testing?

a A random specimen
b A clean-voided specimen
c A 24-hour urine specimen
d A double-voided specimen

20 You are instructed to strain Mr. Powers' urine. You know that straining urine is done to find

a Hematuria
b Stones
c Nocturia
d Urgency

Answers to these questions are on p. 850.

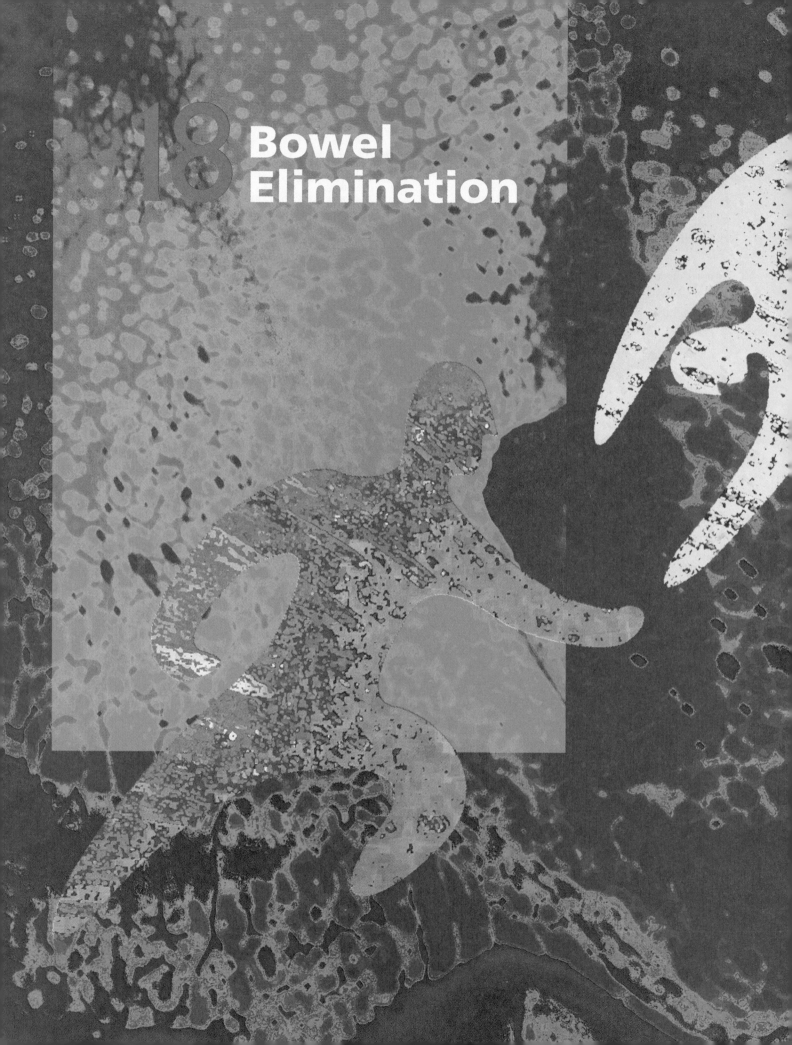

18 Bowel Elimination

OBJECTIVES

- Define the key terms in this chapter
- Describe normal stools and the normal pattern and frequency of bowel movements
- List the observations about defecation to report to the RN
- Identify the factors that affect bowel elimination
- Describe common bowel elimination problems
- Describe the measures that promote comfort and safety during defecation
- Describe bowel training
- Explain why enemas are given
- Know the common enema solutions
- Describe the rules for administering enemas
- Explain the purpose of rectal tubes
- Describe how to care for a person with an ostomy
- Explain why stool specimens are collected
- Perform the procedures described in this chapter

KEY TERMS

anal incontinence The inability to control the passage of feces and gas through the anus; fecal incontinence

bowel movement Defecation

colostomy An artificial opening between the colon and abdominal wall

constipation The passage of a hard, dry stool

defecation The process of excreting feces from the rectum through the anus; a bowel movement

dehydration The excessive loss of water from tissues

diarrhea The frequent passage of liquid stools

enema The introduction of fluid into the rectum and lower colon

fecal impaction The prolonged retention and accumulation of feces in the rectum

fecal incontinence Anal incontinence

feces The semisolid mass of waste products in the colon

flatulence The excessive formation of gas in the stomach and intestines

flatus Gas or air passed through the anus

ileostomy An artificial opening between the ileum (small intestine) and abdominal wall

melena A black, tarry stool

ostomy The surgical creation of an artificial opening

peristalsis The alternating contraction and relaxation of intestinal muscles

stoma An opening; see colostomy and ileostomy

stool Excreted feces

suppository A cone-shaped solid medication that is inserted into a body opening; it melts at body temperature

Like urinary elimination, bowel elimination is a basic physical need. Many factors affect bowel elimination. They include privacy, personal habits, age, diet, exercise and activity, fluids, and drugs. Problems easily occur. Promoting normal bowel elimination is important. You will assist patients in meeting their elimination needs.

NORMAL BOWEL MOVEMENTS

Defecation (bowel movement) is the process of excreting feces from the rectum through the anus. **Feces** refers to the semisolid mass of waste products in the colon. The term **stool** refers to excreted feces.

The frequency of bowel movements varies from person to person. Some have a bowel movement every day. Others have one every 2 to 3 days. Some people have 2 or 3 bowel movements a day. The elimination pattern also involves the time of day. Many people defecate after breakfast, others in the evening.

Stools are normally brown in color. Bleeding in the stomach and small intestine causes black or tarry stools. Bleeding in the lower colon and rectum causes red-colored stools. So do beets. A diet high in green vegetables can cause green stools. Diseases and infection can also cause clay-colored or white, pale, orange-colored, or green-colored stools.

Stools are normally soft, formed, moist, and shaped like the rectum. They have a characteristic odor. The odor is from bacterial action in the intestines. Certain foods and drugs also cause odors.

What to Report to the RN

The RN uses your observations for the nursing process. Therefore stools are carefully observed before disposal. Ask the RN to observe abnormal stools. You need to observe stools and report the following to the RN: color, amount, consistency, odor, shape, size, frequency of defecation, and any complaints of pain.

FACTORS AFFECTING BOWEL ELIMINATION

Normal, regular defecation is affected by many factors. The following factors affect the frequency, consistency, color, and odor of stools. The RN considers these factors when using the nursing process to meet the person's elimination needs. Normal, regular elimination is the goal.

- *Privacy*—Like voiding, bowel elimination is a private act. Lack of privacy prevents many people from defecating despite having the urge. Bowel movement odors and sounds are embarrassing. Ignoring the urge to defecate can lead to constipation.

- *Personal habits*—Many people routinely have a bowel movement after breakfast. Some drink a hot beverage, read a book or newspaper, or take a walk. These activities relax the person. Defecation is easier when a person is relaxed rather than tense.

- *Diet*—A well-balanced diet and bulk are needed. High-fiber foods leave a residue that provides needed bulk. Fruits, vegetables, and whole grain cereals and breads are high in fiber. Certain foods can cause diarrhea or constipation. Milk causes constipation in some people and diarrhea in others. Other milk products and chocolate can cause similar reactions. Spicy foods can irritate the intestines. Frequent stools or diarrhea can result. Gas-forming foods stimulate peristalsis. **Peristalsis** is the alternating contraction and relaxation of intestinal muscles. Increased peristalsis results in defecation. Gas-forming foods include onions, beans, cabbage, cauliflower, radishes, and cucumbers.

- *Fluids*—Feces contain water. Stool consistency depends on the amount of water absorbed in the large intestine. The amount of fluid ingested, urine output, and vomiting are factors. Feces become hard and dry when large amounts of water are absorbed or when fluid intake is poor. Hard, dry feces move through the intestines at a slower rate. Constipation can occur. Drinking 6 to 8 glasses of water every day promotes normal bowel elimination. Warm fluids—coffee, tea, hot cider, and warm water—increase peristalsis.

- *Activity*—Exercise and activity maintain muscle tone and stimulate peristalsis. Irregular elimination and constipation often occur from inactivity and bedrest. Inactivity may result from disease, surgery, injury, and aging.

- *Medications*—Drugs can prevent constipation or control diarrhea. Other drugs have diarrhea or constipation as side effects. Drugs for pain relief often cause constipation. Antibiotics, used to fight or prevent infection, often cause diarrhea. Diarrhea occurs when the antibiotics kill normal flora in the large intestine. Normal flora is necessary in forming stools. (See Focus on Children and Focus on Older Persons.)

COMMON PROBLEMS

Many factors affect normal bowel elimination. Common problems include constipation, fecal impaction, diarrhea, anal incontinence, and flatulence.

Constipation

Constipation is the passage of a hard, dry stool. The person usually strains to have a bowel movement. Stools are large or marble-size. Large stools cause pain as they pass through the anus. Constipation occurs when feces move through the intestine slowly. This allows more time for water absorption. Common causes include a low-fiber diet, ignoring the urge to defecate, decreased fluid intake, inactivity, drugs, aging, and certain diseases. Dietary changes, fluids, activity, enemas, and medications prevent or relieve constipation.

✦ Fecal Impaction

A **fecal impaction** is the prolonged retention and accumulation of feces in the rectum. Feces are hard or putty-like in consistency. Fecal impaction results if constipation is not relieved. The person cannot defecate. More water is absorbed from the already hardened feces. Liquid seeping from the anus is a sign of fecal impaction. Liquid feces pass around the hardened fecal mass in the rectum.

The person tries many times to have a bowel movement. Abdominal discomfort, cramping, and rectal pain are common. A digital examination is done to check for an impaction. This is done by inserting a gloved finger into the rectum and feeling for a hard mass (Fig. 18-1). The mass is felt in the lower rectum. Sometimes it is higher in the colon and out of reach. The digital examination often produces the urge to defecate. The doctor may order drugs and enemas to remove the impaction.

Often it is necessary to remove the fecal mass with a lubricated, gloved finger. This is called *digital removal of an impaction.* A doctor's order is required. A finger is inserted into the rectum and the finger hooked around a piece of feces. Then the finger and stool are removed. The stool is dropped into the bedpan. The process is repeated until the impaction is removed. The procedure is uncomfortable and embarrassing for most people.

Checking for and removing impactions is very dangerous. The vagus nerve in the rectum can be stimulated. This nerve also affects the heart. Stimulation of the vagus nerve slows the heart rate. The heart rate can slow to dangerous levels in some persons. In some agencies, assistive personnel check for and remove impactions. Before you perform these procedures make sure that:

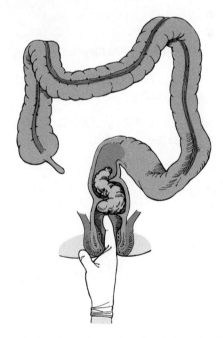

Fig. 18-1 *An index finger is used to check for a fecal impaction.*

- Your state allows assistive personnel to perform them
- They are in your job description
- You have the necessary education and training
- You review the procedure with the RN
- An RN is available to answer questions and to supervise you

You must be very careful and gentle. Rectal bleeding can occur with both procedures. You must follow Standard Precautions and the Bloodborne Pathogen Standard.

Text continued on p. 422

CHECKING FOR A FECAL IMPACTION

PROCEDURE ALERT

- Does your state allow assistive personnel to perform the procedure?
- Is the procedure in your job description?

- Do you have the necessary training and education?
- Is an RN available to answer questions and to supervise you?

PRE-PROCEDURE

1 Explain the procedure to the person.

2 Wash your hands.

3 Collect the following:

- Bedpan and bedpan cover
- Bath blanket
- Toilet tissue
- Gloves
- Lubricant
- Waterproof pad
- Basin of warm water
- Soap
- Washcloth
- Bath towel

4 Identify the person. Check the ID bracelet against the assignment sheet.

5 Provide for privacy.

6 Raise the bed to the best level for body mechanics. Make sure the far bed rail is up.

PROCEDURE

7 Lower the bed rail near you.

8 Cover the person with a bath blanket. Fanfold top linens to the foot of the bed.

9 Position the person in the left Sims' position or in a left side-lying position.

10 Place the waterproof pad under the buttocks.

11 Put on the gloves.

12 Expose the anal area.

13 Lubricate your gloved index finger.

14 Ask the person to take a deep breath through his or her mouth.

15 Insert the gloved finger while the person is taking a deep breath.

16 Check for a fecal mass.

17 Withdraw your finger.

18 Help the person onto the bedpan or to the bathroom or commode if needed. Provide for privacy. See *Giving the Bedpan* (p. 374) or *Assisting the Person to the Commode* (p. 379).

19 Remove and discard the gloves. Wash your hands.

20 Put on clean gloves.

21 Wash the person's anal area with soap and water. Pat dry.

22 Remove the waterproof pad.

23 Help the person assume a comfortable position.

POST-PROCEDURE

24 Return top linens, and remove the bath blanket.

25 Place the call bell within the person's reach.

26 Lower the bed to its lowest position.

27 Raise or lower bed rails as instructed by the RN.

28 Unscreen the person.

29 Clean and return equipment to its proper place. Discard disposable items.

30 Follow agency policy for soiled linen.

31 Remove the gloves, and wash your hands.

32 Report your observations to the RN.

REMOVING A FECAL IMPACTION

PROCEDURE ALERT

- Does your state allow assistive personnel to perform the procedure?
- Is the procedure in your job description?
- Do you have the necessary training and education?
- Is an RN available to answer questions and to supervise you?

PROCEDURE

1. Follow steps 1 through 13 in *Checking for a Fecal Impaction.*

2. Check the person's pulse. Note the rate and rhythm.

3. Ask the person to take a deep breath through the mouth.

4. Insert your lubricated, gloved index finger.

5. Hook your index finger around a small piece of feces.

6. Remove your finger and the feces.

7. Drop the stool into the bedpan.

8. Clean your finger with toilet tissue. Reapply lubricant as needed.

9. Repeat steps 2 through 7 until you no longer feel feces. Check the person's pulse at intervals using your clean gloved hand. Note the rate and rhythm. Stop the procedure if the pulse rate has slowed or if the rhythm is irregular.

10. Wipe the anal area with toilet tissue.

11. Cover the person with the bath blanket.

12. Cover the bedpan.

13. Remove and discard the gloves. Then put on a clean pair of gloves.

14. Raise the bed rail. Take the bedpan to the bathroom.

15. Empty, clean, and disinfect the bedpan.

16. Return the bedpan to the bedside stand.

17. Remove and discard the gloves.

18. Fill the wash basin with warm water.

19. Return to the bedside, and lower the bed rail near you.

20. Put on a clean pair of gloves.

21. Wash the buttocks, and give perineal care.

22. Remove the waterproof pad.

POST-PROCEDURE

23. Help the person assume a comfortable position.

24. Return top linens, and remove the bath blanket.

25. Place the call bell within the person's reach.

26. Lower the bed to its lowest position.

27. Raise or lower bed rails as instructed by the RN.

28. Unscreen the person.

29. Clean and return equipment to its proper place. Discard disposable items.

30. Follow agency policy for soiled linen.

31. Remove the gloves, and wash your hands.

32. Report your observations to the RN.

Diarrhea

Diarrhea is the frequent passage of liquid stools. Feces move through the intestines rapidly. This reduces the time for fluid absorption. The need to defecate is urgent. Some people cannot get to a bathroom in time. Abdominal cramping, nausea, and vomiting also may occur.

Causes of diarrhea include infections, certain drugs, irritating foods, and microbes in food and water. Peristalsis is reduced by diet or medications. Nursing measures include promptly assisting the person to the bathroom or providing the commode or bedpan. Stools require prompt disposal to reduce odors and prevent the spread of microbes. Good skin care is essential. Liquid feces are very irritating to the skin. So is the frequent wiping of the anal area with toilet tissue. Pressure ulcers are a risk if cleanliness and good skin care are not practiced.

Fluid lost through diarrhea is replaced. Otherwise dehydration occurs. **Dehydration** is the excessive loss of water from tissues. Signs and symptoms include pale or flushed skin, dry skin, coated tongue, oliguria (scant amount of urine), thirst, weakness, dizziness, and confusion. Falling blood pressure and increased pulse and respirations are serious signs. The RN uses the nursing process to meet the person's fluid needs. The doctor orders intravenous fluids in severe cases.

Diarrhea is often caused by microbes. Preventing the spread of infection is important. Always practice Standard Precautions when in contact with stools. (See Focus on Children at top right and Focus on Older Persons.)

Fecal Incontinence

Fecal incontinence (anal incontinence) is the inability to control the passage of feces and gas through the anus. Causes include intestinal diseases and nervous system diseases and injuries. Fecal impaction, diarrhea, and some drugs are other causes. Persons with mental health problems or cognitive disorders (Chapters 31 and 32) may not recognize the need or act of defecating. Fecal incontinence also can result from unanswered call bells when the person needs to use the bathroom, commode, or bedpan.

Good skin care is required. A bowel training program may be developed. Providing the bedpan or commode after meals or every 2 to 3 hours may be helpful. Waterproof pads or incontinent pants keep linens and clothes clean. Fecal incontinence affects the person emotionally. Frustration, embarrassment, anger, and humiliation are common emotions. (See Focus on Children at bottom right.)

Flatulence

Gas and air are normally found in the stomach and intestines. They are expelled through the mouth (belching, eructating) and anus. Gas and air passed through the anus

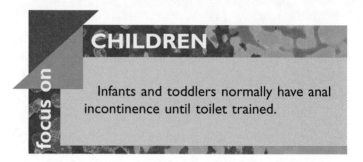

focus on CHILDREN

The bodies of infants and young children contain large amounts of water. They are at risk for dehydration. Death can occur quickly. Report any liquid or watery stool to the RN immediately. Ask the RN to observe the stool. Also note the number of wet diapers. Infants wet less when dehydrated.

focus on OLDER PERSONS

Older persons also are at risk for dehydration. The amount of body water decreases with aging. Many diseases common in older persons also affect body fluids. So do many drugs. Report any signs of diarrhea to the RN immediately. Ask the RN to observe the stool. Death is a risk from unrecognized and untreated dehydration.

focus on CHILDREN

Infants and toddlers normally have anal incontinence until toilet trained.

is called **flatus. Flatulence** is the excessive formation of gas or air in the stomach and intestines. Common causes are:

- Swallowing air while eating and drinking. This includes chewing gum, eating fast, drinking through a straw, and drinking carbonated beverages. Tense or anxious people may swallow large amounts of air when drinking.
- Bacterial action in the intestines
- Gas-forming foods (onions, beans, cabbage, cauliflower, radishes, cucumbers)
- Constipation
- Bowel and abdominal surgeries
- Drugs that decrease peristalsis

BOX 18-1

COMFORT AND SAFETY DURING BOWEL ELIMINATION

- Help the person to the toilet or commode or provide the bedpan as soon as requested.
- Provide for privacy. Ask visitors to leave the room. Close doors, pull curtains around the bed, and pull window curtains or shades. Remember, defecation is a private act. Leave the room if the person can be alone.
- Make sure the bedpan is warm.
- Position the person in a normal sitting or squatting position.
- Cover the person for warmth and privacy.
- Allow enough time for defecation.
- Place the call bell and toilet tissue within the person's reach.
- Stay nearby if the person is weak or unsteady.
- Provide perineal care.
- Dispose of feces promptly. This reduces odors and prevents the spread of microbes.
- Let the person wash the hands after defecating and wiping with toilet tissue.
- Assist the person to the bathroom or commode or offer the bedpan after meals if the person has the problem of incontinence.
- Practice Standard Precautions, and follow the Bloodborne Pathogen Standard.

If flatus is not expelled, the intestines distend. That is, they swell or enlarge from the pressure of the gases. Abdominal cramping or pain, shortness of breath, and a swollen abdomen occur. "Bloating" is a common complaint. Walking and the left side-lying position often produce flatus. Doctors may order enemas, medications, or rectal tubes for relief of flatulence.

COMFORT AND SAFETY DURING ELIMINATION

Certain measures help promote normal bowel elimination. The RN uses the nursing process to meet the person's elimination needs. The nursing care plan may include measures that involve diet, fluids, and exercise. The actions listed in Box 18-1 are routinely practiced to promote comfort and safety during bowel elimination.

BOWEL TRAINING

Bowel training has two goals. One is to gain control of bowel movements. The other is to develop a regular pattern of elimination. Fecal impaction, constipation, and fecal incontinence are prevented.

The urge to defecate is usually felt after a meal, particularly breakfast. Use of the toilet, commode, or bedpan is encouraged at this time. Other factors that promote elimination are included in the nursing care plan and bowel training program. These include a high-

Fig. 18-2 **A,** *A rectal suppository.* **B,** *The suppository is inserted into the rectum.*

fiber diet, increased fluids, warm fluids, activity, and privacy. The RN tells you about a person's bowel training program.

The doctor may order a suppository to stimulate defecation. A **suppository** is a cone-shaped, solid medication that is inserted into a body opening. It melts at body temperature. The rectal suppository is inserted into the rectum by an RN or LPN (Fig. 18-2). A bowel movement occurs about 30 minutes later. Enemas are sometimes ordered.

BOX 18-2

COMFORT AND SAFETY MEASURES FOR GIVING ENEMAS

- Solution temperature for adults is 105° F (40.5° C). The temperature should be 98.6° F (37° C) for children. Measure the temperature with a bath thermometer. Ask the nurse what the temperature should be for the person.
- The amount of solution given depends on the enema's purpose and the person's age. Adults generally receive 500 to 1000 ml. The doctor orders the amount of solution to be given. (See *FOCUS ON CHILDREN*, p. 425.)
- The left Sims' position or a comfortable left side-lying position is preferred.
- For adults, the enema bag is raised 12 inches above the anus. For infants, the bag is raised no more than 3 inches above the anus. Ask the RN how high to raise the bag for the person.
- The nurse and agency procedure manual tell you how far to insert the enema tubing. In the adult, the tubing is usually inserted 3 to 4 inches but never more than 6 inches. (See Focus on Children box, p. 425). Enema tubing can injure the intestine. Stop inserting the tube and call for the nurse if you feel resistance, the person complains of pain, or bleeding occurs.
- The solution is given slowly. Usually it takes 10 to 15 minutes to give 750 to 1000 ml.
- The solution should be retained in the bowel for a certain length of time. The length of time depends on the amount and type of solution. Ask the RN how long the person should retain the enema solution.
- The enema tube is held in place while giving the solution.
- The bathroom must be vacant when the person has the urge to defecate. Make sure that the bathroom will not be used by another person.
- The RN observes the enema results.
- Standard Precautions and the Bloodborne Pathogen Standard are followed.

ENEMAS

An **enema** is the introduction of fluid into the rectum and lower colon. Enemas are ordered by doctors. They are given to remove feces and to relieve constipation or fecal impaction. They are ordered also to clean the bowel of feces before certain surgeries, x-ray procedures, or childbirth. Sometimes enemas are ordered to relieve flatulence and intestinal distention. Bowel training programs can involve enemas.

Enemas are usually safe procedures. Many people give themselves enemas at home. However, enemas are dangerous for older persons and those with certain heart and kidney diseases. Comfort and safety measures are practiced when giving an enema. The rules in Box 18-2 also are followed.

Some states allow assistive personnel to give enemas. Others do not. Before giving an enema, make sure that:

- Your state allows assistive personnel to perform the procedure
- The procedure is in your job description
- You have the necessary education and training
- You review the procedure with the RN
- An RN is available to answer questions and to supervise you

Enema Solutions

The enema solution is ordered by the doctor:

- *Tap-water* enema—obtained from a faucet.
- *Soapsuds enema (SSE)*—add 5 ml of Castile soap to 1000 ml of tap water
- *Saline enema*—a solution of salt and water. Add 2 teaspoons of table salt to 1000 ml of tap water.
- *Oil-retention enema*—mineral oil or a commercial oil-retention enema is used.
- *Commercial enema*—contains about 120 ml (4 ounces) of solution.

Other enema solutions may be ordered. Consult with the RN and use the agency procedure manual to safely prepare and give uncommon enemas. Do not administer enemas that contain medications. Such enemas are given by RNs or LPNs.

✦ The Cleansing Enema

Cleansing enemas clean the bowel of feces and flatus. They are sometimes given before surgery, x-ray procedures, and childbirth. The doctor orders a soapsuds, tap-water, or saline enema. The doctor may order *enemas until clear*. This means that enemas are given until the return solution is clear and free of fecal material. Ask the RN how many enemas to give. Agency policy may allow repeating enemas only 2 or 3 times.

Tap-water enemas can be dangerous. The large intestine may absorb some of the water into the bloodstream. This creates a fluid imbalance in the body. Only one tap-water enema is given. Do not repeat the enema. Repeated enemas increase the risk of excessive fluid absorption.

Soapsuds enemas are very irritating to the bowel's mucous lining. Repeated enemas can damage the bowel. Using more than 5 ml (1 teaspoon) of Castile soap or using stronger soaps can also damage the bowel.

The saline enema solution is similar to body fluid. However, some of the salt solution may be absorbed. This too can cause a fluid imbalance. When there is excess salt in the body, the body retains water. (See Focus on Children.)

Text continued on p. 428

focus on CHILDREN

Only saline enemas are used for children. The amount of enema solution varies for infants and children. Always check with the RN for the amount of solution to give. The following are guidelines:
- Infants—50 to 250 ml
- Toddlers—200 to 300 ml
- School-age children—300 to 500 ml
- Adolescents—500 to 1000 ml

Ask the RN about tube size. The following are size guidelines:
- Infants—#10 to #12 (10 to 12 Fr)
- Toddlers—#14 to #16 (14 to 16 Fr)
- School-age children—#16 to #18 (16 to 18 Fr)

In children, enema solutions are given at body temperature (98.6°F, 37°C). In infants, the tube is inserted 1 inch. In toddlers, the tube is inserted 2 inches. Also, ask the RN how high to raise the enema bag. For infants, the bag should be only 3 inches above the anus.

✦ GIVING A CLEANSING ENEMA

PROCEDURE ALERT

- Does your state allow assistive personnel to perform the procedure?
- Is the procedure in your job description?
- Do you have the necessary training and education?
- Is an RN available to answer questions and to supervise you?

PRE-PROCEDURE

1 Explain the procedure to the person.

2 Wash your hands.

3 Collect the following:

- Bedpan or commode
- Disposable enema kit (enema bag, tube, clamp, and waterproof pad); for adults, the tube size is #22 to #30 (22 to 30 Fr)
- Bath thermometer
- Waterproof pad
- Water-soluble lubricant
- Gloves
- Material for enema solution: 5 ml (1 teaspoon) castile soap or 2 teaspoons salt
- Toilet tissue
- Bath blanket
- IV pole
- Robe and slippers
- Specimen container if needed
- Paper towels

Continued

GIVING A CLEANSING ENEMA—cont'd

PRE-PROCEDURE—cont'd

4 Identify the person. Check the ID bracelet against the assignment sheet.

5 Provide for privacy.

6 Raise the bed to the best level for good body mechanics.

PROCEDURE

7 Lower the bed rail.

8 Cover the person with a bath blanket. Fanfold top linens to the foot of the bed.

9 Position the IV pole so the enema bag is above the anus:

  a Adults—12 inches above the anus

  b Infants—3 inches above the anus

10 Raise the bed rail.

11 Prepare the enema:

  a Close the clamp on the tube.

  b Adjust water flow until it is lukewarm.

  c Fill the enema bag to the 1000 ml mark or as otherwise ordered.

  d Measure water temperature. For adults it should be 105° F (40.5° C).

  e Prepare the enema solution:

    • Saline enema: add 2 teaspoons of salt

    • Soapsuds enema: add 5 ml (1 teaspoon) of Castile soap

    • Tap-water enema: add nothing to the water

  f Stir the solution with the bath thermometer. Scoop off any suds (SSE).

  g Seal the top of the bag.

  h Hang the bag on the IV pole.

12 Lower the bed rail.

13 Position the person in the left Sims' position or in a comfortable left side-lying position.

14 Place a waterproof pad under the buttocks.

15 Put on the gloves.

16 Expose the anal area.

17 Place the bedpan behind the person.

18 Position the enema tube in the bedpan. Open the clamp. Let solution flow through the tube to remove air. Clamp the tube.

19 Lubricate the tube with the lubricant. For adults, lubricate 3 to 4 inches from the tip or as directed by the nurse.

20 Separate the buttocks to see the anus.

21 Ask the person to take a deep breath through the mouth.

22 Insert the tube gently 3 to 4 inches into the adult rectum or to a distance directed by the nurse. Insert the tube when the person is exhaling (Fig. 18-3). Stop and call for the nurse if the person complains of pain, you feel resistance, or bleeding occurs.

23 Check how much solution is in the enema bag.

24 Unclamp the tube, and administer the solution slowly (Fig. 18-4).

25 Ask the person to take slow, deep breaths. This helps the person relax while the enema is given.

26 Clamp the tube if the person needs to defecate, has abdominal cramping, or starts to expel solution. Unclamp when symptoms subside.

27 Give the amount of solution ordered. Stop if the person cannot tolerate the procedure.

28 Clamp the tube before it is empty. This prevents air from entering the bowel.

29 Hold several thicknesses of toilet tissue around the tube and against the anus. Remove the tube.

30 Discard the soiled toilet tissue into the bedpan.

GIVING A CLEANSING ENEMA—cont'd

PROCEDURE—cont'd

31 Wrap the tubing tip with paper towels, and place it inside the enema bag.

32 Help the person onto the bedpan. Raise the head of the bed. Or assist the person to the bathroom or commode. The person wears a robe and slippers when up. The bed is in the lowest position.

33 Place the call bell and toilet tissue within reach. Remind the person not to flush the toilet.

34 Discard disposable items.

35 Remove the gloves, and wash your hands.

36 Leave the room if the person can be left alone.

37 Return when the person signals. Knock before entering.

38 Observe enema results for amount, color, consistency, and odor.

39 Put on the gloves.

40 Obtain a stool specimen if ordered.

41 Provide perineal care as needed.

42 Remove the bed protector.

43 Empty, clean, and disinfect the bedpan or commode. Flush the toilet after the RN observes the results. Return items to their proper place. Remove the gloves, and wash your hands.

44 Help the person wash the hands. Wear gloves for this step if necessary.

45 Return top linens, and remove the bath blanket.

POST-PROCEDURE

46 Make sure the person is comfortable and the call bell is within reach.

47 Lower the bed to its lowest position.

48 Raise or lower bed rails as instructed by the RN. Unscreen the person.

49 Follow agency policy for soiled linen and used supplies.

50 Wash your hands.

51 Report your observations.

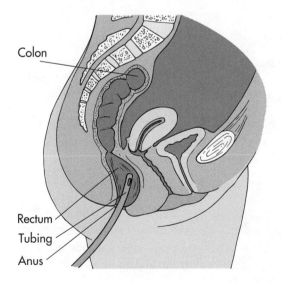

Fig. 18-3 *The enema tubing is inserted into the adult rectum.*

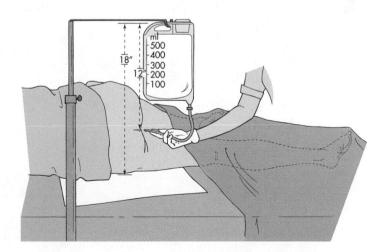

Fig. 18-4 *An enema is given in the left Sims' position. The IV pole is positioned so that the enema bag is 12 inches above the anus and 18 inches above the mattress.*

✦ The Commercial Enema

Commercial enemas cause defecation by irritating and distending the rectum. They are often ordered for constipation or when complete cleansing of the bowel is not indicated.

The commercial enema is prepared and packaged by a manufacturer. It is ready to give. The solution is usually given at room temperature. However, the RN may have you warm the enema in a basin of warm water.

The plastic bottle is squeezed and rolled up from the bottom to give the solution. Do not release pressure on the bottle. If pressure is released, solution is drawn from the rectum back into the bottle. Encourage the person to retain the solution until the urge to defecate is felt. Remaining in the left Sims' or side-lying position helps retain the enema longer.

✦ GIVING A COMMERCIAL ENEMA

PROCEDURE ALERT

- Does your state allow assistive personnel to perform the procedure?

- Is the procedure in your job description?

- Do you have the necessary training and education?

- Is an RN available to answer questions and to supervise you?

PRE-PROCEDURE

1 Explain the procedure to the person.

2 Wash your hands.

3 Collect the following:

- Commercial enema

- Bedpan or commode

- Waterproof pad

- Toilet tissue

- Gloves

- Robe and slippers

- Bath blanket

4 Identify the person. Check the ID bracelet against the assignment sheet.

5 Provide for privacy.

6 Raise the bed to the best level for good body mechanics.

PROCEDURE

7 Lower the bed rail.

8 Cover the person with a bath blanket. Fanfold top linens to the foot of the bed.

9 Position the person in the left Sims' or a comfortable left side-lying position.

10 Place the waterproof pad under the buttocks.

11 Put on the gloves.

12 Expose the anal area.

13 Position the bedpan near the person.

14 Remove the cap from the enema.

15 Separate the buttocks to see the anus.

16 Ask the person to take a deep breath through the mouth.

17 Insert the enema tip 2 inches into the rectum when the person is exhaling (Fig. 18-5). Insert the tip gently.

18 Squeeze and roll the bottle gently. Release pressure on the bottle after you remove the tip from the rectum.

19 Put the bottle into the box, tip first.

20 Help the person onto the bedpan; raise the head of the bed. Or assist the person to the bathroom or commode. The person wears a robe and non-skid slippers when up, and the bed is in the lowest position.

21 Place the call bell and toilet tissue within reach. Remind the person not to flush the toilet.

GIVING A COMMERCIAL ENEMA—cont'd

PROCEDURE—cont'd

22 Discard used disposable items. Remove the gloves, and wash your hands.

23 Leave the room if the person can be left alone.

24 Return when the person signals. Knock before entering.

25 Observe enema results for amount, color, consistency, and odor.

26 Put on gloves.

27 Help the person clean the perineal area if indicated.

28 Remove the bed protector.

29 Empty, clean, and disinfect the bedpan or commode. Flush the toilet after the RN observes the results. Return equipment to its proper place. Remove the gloves, and wash your hands.

30 Help the person wash the hands. Wear gloves for this step if necessary.

POST-PROCEDURE

31 Follow steps 46 through 51 in *Giving a Cleansing Enema.*

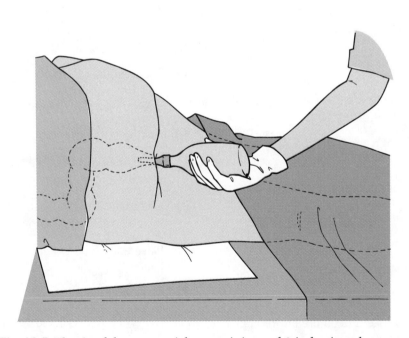

Fig. 18-5 *The tip of the commercial enema is inserted 2 inches into the rectum.*

The Oil-Retention Enema

Oil-retention enemas are given for constipation or fecal impactions. The oil is retained for 30 to 60 minutes to soften feces and lubricate the rectum. This allows feces to pass with ease. Most oil-retention enemas are commercially prepared.

◆ GIVING AN OIL-RETENTION ENEMA

PROCEDURE ALERT

- Does your state allow assistive personnel to perform the procedure?
- Is the procedure in your job description?
- Do you have the necessary training and education?
- Is an RN available to answer questions and to supervise you?

PRE-PROCEDURE

1 Explain the procedure to the person.

2 Wash your hands.

3 Collect the following:

- Commercial oil-retention enema
- Waterproof pad
- Gloves
- Bath blanket

4 Identify the person. Check the ID bracelet against the assignment sheet.

5 Provide for privacy.

6 Raise the bed to the best level for good body mechanics.

PROCEDURE

7 Lower the bed rail.

8 Cover the person with a bath blanket. Fanfold top linens to the foot of the bed.

9 Position the person in the left Sims' or left side-lying position.

10 Place a waterproof pad under the buttocks.

11 Put on the gloves.

12 Expose the anal area.

13 Remove the cap from the enema.

14 Separate the buttocks to see the anus.

15 Ask the person to take a deep breath through the mouth.

16 Insert the tip 2 inches into the rectum when the person is exhaling. Insert the tip gently.

17 Squeeze and roll the bottle slowly and gently. Release pressure on the bottle after you remove the tip from the rectum.

18 Put the bottle in the box, tip first.

19 Cover the person. Leave him or her in the Sims' or side-lying position.

20 Encourage him or her to retain the enema for the time ordered.

21 Place additional waterproof pads on the bed if needed.

22 Remove the gloves.

23 Lower the bed to its lowest position.

24 Raise or lower bed rails as instructed by the RN.

25 Make sure the person is comfortable. Place the call bell within reach.

26 Check the person often.

POST-PROCEDURE

27 Follow steps 46 through 51 in *Giving a Cleansing Enema.*

◆ RECTAL TUBES

A rectal tube is inserted into the rectum to relieve flatulence and intestinal distention. Flatus passes from the body without effort or straining. The rectal tube is inserted 6 inches into the adult rectum. It is left in place for 20 to 30 minutes. This helps prevent rectal irritation. It can be reinserted every 2 to 3 hours. The RN tells you when to insert the tube and how long to leave it in place. *Rectal tubes are not used after rectal surgery.*

Size #22 to #30 (22 to 30 Fr) tubes are used for adults. Often the tube is connected to a flatus bag or to a container with water (Fig. 18-6). The bag inflates as gas passes into it. If connected to a container with water, the water bubbles as gas passes through the tube into the water. For this system, the rectal tube is attached to connecting tubing. The connecting tubing attaches to the water container.

Feces may be expelled along with flatus. If a flatus bag is not used, place the open end of the tube in a folded, waterproof pad. (See Focus on Children.)

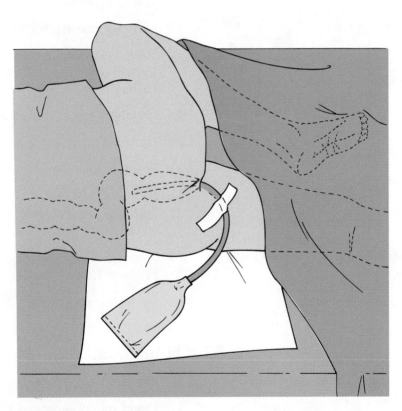

Fig. 18-6 *The tube is inserted 6 inches into the adult rectum. The rectal tube is taped to the buttocks. The flatus bag rests on the bed.*

INSERTING A RECTAL TUBE

PRE-PROCEDURE

1 Explain the procedure to the person.

2 Wash your hands.

3 Collect the following:

- Disposable rectal tube with flatus bag
- Water-soluble lubricant
- Tape
- Gloves
- Waterproof pad

4 Identify the person. Check the ID bracelet against the assignment sheet.

5 Provide for privacy.

6 Raise the bed to the best level for good body mechanics.

PROCEDURE

7 Lower the bed rail.

8 Position the person in the left Sims' or left side-lying position.

9 Place the waterproof pad under the buttocks.

10 Put on the gloves.

11 Expose the anal area.

12 Lubricate the tip of the tube. For adults, lubricate 6 inches.

13 Separate the buttocks to see the anus.

14 Ask the person to take a deep breath through the mouth.

15 Insert the tube 6 inches into the adult rectum when the person is exhaling. Stop if person complains of pain or if you feel resistance. Insert the tube gently.

16 Tape the rectal tube to the buttocks.

17 Position the flatus bag so it rests on the bed protector (see Fig. 18-6).

18 Cover the person.

19 Leave the tube in place no longer than 30 minutes.

20 Lower the bed to its lowest position. Place the call bell within reach. Raise or lower bed rails as instructed by the RN.

21 Remove the gloves, and wash your hands.

22 Leave the room. Check the person often.

23 Return to the room in 30 minutes. Knock before entering the room.

24 Put on gloves, and remove the tube. Wipe the rectal area.

25 Wrap the rectal tube and flatus bag in the bed protector. Remove the bed protector.

26 Ask the person about the amount of gas expelled.

POST-PROCEDURE

27 Make sure the person is comfortable. Place the call bell within reach.

28 Unscreen the person.

29 Discard disposable items. Follow agency policy for soiled linen.

30 Remove the gloves, and wash your hands.

31 Report your observations to the RN.

THE PERSON WITH AN OSTOMY

Sometimes surgical removal of part of the intestines is necessary. Cancer, diseases of the bowel, and trauma (such as stab or bullet wounds) are common reasons for intestinal surgery. An ostomy is sometimes necessary. An **ostomy** is the surgical creation of an artificial opening. The opening is called a **stoma.** The person wears a pouch over the stoma to collect feces and flatus. Stomas do not have nerve endings and are not painful. You will not hurt the person when touching the stoma.

You may assist the RN with the person's postoperative care. Some states let assistive personnel change ostomy pouches. Before changing an ostomy pouch, make sure that:

- Your state allows assistive personnel to perform the procedure
- The procedure is in your job description
- You have the necessary education and training
- You review the procedure with the RN
- An RN is available to answer questions and to supervise you

Colostomy

A **colostomy** is the surgical creation of an artificial opening between the colon and abdominal wall. Part of the colon is brought out onto the abdominal wall and a stoma made. Feces and flatus pass through the stoma rather than the anus. Colostomies are permanent or temporary. If the colostomy is permanent, the diseased part of the colon is removed. A temporary colostomy gives the diseased or injured bowel time to heal. After healing, surgery is done to reconnect the bowel.

The colostomy site depends on the site of colon disease or injury. Figure 18-7 shows common colostomy sites. Stool consistency depends on the colostomy site. Stools are liquid to formed. The more colon remaining to absorb water, the more solid and formed the stool. If the colostomy is near the beginning of the colon, stools are liquid. A colostomy near the end of the large intestine results in formed stools.

Feces irritate the skin. Skin care prevents skin breakdown around the stoma. The skin is washed and dried when the pouch is removed. Then a skin barrier is applied around the stoma. The skin barrier prevents feces from coming in contact with the skin. The skin barrier may be part of the pouch or a separate device.

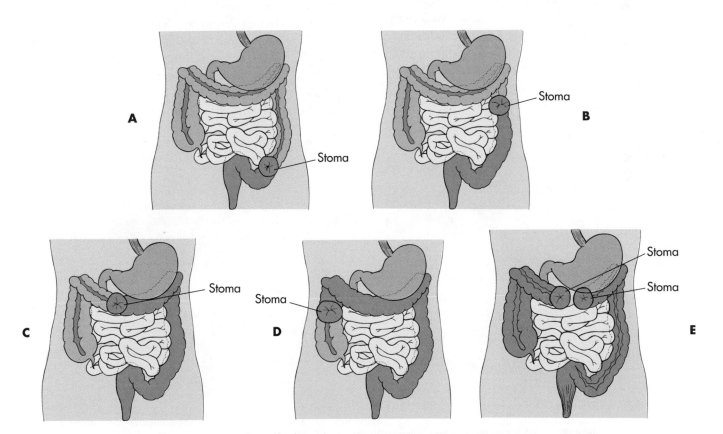

Fig. 18-7 *Colostomy sites. Shading shows the part of the bowel that has been surgically removed.* **A,** *Sigmoid colostomy.* **B,** *Descending colostomy.* **C,** *Transverse colostomy.* **D,** *Ascending colostomy.* **E,** *Double-barrel colostomy. Two stomas are created: one allows for the excretion of fecal material. The other is for the introduction of medicine to help the bowel heal. This type of colostomy is usually temporary.*

Ileostomy

An **ileostomy** is the surgical creation of an artificial opening between the ileum (small intestine) and the abdominal wall. Part of the ileum is brought out onto the abdominal wall and a stoma made. The entire large intestine is removed (Fig. 18-8). Liquid feces drain constantly from an ileostomy. Water is not absorbed because the colon was removed. Feces in the small intestine contain digestive juices that are very irritating to the skin. The ileostomy pouch must fit well so feces do not touch the skin. Good skin care is essential.

✦ Ostomy pouches

The pouch has an adhesive backing that is applied to the skin. Sometimes pouches are secured to ostomy belts (Fig. 18-9). Many pouches have a drain at the bottom that is closed with a clip, clamp, or wire closure. The drain is opened to empty the pouch of feces (see Fig. 18-9). The pouch is emptied when 1/3 to 1/2 full. It is opened also when the bag balloons or bulges with flatus. The drain is wiped with toilet tissue before it is closed.

The pouch is changed every 3 to 7 days. Some people change the pouch whenever soiling occurs. Many people manage their ostomies without help.

Odors are prevented. Good hygiene is essential. The pouch is emptied when feces are present. Avoiding gas-forming foods also controls odors. Special deodorants can be put into the pouch. The RN tells you what to use.

Do not flush pouches down the toilet. Follow agency policy for disposing of used pouches. (See Focus on Children and Focus on Home Care.)

focus on CHILDREN

Children of all ages can have an ostomy, even premature infants. If changing a child's ostomy pouch is delegated to you, the RN will give you the necessary instructions.

focus on HOME CARE

The person can wear regular clothes with an ostomy pouch. However, bulging from feces or flatus is often noticeable with tight clothes. Tight undergarments (girdles and panty hose) can interfere with feces being expelled into the pouch.

Peristalsis continues to move feces through the intestines. As with intact intestines, peristalsis increases after eating. Therefore stomas are usually quieter before breakfast. That is, feces are less like to be expelled at this time. If the person takes a shower or bath with the pouch off, it is best done before breakfast. Showers and baths are delayed 1 or 2 hours after applying a new pouch.

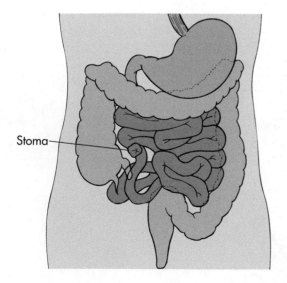

Fig. 18-8 *An ileostomy. The entire large intestine is surgically removed.*

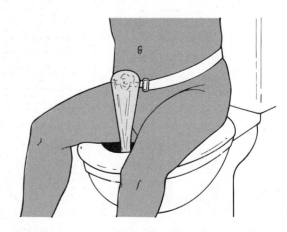

Fig. 18-9 *The ostomy pouch is secured to an ostomy belt. The pouch is emptied by directing it into the toilet and unclamping the end.*

✦ CHANGING AN OSTOMY POUCH

PROCEDURE ALERT

- Does your state allow assistive personnel to perform the procedure?
- Is the procedure in your job description?
- Do you have the necessary training and education?
- Is an RN available to answer questions and to supervise you?

PRE-PROCEDURE

1 Explain the procedure to the person.

2 Wash your hands.

3 Collect the following:
  - Clean pouch with skin barrier
  - Skin barrier (if not part of the pouch)
  - Pouch clamp, clip, or wire closure
  - Clean ostomy belt (if used)
  - Skin barrier as ordered
  - Gauze squares or washcloths
  - Adhesive remover
  - Cotton balls
  - Bedpan with cover
  - Waterproof pad
  - Bath blanket
  - Toilet tissue
  - Wash basin
  - Bath thermometer
  - Prescribed soap or cleansing agent
  - Pouch deodorant
  - Paper towels
  - Gloves
  - Disposable bag

4 Arrange your work area.

5 Identify the person. Check the ID bracelet against the assignment sheet.

6 Provide for privacy.

7 Raise the bed to the best level for good body mechanics.

PROCEDURE

8 Lower the bed rail near you. Make sure the far bed rail is up.

9 Cover the person with a bath blanket. Fanfold linens to the foot of the bed.

10 Place the waterproof pad under the buttocks.

11 Put on the gloves.

12 Disconnect the pouch from the belt if one is worn. Remove the belt.

13 Remove the pouch gently. Gently push the skin down and away from the skin barrier. Place the pouch in the bedpan.

14 Wipe around the stoma with toilet tissue or a gauze square. This removes mucus and feces. Place soiled tissue or gauze in the bedpan.

15 Moisten a cotton ball with adhesive remover. Clean around the stoma to remove any remaining skin barrier. Clean from the stoma outward.

16 Cover the bedpan, and take it to the bathroom. (Raise the bed rail before you leave the bedside.)

17 Measure feces as directed by the RN. Ask the RN to observe abnormal feces. Then empty the pouch and bedpan into the toilet. Note the color, amount, consistency, and odor of feces. Put the pouch in the disposable bag.

18 Remove the gloves, and wash your hands. Put on clean gloves.

19 Fill the wash basin with warm water. Place the basin on the overbed table on top of the paper towels. Lower the bed rail near you.

Continued

✦ CHANGING AN OSTOMY POUCH—cont'd

PROCEDURE—cont'd

20   Clean the skin around the stoma with water. Rinse and pat dry. Use soap or other cleansing agent as directed by the RN.

21   Apply the skin barrier if it is a separate device.

22   Put a clean ostomy belt on the person if a belt is worn.

23   Add deodorant to the new pouch.

24   Remove adhesive backing on the pouch.

25   Center the pouch over the stoma. Make sure the drain points downward.

26   Press around the skin barrier so the pouch seals to the skin. Apply gentle pressure from the stoma outward.

27   Maintain pressure for 1 to 2 minutes.

28   Connect the belt to the pouch (if a belt is worn).

29   Remove the waterproof pad.

30   Cover the person. Remove the bath blanket.

POST-PROCEDURE

31   Make sure the person is comfortable.

32   Raise or lower bed rails as instructed by the RN.

33   Lower the bed to its lowest position. Place the call bell within reach. Unscreen the person.

34   Clean the bedpan, wash basin, and other equipment.

35   Return equipment to its proper place.

36   Discard the disposable bag according to agency policy. Follow agency policy for soiled linen.

37   Remove the gloves, and wash your hands.

38   Report your observations to the RN. Normally the stoma is red like mucous membranes.

✦ STOOL SPECIMENS

When internal bleeding is suspected, feces are checked for blood. Stools are also studied for fat, microbes, worms, and other abnormal contents. The rules for collecting urine specimens (see Chapter 17) apply when collecting stool specimens. Standard Precautions and the Bloodborne Pathogen Standard are followed.

The stool specimen must not be contaminated with urine. Some tests require a warm stool. The specimen is taken to the laboratory immediately if a warm stool is needed.

COLLECTING A STOOL SPECIMEN

PRE-PROCEDURE

1 Explain the procedure to the person.

2 Wash your hands.

3 Collect the following:

- Bedpan and cover (two bedpans if the person needs to urinate) or bedside commode

- Urinal

- Specimen pan for the toilet or commode

- Specimen container and lid

- Tongue blade

- Disposable bag

- Gloves

- Toilet tissue

- Laboratory requisition slip

- Plastic bag

PROCEDURE

4 Label the container with the requested information.

5 Identify the person. Check the ID bracelet against the requisition slip.

6 Provide for privacy.

7 Offer the bedpan or urinal for voiding.

8 Assist the person onto the bedpan or to the toilet or commode. Place the specimen pan under the toilet seat (Fig. 18-10, p. 438). The person wears a robe and nonskid slippers when up.

9 Ask the person not to put toilet tissue in the bedpan, commode, or specimen pan. Provide a disposable bag for toilet tissue.

10 Place the call bell and toilet tissue within reach. Raise or lower bed rails as instructed by the RN.

11 Wash your hands, and leave the room.

12 Return when the person signals. Knock before entering.

13 Lower the bed rail near you.

14 Put on the gloves. Provide perineal care if necessary.

15 Use a tongue blade to take about 2 tablespoons of feces from the bedpan, commode, or specimen pan to the specimen container (Fig. 18-11, p. 438).

16 Put the lid on the specimen container. Do not touch the inside of the lid or container. Place the container in the plastic bag.

17 Place the tongue blade in the disposable bag.

18 Empty, clean, and disinfect the bedpan, commode container, or specimen pan. Remove the gloves, and wash your hands.

19 Return equipment to its proper place.

20 Help the person wash the hands.

POST-PROCEDURE

21 Make sure the person is comfortable. Place the call bell within reach.

22 Make sure the bed is in its lowest position. Raise or lower bed rails as directed by the RN.

23 Unscreen the person.

24 Take the specimen and requisition slip to the laboratory.

25 Wash your hands.

26 Report your observations to the RN.

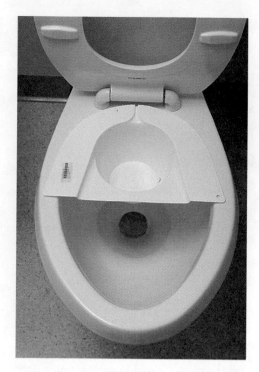

Fig. 18-10 *A specimen pan is placed in the toilet for a stool specimen.*

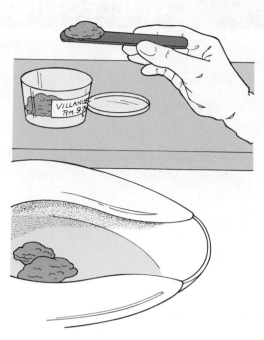

Fig. 18-11 *A tongue blade is used to transfer a small amount of stool from the bedpan to the specimen container.*

✦ Testing Stools for Blood

Blood can appear in stools for many reasons. Ulcers, colon cancer, and hemorrhoids are common causes. Often blood is visible. Blood can usually be seen if bleeding is low in the gastrointestinal tract. Stools are black and tarry if there is bleeding in the stomach or upper GI tract. **Melena** is a black, tarry stool.

Sometimes bleeding occurs in very small amounts. It is difficult to detect such bleeding by just observing the stools. Therefore stools are often tested for the presence of *occult blood*. Occult means hidden or unseen. The test is commonly done to screen for colon cancer.

There are many types of tests. You must follow the manufacturer's instructions for the test ordered. Also follow Standard Precautions and the Bloodborne Pathogen Standard. The RN tells you when to collect the specimen. Many factors can affect the test results. One is eating red meat. Therefore the person cannot eat red meat for 3 days before the test. Bleeding from hemorrhoids and menstrual periods also affect the test results.

TESTING A STOOL SPECIMEN FOR BLOOD

PRE-PROCEDURE

1 Explain the procedure to the person.

2 Wash your hands.

PROCEDURE

3 Collect a stool specimen (see *Collecting a Stool Specimen*).

4 Collect the following:

 • Paper towel

 • Hemoccult test kit (includes developer)

 • Tongue blades

 • Gloves

5 Put on the gloves.

6 Open the test kit.

7 Use a tongue blade to obtain a small amount of stool.

8 Apply a thin smear of stool on box *A* on the test paper (Fig. 18-12, *A*).

9 Use another tongue blade to obtain some feces from another part of the specimen.

10 Apply a thin smear of stool on box *B* on the test paper (Fig. 18-12, *B*).

11 Close the test packet.

12 Turn the test packet to the other side. Open the flap. Apply developer to boxes *A* and *B*. Follow the manufacturer's instructions (Fig. 18-12, *C*).

13 Wait the amount of time noted in the manufacturer's instructions. Time can vary from 10 to 60 seconds.

14 Note and record the color changes (Fig. 18-12, *D*). Follow the manufacturer's instructions.

15 Dispose of the test packet.

16 Discard the tongue blade.

17 Dispose of the specimen.

18 Remove the gloves, and wash your hands.

19 Report the test results and your observations to the RN.

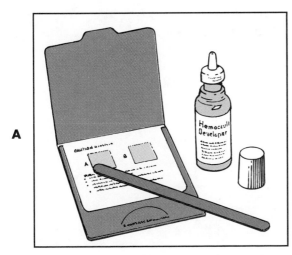
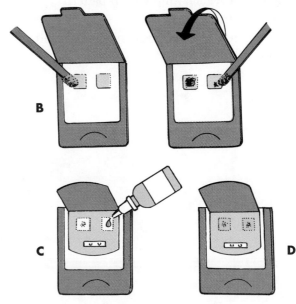

Fig. 18-12 *Testing for occult blood.* **A,** *Stool is smeared on box A.* **B,** *Stool is smeared on box B.* **C,** *Developer is applied to boxes A and B.* **D,** *Color changes are noted.*

REVIEW QUESTIONS

Circle the best answer.

1 Which is *false?*

a A person must have a bowel movement every day.

b Stools are normally brown, soft, and formed.

c Diarrhea occurs when feces move through the intestines rapidly.

d Constipation results when feces move through the large intestine slowly.

2 The prolonged retention and accumulation of feces in the rectum is called

a Constipation

b Fecal impaction

c Diarrhea

d Anal incontinence

3 Which will *not* promote comfort and safety in relation to bowel elimination?

a Asking visitors to leave the room

b Helping the person assume a sitting position

c Offering the bedpan after meals

d Telling the person that you will return very soon

4 Bowel training is aimed at

a Gaining control of bowel movements and developing a regular elimination pattern

b Ostomy control

c Preventing fecal impaction, constipation, and anal incontinence

d All of the above

5 Which is *not* used for a cleansing enema?

a Soap suds

b Saline

c Oil

d Tap water

6 Which is *false?*

a Enema solutions should be 105° F (40.5° C).

b The left Sims' position is used for an enema.

c The enema bag is held 12 inches above the anus.

d The enema solution is administered rapidly.

7 In adults, the enema tube is inserted

a 2 inches

b 4 inches

c 6 inches

d 8 inches

8 The oil-retention enema is retained for

a 10 to 15 minutes

b 15 to 30 minutes

c 30 to 60 minutes

d 60 to 90 minutes

9 Rectal tubes are left in place no longer than

a 60 minutes

b 30 minutes

c 20 minutes

d 10 minutes

REVIEW QUESTIONS—cont'd

10 Which statement about ostomies is *false?*
   a Good skin care around the stoma is essential.
   b Deodorants can control odors.
   c The person wears a pouch.
   d Fecal material is always liquid.

11 A person wears an ostomy pouch. It is usually emptied
   a Every 4 to 6 hours
   b Every morning
   c Every 3 to 7 days
   d When 1/3 to 1/2 full

12 You note a black, tarry stool. This is called
   a Melena
   b Feces
   c Hemostool
   d Occult blood

Answers to these questions are on p. 850.

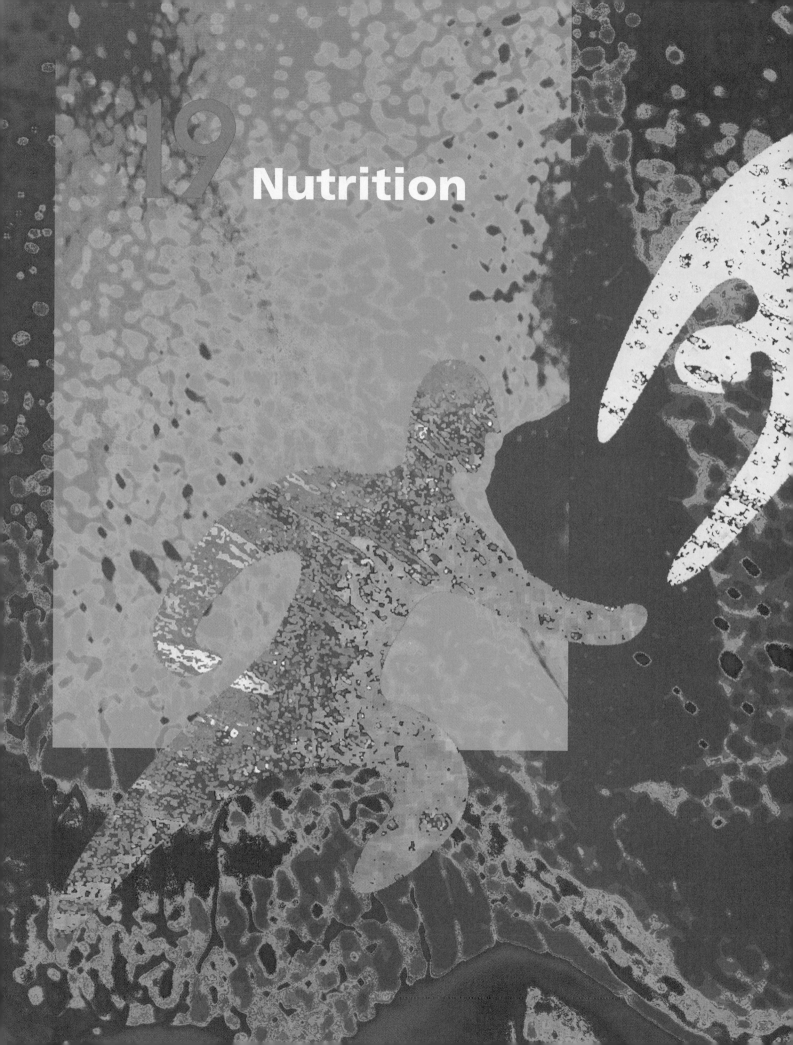

19 Nutrition

- Define the key terms in this chapter
- Explain the purpose and use of the Food Guide Pyramid
- Describe the importance and major sources of protein, carbohydrates, and fats
- Describe the functions and sources of vitamins and minerals
- Explain how to use food labels
- Describe factors that affect eating and nutrition
- Describe the special diets
- Describe between-meal nourishments
- Explain how you can assist with calorie counts
- Explain the purpose of enteral nutrition
- Describe how to handle formula for enteral nutrition
- Explain the difference between scheduled and continuous feedings
- Explain how to prevent aspiration and regurgitation
- Identify the signs and symptoms of aspiration
- Describe the comfort measures that relate to enteral nutrition
- Explain the safety precautions involved in giving tube feedings
- Identify the reasons for removing a nasogastric tube
- Perform the procedures described in this chapter

KEY TERMS

aspiration The breathing of fluid or an object into the lungs

calorie The amount of energy produced from the burning of food by the body

Daily Reference Values (DRVs) The maximum daily intake values for total fat, saturated fat, cholesterol, sodium, carbohydrate, and dietary fiber

Daily Value (DV) How a serving fits into the daily diet; it is expressed in a percentage based on a daily diet of 2000 calories

dysphagia Difficulty or discomfort *(dys)* in swallowing *(phagia)*

enteral nutrition Giving nutrients through the gastrointestinal tract *(enteral)*

gastrostomy A surgically created opening *(stomy)* in the stomach *(gastro)*

gavage Tube feeding

jejunostomy A surgically created opening *(stomy)* into the middle part of the small intestine *(jejunum)*

nasogastric (NG) tube A tube inserted through the nose *(naso)* into the stomach *(gastro)*

nasointestinal tube A tube inserted through the nose into the duodenum or jejunum of the small intestine

nutrient A substance that is ingested, digested, absorbed, and used by the body

nutrition The many processes involved in the ingestion, digestion, absorption, and use of foods and fluids by the body

percutaneous endoscopic gastrostomy (PEG) tube A tube inserted into the stomach *(gastro)* through a stab or puncture wound *(stomy)* made through *(per)* the skin *(cutaneous)*; a lighted instrument *(scope)* allows the doctor to see inside a body cavity or organ *(endo)*

regurgitation The backward flow of food from the stomach into the mouth

Food is a basic physical need necessary for life and health. The amount and quality of foods in the diet are important. They affect a person's current and future well-being. A poor diet and poor eating habits increase a person's risk for infection and acute and chronic diseases. Healing problems and abnormal body functions are also related to poor diet and eating habits. Poor physical and mental functioning increase the risk for accidents and injuries. Besides survival, eating provides pleasure. It is part of social activities with family and friends.

Many factors affect dietary practices. They include culture, finances, and personal choice. Dietary practices also include selecting, preparing, and serving food. The RN considers these factors when using the nursing process to meet the person's nutritional needs.

BASIC NUTRITION

Nutrition is the many processes involved in the ingestion, digestion, absorption, and use of foods and fluids by the body. Good nutrition is needed for growth, healing, and maintaining body functions. Selected foods must provide a well-balanced diet and correct calorie intake. A diet high in fat and calories causes weight gain and obesity. Weight loss occurs when not enough calories are consumed.

Foods and fluids contain nutrients. A **nutrient** is a substance that is ingested, digested, absorbed, and used by the body. Many nutrients are needed for body functions. Nutrients are grouped into fats, proteins, carbohydrates, vitamins, and minerals.

Fats, proteins, and carbohydrates give the body fuel for energy. The amount of energy provided by a nutrient is measured in calories. A **calorie** is the amount of energy produced from the burning of food by the body:
- 1 gram of fat supplies the body with 9 calories
- 1 gram of protein provides 4 calories
- 1 gram of carbohydrate supplies 4 calories

Food Guide Pyramid

In 1992 the U.S. Department of Agriculture (USDA) released its *Food Guide Pyramid*. The Food Guide Pyramid promotes wise food choices (Fig. 19-1). The pyramid has 6 food groups:
- Bread, cereal, rice, and pasta
- Vegetables
- Fruits
- Milk, yogurt, and cheese
- Meat, poultry, fish, dry beans, eggs, and nuts
- Fats, oils, and sweets

The pyramid suggests eating more foods at the bottom level (level 1) and lesser amounts at each level moving to

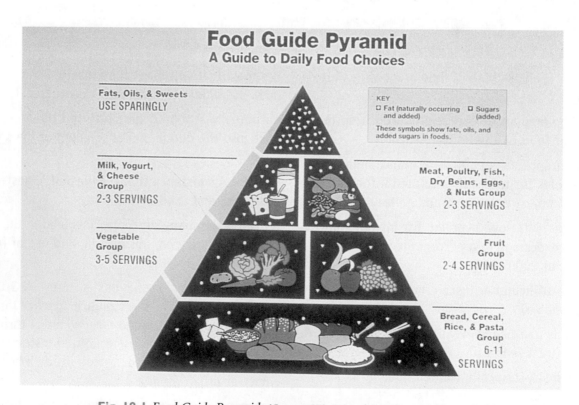

Fig. 19-1 *Food Guide Pyramid. (Courtesy U.S. Dept. of Agriculture, Washington, D.C.)*

DIETARY GUIDELINES FOR AMERICANS

- Eat a variety of foods.
- Maintain a healthy weight.
- Choose a diet low in fat, saturated fat, and cholesterol.
- Choose a diet with plenty of vegetables, fruits, and grain products.
- Use sugars only in moderation.
- Use salt and sodium only in moderation.
- If you drink alcoholic beverages, do so in moderation.

the top (level 4). The Food Guide Pyramid encourages a low-fat diet. More bread, cereal, rice, and pasta (level 1) and more vegetables and fruits (level 2) should be eaten. Food from the milk, yogurt, and cheese group are eaten in moderate amounts. So are foods from the meat, poultry, fish, beans, eggs, and nut group (level 3). Fats, oils, and sweets (level 4) are used sparingly.

Foods from the five food groups in levels 1, 2, and 3 are needed daily. Those foods contain varying amounts of the essential nutrients. No one food or food group contains every nutrient needed by the body.

Note the small circles and triangles in the pyramid (see Fig. 19-1). The circles are for fat and the triangles for sugar. Some sugar and fat naturally occur in all foods. They appear in all levels of the pyramid. There are fewer fats and sugars at levels 1 and 2. The food groups in these levels are low in sugar and fat. More servings are allowed from these groups than the others. The result is a low-fat diet. Level 4 foods contain more fat and calories than do foods at level 1. As you move up the Food Guide Pyramid, fat and calorie amounts increase.

The pyramid is for everyone over 2 years of age. Better health is the goal. Many diseases are related to diet and the kinds of food eaten. They include heart disease, high blood pressure, stroke, diabetes, and certain cancers. Following the Dietary Guidelines for Americans reduces the risk for such diseases. Box 19-1 lists the guidelines developed by the USDA and the U.S. Department of Health and Human Services.

Breads, cereals, rice, and pasta group

This group forms the base of the pyramid. More servings are allowed from this group than any other group. The USDA recommends 6 to 11 servings a day (Box 19-2, p. 446). All foods in the group come from grain (e.g.,

wheat, oats, rice). Protein, carbohydrates, iron, thia-mine, niacin, and riboflavin are the main nutrients in this group. There are small amounts of fats and sugars.

Foods such as pie, cake, cookies, pastries, doughnuts, and muffins are made from grains. However, they are also made with fats and sugars. They are high-fat food choices depending on the amount of fat and sugar added.

Vegetable group

The USDA recommends 3 to 5 servings a day from this group (see Box 19-2). Vegetables provide fiber, vitamins A and C, carbohydrates, and minerals. They are naturally low in fat. A variety of vegetables should be eaten: dark green and yellow vegetables, tomatoes, potatoes, and vegetable juices.

Vegetables can become high in fat from food preparation. French fries are very high in fat compared with a baked or boiled potato. Butter, oil, mayonnaise, salad dressing, sour cream, and sauces are often added to vegetables. These toppings are high in fat. Small amounts of low-fat toppings help keep vegetables low in fat.

Fruit group

Fruits naturally contain some sugar and are low in fat. The USDA recommends 2 to 4 servings of fruit daily (see Box 19-2). Fruits provide carbohydrates, vitamins A and C, potassium, and other minerals. This group includes all fruits and fruit juices. Fresh fruits and juices are best. Frozen or canned fruits should be unsweetened. Often they are sweetened or syrupy and therefore higher in sugar and calories.

Milk, yogurt, and cheese group

Milk and milk products are high in protein, carbohydrates, fat, calcium, and riboflavin. The USDA recommends 2 to 3 daily servings from the milk group—milk, cheese, and yogurt (see Box 19-2). Children and breastfeeding mothers need 3 servings a day.

Skim milk has less fat than whole milk. One cup of skim milk has only a trace of fat; 1 cup of whole milk has 8 grams of fat. One cup of skim milk has about 86 calories. One cup of whole milk has about 150 calories—72 of the calories come from fat. Other low-fat foods in this group include cheeses made with skim milk, low or nonfat yogurt, and ice milk ice cream.

Meat, poultry, fish, dry beans, eggs, and nuts group

This food group is higher in fat than the milk, fruit, vegetable, and bread groups. The USDA recommends 2 to 3 servings a day (see Box 19-2). Protein, fat, iron, and thiamine are the main nutrients found in this group.

BOX 19-2

FOOD GUIDE PYRAMID SERVING SIZES

Bread, Cereals, Rice, and Pasta Group
I slice of bread = I serving
I ounce of ready-to-eat cereal = I serving
$1/2$ cup of cooked cereal, rice, or pasta = I serving

Vegetable Group
I cup raw leafy vegetables = I serving
$1/2$ cup other cooked or chopped raw vegetables = I serving
$3/4$ cup vegetable juice = I serving

Fruit Group
I medium apple, orange, or banana = I serving
$1/2$ cup chopped, cooked, or canned fruit = I serving
$3/4$ cup fruit juice = I serving

Milk, Cheese, and Yogurt Group
I cup of milk or yogurt = I serving
$1/2$ to I ounce cheese = I serving
2 ounces process cheese = I serving

Meat, Poultry, Fish, Dry Beans, Eggs, and Nuts Group
2 to 3 ounces cooked lean meat, poultry, or fish = I serving
$1/2$ cup cooked dry beans = I serving
I egg = I serving
2 tablespoons peanut butter = I serving

Fats, Oils, and Sweets Group
Use sparingly

Serving size is very important for a well-balanced diet. This is very important for meat, poultry, and fish because they contain many calories. Culture, appetite, personal choice, and the recipe used are some factors affecting serving size. A quarter-pound hamburger, a 12-ounce steak, a 10-ounce lobster tail, and a quarter of a chicken are servings offered by restaurants. *One serving* in this group is 2 to 3 ounces of boned meat, fish, or poultry. A 12-ounce steak is 4 to 6 servings from this group!

Remember, foods in this group are high in fat. The more fat, the greater the number of calories. Wise food choices lower fat intake from this group. Fish and shellfish are low in fat. Chicken and turkey have less fat than veal, beef, pork, and lamb. Skinless chicken and turkey are even lower in fat. Veal is lower in fat than beef. Lean cuts of beef and pork should be used. Egg yolks have more fat than egg whites. Low-fat egg substitutes can be used for cooking and baking.

Food preparation is also important. Trim fat from meat and poultry. Remove skin from poultry. Roasting, broiling, and baking are better than frying. Gravies and sauces also add fat.

Nuts and peanut butter have the most fat in this group. Use them wisely. As shown in Figure 19-2, 1 serving of peanut butter (2 tablespoons) equals 1 meat serving (2 to 3 ounces)! Peas and cooked dry beans are very low in fat. Use them often.

Fats, oils, and sweets group

This group is at the top of the pyramid. The USDA recommends that it be used sparingly and as little as possible. Fats, oils, and sweets (foods with added sugar) have little nutritional value. However, they are very high in calories. Foods in this group include cooking oils, shortening, butter, margarine, salad dressing, soft drinks, sour cream, cream cheese, and frosting. They also include all

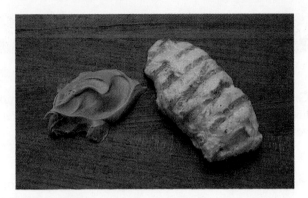

Fig. 19-2 *Two tablespoons of peanut butter (1 serving) equals this 3-ounce chicken breast (1 serving).*

candy, many desserts (cookies, cake, pie, ice cream), jelly and jam, syrup, and alcohol.

Many low-fat or nonfat foods can be bought. Food labels are used to determine fat content.

Nutrients

No one food or food group has every essential nutrient. A well-balanced diet consists of servings from the five food groups in levels 1, 2, and 3 of the Food Guide Pyramid. It ensures an adequate intake of the essential nutrients:

- *Protein*—the most important nutrient, is needed for tissue growth and repair. Protein sources include meat, fish, poultry, eggs, milk and milk products, cereals, beans, peas, and nuts. High-protein foods are costly. Persons with low incomes often lack protein in their diets.
- *Carbohydrates*—provide energy and fiber for bowel elimination. They are found in fruits, vegetables, breads, cereals, and sugar. Carbohydrates are broken down into sugars during digestion. The sugars are then absorbed into the bloodstream. The fiber is not digested. It provides the bulky part of chyme for elimination.
- *Fats*—provide energy and add flavor to food and help the body use certain vitamins. Fat sources include the fat in meats, lard, butter, shortening, salad and vegetable oils, milk, cheese, egg yolks, and nuts. Dietary fat not needed by the body is stored as body fat (adipose tissue).
- *Vitamins*—do not provide calories but are essential nutrients. The body stores vitamins A, D, E, and K. Vitamin C and the B complex vitamins are not stored. They must be ingested daily. Each vitamin is needed for certain body functions. The lack of a specific vitamin results in signs and symptoms of an illness. Table 19-1 on p. 448 lists the sources and major functions of common vitamins.

- *Minerals*—are used for many body processes. They are needed for bone and tooth formation, nerve and muscle function, fluid balance, and other body processes. Table 19-2 on p. 449 lists the major functions and dietary sources of common minerals.

Food Labels

The Nutrition Labeling and Education Act of 1990 (NLEA) requires food labeling for almost all foods (Fig. 19-3 on p. 449). Food labels are useful for planning a healthy diet and for following special diets ordered by the doctor (see p. 454). The food label (Fig. 19-4, p. 450) has information about:

- Serving size and how the serving fits into the daily diet
- Total number of calories per serving and the number of calories from fat
- The total amount of fat and the amount of saturated fat
- Amount of cholesterol, sodium, and protein
- Total amount of carbohydrates and the amount of dietary fiber and sugars
- Amount of vitamins A and C
- Amount of calcium and iron

How a serving fits into the daily diet is called the **Daily Value (DV)**. The Daily Value is expressed in a percent (%). The percent is based on a daily diet of 2000 calories. Some food labels show the maximum daily intake values for total fat, saturated fat, cholesterol, sodium, carbohydrate, and dietary fiber. These are **Daily Reference Values (DRVs)**. The DV and DRVs are used as follows:

- No more than 30% of the calories in the daily diet should come from fat.
- Based on a 2000-calorie diet, the diet should have no more than 65 grams of fat.
- The food label in Figure 19-4 shows that one serving has 13 grams of fat, or 20% of the Daily Value.
- The person can have 52 more grams of fat (80%) that day.

Text continued on p. 450

TABLE 19-1

FUNCTIONS AND SOURCES OF COMMON VITAMINS

Vitamin A
Major functions: Growth; vision; healthy hair, skin, and mucous membranes; resistance to infection
Sources: Liver, spinach, green leafy and yellow vegetables, yellow fruits, fish liver oils, egg yolk, butter, cream, whole milk

Vitamin B_1 (Thiamine)
Major functions: Muscle tone; nerve function; digestion; appetite; normal elimination; carbohydrate use
Sources: Pork, fish, poultry, eggs, liver, breads, pastas, cereals, oatmeal, potatoes, peas, beans, soybeans, peanuts

Vitamin B_2 (Riboflavin)
Major functions: Growth; healthy eyes; protein and carbohydrate metabolism; healthy skin and mucous membranes
Sources: Milk and milk products, liver, green leafy vegetables, eggs, breads, cereals

Vitamin B_3 (Niacin)
Major functions: Protein, fat, and carbohydrate metabolism; nervous system function; appetite; digestive system function
Sources: Meat, pork, liver, fish, peanuts, breads and cereals, green vegetables, dairy products

Vitamin B_{12}
Major functions: Formation of red blood cells; protein metabolism; nervous system functioning
Sources: Liver, meats, poultry, fish, eggs, milk, cheese

Folic Acid
Major functions: Formation of red blood cells; functioning of the intestines; protein metabolism
Sources: Liver, meats, fish, poultry, green leafy vegetables, whole grains

Vitamin C (Ascorbic Acid)
Major functions: Formation of substances that hold tissues together; healthy blood vessels, skin, gums, bones, and teeth; wound healing; prevention of bleeding; resistance to infection
Sources: Citrus fruits, tomatoes, potatoes, cabbage, strawberries, green vegetables, melons

Vitamin D
Major functions: Absorption and metabolism of calcium and phosphorus; healthy bones
Sources: Fish liver oils, milk, butter, liver, exposure to sunlight

Vitamin E
Major functions: Normal reproduction; formation of red blood cells; muscle function
Sources: Vegetable oils, milk, eggs, meats, cereals, green leafy vegetables

Vitamin K
Major functions: Blood clotting
Sources: Liver, green leafy vegetables, egg yolk, cheese

TABLE 19-2 FUNCTIONS AND SOURCES OF COMMON MINERALS

Calcium

Major functions: Formation of teeth and bones; blood clotting; muscle contraction; heart function; nerve function

Sources: Milk and milk products, green leafy vegetables, whole grains, egg yolks, dried peas and beans, nuts

Phosphorus

Major functions: Formation of bones and teeth; use of proteins, fats, and carbohydrates; nerve and muscle function

Sources: Meat, fish, poultry, milk and milk products, nuts, egg yolks, dried peas and beans

Iron

Major functions: Allows red blood cells to carry oxygen

Sources: Liver, meat, eggs, green leafy vegetables, breads and cereals, dried peas and beans, nuts

Iodine

Major functions: Thyroid gland function; growth; and metabolism

Sources: Iodized salt, seafood, and shellfish

Sodium

Major functions: Fluid balance; nerve and muscle function

Sources: Almost all foods

Potassium

Major functions: Nerve function; muscle contraction; heart function

Sources: Fruits, vegetables, cereals, meats, dried peas and beans

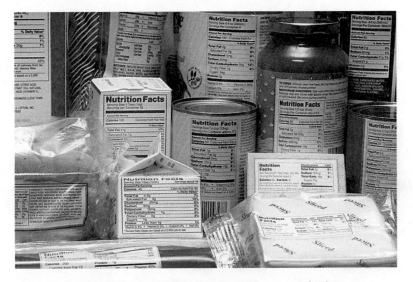

Fig. 19-3 *Food labels are required on most foods.*

Nutrition Facts

Serving Size 1 cup (228g)
Servings Per Container 2

Amount Per Serving

Calories 260 Calories from Fat 120

	% Daily Value*
Total Fat 13g	**20%**
Saturated Fat 5g	**25%**
Cholesterol 30mg	**10%**
Sodium 660mg	**28%**
Total Carbohydrate 31g	**10%**
Dietary Fiber 0g	**0%**
Sugars 5g	
Protein 5g	

Vitamin A 4%	•	Vitamin C 2%	
Calcium 15%	•	Iron 4%	

* Percent Daily Values are based on a 2,000 calorie diet. Your daily values may be higher or lower depending on your calorie needs:

	Calories:	2,000	2,500
Total Fat	Less than	65g	80g
Sat Fat	Less than	20g	25g
Cholesterol	Less than	300mg	300mg
Sodium	Less than	2,400mg	2,400mg
Total Carbohydrate		300g	375g
Dietary Fiber		25g	30g

Calories per gram:
Fat 9 • Carbohydrate 4 • Protein 4

Fig. 19-4 *Information contained on a food label. (From U.S. Food and Drug Administration:* FDA consumer: an FDA consumer special report, *May 1993.)*

FACTORS AFFECTING EATING AND NUTRITION

Many factors affect nutrition and eating habits. Some begin during infancy and continue throughout life. Others develop later.

- *Culture*—Culture influences dietary practices, food choices, and food preparation. Frying, baking, smoking, or roasting food and eating raw food are cultural practices. The use of sauces and spices is also related to culture.
- *Religion*—Selecting, preparing, and eating food often involve religious practices. Members of a religious group may follow all, some, or none of the dietary practice of their faith. You need to respect the person's religious practices. Box 19-3 lists the dietary practices of the major religious groups.
- *Finances*—People with limited incomes often buy the cheaper carbohydrate foods. Their diets often lack protein and certain vitamins and minerals.
- *Appetite*—Appetite relates to the desire for food. When hungry, a person seeks food and eats until the appetite is satisfied. Aromas and thoughts of food can also stimulate the appetite.
- *Personal choice*—The like or dislike of certain foods is a personal matter. Food likes begin in childhood. They are influenced by the way food looks, how it is prepared, its smell, or the recipe. Body reactions affect food choices. People usually avoid foods that cause allergic reactions, nausea, vomiting, diarrhea, indigestion, or headaches.

BOX 19-3

RELIGION AND DIETARY PRACTICES

Adventist (Seventh Day Adventist)
- Coffee, tea, and alcohol are not allowed.
- Beverages with caffeine (colas) are not allowed.
- Some groups forbid the eating of meat.

Baptist
- Some groups forbid coffee, tea, and alcohol.

Christian Scientist
- Alcohol and coffee are not allowed.

Church of Jesus Christ of Latter Day Saints (Mormon)
- Alcohol and hot drinks, such as coffee and tea, are not allowed.
- Meat is not forbidden, but members are encouraged to eat meat infrequently.

Greek Orthodox Church
- Wednesdays, Fridays, and Lent are days of fasting.
- Meat and dairy products are usually avoided during days of fast.

Islam (Muslim or Moslem)
- All pork and pork products are forbidden.
- Alcohol is not allowed except for medical reasons.

Judaism (Jewish faith)
- Foods must be kosher (prepared according to Jewish law).
- Meat of kosher animals (cows, goats, and sheep) can be eaten.
- Chickens, ducks, and geese are kosher fowls.
- Kosher fish have scales and fins, such as tuna, sardines, carp, and salmon.
- Shellfish cannot be eaten.
- Milk, milk products, and eggs from kosher animals and fowl are acceptable.
- Milk and milk products cannot be eaten with or immediately after eating meat.
- Milk and milk products can be eaten 6 hours after eating meat.
- Milk and milk products can be a part of the same meal with meat—they are served separately and before the meat.
- Kosher foods are not prepared in utensils used to prepare nonkosher foods.
- Breads, cakes, cookies, noodles, and alcoholic beverages are not consumed during Passover.

Roman Catholic
- Fasting for 1 hour before receiving Holy Communion.
- Fasting from meat on Ash Wednesday and Good Friday—some may continue to fast from meat on Fridays.   .

- *Illness*—Appetite usually decreases during illness and recovery from injuries. However, nutritional needs increase at these times. The body must fight infection, heal tissue, and replace lost blood cells. Nutrients lost through vomiting and diarrhea must be replaced.

- *Health*—Some diseases and drugs cause a sore mouth, which makes eating painful. Loss of teeth affects chewing, especially protein foods. Some illness and medications cause loss of appetite.

(See Focus on Children and Focus on Older Persons on p. 452 and Focus on Home Care and Focus on Long-Term Care on p. 453.)

Text continued on p. 454

CHILDREN

Infants are breast fed or bottle fed. For bottle-fed babies, the doctor prescribes the formula to use. Solid foods are introduced at about 5 months of age. Usually cereal is the first solid food given. Others are added as the infant grows. The RN tells you what foods the infant can have.

The Food Guide Pyramid applies to children 2 years of age and older. The RN tells you about the child's special needs.

OLDER PERSONS

Many changes occur in the gastrointestinal system. Difficulty swallowing often occurs from decreases in the amount of saliva. **Dysphagia** is difficulty or discomfort (dys) in swallowing (phagia). Taste and smell dull, and appetite decreases. Secretion of digestive juices decreases. As a result, fried and fatty foods are hard to digest and may cause indigestion. Loss of teeth and ill-fitting dentures affect chewing. This results in digestion problems. Hard to chew foods, such as high-protein foods, are avoided. Decreased peristalsis results in slower emptying of the stomach and colon. Flatulence and constipation are common because of decreased peristalsis (see Chapter 18).

Dry, fried, and fatty foods should be avoided. This helps swallowing and digestion problems. Good oral hygiene and denture care improve the ability to taste. People may not have natural teeth or dentures. Their food is pureed or ground. Avoiding high-fiber foods may be necessary even though they help prevent constipation. Foods high in fiber are hard to chew and can irritate the intestines. High-fiber foods include apricots, celery, and fruits and vegetables with skins and seeds. Foods that provide soft bulk are often ordered for those with chewing difficulties or constipation. These foods include whole-grain cereals and cooked fruits and vegetables.

Older persons need fewer calories than younger persons. Energy levels and daily activity levels are lower. The diet must include foods that contain calcium to prevent musculoskeletal changes. Protein is needed for tissue growth and repair. However, the diets of some older persons may lack protein. High-protein foods are generally the most expensive.

focus on HOME CARE

A home care assignment may involve shopping for groceries, planning meals, and cooking. These require knowledge of the Food Guide Pyramid, basic nutrition, and food labels. Also know the person's food preferences and eating habits. For example, some people have their large meal in the evening, others at noon. Some people eat the same thing for breakfast every day. Also review what foods are allowed on the person's diet (see p. 454). Special eating and digestive problems caused by illness, injury, or aging are considered when preparing and serving meals. The person's finances are another factor when planning meals. The RN and dietitian advise you about what to prepare. A good cookbook is a helpful guide for planning and preparing meals.

Plan menus for a full week. Check recipes to make sure all ingredients are on hand or are on the shopping list. You can save money by checking newspapers for sales and using coupons. Save all grocery receipts for the person or family member.

Properly store foods when you return from the store. Refrigerate dairy products and most fresh fruits and vegetables right away. Freeze meat, poultry, fish, and frozen foods unless they are used that day. Dried, packaged, canned, and bottled foods keep well in cabinets. See p. 201 for how to safely handle food.

focus on LONG-TERM CARE

The Omnibus Budget Reconciliation Act of 1987 (OBRA) has the following requirements for food served in long-term care centers:

- The nutritional and special dietary needs of each person must be met.
- Residents must receive a well-balanced diet. The diet must be nourishing and taste good. Food must be well seasoned. It must not be too salty or too sweet.
- Food must be appetizing. It must have an appealing aroma and be attractive.
- Hot food must be served hot and cold food served cold. Centers have special food servers to keep food at the correct temperature. Food is served promptly. Otherwise, hot food will cool and cold food will warm.
- Food must be prepared to meet the person's individual needs. Some persons need food cut, ground, or chopped. Others have special diets ordered by the doctor.
- Each person must receive at least three meals per day and be offered a bedtime snack.
- The center must provide any special eating equipment and utensils that are needed (Fig. 19-5, p. 454). Hands, wrists, and arms may be affected by disease or injury. Special equipment may be needed so the person can eat independently. You must make sure needed equipment is used by the person.

Some centers have dining areas where residents can dine with guests. The resident can have a family meal with a spouse, children, grandchildren, other relatives, or friends. The dietary department provides the meal, or it may be brought by the family. Holidays, birthdays, anniversaries, and other special events can be celebrated.

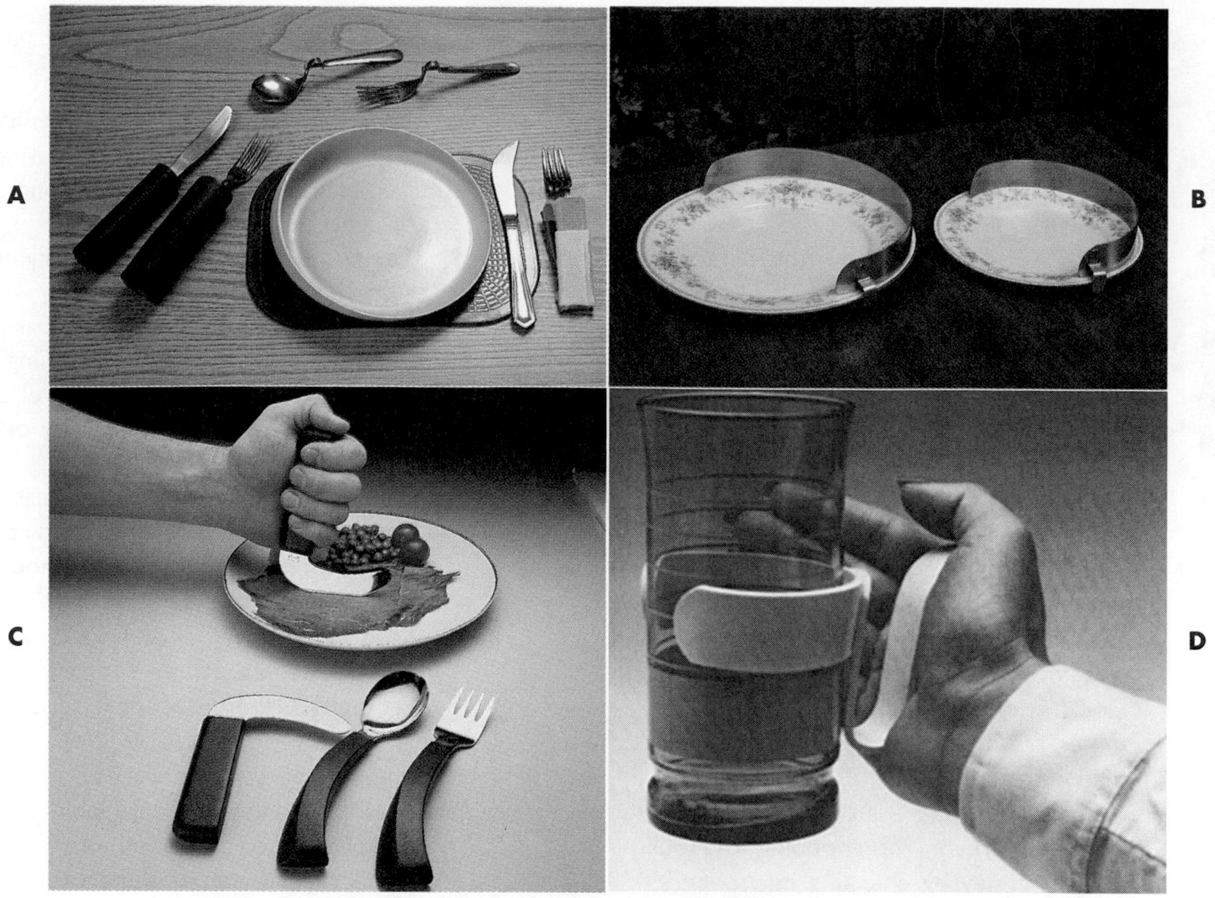

Fig. 19-5 *Eating utensils for persons with special needs.* **A,** *The curved fork fits over the hand. The rounded plate helps keep food on the plate. Special grips and swivel handles are helpful for some persons.* **B,** *Plate guards help keep food on the plate.* **C,** *Knives with rounded blades are rocked back and forth to cut food. The person does not need a fork in one hand and a knife in the other.* **D,** *Glass or cup holder. (Courtesy Bissell Healthcare Corp; Fred Sammons, Inc.)*

SPECIAL DIETS

Doctors order special diets for a nutritional deficiency or a disease, to eliminate or decrease certain substances in the diet, or for weight control (Table 19-3, pp. 455-456). Special diets are common before and after surgery and for persons with diabetes. Persons with diseases of the heart, kidneys, gallbladder, liver, stomach, or intestines may receive special diets. Allergies, obesity, and other disorders also require special diets.

Regular diet, general diet, and house diet have no dietary limits or restrictions. The sodium-restricted diet and diabetic diet are often ordered. They are described in greater detail.

The Sodium-Restricted Diet

The average amount of sodium in the daily diet is 3000 to 7000 mg. The body needs half this amount daily. Healthy people excrete excess sodium in the urine. Heart and kidney diseases cause the body to retain the extra sodium. So do some drugs and some complications of pregnancy.

Sodium causes the body to retain water. If there is too much sodium, the body retains more water. Tissues swell with water, and there are excess amounts of fluid in the blood vessels. The heart has to work harder. That is, the workload of the heart increases. The extra workload can cause serious complications or death. Restricting sodium in the diet decreases the amount of sodium in the body. The body retains less water. Less water in the tissues and blood vessels reduces the amount of work for the heart.

TABLE 19-3

SPECIAL DIETS

Diet:	Clear-liquid
Description:	Clear liquids that do not leave a residue; nonirritating and nongas-forming
Use:	Postoperatively, acute illness, infection, and nausea and vomiting
Foods alllowed:	Water, tea, and coffee (without milk or cream); carbonated beverages; gelatin; clear fruit juices (apple, grape, cranberry); fat-free clear broth; hard candy, sugar, and popsicles
Diet:	Full-liquid
Description:	Foods that are liquid at room temperature or that melt at body temperature
Use:	Advance from clear-liquid diet postoperatively; for stomach irritation, fever, and nausea and vomiting
Foods allowed:	All foods allowed on a clear-liquid diet; custard; eggnog; strained soups; strained fruit and vegetable juices; milk; creamed cereals; plain ice cream and sherbet
Diet:	Soft
Description:	Semisolid foods that are easily digested
Use:	Advance from full-liquid diet; chewing difficulties, gastrointestinal disorders, and infections
Foods allowed:	All liquids; eggs (not fried); broiled, baked, or roasted meat, fish, or poultry that is chopped or shredded; mild cheeses (American, Swiss, cheddar, cream, cottage); strained fruit juices; refined bread (no crust) and crackers; cooked cereal; cooked or pureed vegetables; cooked or canned fruit without skin or seeds; pudding; plain cakes
Diet:	Low-residue
Description:	Food that leaves a small amount of residue in the colon
Use:	Diseases of the colon and diarrhea
Foods allowed:	Coffee, tea, milk, carbonated beverages, strained fruit juices; refined bread and crackers; creamed and refined cereal; rice; cottage and cream cheese; eggs (not fried); plain puddings and cakes; gelatin; custard; sherbet and ice cream; strained vegetable juices; canned or cooked fruit without skin or seeds; potatoes (not fried); strained cooked vegetables; plain pasta; *no raw fruits and vegetables*
Diet:	High-fiber
Description:	Foods that increase the amount of residue in the colon to stimulate peristalsis
Use:	Constipation and colon disorders
Foods allowed:	All fruits and vegetables; whole wheat bread; whole grain cereals; fried foods; whole grain rice; milk, cream, butter, and cheese; meats
Diet:	Bland
Description:	Foods that are mechanically and chemically nonirritating and low in roughage; foods served at moderate temperatures; no strong spices or condiments
Use:	Ulcers, gallbladder disorders, and some intestinal disorders; postoperatively after abdominal surgery
Foods allowed:	Lean meats; white bread; creamed and refined cereals; cream or cottage cheese; gelatin, plain puddings, cakes, and cookies; eggs (not fried); butter and cream; canned fruits and vegetables without skin and seeds; strained fruit juices; potatoes (not fried); pastas and rice; strained or soft cooked carrots, peas, beets, spinach, squash, and asparagus tips; creamed soups from allowed vegetables; no fried foods

TABLE 19-3

SPECIAL DIETS—cont'd

Diet: High-calorie
Description: Calorie intake is increased to about 4000 per day; includes three full meals and between-meal snacks
Use: Weight gain and some thyroid imbalances
Foods allowed: Dietary increases in all foods

Diet: Low-calorie
Description: Calorie intake is reduced below the minimum daily requirements
Use: Weight reduction
Foods allowed: Foods low in fats and carbohydrates and lean meats; avoid butter, cream, rice, gravies, salad oils, noodles, cakes, pastries, carbonated and alcoholic beverages, candy, potato chips, and similar foods

Diet: High-iron
Description: Foods that are high in iron
Use: Anemia; following blood loss; for women during the reproductive years
Foods allowed: Liver and other organ meats; lean meats; egg yolks; shellfish; dried fruits; dried beans; green leafy vegetables; lima beans; peanut butter; enriched breads and cereals

Diet: Low-fat (low-cholesterol)
Description: Foods low in fat and foods prepared without adding fat
Use: Heart disease, gallbladder disease, disorders of fat digestion, and liver disease
Foods allowed: Skim milk or buttermilk; cottage cheese (no other cheeses allowed); gelatin; sherbet; fruit; lean meat, poultry, and fish (baked, broiled, or roasted); fat-free broth; soups made with skim milk; margarine; rice, pasta, breads and cereals; vegetables; potatoes

Diet: High-protein
Description: Aid and promote tissue healing
Use: For burns, high fever, infection, and some liver diseases
Foods allowed: Meat, milk, eggs, cheese, fish, poultry; breads and cereals; green leafy vegetables

Diet: Sodium-restricted
Description: A certain amount of sodium is allowed; sodium restriction ranges from mild to severe
Use: Heart disease, fluid retention, and some kidney diseases
Foods allowed: Fruits and vegetables and unsalted butter are allowed; adding salt at the table is not allowed; highly salted foods and foods high in sodium are not allowed; the use of salt during cooking may be restricted

Diet: Diabetic
Description: The amount of carbohydrates and number of calories are regulated; protein and fat are also regulated
Use: Diabetes mellitus
Foods allowed: Determined by nutritional and energy requirements

The doctor orders the amount of restriction for the person. Many low-salt or salt-free foods can be bought. Food labels are used to determine salt content.

- *2000 mg to 3000 mg sodium diet*—this is called the *low-salt diet.* Sodium restriction is mild. All high-sodium foods are omitted (Box 19-4, p. 458). A minimum amount of salt is used for cooking. Salt is not added to foods at the table.
- *1000 mg sodium diet*—sodium restriction is moderate. Food is cooked without salt. Foods high in sodium are omitted. Vegetables high in sodium are restricted in amount. Salt-free products, such as salt-free bread, are used. Diet planning is necessary.
- *500 mg sodium diet*—sodium restriction is severe. Restrictions for the mild and moderate sodium diets are followed. In addition, vegetables high in sodium are omitted. Milk is limited to 1 cup per day. Only 1 egg per day is allowed. Meat is limited to 4 ounces per day. Diet planning is essential.

The Diabetic Diet

The diabetic diet is ordered for people with diabetes mellitus. Diabetes mellitus is a chronic disease from a lack of insulin (see Chapter 30). The pancreas produces and secretes insulin. Insulin allows the body to use sugar. If there is not enough insulin, sugar builds up in the bloodstream rather than being used by cells for energy. Diabetes is usually treated with insulin or medications, diet, and exercise.

Carbohydrates are broken down into sugar during digestion. The amount of carbohydrates is controlled with the diabetic diet. Only the amount of carbohydrates needed is ingested. The doctor determines the amount of carbohydrate, fat, protein, and calories a person should have. The person's age, gender, activity, and weight are considered.

Allowed calories and nutrients are divided among three meals and between-meal nourishments (see p. 461). The person must eat only what is allowed and all that is allowed. Otherwise the person gets too many or too few carbohydrates. The American Diabetes Association has food lists that have equal amounts of nutrients and calories. The lists are called *exchanges.* The exchanges allow variety in menu planning. For example, a person does not want grapefruit. The exchange list is checked for other fruits. The person sees that one small orange equals one-half grapefruit. Therefore the person knows how much to eat. The RN and dietitian help the person and family learn how to use the exchange lists.

You must serve the person's meal on time. The person must eat at regular times to maintain a certain blood sugar level. Always check the tray to see what the person ate. Report to the RN what the person did and did not eat. If all food was not eaten, a between-meal nourishment is needed. The nourishment makes up for what was not eaten at the regular meal. The amount of insulin given also depends on the person's daily food intake.

ASSISTING THE PERSON WITH EATING

Weakness and illness can affect a person's appetite and ability to eat. Odors, unpleasant equipment, an uncomfortable position, the need for oral hygiene, the need to void, and pain are some factors that affect appetite. Nursing staff can control these factors by getting the person ready for meals:

- Assist the person with oral hygiene. Be sure dentures are in place.
- Provide for elimination needs. Assist the person to the bathroom or bedside commode. Or offer the bedpan or urinal.
- Change clothing, and provide clean linens for incontinent persons.
- Assist the person in washing his or her hands.
- Position the person for eating:
  - For persons in bed—raise the head of the bed to a comfortable sitting position.
  - For persons in chairs—assist the person in transferring from the bed to a chair. Position the overbed table in front of the person.
- Assist persons to the dining room.

✧ Serving Meal Trays

In hospitals, food is usually served in the person's room. Some persons eat in dining rooms, the cafeteria, or lounges. Food is served in containers that keep hot and cold foods at the correct temperature. You will serve meal trays after preparing persons for meals. You can serve trays promptly if patients are ready to eat. Serving trays promptly keeps food at the right temperature. (See Focus on Long-Term Care on p. 459.)

Text continued on p. 460

BOX 19-4

HIGH-SODIUM FOODS

Bread, Cereal, Rice, and Pasta Group
Saltine crackers
Baking powder biscuits
Muffins
Bisquick
Pretzels
Salted crackers
Quick breads (corn bread, nut bread)
Pancakes
Waffles
Instant cooked cereal
Processed bran cereals
Rice
Noodle mixes
Corn chips and other salted snacks

Vegetable Group
Sauerkraut
Tomato juice
V-8 juice
Vegetables in creams or sauces
Frozen vegetables processed with salt or sodium
Bloody Mary mixes
Potato chips
French fries
Instant potatoes
Pickles
Relishes

Fruit Group
No restrictions

Milk, Yogurt, and Cheese Group
Buttermilk
Cheese
Commercial dips made with sour cream

Meat, Poultry, Fish, Dry Beans, Eggs, and Nuts Group
Bacon
Ham
Sausage
Salt pork

Meat, Poultry, Fish, Dry Beans, Eggs, and Nuts Group—cont'd
Hot dogs
Luncheon meats
Corned or chopped beef
Organ meats
Shellfish
Sardines
Herring
Anchovies
Caviar
Kosher meats
Canned tuna
Canned salmon
Mackerel
Salted nuts or seeds
Peanut butter

Fats, Oils, and Sweets
Salad dressings
Mayonnaise
Baked desserts

Other
Mineral water
Club soda
Canned soups
Bouillon cubes
Dried soup mixes
Olives
Salted popcorn
Frozen or canned dinners
Salt
Baking powder
Baking soda
Celery, onion, garlic, and other seasoning salts
Meat tenderizers
Worcestershire sauce
Soy sauce
Mustard
Catsup
Horseradish
Sauces: chili, tomato, steak, barbecue

Modified from Lewis SM, Collier IC, Heitkemper MM: *Medical-surgical nursing: assessment and management of clinical problems,* ed 4, St Louis, 1996, Mosby.

focus on

LONG-TERM CARE

Long-term care centers have special dining and feeding programs:

- *Social dining*—residents eat in a dining room. Each table has 4 to 6 residents. Tables have tablecloths or placemats. Food is served as in a restaurant. This program is for persons who are oriented and can feed themselves.
- *Family dining*—food is placed in bowls and on platters. Residents serve themselves as they would at home.
- *Assistive dining*—the dining room has circular or horseshoe-shaped tables. Residents who need assistance with eating are seated around these tables. An assistive person sits at the center of the table and feeds as many as four residents.

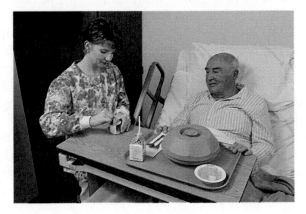

Fig. 19-6 *Open cartons and other containers for the patient.*

SERVING MEAL TRAYS

PROCEDURE

1. Wash your hands.

2. Make sure the tray is complete. Check items on the tray with the dietary card.

3. Identify the person. Check the ID bracelet against the dietary card.

4. Have the person in a sitting position if possible.

5. Place the tray on the overbed table within the person's reach. Adjust table height as necessary.

6. Remove food covers. Open milk cartons and cereal boxes, cut meat, and butter bread if indicated (Fig. 19-6).

7. Place the napkin and silverware within reach.

8. Measure and record intake if ordered (see Chapter 20). Note the amount and type of foods eaten (see p. 461).

9. Remove the tray.

10. Assist the person with oral hygiene. (Wear gloves for this step.)

11. Clean any spills, and change soiled linen.

12. Help the person return to bed if indicated.

POST-PROCEDURE

13. Make sure the person is comfortable

14. Place the call bell within reach.

15. Raise or lower bed rails as instructed by the RN.

16. Wash your hands.

17. Report your observations to the RN.

✦ Feeding the Person

Some persons cannot feed themselves. Weakness, paralysis, casts, and other physical limitations may make self-feeding impossible. These persons are fed.

Provide a relaxed mood so that the person does not feel rushed. Many people pray before eating. Provide time and privacy for a prayer. This shows caring and respect for the person. Ask the person about the order in which to offer foods and fluids. Spoons are used. They are less likely to cause injury than forks. The spoon should be only one-third full. The portion is easily chewed and swallowed.

Persons who cannot feed themselves may be angry, humiliated, and embarrassed. They do not like depending on others. Some are depressed or resentful. Others refuse to eat. These persons should try to feed themselves as much as possible. However, they should not exceed activity limits ordered by the doctor. Be supportive and encouraging.

Visually impaired persons are often keenly aware of food aromas. Often they can identify some foods served. Always tell the person what foods and fluids are on the tray. When feeding a visually impaired person, always identify what you are offering. For persons who feed themselves, identify foods and fluids and their location on the tray. Use the numbers on a clock to identify the location of foods (Fig. 19-7).

Meals provide social contact with others. Engage the person in pleasant conversation. However, give the person enough time to chew and swallow food. Also, sit so that you face the person. Sitting is more relaxing. It shows the person that you have time to feed the person. Standing communicates nonverbally that you do not have time and that you are in a hurry. By facing the person, you can see how well the person is eating. You can also see if the person has problems swallowing.

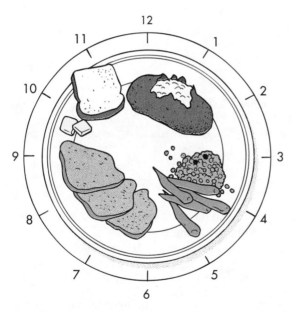

Fig. 19-7 *The numbers on a clock are used to help a visually impaired person locate food on the tray.*

Fig. 19-8 *A spoon is used to feed the person. The spoon is no more than one-third full.*

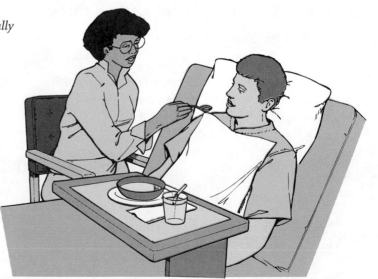

FEEDING A PERSON

PROCEDURE

1 Explain the procedure to the person.

2 Wash your hands.

3 Position the person in a comfortable sitting position.

4 Bring the tray into the room. Place it on the overbed table.

5 Identify the person. Check the ID bracelet against the dietary card.

6 Drape a napkin across the person's chest and underneath the chin.

7 Prepare the food for eating.

8 Tell the person what foods are on the tray.

9 Serve foods in the order the person prefers. Alternate between solid and liquid foods. Use a spoon for safety as in Figure 19-8. Allow enough time for chewing. Do not rush the person.

10 Use straws for liquids if the person cannot drink out of a glass or cup. Have one straw for each liquid. Provide a short straw for weak persons.

11 Converse with the person in a pleasant manner.

12 Encourage him or her to eat as much as possible.

13 Wipe the person's mouth with a napkin.

14 Note how much and which foods were eaten.

15 Measure and record intake if ordered (see Chapter 20).

16 Remove the tray.

17 Provide oral hygiene. (Wear gloves for this step.)

POST-PROCEDURE

18 Make sure the person is comfortable.

19 Place the call bell within reach.

20 Raise or lower bed rails as instructed by the RN.

21 Wash your hands.

22 Report your observations to the RN:

- The amount and kind of food eaten

- Complaints of nausea or dysphagia (difficulty or discomfort in swallowing)

Between-Meal Nourishments

Many special diets involve between-meal nourishments. Commonly served nourishments are crackers, milk, juice, a milkshake, cake, wafers, a sandwich, gelatin, and custard. Serve nourishments as soon as they arrive on the nursing unit. Provide needed eating utensils, a straw, and a napkin. Follow the same considerations and procedures described for serving meal trays and feeding persons.

Calorie Counts

For some patients it is important to keep track of calorie intake. A flow sheet is provided for this purpose. Your role is to note what the person ate and how much. For example, a patient is served a chicken breast, a baked potato, beans, a roll, pudding, and two pats of butter. You note that the person ate all the chicken, half the potato, and the roll. One pat of butter was used. The beans and pudding were not eaten. You note these on the form. An RN or dietitian then converts these portions into calories. The RN tells you what patients require calorie counts.

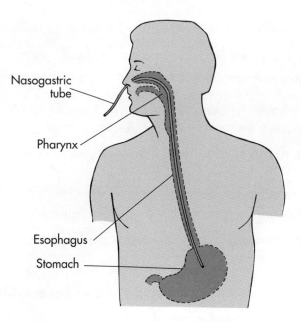

Fig. 19-9 *A nasogastric tube is inserted through the nose and esophagus into the stomach.*

Nasogastric tube

Pharynx

Esophagus

Stomach

ENTERAL NUTRITION

Persons who cannot chew or swallow often require enteral nutrition. **Enteral nutrition** is giving nutrients through the gastrointestinal tract *(enteral)*. Formula is given through a feeding tube inserted into the stomach or small intestine. (**Gavage** is another term for tube feeding.)

- A **nasogastric (NG) tube** is inserted through the nose *(naso)* into the stomach *(gastro)* (Fig. 19-9). A doctor or an RN performs the procedure.
- A **nasointestinal tube** is inserted through the nose into the duodenum or jejunum of the small intestine (Fig. 19-10). A doctor or an RN performs the procedure.
- A **gastrostomy** is an opening *(stomy)* in the stomach *(gastro)* (Fig. 19-11). The opening is created surgically.
- A **jejunostomy** is an opening *(stomy)* into the middle part of the small intestine *(jejunum)* (Fig. 19-12). The opening is created surgically.

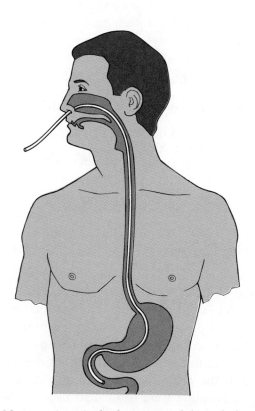

Fig. 19-10 *A nasointestinal tube is inserted through the nose into the duodenum or jejunum of the small intestine.*

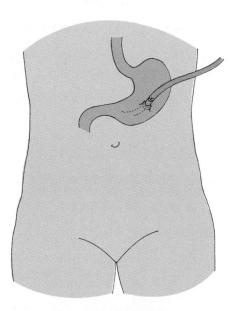

Fig. 19-11 *A gastrostomy tube.*

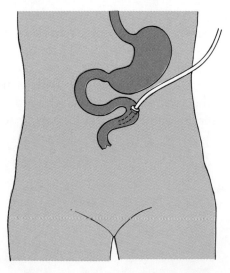

Fig. 19-12 *A jejunostomy tube.*

- A **percutaneous endoscopic gastrostomy (PEG) tube** is inserted with an endoscope. An endoscope is a lighted instrument *(scope)*. It allows the doctor to see inside a body cavity or organ *(endo)*. The endoscope allows the doctor to see inside the stomach. The doctor inserts the endoscope through the person's mouth and esophagus and into the stomach. A stab or puncture wound *(stomy)* is made through *(per)* the skin *(cutaneous)* and into the stomach *(gastro)*. A tube is inserted into the stomach through the stab wound (Fig. 19-13).

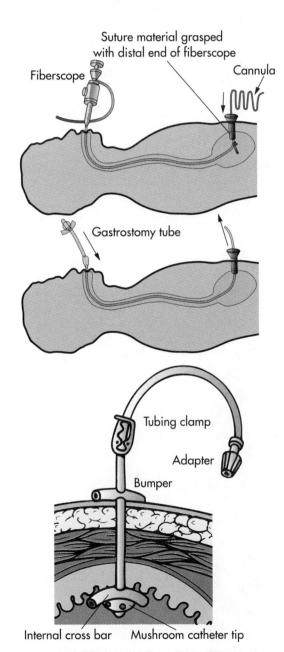

Suture material grasped with distal end of fiberscope

Fiberscope

Cannula

Gastrostomy tube

Tubing clamp

Adapter

Bumper

Internal cross bar   Mushroom catheter tip

Fig. 19-13 *A percutaneous endoscopic gastrostomy. (From Lewis SM, Collier IC, Heitkemper MM: Medical-surgical nursing: assessment and management of clinical problems, ed 4, St Louis, 1996, Mosby.)*

Feeding tubes are used when food cannot pass normally from the mouth into the esophagus and then into the stomach. Cancer of the head, neck, or esophagus is a common cause. So is trauma or surgery to the face, mouth, head, or neck. Coma is another reason for tube feedings. So is dysphagia caused by paralysis. Some persons with dementia no longer know how to eat and may require tube feedings. Gastrostomy, jejunostomy, and PEG feedings are used for long-term enteral nutrition. The ostomy may be temporary or permanent.

Formulas

The doctor orders the type of formula and the amount to give. Most formulas contain protein, carbohydrates, fat, vitamins, and minerals. Commercial formulas are common. Sometimes formula is prepared by the dietary department.

Formulas provide an environment for the growth of microbes. Contamination can occur when preparing, storing, or giving tube feedings. To prevent contamination:

- Wear gloves when preparing or handling formula. Replace soiled gloves as necessary.
- Do not use dented or damaged cans.
- Check the expiration date on commercial formulas. Return expired products to the supply area.
- Check the date on formulas prepared by the dietary department. Discard any formula more than 24 hours old.
- Wash cans or bottles before opening them.
- Label cans or bottles with the time and date opened.
- Refrigerate open cans, bottles, or prepared formula. Place a tight cover or lid over the container. Use the formula within 24 hours. Discard formula more than 24 hours old.
- Clear the tube before and after the feeding. Use 30 to 50 ml of water or other fluid according to agency policy. (This is part of the person's intake. Total intake for a feeding is often limited to 450 ml.)

Scheduled and Continuous Feedings

The doctor orders scheduled or continuous feedings. Scheduled feedings usually are given four times a day with a syringe or feeding bag (Fig. 19-14, p. 464). Usually about 400 ml is given over 20 minutes during a scheduled feeding. The amount and rate are like eating a regular meal.

Continuous feedings require electronic feeding pumps (Fig. 19-15, p. 464). Nasointestinal and jejunostomy tube feedings are always continuous.

Formula is given at room temperature. Cold fluids can cause cramping. Sometimes continuous feedings are

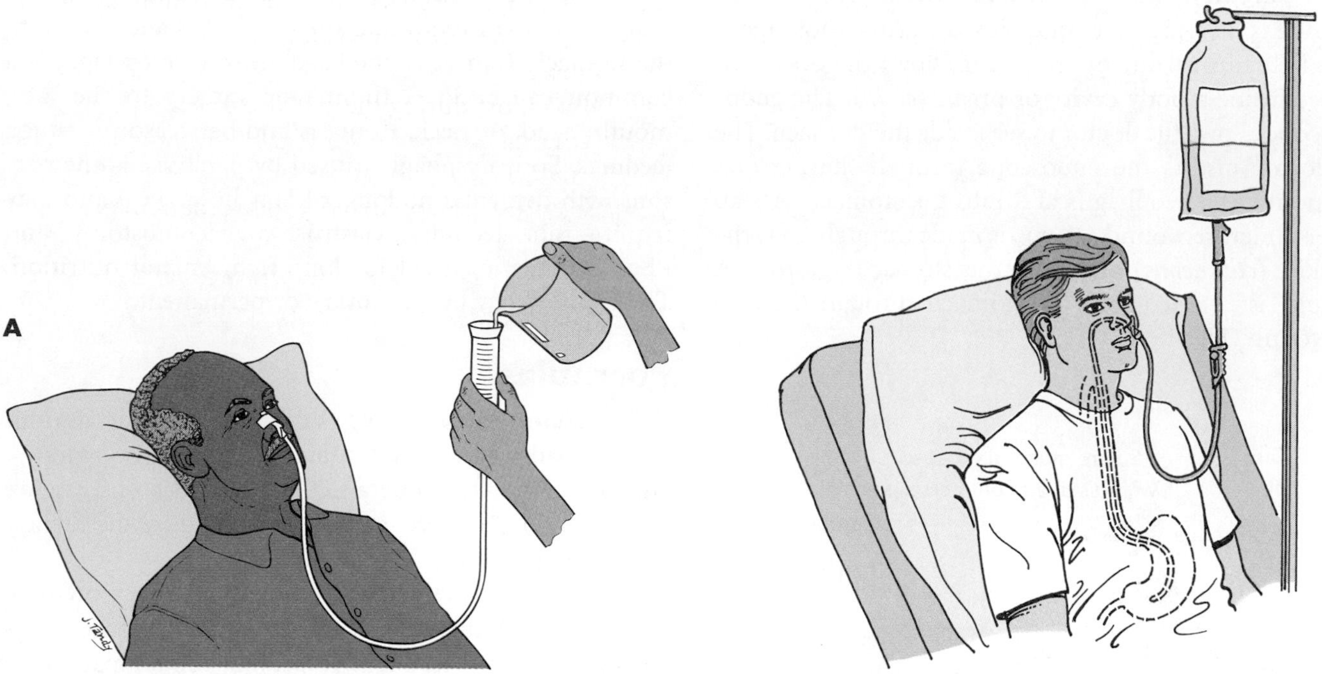

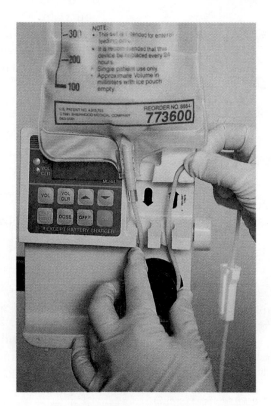

Fig. 19-14 A, *A tube feeding is given with a syringe.* **B,** *Formula drips from a feeding bag into the feeding tube.* (**B** *from Potter PA, Perry AG:* Fundamentals of nursing: concepts, process, and practice, *ed 4, St Louis, 1997, Mosby.*)

Fig. 19-15 *Feeding pump.* (*From Potter PA, Perry AG:* Fundamentals of nursing: concepts, process, and practice, *ed 4, St Louis, 1997, Mosby.*)

kept cold with ice chips around the container. Otherwise microbes grow in warm formula. The formula warms to room temperature as it drips from the bag and passes through the connecting tubing to the feeding tube.

Formula is added to continuous feedings every 3 to 4 hours. However, do not add new formula to formula in the bag. Otherwise new formula is added to old formula that may be contaminated with microbes. Formula should not hang longer than 4 hours to prevent the growth of microbes. Some formulas have preservatives. They can hang longer. The RN tells you how long the formula can hang.

Preventing Aspiration

Aspiration is a major complication of nasogastric and nasointestinal tubes. Remember, **aspiration** is the breathing of fluid or an object into the lungs. These tubes are passed through the esophagus and then into the stomach or small intestine. During insertion, the tube can slip into the respiratory tract. This causes aspiration. An x-ray film is the best way to determine tube placement. One is taken after the doctor or RN inserts the tube.

After insertion, the tube can move out of place from coughing, sneezing, vomiting, suctioning, and poor positioning. The tube can move from the stomach or intestines into the esophagus and then into the respiratory tract. *Therefore the RN checks tube placement before every scheduled tube feeding.* With continuous tube feedings, the RN checks tube placement every 4 to 8 hours. To assess tube placement, the RN attaches a syringe to the tube and aspirates gastrointestinal secretions. Then the RN measures the pH of the secretions.

Aspiration also occurs from regurgitation. **Regurgitation** is the backward flow of food from the stomach into the mouth. This can occur with nasogastric, gastrostomy, and PEG tubes. Delayed stomach emptying and overfeeding are common causes of regurgitation. To prevent regurgitation, the person sits or is in semi-Fowler's position for the feeding. The person remains in this position for at least 1 hour after the feeding. This promotes movement of the formula through the gastrointestinal system and prevents aspiration. The left side-lying position is avoided. This position prevents the stomach from emptying.

The risk of regurgitation is less with nasointestinal and jejunostomy tubes. Formula passes directly into the small intestine. Also, formula is given at a slow rate. Remember, during digestion, food slowly passes from the stomach to the small intestine. The stomach handles larger amounts of food at one time than does the small intestine.

Observations

The RN must be alert to signs and symptoms of aspiration. Other complications include diarrhea, constipation, and delayed stomach emptying. You must report the following to the RN immediately:

- Nausea
- Discomfort during the tube feeding
- Vomiting
- Diarrhea
- Distended (enlarged and swollen) abdomen
- Coughing
- Complaints of indigestion or heart burn
- Redness, swelling, drainage, odor, or pain at the ostomy site
- Elevated temperature
- Signs and symptoms of respiratory distress (see Chapter 21)
- Increased pulse rate
- Complaints of flatulence

Comfort Measures

The person with a feeding tube is usually NPO. *NPO* is the abbreviation for the Latin term *nils per os*, which means nothing by mouth. Dry mouth, dry lips, and sore throat are sources of discomfort. Some persons are allowed hard candy or gum. The person's nursing care plan will likely include frequent oral hygiene, lubricant for the lips, and mouth rinses. The nose and nostrils also are cleaned every 4 to 8 hours as directed by the RN.

Nasogastric and nasointestinal tubes can irritate and cause pressure on the nose. Sometimes they alter the shape of the nostrils or cause pressure ulcers. Securing the tube helps prevent these problems. Use tape or a tube holder to secure the tube to the nose (Fig. 19-16, p. 466). Tube holders have foam cushions that prevent pressure on the nose. They also eliminate the need for retaping, which irritates the nose. The tube also is secured to the person's gown. Loop a rubber band around the tube. Then pin the rubber band to the person's gown with a safety pin. Or tape the tube to the gown.

✦ Giving Tube Feedings

You assist the RN with tube feedings. Some states allow assistive personnel to give tube feedings through the nasogastric and nasointestinal routes. Some also allow assistive personnel to give tube feedings through established (healed) gastrostomy and jejunostomy sites. Before you give a tube feeding make sure that:

- The procedure is allowed by your state.
- The procedure is in your job description.
- You have the necessary education and training.
- You are familiar with the agency's equipment and supplies.
- You review the procedure with the RN.
- An RN is available for questions and supervision.
- The RN checks tube placement.

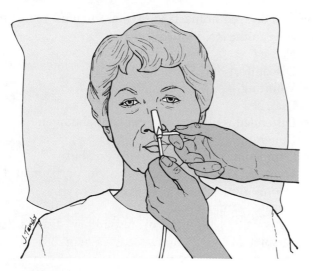

Fig. 19-16 *The feeding tube is taped to the nose.*

The person may have intravenous infusions, drainage tubes, and a breathing tube (see Chapter 21). You must know the purpose of each tube. *Formula must enter only the feeding tube.* Otherwise the person can die. Always check and inspect the feeding tube with the RN before giving a tube feeding. Often RNs will label the person's tubes to identify their purpose. Even if tubes are labeled, you should still check and inspect the feeding tube with the RN. (See Focus on Children, Focus on Older Persons, and Focus on Home Care.)

focus on CHILDREN

Nasogastric, gastrostomy, and PEG tube feedings are more common in infants and children than intestinal feeding tubes. Feedings are usually scheduled.

The RN tells you how to position the child. Holding the infant or small child in your lap is the preferred position. This helps comfort the child and elevates the head and chest. If the child cannot be held, the child is placed in a right side-lying position with the head and chest elevated. After the feeding, the child is positioned on the right side or in Fowler's position for 1 hour.

The RN also tells you how much formula to give. The flow rate usually is 5 ml every 5 to 10 minutes in small infants. In older infants and children, it is 10 ml per minute. Feedings take 15 to 30 minutes. A slow feeding prevents cramping, nausea, and vomiting. After the feeding, the tube is flushed with 5 to 15 ml of sterile water.

Give infants pacifiers to suck on during the feeding. This allows the normal sucking reflex for feeding (see Chapter 8). Also, pacifiers are comforting and reduce crying.

focus on OLDER PERSONS

The digestive process slows with aging. Stomach emptying also slows. Therefore the older person is at risk for regurgitation. Older persons may require less formula and a longer feeding time to prevent overfeeding.

focus on HOME CARE

An RN is not present in the home to check tube placement. Family members are often taught to check tube placement and to give tube feedings. Follow state and agency policies for giving tube feedings in the home setting.

GIVING A TUBE FEEDING

PROCEDURE ALERT

- Does your state allow assistive personnel to perform the procedure?
- Is the procedure in your job description?
- Do you have the necessary training and education?
- Is an RN available to answer questions and to supervise you?

PRE-PROCEDURE

1 Review the procedure with the RN. Ask what feeding method to use: syringe, feeding bag, or feeding pump.

2 Review the manufacturer's instructions for the feeding pump.

3 Ask the RN to verify tube placement. Check and inspect the tube with the RN to make sure you are using the right tube.

4 Explain the procedure to the person.

5 Collect the following:

- 30 or 50 ml bulb syringe or feeding bag with tubing

- Feeding pump

- IV pole for the feeding bag or ready-to-hang bottle

- Formula as directed by the RN

- 30 to 50 ml water or other flushing solution

- Gloves

6 Check the date on the formula. Do not use formula if the expiration date has passed.

7 Make sure the formula is at room temperature.

8 Clean the formula can or bottle.

9 Identify the person. Check the ID bracelet against the assignment sheet.

10 Provide for privacy.

PROCEDURE

11 Position the person in a sitting or semi-Fowler's position. The RN tells you how to position the person.

12 Put on the gloves.

13 Open the can or bottle.

14 *Give a scheduled NASOGASTRIC or GASTROSTOMY feeding using a syringe:*

a Pinch or clamp the feeding tube. This prevents air from entering the tube and then the stomach.

b Attach the syringe to the feeding tube.

c Fill the syringe with formula (see Fig. 19-14, *A*).

d Unpinch or unclamp the feeding tube.

e Let the formula slowly pass from the syringe into the feeding tube. Raise or lower the syringe to adjust the flow rate. The higher the syringe, the faster the flow rate.

f Add formula as necessary. Do not let the syringe empty. Otherwise air enters the feeding tube.

g Ask the person about feelings of fullness or cramping. Pinch or clamp tubing if one or both of these occur.

h Give formula over 20 minutes or as directed by the RN.

i Pinch the feeding tube as the syringe empties.

j Add the water or flushing solution to the syringe.

k Release the feeding tube, and let the water or flushing solution clear the tube.

l Pinch or clamp the feeding tube as the syringe empties. Do not let air enter the feeding tube.

m Remove the syringe.

n Cap or clamp the feeding tube.

15 *Give a scheduled NASOGASTRIC, GASTROSTOMY, or PEG feeding using a feeding bag:*

a Close the clamp on the connecting tubing.

b Fill the feeding bag with formula.

Continued

GIVING A TUBE FEEDING—cont'd

PROCEDURE—cont'd

c Squeeze the drip chamber so it partially fills with formula.

d Open the clamp on the connecting tubing slowly.

e Let formula flow through the connecting tubing to clear it of air.

f Clamp the tubing.

g Hang the feeding bag from the IV pole.

h Attach the connecting tubing to the feeding tube (see Fig. 19-14, *B*).

i Adjust the clamp on the connecting tubing to regulate the flow rate. The RN tells you the number of drops per minute. Formula is usually given over 20 minutes.

j Clamp the connecting tubing before the bag empties of formula.

k Add water or flushing solution to the bag.

l Unclamp the tubing, and let the water or flushing solution clear the feeding tube.

m Clamp the connecting tubing as it empties. Do not let air enter the feeding tube.

n Pinch or clamp the feeding tube.

o Disconnect the connecting tube from the feeding tube.

p Cap or clamp the feeding tube.

16 *Give a continuous NASOGASTRIC, NASO-INTESTINAL, GASTROSTOMY, PEG, or JEJUNOSTOMY feeding using a pump:*

a Follows step 15 a–h.

b Follow the manufacturer's instructions for threading the connecting tubing on through the pump (see Fig. 19-15).

c Set the flow rate as directed by the RN.

d Add ice around the bag as directed by the RN.

e Tell the RN when the bag is emptying. The RN assesses the person, checks for tube placement, and flushes the tube before adding more formula.

POST-PROCEDURE

17 Record the amount of formula given on the intake and output record. Also record the amount of water or flushing solution used to clear the tube.

18 Position the person as directed by the RN. The person sits or is in semi-Fowler's position. Or position the person in the right side-lying position with the head of the bed raised about 30 degrees. The position is maintained for 1 hour after the feeding.

19 Make sure the person is comfortable.

20 Place the call bell within the person's reach.

21 Make sure the bed is in its lowest position.

22 Raise or lower bed rails as instructed by the RN.

23 Unscreen the person.

24 Clean and return equipment to its proper place.

25 Remove and discard the gloves.

26 Wash your hands.

27 Report your observations to the RN.

✦ Removing a Nasogastric Tube

The nasogastric tube is removed when the person can eat and swallow. The person must not have nausea and vomiting. The doctor gives the order to remove the tube.

Your state and job description may allow you to remove nasogastric tubes. Make sure you have the necessary training and education. Also, review the procedure with the RN. Standard Precautions and the Bloodborne Pathogen Standard are followed.

REMOVING A NASOGASTRIC TUBE

PROCEDURE ALERT

- Does your state allow assistive personnel to perform the procedure?
- Is the procedure in your job description?

- Do you have the necessary training and education?
- Is an RN available to answer questions and to supervise you?

PRE-PROCEDURE

1 Review the procedure with the RN.

2 Explain the procedure to the person.

3 Collect the following:

- Towel
- Tissues
- Gloves
- Equipment for oral hygiene

4 Identify the person. Check the ID bracelet against the assignment sheet.

5 Provide for privacy.

PROCEDURE

6 Position the person in a sitting or semi-Fowler's position.

7 Put on the gloves.

8 Place the towel across the person's chest.

9 Give the person tissues so he or she can wipe the nose after the tube is removed.

10 Unpin or untape the tube from the person's gown.

11 Remove tape or the tube holder.

12 Disconnect the tube if it is attached to suction.

13 Pinch the tube shut. This prevents tube contents from draining out during removal.

14 Ask the person to take a deep breath. Ask the person to hold that breath. (This closes the epiglottis, which acts like a lid over the larynx. It prevents food from entering the airway. During this procedure, it prevents aspiration of stomach contents.)

15 Withdraw the tube. Use quick, smooth motions.

16 Place the tube in a biohazard bag.

17 Assist the person with oral hygiene.

18 Remove the towel.

19 Remove the gloves.

POST-PROCEDURE

20 Make sure the person is comfortable.

21 Place the call bell within reach.

22 Make sure the bed is in its lowest position.

23 Raise or lower bed rails as instructed by the RN.

24 Unscreen the person.

25 Put on clean gloves.

26 Clean and return equipment to its proper place.

27 Follow agency policy for soiled linens.

28 Remove the gloves, and wash your hands.

29 Report your observations to the RN.

OTHER METHODS FOR MEETING NUTRITIONAL NEEDS

Sometimes other methods are used to meet a person's nutritional needs. Intravenous (IV) therapy and hyperalimentation are common:

- **Intravenous therapy**—Many persons receive fluid through a needle inserted into a vein. The fluid may contain sugar, minerals, and vitamins. IV therapy does not provide fat and protein. It provides fluids and sugar for energy. IV therapy is not used for long-term nutritional therapy. IV therapy is presented in Chapter 20.

- **Hyperalimentation**—This is the intravenous administration of a solution highly concentrated with proteins, carbohydrates, vitamins, and minerals. Fat can be added also. The solution is far more nutritious than a regular IV solution. Hyperalimentation is used for seriously ill and injured persons. *Assistive personnel are never responsible for administering or regulating hyperalimentation solutions.*

REVIEW QUESTIONS

Circle T *if the statement is true or* F *if the statement is false.*

1 T F Mr. Bonner is on a sodium-restricted diet. He asks for some salt for his chicken. You should bring him the salt.

2 T F Nasointestinal tube feedings are continuous.

3 T F Jejunostomy tube feedings are scheduled.

4 T F Jejunostomy tube feedings are given with a syringe.

5 T F Feeding formulas provide an environment for the growth of microbes.

6 T F Sterile technique is required when removing a nasogastric tube.

7 T F Open formula must be used within 24 hours.

Circle the best *answer.*

8 Nutrition is
 a Fats, proteins, carbohydrates, vitamins, and minerals
 b The many processes involved in the ingestion, digestion, absorption, and use of food and fluids by the body
 c The Food Guide Pyramid
 d The balance between calories taken in and used by the body

9 The Food Guide Pyramid encourages
 a A low-fat diet c A low-fiber diet
 b A high-fat diet d A low-salt diet

10 How many daily servings of breads, cereals, rice, and pasta are recommended?
 a 6 to 11 c 2 to 4
 b 3 to 5 d 2 to 3

11 How many daily servings of the meat group are recommended?
 a 6 to 11
 b 3 to 5
 c 2 to 4
 d 2 to 3

12 Which food groups contain the most fat?
 a Breads, cereal, rice, and pasta
 b Fruits
 c Milk, yogurt, and cheese
 d Meat, poultry, fish, dry beans, eggs, and nuts

13 Fats, oils, and sweets
 a Should be used in moderate amounts
 b Are low in calories
 c Should be used sparingly
 d Have great nutritional value

14 Protein is needed for
 a Tissue growth and repair
 b Energy and the fiber for bowel elimination
 c Body heat and the protection of organs from injury
 d Improving the taste of food

15 Which foods provide the *most* protein?
 a Butter and cream
 b Tomatoes and potatoes
 c Meats and fish
 d Corn and lettuce

16 Which person does not require a sodium-restricted diet? The person with
 a Diabetes mellitus   c Kidney disease
 b Heart disease   d Liver disease

17 The diabetic diet controls the amount of
 a Water   c Carbohydrates
 b Sodium   d Nutrients

18 Diet planning for the diabetic diet involves
 a Calculating the amount of sodium
 b Exchange lists
 c Measuring fluid intake
 d Giving insulin with meals

19 Which statement about feeding a person is *false?*
 a You should ask if he or she wants to pray before eating.
 b You should use a fork to feed the person.
 c You should ask the person the order in which foods should be served.
 d You should engage the person in a pleasant conversation.

20 You are going to give a gastrostomy tube feeding. The person is positioned in
 a Semi-Fowler's position
 b The left side-lying position
 c The right side-lying position
 d The prone position

21 What is the preferred position for giving a tube feeding to an infant or small child?
 a Elevating the head of the bed 30 degrees
 b Holding the child in your lap
 c The right side-lying position
 d Fowler's position

22 Before giving a tube feeding, you must do the following *except*
 a Review the procedure with the RN
 b Explain the procedure to the person
 c Provide for the person's privacy
 d Check tube placement

23 Formula for tube feedings is given
 a At body temperature   c Hot
 b At room temperature   d Cold

24 You are to give a scheduled tube feeding to an adult. How much formula is usually given during the feeding?
 a 100 ml   c 300 ml
 b 200 ml   d 400 ml

25 Continuous feedings are given with a
 a Syringe   c PEG tube
 b Feeding bag   d Feeding pump

26 Tube placement is checked to prevent
 a Aspiration   c Overfeeding
 b Regurgitation   d Cramping

27 To prevent regurgitation, the person is positioned
 a In semi-Fowler's position for 30 minutes after the feeding
 b In semi-Fowler's position for 1 hour after the feeding
 c In the left side-lying position for 30 minutes after the feeding
 d In the left side-lying position for 1 hour after the feeding

28 A person with a feeding tube is usually
 a Allowed a regular diet   c NPO
 b On bedrest   d In a coma

Answers to these questions are on p. 850.

20 Fluids and Blood

- Define the key terms in this chapter
- Describe normal adult fluid requirements and the common causes of dehydration
- Explain your responsibilities when encourage fluids, restricted fluids, and NPO are ordered
- Explain the purpose of measuring intake and output
- Identify foods that are counted as fluid intake
- Know the types of IV solutions
- Explain the difference between peripheral IV sites and central venous sites
- Describe the equipment used in IV therapy
- Describe how you assist the RN in maintaining the IV flow rate
- Explain the safety measures necessary for IV therapy
- Identify the signs and symptoms of IV therapy complications
- Know the four blood groups in the ABO system
- Know the difference between Rh-positive and Rh-negative blood
- Know the common blood products used for transfusions
- Explain how to obtain blood from the blood bank
- Explain how to assist the RN with the administration of blood
- Identify the signs and symptoms of a transfusion reaction
- Perform the procedures described in this chapter

KEY TERMS

air embolism Air that enters the cardiovascular system and travels to the lungs where it obstructs blood flow

antibody A substance in the blood plasma that fights or attacks *(anti)* antigens

antigen A substance that the body reacts to

blood transfusion The intravenous administration of blood or its products

dehydration A decrease in the amount of water in body tissues

edema The swelling of body tissues with water

erythrocyte Red *(erythro)* blood cell *(cyte);* carries oxygen to the cells

flow rate The number of drops per minute (gtt/min)

graduate A calibrated container used to measure fluid

hemoglobin The substance in red blood cells that picks up oxygen in the lungs and carries it to the cells; it gives blood its red color

hemolysis The destruction *(lysis)* of blood *(hemo)*

intake The amount of fluid taken in by the body

intravenous (IV) therapy The administration of fluids into a vein; IV, IV therapy, and IV infusion

leukocyte White *(leuko)* blood cell *(cyte);* protects the body against infection

output The amount of fluid lost by the body

phlebitis Inflammation *(itis)* of a vein *(phleb)*

plasma The liquid portion of the blood; it carries blood cells to other body cells

platelet Thrombocyte

red blood cells (RBCs) Erythrocytes

thrombocyte A cell *(cyte)* necessary for the clotting *(thrombo)* of blood

After oxygen, water is the most important physical need for survival. Death can result from an inadequate water intake or from excessive fluid loss. Water enters the body through fluids and foods. Water is lost through the urine and feces, through the skin as perspiration, and through the lungs with expiration. Fluid balance must be maintained for health. There must be a balance between the amount of fluid taken in and the amount lost.

The blood is a body fluid. The body needs adequate amounts of blood to function and survive. Blood carries nutrients, chemicals, and oxygen to the cells. Without adequate nutrition and necessary chemicals, body cells do not function properly. Cells die without oxygen. Cellular death affects organ function. The person can die.

FLUID BALANCE

The amount of fluid taken in (**intake**) and the amount lost (**output**) must be equal. If fluid intake exceeds fluid output, body tissues swell with water. This is called **edema.** Edema is common in people with heart and kidney diseases. **Dehydration** is a decrease in the amount of water in the tissues. It results when fluid output exceeds intake. Inadequate fluid intake, vomiting, diarrhea, bleeding, excessive sweating, and increased urine production are common causes of dehydration.

Normal Requirements

An adult needs 1500 ml of water daily to survive. Approximately 2000 to 2500 ml of fluid per day is required to maintain a normal fluid balance. The water requirement increases with hot weather, exercise, fever, and illness. Excessive fluid losses also increase the water requirement. (See Focus on Children and Focus on Older Persons.)

Special Orders

The doctor may order the amount of fluid a person can have during a 24-hour period. This is done to maintain fluid balance. Special orders include *encourage fluids, restrict fluids, and nothing by mouth:*

- *Encourage fluids*—the person drinks increased amounts of fluid. The force fluids order may be general or for a specific amount. Records are kept of the intake. A variety of allowed fluids are provided. They must be within the person's reach and served at the correct temperature. Frequently offer fluids to persons who cannot feed themselves.
- *Restrict fluids*—fluids are limited to a certain amount. Fluids are offered in small amounts and in small containers. The water pitcher is removed from the room or kept out of sight. Accurate intake

focus on CHILDREN

Minimum daily water requirements vary with age. Infants and young children have more body water. They need more fluids than do adults. Excessive fluid losses cannot be tolerated and will quickly cause death in an infant or child.

focus on OLDER PERSONS

The amount of body water decreases with age. Older persons also are at risk for diseases that affect fluid balance. Examples include heart disease, kidney disease, cancer, and diabetes mellitus. Many older persons also take drugs that affect fluid balance. Some drugs cause the body to lose fluids. Others cause the body to retain water. The older person is at risk for dehydration and edema.

records are kept. The person needs frequent oral hygiene. Oral hygiene helps keep mucous membranes of the mouth moist.
- *Nothing by mouth*—the person cannot eat or drink anything. *NPO* is the abbreviation for the Latin term *nils per os,* which means nothing by mouth. Persons are usually NPO before and after surgery, before some laboratory tests and x-ray procedures, and in the treatment of certain illnesses. The water pitcher and glass are removed. Frequent oral hygiene is allowed, but the person cannot swallow any fluid. The person is kept NPO 6 to 8 hours before surgery, laboratory tests, or x-ray procedures.

Intake and Output Records

The doctor or RN may want a person's fluid intake and output measured. This involves keeping intake and output (I&O) records. I&O records are used to evaluate fluid balance and kidney function. They are used also to determine and evaluate medical treatment. I&O records are kept when the person is NPO and when fluids are being encouraged or restricted. Many diseases and injuries also require measuring output.

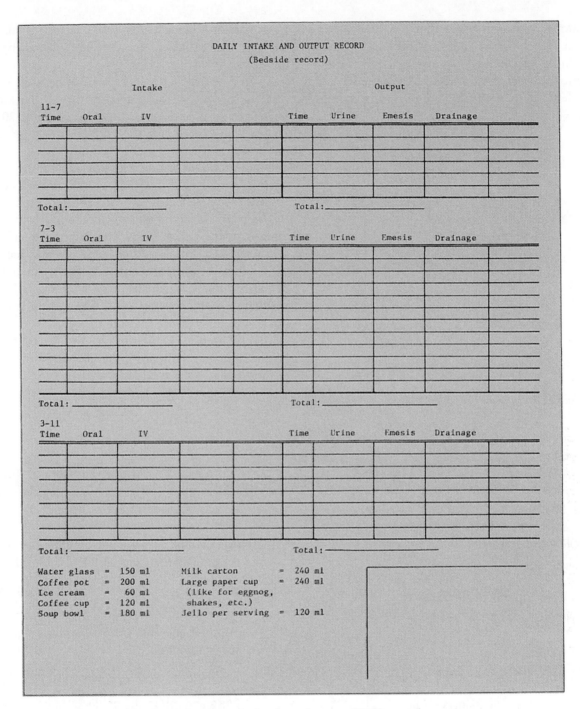

DAILY INTAKE AND OUTPUT RECORD
(Bedside record)

Intake   Output

11–7 Time	Oral	IV			Time	Urine	Emesis	Drainage	

Total: _____   Total: _____

7–3 Time	Oral	IV			Time	Urine	Emesis	Drainage	

Total: _____   Total: _____

3–11 Time	Oral	IV			Time	Urine	Emesis	Drainage	

Total: _____   Total: _____

Water glass	=	150 ml	Milk carton	= 240 ml
Coffee pot	=	200 ml	Large paper cup	= 240 ml
Ice cream	=	60 ml	(like for eggnog,	
Coffee cup	=	120 ml	shakes, etc.)	
Soup bowl	=	180 ml	Jello per serving	= 120 ml

Fig. 20-1 *An intake and output (I&O) record.*

To measure fluid intake, all liquid ingested by the person through the mouth is measured. So are fluids given in IV therapy and tube feedings. The obvious fluids are measured: water, milk, coffee, tea, juices, soups, and soft drinks. So are soft and semisolid foods such as ice cream, sherbet, custard, pudding, creamed cereals, gelatin, and popsicles. Output to be measured includes urine, vomitus, diarrhea, and wound drainage.

✦ Measuring Intake and Output

Intake and output are measured in milliliters (ml) or in cubic centimeters (cc). These metric system measurements are equal in amount. One ounce equals 30 ml. A pint is about 500 ml. There are about 1000 ml in a quart. You need to know the fluid capacity of bowls, dishes, cups, pitchers, glasses, and other containers used to serve fluids. Most I&O records have tables for use in measuring intake (Fig. 20-1).

A **graduate** is used to measure fluids. A graduate is a measuring container. It is like a measuring cup but larger. Some graduates are marked in ounces and in milliliters or cubic centimeters (Fig. 20-2). A graduate is used to measure leftover fluids, urine, vomitus, and drainage from suction (see Chapter 28). Plastic urinals, kidney basins, and other receptacles are often marked in amounts.

An I&O record is usually kept at the bedside. Whenever fluid is ingested or output is measured, the amount is recorded in the appropriate column (see Fig. 20-1). The amounts are totaled at the end of the shift. The total amount for the shift is recorded in the person's chart. The person's I&O are also communicated to the next shift during the end-of-shift report. Intake through IV therapy or tube feedings is also recorded and reported.

The purpose of measuring intake and output is explained to the person. How the person can take part is also explained. Some persons measure and record their own intake. Family members may be involved. The urinal, commode, bedpan, or specimen pan is used for voiding. The toilet is not used. The person is reminded not to put toilet tissue into the receptacle.

Medical asepsis, Standard Precautions, and the Bloodborne Pathogen Standard are followed when measuring output.

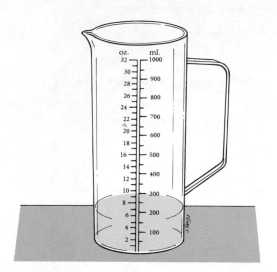

Fig. 20-2 *A graduate (measuring container) calibrated in milliliters.*

MEASURING INTAKE AND OUTPUT

PROCEDURE

1 Explain the procedure to the person.

2 Collect the following:

   • Intake and output (I&O) record

   • Graduate

   • Gloves

3 Place the I&O record at the bedside.

4 Measure intake as follows:

   a Pour liquid remaining in a container into the graduate used to measure intake.

   b Measure the amount at eye level.

   c Check the amount of the serving on the I&O record.

   d Subtract the remaining amount from the full serving amount.

   e Repeat steps 5a through 5d for each liquid.

   f Add the amounts from 5e together. Record the time and amount on the I&O record.

5 Measure output as follows: (Wear gloves for this step.)

   a Pour the fluid into the graduate used to measure output.

   b Measure the amount at eye level.

   c Rinse and return the graduate to its proper place.

   d Clean and rinse the bedpan, urinal, kidney basin, or other drainage container. Return it to its proper place.

6 Remove the gloves, and wash your hands.

7 Record output on the I&O record. Also note the time.

8 Report your observations to the RN.

✦ Providing Drinking Water

Patients need fresh drinking water. Fresh water is usually provided during the day and evening and whenever the water pitcher is empty. Before passing water you need to know about any special orders. Some persons are NPO, on restricted fluids, or not allowed ice. The rules of medical asepsis are practiced when passing drinking water.

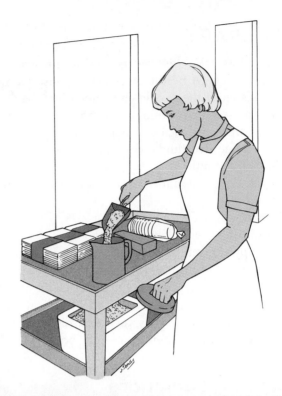

Fig. 20-3 *Follow the rules of medical asepsis when passing drinking water. Do not let the scoop touch any part of the water pitcher when adding ice.*

PROVIDING FRESH DRINKING WATER

PROCEDURE

1   Get a list of persons who have special fluid orders (NPO, fluid restriction, or no ice). The list is obtained from the RN.

2   Wash your hands.

3   Collect the following:
- Cart
- Ice chest filled with ice and a cover for the chest
- Scoop
- Disposable cups
- Straws
- Paper towels
- Large water pitcher filled with cold water (optional, depending on agency procedure)

4   Arrange items on the cart on top of the paper towels.

5   Move the cart until you are just outside a person's room. Check the list to see if the person has special orders.

6   Check the ID bracelet, and call the person by name.

7   Take the water pitcher from the overbed table. Empty it into the sink in the bathroom.

8   Fill the pitcher half full with water. Get water from the tap or pitcher on the cart.

9   Fill the water pitcher with ice if it is allowed. Use the scoop for the ice (Fig. 20-3).

10   Place the pitcher, disposable cup, and straw on the overbed table. Make sure the person can easily reach the items.

11   Fill the disposable cup with fresh water.

12   Repeat steps 5 through 11 for each person.

13   Return the equipment to the utility room. Clean and return equipment to its proper place.

14   Wash your hands.

IV THERAPY

Intravenous (IV) therapy is the administration of fluids into a vein. A needle or catheter is inserted into a vein. Fluids enter the needle or catheter and go directly into the person's circulation. *IV* and *IV infusion* also refer to IV therapy. Doctors order IV therapy to:

- Provide needed fluids when the person cannot take fluids by mouth.
- Replace minerals and vitamins lost because of illness or injury.
- Provide sugar for energy.
- Administer medications and blood.

IV therapy is given in hospital, out-patient, long-term care, and home settings. RNs are responsible for IV therapy. They start and maintain the infusion according to the doctor's orders. RNs also give IV medications and administer blood. State laws vary regarding the role of LPNs in IV therapy. They also vary about the role of assistive personnel.

Intravenous Solutions

The doctor orders the type of IV solution to use. The solution ordered depends on the purpose of the IV therapy:

- *Nutrient solutions* are given for energy and fluid replacement. They contain carbohydrates in the form of sugar. Dextrose solutions are common.
- *Electrolyte solutions* contain minerals such as sodium, chloride, and potassium. These minerals help maintain the body's fluid balance. They are needed also for many body functions. These solutions are given when the body needs water. They also correct mineral (electrolyte) imbalances.
- *Blood volume expanders* increase the blood volume. They are used to treat hemorrhage (severe blood loss) and plasma loss. Plasma is the fluid portion of blood. Plasma loss occurs with severe burns.

Box 20-1 lists the common IV solutions. Medications and minerals often are added to IV solutions. The pharmacist or RN adds them as ordered by the doctor. Sometimes IV solutions contain medications added by the manufacturer.

SITES
Peripheral Sites

Arm and hand veins are common IV sites for adults. The back of the hand and forearm provide useful sites (Fig. 20-4, *A*). Veins in the antecubital space (crease of the elbow) are sometimes used (Fig. 20-4, *B*). Foot veins also are sites but are avoided if possible. They are small and

BOX 20-1 **INTRAVENOUS SOLUTIONS**

Nutrient Solutions
- D5W—dextrose 5% in water
- Dextrose 5% in 0.45% sodium chloride—5% dextrose in half-strength saline; dextrose in half-strength saline

Electrolyte Solutions
- 0.9% sodium chloride—normal saline
- Lactated Ringer's
- Ringer's solution

Blood Volume Expanders
- Dextran
- Plasma
- Human serum albumin

focus on CHILDREN

Scalp and dorsal foot veins (Fig. 20-5) are the peripheral sites for infants. *Dorsal* means on the back of something. Dorsal foot veins are on the back of the foot. Hand and arm veins also are used.

easily irritated. Arm and foot sites are called *peripheral IV sites*. Periphery comes from the Greek words that mean around *(peri)* a boundary *(phery)*. The boundary is the center of the body near the heart. Therefore peripheral IV sites are located away from the center of the body.

RNs insert peripheral IVs. The site selected depends on the expected length of IV therapy, the solution, and the condition of the person's veins.

The RN tries to select a site in the person's nondominant hand or arm. Using the dominant hand interferes with some activities of daily living. Certain sites are avoided to prevent injury to the arm. For example, in women, the arm on the side of a mastectomy (removal *[ectomy]* of a breast *[mast]*) is avoided. In persons with hemiplegia (paralysis *[plegia]* on one side of the body *[hemi]*), sites on the paralyzed side are avoided. For dialysis patients, the arm with a hemodialysis access site is also avoided. (See Focus on Children.)

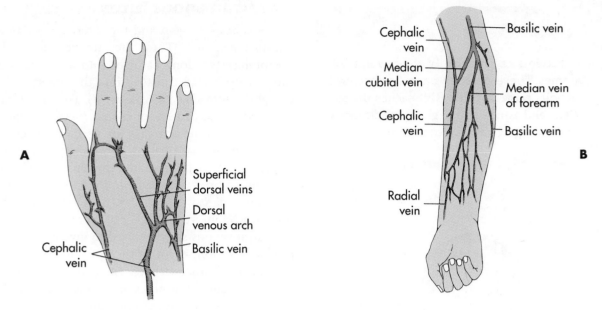

Fig. 20-4 *Sites for IV therapy in adults.* **A,** *Back of the hand.* **B,** *Forearm and antecubital space. (From Potter PA, Perry AG: Fundamentals of nursing: concepts, process, and practice, ed 4, St Louis, 1997, Mosby.)*

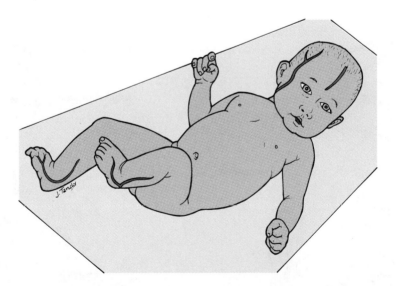

Fig. 20-5 *The scalp and foot provide IV sites in infants.*

Central Venous Sites

The subclavian vein and the internal jugular vein are *central venous sites*. These sites are close to the heart. A doctor inserts a long catheter into a central vein. The catheter tip is then threaded into the superior vena cava or right atrium (Fig. 20-6, *A* and *B*). The catheter is called a *central venous catheter* or *central line*. The cephalic and basilic veins in the arm also are used. Catheters inserted into these sites are called *peripherally inserted central catheters (PICC)*. Inserted into the cephalic or basilic vein, the catheter tip is threaded into the subclavian vein or the superior vena cava (Fig. 20-6, *C*). Doctors and specially trained RNs insert PICCs.

Central venous sites are used to give large amounts of fluid and for long-term IV therapy. They also are used to give IV medications that irritate the peripheral veins. Sometimes surgery is necessary to insert a central venous catheter. (See Focus on Home Care.)

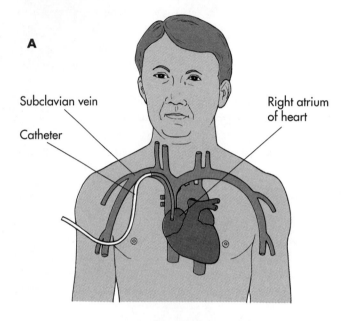

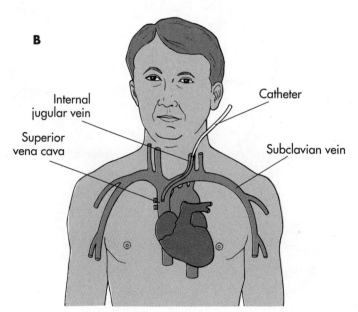

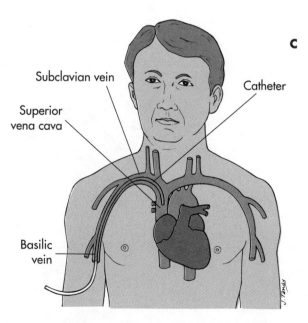

Fig. 20-6 *Central venous sites.* **A,** *Subclavian vein. The catheter tip is in the right atrium.* **B,** *Internal jugular vein. The catheter tip is in the superior vena cava.* **C,** *Basilic vein. This is a peripherally inserted central catheter (PICC).*

Equipment

The basic equipment used in IV therapy includes the solution container, IV needle or catheter, infusion set (tubing), and IV pole (Fig. 20-7). Your state and agency may allow you to assist the RN in collecting and setting up equipment.

Solution container

The solution container is a plastic bag or glass bottle. Plastic bags are common. The outside of the bag is clean. The inside and the solution are sterile. Always inspect the bag for contamination (Fig. 20-8). The solution must be clear and free of particles. Cloudy solutions are not used. The bag's expiration date is another sign of sterility. If the expiration date has passed, the bag is not used. Leaking, cracked, and open bags are not used. Return contaminated bags to the central supply area. Place a note about the problem on the bag.

IV fluid bags come in different sizes: 50, 100, 250, 500, or 1000 ml (milliliters). The size used depends on the amount of fluid ordered.

The RN tells you what type of solution to get (see Box 20-1). Doctors and RNs often use abbreviations and other names for the various IV solutions. You must clearly understand what the RN asks you to get. Always repeat the information back to the RN to make sure you understand correctly. After collecting the bag, ask the RN to check the bag to make sure it is the right one. If a solution contains medicine, the RN collects the container.

Catheters and needles

A catheter or needle is inserted into a vein. An intravenous catheter is a plastic tube (Fig. 20-9, *A*, p. 482). A needle fits over or is inside the catheter for insertion. After insertion, the needle is removed. Butterfly needles also are used (Fig. 20-9, *B*, p. 482). However, short catheters are more commonly used.

Catheters and needles come in different sizes. The RN selects the size based on the reasons for the IV therapy and the person's age. Smaller sizes are used for infants and children.

Infusion sets

The infusion set (tubing) connects the solution bag to the catheter or needle (see Fig. 20-7). The parts of the infusion set are shown in Figure 20-10 on p. 482. The *insertion spike* is sterile. A protector cap keeps the spike sterile. The cap is removed to insert the spike into the solution bag.

The *needle adapter* also is sterile. A protector cap keeps it sterile. The RN removes the cap to connect the needle adapter to the IV catheter or needle.

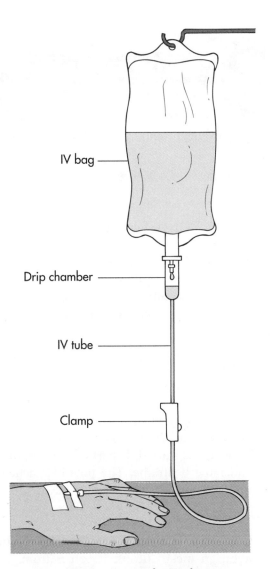

IV bag —

Drip chamber —

IV tube —

Clamp —

Fig. 20-7 *Equipment for IV therapy.*

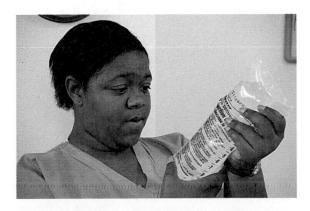

Fig. 20-8 *The IV bag is inspected for contamination.*

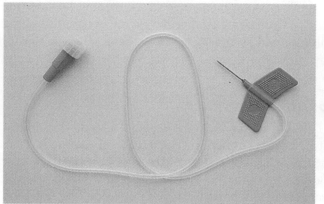

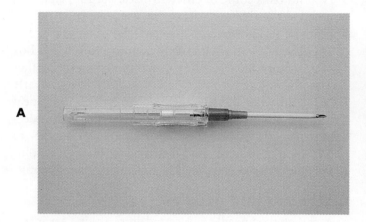

A

B

Fig. 20-9 **A,** *Intravenous catheter.* **B,** *Butterfly needle.*

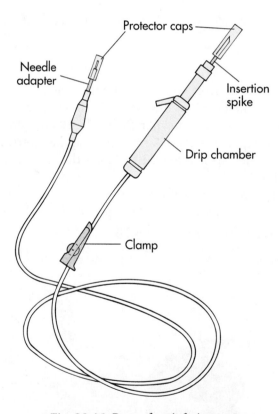

Fig. 20-10 *Parts of an infusion set.*

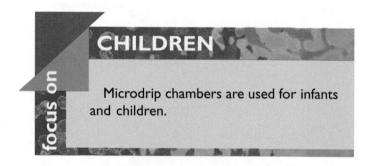

CHILDREN

focus on

Microdrip chambers are used for infants and children.

Fluid drips from the solution bag into the *drip chamber*. Drip chambers have macrodrips or microdrips. Depending on the manufacturer, macrodrip sets (*macro* means large) have 10 to 20 drops per milliliter (ml). Microdrip sets (*micro* means small) have 60 drops per ml. The RN uses the *clamp* to regulate the flow rate. (See Focus on Children.)

The IV pole

The fluid bag hangs from the IV pole or ceiling hook. *IV standard* is another name for an IV pole. IV poles are portable or part of the bed. If portable, they are kept in the supply area. An IV pole is brought to the bedside when IV therapy is started. If part of the bed, the pole is stored under the bedframe. The pole is attached to the head, foot, or side of the bed when needed.

Flow Rate

The flow rate is measured in drops per minute. The abbreviation *gtt* means drops. It comes from the Latin word *guttae,* which means *drops*.

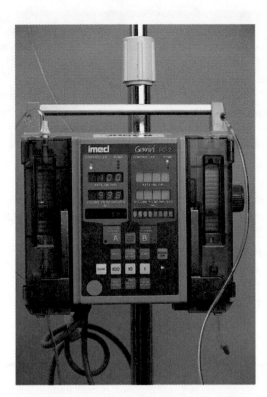

Fig. 20-11 *Electronic infusion device.* (*From Elkin MK, Perry AG, Potter PA: Nursing interventions and clinical skills, St Louis, 1996, Mosby.*)

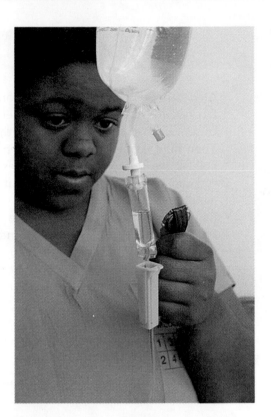

Fig. 20-12 *The flow rate is checked by counting the number of drops per minute.*

The doctor orders the amount of fluid to give and amount of time in which to give it in. With this information, the RN decides to use a macrodrip or a microdrip chamber. The RN then calculates the flow rate. The **flow rate** is the number of drops per minute (gtt/min).

The RN sets the clamp for the flow rate. Electronic infusion devices often are used to control the flow rate (Fig. 20-11). An alarm sounds if a problem occurs with the flow rate. Tell the nurse immediately if you hear the alarm. *Never change the position of the clamp or adjust any controls on infusion pumps.*

You assist the RN with IV therapy by checking the flow rate. The RN tells you the number of drops per minute. Check the flow rate by counting the number of drops in 1 full minute (Fig. 20-12). Tell the RN immediately:

- If no fluid is dripping
- If the rate is too fast
- If the rate is too slow

Also, check the time tape on the IV bag (Fig. 20-13). The time tape shows how much fluid is to be given over a period of time. For example, the doctor orders 1000 ml of fluid to be given over 8 hours. The RN marks the tape in 8 one-hour intervals. To check if fluid is being given on time, the fluid line is compared with the time line on the tape. If the fluid line is above or below the time line,

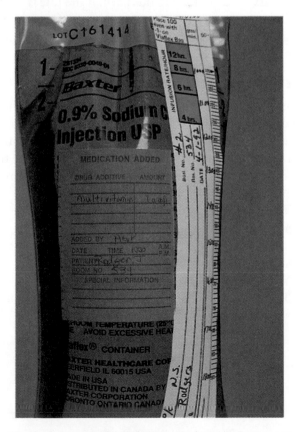

Fig. 20-13 *Time tape applied to an IV bag.* (*From Elkin MK, Perry AG, Potter PA: Nursing interventions and clinical skills, St Louis, 1996, Mosby.*)

SAFETY MEASURES FOR IV THERAPY

- Always practice Standard Precautions and follow the Bloodborne Pathogen Standard.
- Do not move the needle or catheter. The position of the IV needle or catheter must be maintained when assisting a person. If the needle or catheter is moved, it may come out of the vein. Then fluid flows into the tissues (infiltration), or the flow stops.
- Follow the safety measures for restraints if a restraint is used. Sometimes the nurse splints or restrains the extremity to prevent movement of the part (Fig. 20-14). This helps prevent the needle or catheter from moving.
- Be careful not to move the needle or catheter when changing a gown.
- Protect the IV container, tubing, and needle or catheter when ambulating the person. A portable IV standard is rolled along next to the person (Fig. 20-15).
- Assist the person with turning and repositioning. The IV bag is moved to the side of the bed on which the person is lying. Always allow enough slack in the tubing. The needle dislodges if pressure is exerted by the tubing.
- Notify the RN immediately if bleeding occurs from the insertion site. Follow Standard Precautions and the Bloodborne Pathogen Standard.
- Notify the RN immediately of any signs and symptoms listed in Box 20-3.

the flow rate is too slow or too fast. Tell the RN immediately if too much or too little fluid was given.

The person can suffer serious harm if the rate is too fast or too slow. Changes in flow rate can occur from position changes. Kinked tubes and lying on the tubing also are common problems.

Assisting the RN

You assist the RN with meeting the hygiene and activity needs of persons with IVs. You may be allowed to prime IV tubing, change IV dressings, and discontinue IVs. Before you perform these procedures, make sure that:

- Your state allows assistive personnel to perform the procedure
- The procedure is in your job description
- You have the necessary training
- You know how to use the agency's equipment and supplies
- You review the procedure with an RN
- The RN is available to answer questions and to supervise you

You are never responsible for starting or maintaining an IV infusion. Nor do you regulate the flow rate or change IV solution containers. Assistive personnel never administer blood or IV medications. However, you assist the RN in providing safe care. The safety measures in Box 20-2 are important. Complications can occur from IV therapy. Report any of the signs and symptoms listed in Box 20-3 to the RN immediately.

Remember, contact with blood is likely. Always practice Standard Precautions and follow the Bloodborne Pathogen Standard.

✦ *Priming IV tubing*

To *prime* IV tubing means to prepare it for the administration of IV fluids. The infusion set is attached to the IV bag. Fluid is allowed to flow through the tubing. This removes air from the tubing. All air is removed before the tubing is attached to the IV catheter or tubing. Removing air includes removing bubbles. If the tubing is not primed, air enters the cardiovascular system and travels to the lungs where it obstructs blood flow. This is called an **air embolism.** An air embolism is a life-threatening event. The person can die.

After the tubing is primed, the RN connects it to the IV catheter or needle. The RN sets the flow rate. If an infusion pump is used, the RN inserts the tubing into the pump and sets the rate.

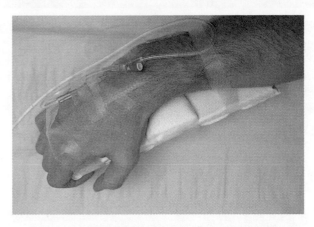

Fig. 20-14 *An armboard prevents movement at the IV site. (From Elkin MK, Perry AG, Potter PA:* Nursing interventions and clinical skills, *St Louis, 1996, Mosby.)*

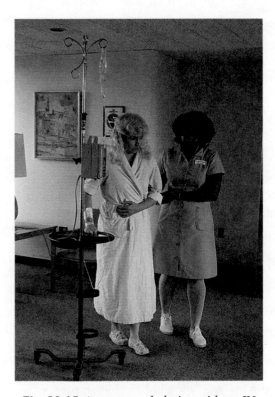

Fig. 20-15 *A person ambulating with an IV.*

SIGNS AND SYMPTOMS OF IV THERAPY COMPLICATIONS

Local—at the IV Site
- Bleeding
- Puffiness or swelling
- Pale or reddened skin
- Complaints of pain at or above the IV site
- Hot or cold skin near the site

Systemic—Involving the Whole Body
- Fever
- Itching
- Drop in blood pressure
- Tachycardia (pulse rate greater than 100 beats per minute)
- Irregular pulse
- Cyanosis
- Changes in mental function
- Loss of consciousness
- Difficulty breathing (dyspnea)
- Shortness of breath
- Decreasing or no urine output
- Chest pain
- Nausea
- Confusion

PRIMING IV TUBING

PROCEDURE ALERT

- Does your state allow assistive personnel to perform the procedure?
- Is the procedure in your job description?
- Do you have the necessary training and education?
- Is an RN available to answer questions and to supervise you?

PRE-PROCEDURE

1 Review the procedure with the RN.

2 Wash your hands.

3 Collect the following as directed by the RN:

- IV solution (get this from the RN if it contains medications)
- Infusion set
- IV pole
- Alcohol swabs
- IV gown (has sleeves that snap close)
- IV label
- Gloves

4 Check the solution bag:

a Check to see that the solution is clear and free of particles.

b Make sure the bag is unopened.

c Make sure the bag does not leak.

d Check the bag for cracks.

e Check the expiration date.

5 Ask the RN to check the IV solution. You must make sure that you have the right solution.

6 Arrange equipment on a clean work area.

7 Identify the patient. Check the ID bracelet against the assignment sheet.

8 Explain what you are going to do.

9 Provide for privacy.

PROCEDURE

10 Help the person tend to any personal hygiene or elimination needs. Wear gloves. Clean and return equipment to its proper place. Wash your hands.

11 Help the person change into the IV gown.

12 Write the person's name and the date and time on the IV label.

13 Apply the IV label to the bag. Apply it so that it can be read after hanging the bag (see Fig. 20-13).

14 Open the sterile infusion set. Make sure the protective caps are on the spike and the needle adapter.

15 Open the clamp, and move it to the end of the drip chamber.

16 Close the clamp all the way.

17 Remove the protective cap from the bag (Fig. 20-16). The opening is sterile. Do not touch the opening.

18 Clean the rubber stopper on a bottle with an alcohol swab.

19 Remove the protective cap from the spike. The spike is sterile. Do not touch the spike. *Do not let anything touch the spike.*

20 Insert the spike into the bag (Fig. 20-17). If a bottle is used, insert the spike into the rubber stopper.

21 Hang the bag on the IV pole.

22 Squeeze the drip chamber gently. Squeeze until the drip chamber is about $1/2$ full (Fig. 20-18).

23 Remove the protective cap from the needle adapter. Save the cap for step 28. *The adapter is sterile. Do not touch the adapter. Do not let anything touch the adapter.*

24 Hold the needle end of the tubing over a sink or container.

25 Open the clamp slowly. Open it only half way.

26 Allow fluid to flow through the tubing until it is free of air and bubbles.

27 Close the clamp.

28 Put the protective cap on the needle adapter. *Do not touch the adapter.*

29 Check the tube for bubbles. Gently tap tubing at a bubble site to remove the bubble (Fig. 20-19).

POST-PROCEDURE

30 Make sure the person is comfortable.

31 Make sure the call bell is within reach.

32 Raise or lower bed rails as instructed by the RN.

33 Tell the patient that the RN will start the IV.

34 Unscreen the person.

35 Tell the RN that the tubing is primed. Report any patient observations.

36 Wash your hands.

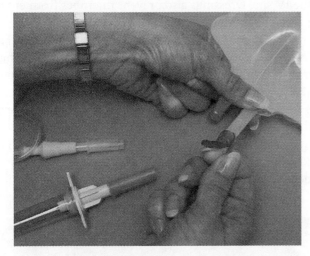

Fig. 20-16 *Removing the protective cap from the entry site of solution bag. (From Potter PA, Perry AG:* Fundamentals of nursing: concepts, process, and practice, *ed 4, St Louis, 1997, Mosby.)*

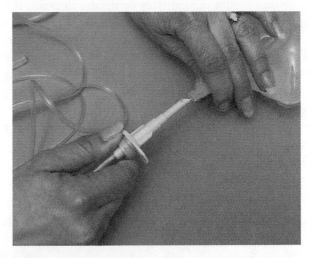

Fig. 20-17 *Inserting the spike into the entry site of the solution bag. (From Potter PA, Perry AG:* Fundamentals of nursing: concepts, process, and practice, *ed 4, St Louis, 1997, Mosby.)*

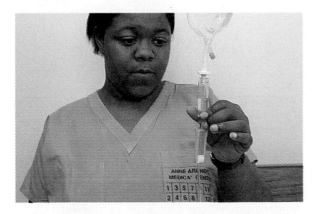

Fig. 20-18 *Squeezing the drip chamber.*

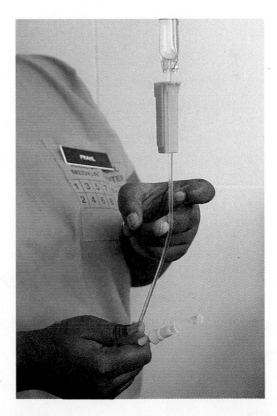

Fig. 20-19 *IV tubing is tapped to remove bubbles.*

✦ *Changing IV dressings*

After starting an IV, the RN applies a dressing to the IV site. When the IV site is changed in 2 or 3 days, the RN applies a new dressing. Sometimes IV dressings become wet, soiled, or loose. A new dressing is required. Your state and job description may allow you to change dressings at *peripheral IV sites*. The RN tells you when to change the dressing. *Do not change dressings on central venous catheters or PICCs unless allowed by your state and agency. You will need special training for the procedure.*

Dressings secure the catheter or needle in place. If not secured, the catheter or needle can easily slip out of the vein. With loose dressings, the catheter or needle can move. The flow rate is affected when the catheter or needle is out of position. Also, the catheter or needle can puncture the vein. IV fluid flows into surrounding tissues. This is called *infiltration*. That is, the fluid infiltrates (goes into) other tissues. The flow rate slows. Swelling occurs at the IV site and surrounding area.

Dressings also prevent phlebitis and infection at the venipuncture site. **Phlebitis** is an inflammation *(itis)* of

focus on OLDER PERSONS

Remember, older persons have fragile skin. Be careful when removing tape. You must prevent skin tears.

the vein *(phleb)*. The person has pain, redness, and swelling at the IV site. Dressings also prevent microbes from entering the vein and bloodstream.

Gauze or transparent dressings are usually used. The IV site is easy to observe with transparent dressings. Sterile technique is used (see Chapter 11). Also, see Chapter 28 for assisting with wound care. Remember to practice Standard Precautions and to follow the Bloodborne Pathogen Standard. Contact with blood is likely.

Agency procedures vary for changing IV dressings. The following procedure serves as a guideline. (See Focus on Older Persons.)

✦ CHANGING A PERIPHERAL IV DRESSING

PROCEDURE ALERT

- Does your state allow assistive personnel to perform the procedure?

- Is the procedure in your job description?

- Do you have the necessary training and education?

- Is an RN available to answer questions and to supervise you?

PRE-PROCEDURE

1 Review the procedure with the RN.

2 Explain the procedure to the person.

3 Wash your hands.

4 Collect the following:

- Betadine swab (check with the RN for patient allergies)

- Alcohol swab

- Sterile 4 × 4 or 2 × 2 gauze dressing or a transparent dressing

- ½-inch transparent tape (if using a transparent dressing)

- ½-inch and 1-inch nonallergenic tape (if using a gauze dressing)

- Adhesive remover

- Cotton balls

- Gloves

- Towel

- Leakproof plastic bag

5 Arrange equipment on the overbed table.

6 Identify the patient. Check the ID bracelet against the assignment sheet.

7 Provide for privacy.

8 Raise the bed to a level for good body mechanics.

9 Make sure you have good lighting.

✛ CHANGING A PERIPHERAL IV DRESSING—cont'd

PROCEDURE

10 Cut two strips of 1/2-inch tape. If using a gauze dressing, also cut two strips of 1-inch tape. Hang the tape from the edge of the overbed table for later use.

11 Open the dressings and the Betadine and alcohol swabs.

12 Expose the IV site. Place the towel under the person's arm.

13 Put on the gloves.

14 Remove the soiled dressing. Be careful not to move the catheter or needle:

   a Remove the tape. Pull tape toward the IV site. Discard the tape into the plastic bag.

   b Remove the dressing. Remove one layer of gauze at a time. Touch only the outer edge of the dressing.

   c Discard the dressing into the plastic bag.

15 Observe the IV site. Check for redness, swelling, and drainage. Call for the RN to assess the site.

16 Hold the hub of the needle or catheter to keep it in place. (The hub is the plastic colored part. See Fig. 20-9.) Use your nondominant hand. Hold the hub through step 21.

17 Remove the tape securing the catheter or needle. Discard the tape into the plastic bag.

18 Remove any adhesive left from the tape. Use cotton balls moistened with adhesive remover. Clean away from the IV site. Discard cotton balls into the plastic bag.

19 Clean the IV site with the alcohol swab. Use a circular motion starting at the IV site. Work outward about 2 inches. Let the alcohol dry. Discard used swabs into the plastic bag.

20 Clean the IV site with the Betadine swab. Clean as in step 19. Discard used swabs into the plastic bag.

21 Let the site dry for 2 minutes.

22 Secure the catheter in place with 1/2-inch tape (Fig. 20-20, p. 490). Your agency's procedure may omit this step for transparent dressings. If so, go to step 24.

   a Slide a tape strip—sticky side up—under the catheter hub.

   b Cross the left side of the tape over the hub to the right side.

   c Cross the right side of the tape over the hub to the left side.

   d Place a second tape strip—sticky side down—across the catheter hub.

23 Apply a gauze dressing over the catheter hub. (Do not cover the needle adapter.) Secure the dressing in place with 1-inch tape. Place the tape across the dressing.

24 Apply a transparent dressing (Fig. 20-21, p. 490). Do not cover the needle adapter.

   a Apply a piece of 1/2-inch transparent tape across the catheter hub.

   b Apply the transparent dressing over the IV site.

   c Smooth and seal the dressing over the IV site.

25 Make a loop in the IV tubing over the dressing. Make sure the needle adapter is securely attached to the catheter hub.

26 Secure the loop to the dressing with tape. Apply the tape over the tape already on the dressing.

27 Write the date and time of the dressing change on the tape (Fig. 20-22, p. 490). Also note the size of the catheter. (Get this information from the RN.)

28 Remove the towel.

29 Remove the gloves. Discard into the plastic bag.

30 Check the flow rate. Ask the RN to adjust the flow rate if needed.

Continued

✦ CHANGING A PERIPHERAL IV DRESSING—cont'd

POST-PROCEDURE

31 Make sure the person is comfortable.

32 Place the call bell within reach.

33 Raise or lower bed rails as instructed by the RN.

34 Lower the bed to its lowest horizontal position.

35 Unscreen the person.

36 Discard the plastic bag, used supplies, and soiled linen according to agency policy. (Wear gloves if contact with blood is likely.)

37 Wash your hands.

38 Report your observations of the IV site and old dressing to the RN. Also report any other observations or patient complaints.

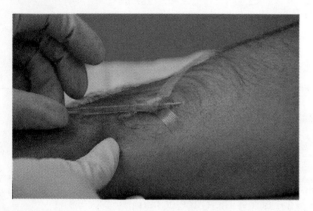

Fig. 20-20 *The catheter is secured in place with ½-inch tape.* (From Elkin MK, Perry AG, Potter PA: Nursing interventions and clinical skills, St Louis, 1996, Mosby.)

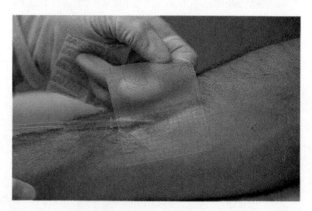

Fig. 20-21 *Transparent dressing applied over the catheter hub.* (From Elkin MK, Perry AG, Potter PA: Nursing interventions and clinical skills, St Louis, 1996, Mosby.)

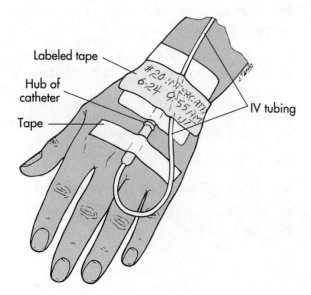

Fig. 20-22 *The dressing is labeled with date and time of the dressing change. The catheter size is also noted.*

✦ Discontinuing peripheral IVs

The doctor decides when to stop IV therapy. The doctor ends IV therapy when the person is no longer NPO, fluid balance is normal, or IV medications are no longer needed.

Peripheral IV sites are changed every 2 or 3 days. This reduces the risk of infection at the IV site. The RN starts the IV at a new site. The needle or catheter is removed from the old site.

The RN tells you when to discontinue an IV. The procedure should not cause the person pain or discomfort. Agency procedures vary. The following procedure is a guideline. Remember to practice Standard Precautions and follow the Bloodborne Pathogen Standard. Contact with blood is likely.

DISCONTINUING A PERIPHERAL IV

PROCEDURE ALERT

- Does your state allow assistive personnel to perform the procedure?

- Is the procedure in your job description?

- Do you have the necessary training and education?

- Is an RN available to answer questions and to supervise you?

PRE-PROCEDURE

1 Review the procedure with the RN.

2 Explain the procedure to the person.

3 Wash your hands.

4 Collect the following:

- Two sterile 2 × 2 or 4 × 4 gauze dressings

- Adhesive remover

- Cotton balls

- Alcohol swabs

- Betadine swabs (check with the RN for patient allergies)

- Tape

- Towel

- Gloves

- Leakproof plastic bag

5 Arrange supplies on the overbed table.

6 Identify the person. Check the ID bracelet against the assignment sheet.

7 Provide for privacy.

8 Raise the bed to the best level for good body mechanics.

PROCEDURE

9 Open the dressings, cotton balls, and alcohol and Betadine swabs.

10 Put on the gloves.

11 Expose the IV site.

12 Put the towel under the site.

13 Stop the flow of IV fluids. Close the clamp, or move it to the OFF position.

14 Note the amount of fluid remaining in the IV solution container.

15 Hold the hub of the catheter or needle through step 17. This prevents movement of the catheter or needle and injury to the vein.

16 Remove the tape from the dressing. Discard it into the plastic bag.

17 Remove the dressing. Discard it into the plastic bag.

18 Remove any adhesive. Use cotton balls moistened with adhesive remover. Discard cotton balls into the plastic bag.

19 Clean the IV site with an alcohol swab. Discard the swab into the plastic bag.

20 Clean the IV site with a Betadine swab. Discard the swab into the plastic bag.

21 Place a gauze square over the IV site. Hold it in place.

22 Remove the needle or catheter. Holding the hub, slowly pull the needle or catheter straight out of the vein.

23 Check the needle or catheter to make sure it is intact. This is done to make sure the needle or catheter is not left in the vein where it can travel to the lung. *Call for the RN immediately if it is not intact.*

24 Discard the catheter or needle into the sharps container in the room.

25 Apply pressure to the IV site with the gauze dressing. Apply pressure for 2 to 3 minutes. This stops bleeding from the IV site.

26 Remove the gauze dressing. Discard it into the plastic bag.

27 Apply a sterile gauze dressing to the IV site.

28 Tape the dressing in place.

29 Remove the towel.

30 Discard used supplies into the plastic bag.

31 Remove the gloves.

Continued

DISCONTINUING A PERIPHERAL IV—cont'd

POST-PROCEDURE

32 Make sure the person is comfortable.

33 Place the call bell within reach.

34 Raise or lower bed rails as instructed by the RN.

35 Lower the bed to its lowest horizontal position.

36 Unscreen the person.

37 Discard used supplies, the plastic bag, the IV bag, and soiled linen according to agency policy. (Wear gloves for this step if contact with blood is likely.)

38 Wash your hands.

39 Report the following to the RN:

- The amount of fluid remaining in the IV bag
- Observations of the IV site
- Other observations or patient complaints

BLOOD ADMINISTRATION

Causes of inadequate amounts of blood are many. Blood loss often occurs from injury, disease, and surgery. When bleeding occurs, the blood normally clots to stop the bleeding. If the blood cannot clot, bleeding continues. This causes more blood loss.

As blood cells normally die off, the body must replace them. Poor nutrition affects the body's ability to produce blood cells. Also, the bone marrow must be able to produce new blood cells.

To restore normal amounts of blood and blood cells, the doctor orders the intravenous administration of blood or its products (parts). This is called a **blood transfusion.** The RN carries out the order. Blood administration is complex. The *right blood* must be given *to the right person.* Transfusion reactions are serious and life-threatening. Close observation of the person is important. So is preventing the spread of bloodborne diseases.

Your role in blood administration is to assist the RN in providing safe care to the person. You must be alert for the signs and symptoms of a transfusion reaction.

Blood and Blood Products

The blood consists of cells and a liquid called **plasma**. Plasma is mostly water. It carries blood cells to other body cells. Plasma also carries other substances needed by cells for proper functioning. These include nutrients (proteins, fats, and carbohydrates), hormones, and chemicals. Plasma also carries waste products to the skin and kidneys for removal from the body.

Red blood cells (RBCs) are called **erythrocytes**. Erythrocyte means red *(erythro)* cell *(cyte)*. RBCs carry oxygen to the cells. The blood gets its red color from a substance in the RBC called **hemoglobin**. As red blood cells circulate through the lungs, hemoglobin picks up oxygen. The hemoglobin carries oxygen to the cells.

The body has about 25 trillion (25,000,000,000,000) red blood cells. About 4.5 to 5 million cells are in a cubic millimeter of blood (the size of a tiny drop). These cells live for 3 or 4 months. They are destroyed by the liver and spleen as they wear out. Bone marrow produces new red blood cells. About 1 million new red blood cells are produced every second.

White blood cells (WBCs), called **leukocytes,** are colorless. (*Leuko* means white; *cyte* means cell). They protect the body against infection. There are 5,000 to 10,000 white blood cells in a cubic millimeter of blood. At the first sign of infection, WBCs rush to the site of the infection and multiply rapidly. The number of WBCs increases when there is an infection in the body. WBCs also are produced by the bone marrow. They live about 9 days.

Platelets (thrombocytes) are cells *(cyte)* necessary for the clotting *(thrombo)* of blood. They are also produced by the bone marrow. There are about 200,000 to 400,000 platelets in a cubic millimeter of blood. A platelet lives about 4 days.

The doctor orders blood or blood products (components) for the person (Fig. 20-23). The person's condition and the availability of compatible blood affect the doctor's decision. The following are often ordered:

- Whole blood
- Packed red blood cells
- Fresh frozen plasma
- Platelets
- Albumin

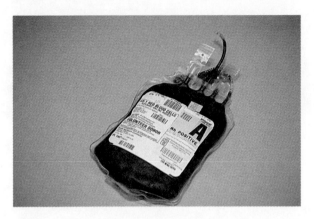

Fig. 20-23 *Blood products are packaged for administration.*

Blood Groups and Types

Blood groups and types involve the ABO system and the Rh system. These systems are important when matching blood for transfusions. If the donor blood does not match the person's blood, life-threatening reactions occur.

The ABO system

An **antigen** is a substance that the body reacts to. That is, the body attacks or fights the substance. Two types of antigens, type A and type B, are on the surface of red blood cells. If the type A antigen is in the person's blood, the person's blood group is called *type A*. If the type B antigen is present, the blood group is *type B*. Some people have both the type A and the type B antigen in their blood. This blood group is called *type AB*. The blood group *type O* is when neither the type A nor the type B antigens are present.

In summary, the four blood groups are:
- Type A—the type A antigen is present
- Type B—the type B antigen is present
- Type AB—the type A and the type B antigens are present
- Type O—the type A and the type B antigens are *not* present

Antibodies are substances in the blood plasma that fight or attack (*anti*) antigens. They are normally present in the blood. Antibodies attack antigens not normally present in the person's blood. There are anti-A antibodies and anti-B antibodies:
- Blood group type A—contains anti-B antibodies
- Blood group type B—contains anti-A antibodies
- Blood group type AB—contains no antibodies
- Blood group type O—contains anti-A and anti-B antibodies

When a blood transfusion is ordered, the person must receive a compatible blood type. Otherwise, the antibodies attack the antigens. For example, a person with type A blood (type A antigens), has anti-B antibodies. If type B blood enters the person's bloodstream, the anti-B antibodies attack the type B blood. **Hemolysis** occurs. The blood *(hemo)* is destroyed *(lysis)*. This is a life-threatening reaction.

Type O blood does not contain the type A or type B antigen. Therefore it is called the *universal donor*. Persons with any blood type can receive type O blood. Even if the anti-A or anti-B antibodies are present, there are no type A or type B antigens to attack in type O blood.

The Rh system

The Rh factor was first found in the rhesus (Rh) monkey. It is an antigen on the surface of red blood cells. Persons with the Rh factor are *Rh positive (Rh+)*. Persons without the Rh factor are *Rh negative (Rh−)*.

A person without the antigen (Rh negative; Rh−) must not receive blood with the antigen (Rh positive; Rh+). Otherwise, hemolysis occurs. However, a person with Rh+ blood can receive Rh− blood. This is because the antigen is not present. Antibodies have no antigen to attack.

Cross-matching

When a person needs blood, the doctor orders laboratory *type and cross-matching* tests. Tests are done to determine the person's blood type. Then the person's blood is matched with the donor blood. This is called cross-matching. The tests determine if the person's blood is compatible with the donor's blood.

Assisting the RN

The RN is responsible for starting, maintaining, and ending blood transfusions. This includes assessing the person for transfusion reactions. The RN may ask you to assist in observing the person for transfusion reactions. Your state and agency may allow you to obtain blood from the blood bank.

✦ Obtaining blood from the blood bank

When type and cross-matching are complete, the laboratory notifies the RN that the blood is ready in the blood bank. The blood bank is located in the laboratory (Fig. 20-24, p. 494). Remember, *the right blood must be given to the right person.* You must obtain the right blood from the blood bank. Strict identification measures are practiced.

Time is critical when a person needs blood. You must go straight to the blood bank and immediately report back to the RN. Do not stop on the way to and from the blood bank. Do not stop to visit, do other errands, use the restroom, have a break, or to do any other activity. Minutes count.

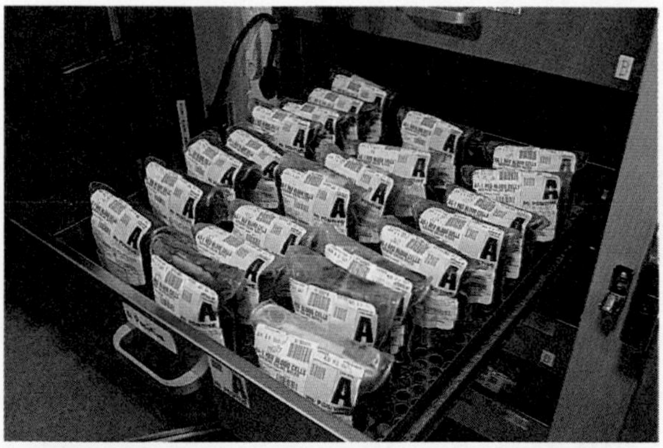

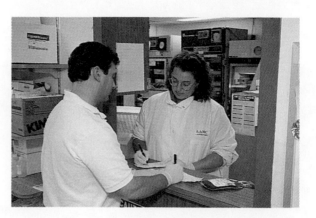

Fig. 20-24 *Blood is stored in refrigerators in the blood bank.*

Fig. 20-25 *Blood is checked with the laboratory technician.*

◆ OBTAINING BLOOD FROM THE BLOOD BANK

PROCEDURE ALERT

- Does your state allow assistive personnel to perform the procedure?

- Is the procedure in your job description?

- Do you have the necessary training and education?

- Is an RN available to answer questions and to supervise you?

PROCEDURE

1 Review the procedure with the RN.

2 Wash your hands.

3 Take the blood requisition form to the blood bank.

4 Tell the following to the laboratory technician:

- Who you are

- What you want

- That you have a requisition for blood or a blood product

5 Check the requisition form and the blood bag label with the laboratory technician (Fig. 20-25). Follow agency policy. Read the following out loud:

a The person's name—last name, first name, and middle initial

b The person's ID number

c The person's blood type—A, B, AB, or O

d The person's Rh factor—Rh+ or Rh−

e The blood donor number

f Expiration date on the blood

6 Thank the technician for helping you.

7 Return immediately to the nursing unit.

8 Give the blood to the RN.

9 Wash your hands.

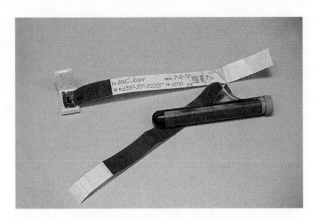

Fig. 20-26 *The patient is given an ID bracelet for blood administration when the specimen is drawn for type and cross-matching. All blood products for the patient have a number that matches the ID bracelet.*

Transfusion reactions

Transfusion reactions occur when the person's blood does not match with donor blood. Antibodies in the person's blood attack and destroy antigens in the donor blood. Blood cells are destroyed in the process (hemolysis). The person's life is seriously threatened. Death can occur.

Giving the wrong blood to the wrong person is a common cause of transfusion reactions. To prevent this, the blood bag tag is again checked with the blood requisition form before the blood is administered. Identifying information is also checked with the person's ID bracelet (Fig. 20-26). This is usually done by two RNs at the person's bedside. Agency policy may allow you to check the blood with the RN. You must be very careful. If the information does not match exactly, tell the RN.

Before starting the transfusion, the person's vital signs are measured. The RN may ask you to do this. These vital signs serve as a baseline. The RN compares vital signs taken during the transfusion with the baseline vital signs. A change in any vital sign signals a transfusion reaction.

The first 15 minutes of the transfusion is the most critical time for the person. The RN carefully assesses the person for signs and symptoms of a transfusion reaction. The person's vital signs are measured often.

Vital signs are measured during the transfusion and for 1 hour after the transfusion. It usually takes about 2 hours to transfuse 1 unit (1 bag) of blood. The RN may ask you

to assist with measuring vital signs. The RN tells you how often to measure them—usually every 15 or 30 minutes. These vital signs are recorded on a flow sheet. You must measure vital signs on time and accurately.

When you measure vital signs, also check the flow rate. The RN tells you the number of drops per minute. Immediately tell the RN if:

- The flow rate is too fast
- The flow rate is too slow
- The transfusion has stopped
- The bag is close to empty

You also must be alert for signs and symptoms of transfusion reactions (Box 20-4). Report any sign or symptom immediately to the RN. The RN will stop the transfusion.

BOX 20-4

SIGNS AND SYMPTOMS OF TRANSFUSION REACTIONS

- Chills
- Fever
- Headache
- Back pain or backache
- Chest pain
- Dyspnea (difficulty breathing)
- Tachypnea (rapid breathing)
- Coughing
- Tachycardia (rapid pulse)
- Hypotension (low blood pressure)
- Loss of consciousness
- Cardiac arrest
- Flushing
- Blood in the urine
- Itching
- Hives (urticaria)
- Wheezing
- Warm, flushed skin
- Anxiety
- Muscle pain
- Nausea
- Vomiting
- Abdominal cramping
- Diarrhea

REVIEW QUESTIONS

Circle the best answer.

1 Fluid intake and output should be equal.
   a True
   b False

2 Adult fluid requirements for normal fluid balance are about
   a 1000 to 1500 ml daily
   b 1500 to 2000 ml daily
   c 2000 to 2500 ml daily
   d 2500 to 3000 ml daily

3 A person is NPO. You should
   a Provide a variety of fluids
   b Offer fluids in small amounts and small containers
   c Remove the water pitcher and glass
   d Prevent the person from having oral hygiene

4 Which are *not* counted as liquid foods?
   a Coffee, tea, juices, and soft drinks
   b Butter, spaghetti sauce, and melted cheese
   c Ice cream, sherbet, custard, and pudding
   d Jello, popsicles, soup, and creamed cereals

5 Which IV solution is given for energy and fluid replacement?
   a Electrolyte solutions
   b Normal saline solutions
   c Blood volume expanders
   d Nutrient solutions

6 The following are peripheral IV sites *except*
   a Scalp veins
   b Neck veins
   c Arm veins
   d Foot veins

7 When selecting a peripheral IV site, the RN avoids the following *except*
   a The person's dominant side
   b The person's nondominant side
   c The side of a mastectomy
   d The side of paralysis

8 You collect an IV bag. You check the following *except*
   a For clearness and particles
   b The expiration date
   c For leaks and cracks
   d The medications added

9 Which parts of the IV infusion set are sterile?
   a The clamp and tubing
   b The clamp and spike
   c Tubing and drip chamber
   d The spike and needle adapter

10 The IV flow rate is
   a The number of gtt/ml
   b The number of gtt/min
   c The number of drops in a microdrip
   d The number of drops in a macrodrip

11 You note that the IV flow rate is too slow. You must
   a Tell the RN immediately
   b Adjust the flow rate
   c Reposition the person
   d Clamp the tubing

12 Air is removed from IV tubing to prevent
   a Phlebitis
   b An air embolism
   c PICC
   d All of the above

REVIEW QUESTIONS—cont'd

13 You are changing an IV dressing. Which is *false?*

   a Standard Precautions and the Bloodborne Pathogen Standard are followed.

   b A transparent dressing allows easy observation of the IV site.

   c Tape is placed over the needle adapter.

   d You check the flow rate after applying the dressing.

14 You are discontinuing an IV catheter. You remove the catheter by

   a Pulling it straight out

   b Pulling it out as you remove the dressing

   c Moving it to the left and then the right

   d Deflating the balloon

15 Which carry oxygen to the cells?

   a Antibodies

   b Antigens

   c Erythrocytes

   d Platelets

16 The liquid portion of blood is called

   a Plasma

   b Erythrocytes

   c Hemoglobin

   d Hemolysis

17 Which is necessary for blood clotting?

   a Plasma

   b Erythrocytes

   c Hemoglobin

   d Platelets

18 A person's blood has the type B antigen. The person's blood type is

   a Type A

   b Type B

   c Type AB

   d Type O

19 A person with type O blood

   a Has the type A and type B antigens

   b Is Rh+

   c Has no antigens

   d Is Rh−

20 Who can receive type O blood?

   a Persons with type A blood or type B blood

   b Persons with type AB blood

   c Persons with type O blood

   d All of the above

21 You are asked to obtain blood from the blood bank. The following are checked with the laboratory technician *except*

   a The person's blood type

   b The person's Rh factor

   c The person's ID bracelet

   d The blood's expiration date

22 The most critical time for a transfusion reaction is

   a The first 15 minutes of the infusion

   b The first hour of the infusion

   c The last hour of the infusion

   d The first hour after the infusion

23 A patient is receiving a blood transfusion. The person complains of a backache and chills. What should you do?

   a Measure the person's vital signs.

   b Tell the RN immediately.

   c Stop the transfusion.

   d Ask about other signs and symptoms.

24 The following are signs and symptoms of a transfusion reaction *except*

   a Wound drainage

   b Hypotension

   c Tachycardia

   d Chest pain

Answers to these questions are on p. 852.

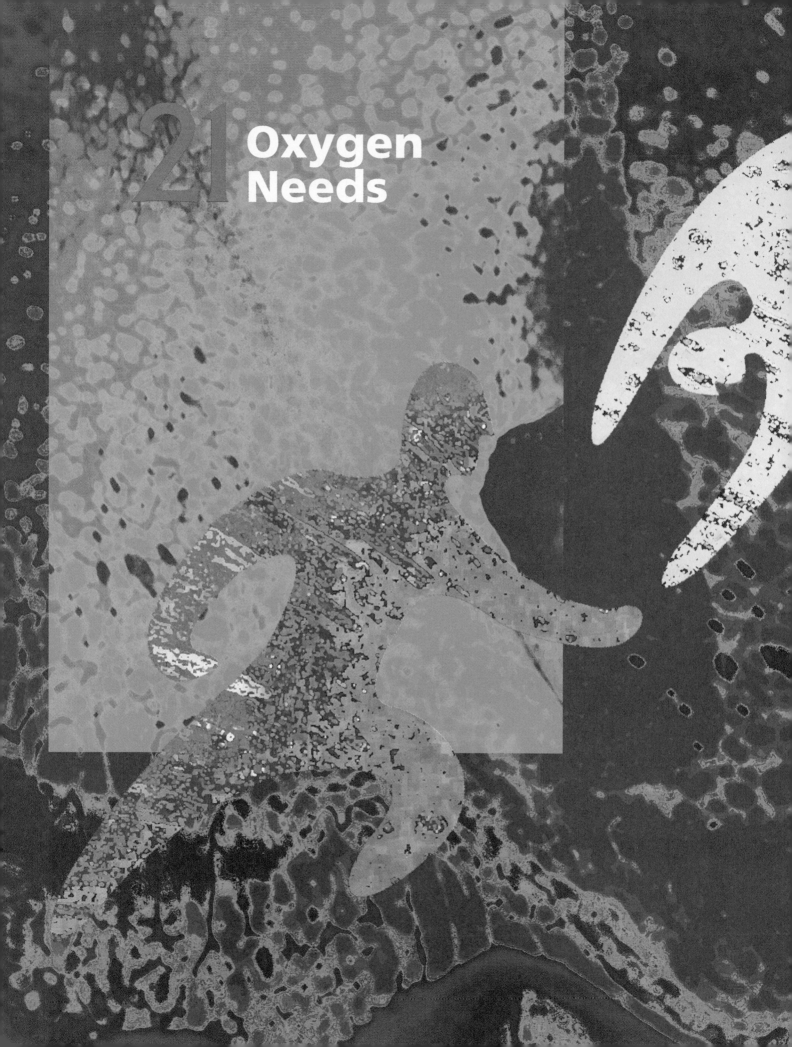

21 **Oxygen Needs**

- Define the key terms in this chapter
- Describe the factors affecting oxygen needs
- Identify the signs and symptoms of hypoxia and altered respiratory function
- Described the tests used to diagnose respiratory problems
- Explain how positioning, coughing and deep breathing, and incentive spirometry promote oxygenation
- Describe the devices used to administer oxygen
- Explain how to safely assist with oxygen therapy
- Explain how to assist in the care of persons with an artificial airway
- Describe the safety measures for oral suctioning
- Explain how to assist in the care of persons on mechanical ventilation
- Explain how to assist in the care of persons with chest tubes
- Perform the procedures described in this chapter

allergy A sensitivity to a substance that causes the body to react with signs and symptoms

apnea The lack or absence *(a)* of breathing *(pnea)*

Biot's respirations Irregular breathing with periods of apnea; respirations may be slow and deep or rapid and shallow

bradypnea Slow *(brady)* breathing *(pnea)*; respirations are fewer than 10 per minute

Cheyne-Stokes Respirations gradually increase in rate and depth and then become shallow and slow; breathing may stop *(apnea)* for 10 to 20 seconds

dyspnea Difficult, labored, or painful *(dys)* breathing *(pnea)*

hemoptysis Bloody *(hemo)* sputum (*ptysis* meaning "to spit")

hemothorax The collection of blood *(hemo)* in the pleural space *(thorax)*

hyperventilation Respirations that are rapid *(hyper)* and deeper than normal

hypoventilation Respirations that are slow *(hypo)*, shallow, and sometimes irregular

hypoxemia A reduced amount *(hypo)* of oxygen *(ox)* in the blood *(emia)*

hypoxia A deficiency *(hypo)* of oxygen *(oxia)* in the cells

intubation The process of inserting an artificial airway

Kussmaul's respirations Very deep and rapid respirations; a sign of diabetic coma

mechanical ventilation Using a machine to move air into and out of the lungs

orthopnea Being able to breathe *(pnea)* deeply and comfortably only while sitting or standing *(ortho)*

orthopneic position Sitting up in bed *(ortho)* and leaning forward over the bedside table

oxygen concentration The amount of hemoglobin that contains oxygen (O_2)

pleural effusion The escape and collection of fluid *(effusion)* in the pleural space

pneumothorax The collection of air *(pneumo)* in the pleural space *(thorax)*

pollutant A harmful chemical or substance in the air or water

respiratory arrest Breathing stops

respiratory depression Slow, weak respirations that occur at a rate of fewer than 12 per minute; respirations are not deep enough to bring enough air into the lungs

sputum Expectorated mucus

suction The process of withdrawing or sucking up fluid (secretions)

tachypnea Rapid *(tachy)* breathing *(pnea)*; respirations are usually more than 24 per minute

Oxygen (O_2) is a tasteless, odorless, and colorless gas. It is a basic need and is necessary for survival. Death occurs within minutes if a person stops breathing. Serious illnesses occur without enough oxygen. Illness, surgery, and injuries affect the amount of oxygen in the blood and cells.

FACTORS AFFECTING OXYGEN NEEDS

The respiratory and cardiovascular systems must function properly for cells to get enough oxygen. Any disease, injury, or surgery involving these systems affects the body's ability to take in oxygen and deliver it to the cells. Each body system depends on the other. Altered function of any system (e.g., the nervous, musculoskeletal, or urinary system) affects the body's ability to meet its oxygen needs. Major factors affecting oxygen needs are:

- *Respiratory system status*—Structures must be intact and functioning. The airway must be open (patent). Alveoli must exchange O_2 and carbon dioxide (CO_2).
- *Cardiovascular system function*—Blood must flow freely to and from the heart. Narrowed vessels affect the delivery of oxygen-rich blood to the cells and blood return to the heart. Capillaries and cells must exchange O_2 and CO_2.
- *Red blood cell count*—The blood must have enough red blood cells (RBCs). RBCs contain hemoglobin, which picks up oxygen in the lungs and carries it to the cells. The bone marrow must produce enough RBCs. Poor diet, chemotherapy, and leukemia affect bone marrow function. Blood loss also reduces the number of RBCs.
- *Intact nervous system*—Nervous system diseases and injuries can affect respiratory muscle function. Breathing may be difficult or impossible. Brain damage affects respiratory rate, rhythm, and depth. Narcotics and depressant drugs are chemicals that affect the brain. They slow respirations. The amount of O_2 and CO_2 in the blood also affects brain function. Respirations increase when O_2 is lacking. The body tries to bring in more oxygen. Respirations also increase when CO_2 increases. The body tries to get rid of CO_2.
- *Aging*—Respiratory muscles weaken, and lung tissue becomes less elastic. There is decreased strength for coughing. Coughing and removing secretions from the upper airway are important. Otherwise, upper respiratory tract infections can lead to *pneumonia* (inflammation of the lung). Older persons are at risk for respiratory complications after surgery.

- *Exercise*—Oxygen needs increase with exercise. Normally, respiratory rate and depth increase to bring enough O_2 into the lungs. Persons with heart and respiratory diseases may have enough oxygen at rest. However, even slight activity can increase their oxygen needs. Their bodies may not be able to bring in oxygen and to deliver it to cells.
- *Fever*—Oxygen needs increase. As with exercise, respiratory rate and depth must increase to meet the body's needs.
- *Pain*—Pain increases the need for oxygen. Respirations increase to meet this need. However, chest and abdominal injuries and surgeries often involve the respiratory muscles. This interferes with breathing in and out.
- *Medications*—Some drugs depress the respiratory center in the brain. **Respiratory depression** is slow, weak respirations at a rate of fewer than 12 per minute. Respirations are too shallow to bring enough air into the lungs. **Respiratory arrest** is when breathing stops. Narcotics such as morphine and Demerol can have these effects. (The word narcotic comes from the Greek word *narkoun*. It means stupor or to be numb.) These drugs are given in safe amounts for severe pain. Substance abusers are at risk for respiratory depression and respiratory arrest from overdoses of narcotics and depressants. Narcotics include opium, heroin, and methadone. Depressant drugs include barbiturates (Nembutal, phenobarbital, secobarbital, Tuinal, and others) and the benzodiazepines (Dalmane, diazepam, Halcion, Librium, Tranxene, Valium, Xanax, and others).
- *Smoking*—Smoking causes lung cancer and chronic obstructive pulmonary disease (COPD). It is a risk factor for coronary artery disease.
- *Allergies*—An **allergy** is a sensitivity to a substance that causes the body to react with signs and symptoms. Respiratory signs and symptoms include runny nose, wheezing, and congestion. Mucous membranes in the upper airway swell. With severe swelling, the airway closes. Shock and death are risks. Pollens, dust, foods, drugs, and cigarette smoke often cause allergies. Persons with allergies are at risk for chronic bronchitis and asthma.
- *Pollutant exposure*—A **pollutant** is a harmful chemical or substance in the air or water. Dust, fumes, toxins, asbestos, coal dust, and sawdust are some air pollutants. They damage the lungs. Pollutant exposure occurs in home, work, and community settings.
- *Nutrition*—Good nutrition is needed for red blood cell production. RBCs live about 3 or 4 months. New ones must replace those that die off. The body needs iron and vitamins (vitamin B_{12}, vitamin C, and folic acid) to produce RBCs.

- *Substance abuse*—Alcohol depresses the brain. Excessive amounts reduce the cough reflex and increase the risk of aspiration. Obstructed airway and pneumonia are risks from aspiration. Respiratory depression and respiratory arrest are risks when narcotics and depressant drugs are abused.

ALTERED RESPIRATORY FUNCTION

Respiratory system function involves three processes. Air moves into and out of the lungs. Oxygen and carbon dioxide are exchanged at the alveoli. The blood transports O_2 to the cells and removes CO_2 from them. Respiratory function is altered if even one process is affected.

Hypoxia

Hypoxia is a deficiency *(hypo)* of oxygen *(oxia)* in the cells. Cells do not receive enough oxygen. Therefore they do not function properly. Hypoxia is caused by any illness, disease, injury, or surgery affecting respiratory function. The brain is very sensitive to inadequate oxygen. Restlessness is an early sign of hypoxia. So are dizziness and disorientation. Report signs and symptoms of hypoxia to the RN immediately (Box 21-1).

Hypoxia is life-threatening. The heart, brain, and other organs must receive enough oxygen to function. Oxygen is given, and treatment is directed at the cause of the hypoxia.

Abnormal Respirations

Normal respirations occur between 12 and 20 times per minute in the adult. Infants and children have faster rates. Respirations are normally quiet, effortless, and regular. Both sides of the chest rise and fall equally. The following breathing patterns are abnormal:

- **Tachypnea**—rapid *(tachy)* breathing *(pnea)*. Respirations are usually more than 24 per minute. Fever, exercise, pain, pregnancy, airway obstruction, and hypoxemia are common causes. **Hypoxemia** is a reduced amount *(hypo)* of oxygen *(ox)* in the blood *(emia)*.
- **Bradypnea**—slow *(brady)* breathing *(pnea)*. Respirations are fewer than 10 per minute. Bradypnea is seen with drug overdoses and central nervous system disorders.
- **Apnea**—the lack or absence *(a)* of breathing *(pnea)*. It occurs in cardiac arrest and respiratory arrest.
- **Dyspnea**—difficult, labored, or painful *(dys)* breathing *(pnea)*. Heart disease, exercise, and anxiety are common causes.

BOX 21-1

SIGNS AND SYMPTOMS OF HYPOXIA

- Restlessness
- Dizziness
- Disorientation
- Confusion
- Behavior and personality changes
- Difficulty concentrating and following directions
- Apprehension
- Anxiety
- Fatigue
- Agitation
- Increased pulse rate
- Increased rate and depth of respirations
- Sitting position, often leaning forward
- Cyanosis (bluish color to the skin, lips, mucous membranes, and nail beds)
- Dyspnea

- **Hypoventilation**—respirations that are slow *(hypo)*, shallow, and sometimes irregular. Lung disorders affecting the alveoli are common causes. Pneumonia is an example. Other causes include obesity, airway obstruction, drug side effects, and nervous system and musculoskeletal disorders affecting the respiratory muscles.
- **Hyperventilation**—respirations that are rapid *(hyper)* and deeper than normal. Its many causes include asthma, emphysema, infection, fever, central nervous system disorders, hypoxia, anxiety, pain, and some drugs.
- **Cheyne-Stokes**—respirations gradually increase in rate and depth and then become shallow and slow. Breathing may stop (apnea) for 10 to 20 seconds. Drug overdose, heart failure, renal failure, and brain disorders are common causes. These respirations are common when death is near.
- **Orthopnea**—breathing *(pnea)* deeply and comfortably only while sitting or standing *(ortho)*. Common causes include emphysema, asthma, pneumonia, angina pectoris, and other heart and respiratory disorders.
- **Biot's respirations**—irregular breathing with periods of apnea. Respirations are slow and deep or rapid and shallow. They occur with central nervous system disorders.
- **Kussmaul's respirations**—very deep and rapid respirations. They are a sign of diabetic coma.

BOX 21-2

SIGNS AND SYMPTOMS OF ALTERED RESPIRATORY FUNCTION

- Signs and symptoms of hypoxia (see Box 21-1)
- Any abnormal breathing pattern (see p. 501)
- Complaints of shortness of breath or being "winded" or "short-winded"
- Cough (note frequency and time of day)
  - Dry and hacking
  - Harsh and barking
  - Productive (produces sputum) or nonproductive
- Sputum
  - Color—clear, white, yellow, green, brown, or red
  - Odor—none or foul odor
  - Consistency—thick, watery, or frothy (with bubbles or foam)
  - **Hemoptysis**—bloody (hemo) sputum (ptysis meaning "to spit"); note if the sputum is bright red, dark red, blood-tinged, or streaked with blood
- Noisy respirations
  - Wheezing
  - Wet sounding respirations
  - Crowing sounds
- Chest pain (note location)
  - Constant
  - Person's description (stabbing, knife-like, aching)
  - What makes it worse (movement, coughing, yawning, sneezing, sighing, deep breathing)
- Cyanosis
  - Skin
  - Mucous membranes
  - Lips
  - Nail beds
- Changes in vital signs
- Body position
  - Sitting upright
  - Leaning forward or hunched over a table

Assisting With Assessment and Diagnostic Testing

Altered respiratory function may be an acute or chronic problem. Doctors and nurses are always alert for altered respiratory function. Report your observations to the RN promptly and accurately (Box 21-2). Quick action is necessary to meet the person's oxygen needs. Measures are taken to correct the situation and prevent the problem from getting worse.

The doctor orders tests to determine the cause of altered respiratory function. The following tests are common. You are likely to assist with pulse oximetry and collecting sputum specimens.

- *Chest x-ray (CXR)*—An x-ray is taken of the chest. It is used to evaluate changes in the lungs. All clothing and jewelry from the waist to the neck are removed. The person wears a hospital gown.
- *Lung scan*—The lungs are scanned to see what areas are not getting air or blood. The person inhales radioactive gas and is injected with a radioisotope. *Radioactive* means to give off radiation. A *radioisotope* is an element that gives off radiation. Lung tissue getting air and blood flow "take up" the radioactive substances. A scanner senses areas with radioactive substances. As when having a chest x-ray, the person removes all clothing and jewelry from the waist to the neck. A hospital gown is worn.

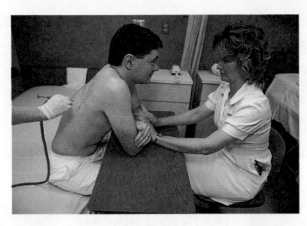

Fig. 21-1 *The person is positioned for a thoracentesis.* (From Elkin MK, Perry AG, Potter PA: Nursing interventions and clinical skills, St Louis, 1996, Mosby.)

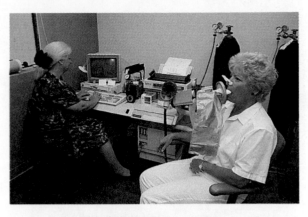

Fig. 21-2 *Pulmonary function testing.*

- *Bronchoscopy*—A scope *(scopy)* is passed into the trachea and bronchi *(broncho)*. The doctor inspects the larynx, trachea, and bronchi for bleeding and tumors. The doctor can take tissue samples (biopsy) or remove mucous plugs and foreign objects. The person takes nothing by mouth (NPO) for 6 to 8 hours before the procedure. This reduces the danger of vomiting and aspiration. A local or general anesthetic is given. After the procedure, the person is NPO and watched carefully until the gag and swallow reflexes return. They usually return in about 2 hours. Preoperative care and postoperative care are given as directed by the RN.

- *Thoracentesis*—The pleura *(thora)* is punctured, and air or fluid is aspirated *(centesis)* from it. The doctor inserts a needle through the chest wall into the pleural sac. Injury or disease can cause the pleural sac to fill with air, blood, or fluid. This affects respiratory function. The procedure also is done to remove fluid for laboratory study or to inject anticancer drugs into the pleural sac. The procedure takes a few minutes. Vital signs are taken before a local anesthetic is given. The person sits up and leans forward and is asked not to talk, cough, or move suddenly (Fig. 21-1). Postprocedure care involves applying a dressing to the puncture site and taking vital signs. A chest x-ray is taken to check for lung damage. The person is checked often for shortness of breath, dyspnea, cough, sputum, chest pain, cyanosis, vital sign changes, and other respiratory signs and symptoms.

- *Pulmonary function tests*—Tests measure the amount of air moving into and out of the lungs (volume) and how much air the lungs can hold (capacity). The person takes as deep a breath as possible. Using a mouthpiece, the person blows into a machine (Fig.

21-2). The tests are used to evaluate persons at risk for lung diseases or postoperative pulmonary complications. They are used also to measure the progress of lung disease and its treatment. Fatigue is common after the tests. The person should rest after the procedure.

- *Arterial blood gases (ABGs)*—A radial or femoral artery is punctured to obtain arterial blood. Laboratory tests measure the amount of oxygen in the blood. Hemorrhage from the artery must be prevented. Pressure is applied to the artery for at least 5 minutes after the procedure. Pressure is applied longer if the person has blood clotting problems.

✦ Pulse oximetry

Pulse oximetry measures *(metry)* oxygen *(oxi)* concentration in arterial blood. **Oxygen concentration** is the amount (percent) of hemoglobin that contains oxygen. The normal range is 95% to 100%. For example, if 97% of all the hemoglobin (100%) carries O_2, tissues get enough oxygen. If only 90% of the hemoglobin contains O_2, tissues do not get enough oxygen to function. Measurements are used to prevent hypoxia and to evaluate treatment.

A sensor (or probe) is attached to the person's finger, toe, earlobe, nose, or forehead (Fig. 21-3, p. 504). Two light beams on one side of the sensor pass through the tissues. A detector on the other side measures the amount of light passing through the tissues. The oximeter receives this information and measures the oxygen concentration. The value and the person's pulse rate are displayed on the monitor. Oximeters have alarms. The alarms sound if oxygen concentration is low, the pulse is too fast or slow, or other problems occur.

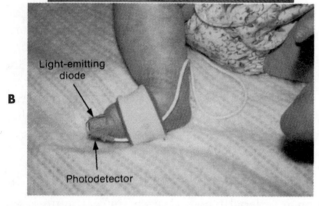

Fig. 21-3 A, *A pulse oximetry sensor is attached to a person's finger.* **B,** *The sensor is attached to an infant's great toe.* (B from Wong DL: Whaley & Wong's nursing care of infants and children, ed 5, St Louis, 1995, Mosby.)

A good sensor site is needed. The RN tells you what site to use based on the person's condition. Swollen sites are avoided. So are sites with breaks in the skin. Finger and toe sites are avoided in persons with poor circulation.

Bright light, dark nail polish, and movements affect measurements. Place a towel over the sensor to block bright light. Remove nail polish, or use another site. Movements from shivering, seizures, or tremors affect finger sensors. The earlobe is a better site for these problems. Blood pressure cuffs affect blood flow. If using a finger site, do not measure blood pressure on that side.

Report and record measurements accurately. Use the abbreviation SpO_2 when recording the oxygen concentra-

tion value (S=saturation, p=pulse, O_2=oxygen). Also report and record:

- The date and time
- What the person was doing at the time of the measurement
- Oxygen flow rate and the device used (p. 514)
- Reason for the measurement (routine or change in the person's condition)
- Other observations

Pulse oximetry does not lessen the need for good observations. The person's condition can change rapidly. You assist the RN in observing for signs and symptoms of hypoxia. (See Focus on Children, Focus on Older Persons, and Focus on Home Care.)

USING A PULSE OXIMETER

PROCEDURE ALERT

- Does your state allow assistive personnel to perform the procedure?

- Is the procedure in your job description?

- Do you have the necessary training and education?

- Is an RN available to answer questions and to supervise you?

PRE-PROCEDURE

1 Review the procedure with the RN.

2 Ask the RN what site to use.

3 Explain the procedure to the person.

4 Collect the following:

- Oximeter and sensor

- Nail polish remover

- Cotton balls

- SpO$_2$ flow sheet

- Tape

- Towel

5 Identify the person. Check the ID bracelet against your assignment sheet.

6 Provide for privacy.

PROCEDURE

7 Make sure the person is comfortable.

8 Remove nail polish using a cotton ball. (If a toe site is used, remove any nail polish).

9 Dry the site with a towel.

10 Clip or tape the sensor to the site. Make sure the site is dry.

11 Turn on the oximeter.

12 Check the person's pulse (apical or radial) with the pulse on the display. The pulses should be equal. Tell the RN if the pulses are not equal.

13 Read the SpO$_2$ on the display. Note the value on the flow sheet.

14 Leave the sensor in place for continuous monitoring. Otherwise, turn off the oximeter and remove the sensor.

POST-PROCEDURE

15 Make sure the person is comfortable.

16 Place the call bell within the person's reach.

17 Raise or lower bed rails as instructed by the RN.

18 Unscreen the person.

19 Return the pulse oximeter to its proper place if continuous monitoring is not ordered.

20 Wash your hands.

21 Report the SpO$_2$ and your other observations to the RN.

✦ *Collecting sputum specimens*

Respiratory disorders cause the lungs, bronchi, and trachea to secrete mucus. The mucus is called **sputum** when expectorated (expelled) through the mouth. Sputum is different from saliva. Saliva is a thin, clear liquid produced by the salivary glands in the mouth. Saliva is often called "spit."

Sputum specimens are studied for blood, microbes, and abnormal cells. The person coughs up sputum from the bronchi and trachea. This is often painful and difficult. Specimen collection is easier in the early morning when secretions are coughed up upon awakening. The person rinses the mouth with water. Rinsing decreases saliva and removes food particles. Mouthwash is not used before the procedure. It destroys some of the microbes in the mouth.

Collecting a sputum specimen can embarrass the person. Coughing and expectorating sounds can upset or nauseate other persons nearby. Also, sputum is unpleasant to look at. For these reasons, privacy is important. The specimen container is covered and placed in a bag. Some agencies use sputum containers that conceal the contents. (See Focus on Children and Focus on Older Persons.)

CHILDREN

focus on

Breathing treatments and suctioning are often needed to produce a sputum specimen in infants and small children. The RN or respiratory therapist gives the breathing treatment. The RN suctions the trachea for the sputum specimen. The infant or child is likely to be uncooperative during suctioning. You can assist by holding the child's head and arms still.

OLDER PERSONS

focus on

Older persons may not have the strength to cough up sputum. Coughing is easier after postural drainage. Postural drainage involves draining secretions by gravity. Gravity causes fluids to flow down. Therefore the person is positioned so a lung part is lower than the airway (Fig. 21-4). Different positions are used depending on what part of the lungs to drain. The RN or respiratory therapist is responsible for postural drainage.

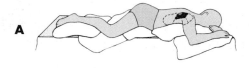

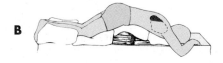

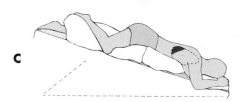

Fig. 21-4 *Some positions used for postural drainage.* **A,** *Draining the right upper lobe.* **B,** *Draining the right middle lobe.* **C,** *Draining the right lower lobe.* (*From Potter PA, Perry AG:* Fundamentals of nursing: concepts, process, and practice, *ed 4, St Louis, 1997, Mosby.*)

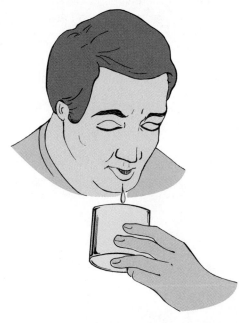

Fig. 21-5 *The person expectorates into the center of the specimen container.*

COLLECTING A SPUTUM SPECIMEN

PRE-PROCEDURE

1 Explain the procedure to the person.

2 Wash your hands.

3 Collect the following:

- Sputum specimen container
- Tissues
- Label
- Laboratory requisition
- Disposable bag
- Gloves

PROCEDURE

4 Label the container.

5 Identify the person. Check the ID bracelet against the requisition slip.

6 Provide for privacy. If able, the person goes into the bathroom to obtain the specimen.

7 Ask the person to rinse the mouth out with clear water.

8 Put on the gloves.

9 Have the person hold the container. Only the outside of the container is touched.

10 Ask the person to cover the mouth and nose with tissues when coughing.

11 Ask him or her to take two or three deep breaths and cough up the sputum.

12 Have the person expectorate directly into the container (Fig. 21-5). Sputum should not touch the outside of the container.

13 Collect 1 to 2 tablespoons of sputum unless told to collect more.

14 Put the lid on the container immediately.

15 Place the container in the bag. Attach the requisition to the bag.

16 Remove the gloves.

POST-PROCEDURE

17 Make sure the person is comfortable and unscreened. Place the call bell within reach.

18 Wash your hands.

19 Take the bag to the laboratory.

20 Wash your hands.

21 Report the following to the RN:

- The time the specimen was collected and taken to the laboratory
- The amount of sputum collected
- How easily the person raised the sputum
- The consistency and appearance of sputum (see Box 21-2)
- Any other observations

PROMOTING OXYGENATION

For the body to get enough oxygen, air must move deeply into the lungs. Air must reach the alveoli for the exchange of oxygen and carbon dioxide with the blood. Disease and injury can prevent air from reaching the alveoli. Secretions can congest lung tissue and the airway. Pain, immobility, and narcotics interfere with deep breathing and coughing up secretions. Therefore secretions collect in the respiratory system. They interfere with air movement and alveolar function in the affected part of the lung. Secretions also provide an environment for microbes. Infection is a threat.

The RN plans measures to meet the person's oxygen needs. The following measures are often included in nursing care plans.

Positioning

Breathing is usually easier in semi-Fowler's and Fowler's position. Persons with difficulty breathing often prefer to sit up in bed and lean forward over the overbed table. This is called the **orthopneic position.** *Ortho* means sitting or standing; *pnea* means breathing. You can increase the person's comfort by placing a pillow on the overbed table (Fig. 21-6).

Frequent position changes are important. Unless the doctor limits positioning, the person must not lie on one side for a long time. This prevents lung expansion on that side and allows secretions to pool. Position changes are usually done at least every 2 hours.

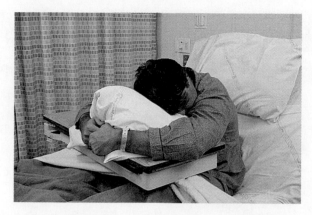

Fig. 21-6 *The person is in the orthopneic position. Note that a pillow is on the overbed table for the person's comfort.*

✦ Coughing and Deep Breathing

Mucus is removed by coughing. Deep breathing promotes air movement into most parts of the lungs. Coughing and deep breathing exercises are helpful for persons with respiratory disorders. They are routinely done after surgery and are important for persons on bedrest. The exercises are painful after injury or surgery. The person may be afraid of breaking open an incision while coughing.

Coughing and deep breathing help prevent pneumonia and atelectasis. *Atelectasis* is the collapse of a portion of the lung. It occurs when mucus collects in the airway. Air cannot get to a part of the lung, and the lung collapses.

The frequency of coughing and deep breathing varies. Some doctors order the exercises every 1 or 2 hours while the person is awake. Others want them done 4 times a day. The RN tells you when coughing and deep breathing are done. You are told how many deep breaths and coughs the person should do.

ASSISTING THE PERSON WITH COUGHING AND DEEP-BREATHING EXERCISES

PRE-PROCEDURE

1 Explain the procedure to the person.

2 Identify the person. Check the ID bracelet against your assignment sheet.

3 Provide for privacy.

PROCEDURE

4 Help the person to a comfortable sitting position: dangling, semi-Fowler's, or Fowler's.

5 Have the person deep breathe:

   a Have the person place the hands over the rib cage (Fig. 21-7, p. 510).

   b Ask the person to exhale. Explain that when exhaling, the ribs should move as far down as possible.

   c Have the person take a deep breath. It should be as deep as possible. Remind the person to inhale through the nose.

   d Ask the person to hold the breath for 3 seconds.

   e Ask the person to exhale slowly through pursed lips (Fig. 21-8, p. 510). The person should exhale until the ribs move as far down as possible.

   f Repeat this step four more times.

6 Ask the person to cough:

   a Have the person interlace the fingers over the incision (Fig. 21-9, A, p. 510). The person can also hold a small pillow or folded towel over the incision (Fig. 21-9, B, p. 510).

   b Have the person take in a deep breath as in step 5.

   c Ask the person to cough strongly twice with the mouth open.

POST-PROCEDURE

7 Assist the person to a comfortable position.

8 Raise or lower bed rails as instructed by the RN.

9 Place the call bell within reach.

10 Unscreen the person.

11 Report your observations to the RN:

   • The number of times the person coughed and deep breathed

   • How the person tolerated the procedure

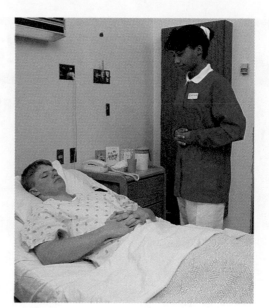

Fig. 21-7 *The hands are over the rib cage for deep breathing.*

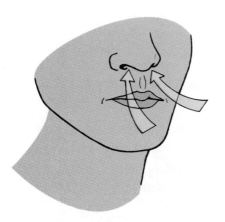 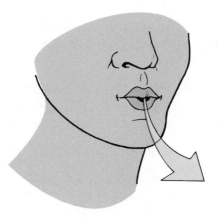

Fig. 21-8 *The person inhales through the nose and exhales through pursed lips during the deep-breathing exercise.*

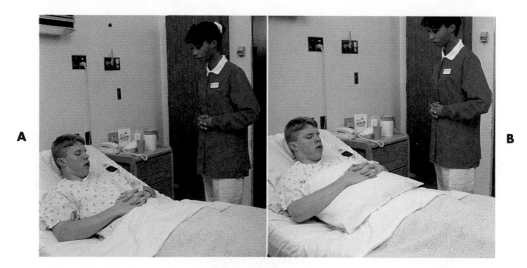

A   B

Fig. 21-9 *The person supports an incision for the coughing exercise.* **A,** *Fingers are interlaced over the incision.* **B,** *A small pillow is held over the incision.*

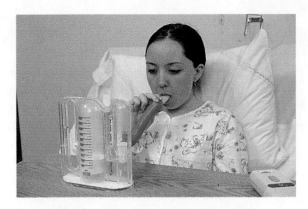

Fig. 21-10 *The person uses a spirometer.*

Incentive Spirometry

Incentive means to give encouragement. A *spirometer* is a machine that measures the amount (volume) of air inhaled. Thus incentive spirometry involves encouraging the person to inhale until reaching a preset volume of air. Balls or bars in the spirometer allow the person to see the movement of air when inhaling (Fig. 21-10).

The spirometer is placed upright. The person exhales normally and then seals the lips around a mouthpiece. The person takes in a slow, deep breath until the balls rise to the desired height. The breath is held for 2 to 6 seconds to keep the balls floating. Then the person removes the mouthpiece and exhales slowly. The person may cough at this time. The RN tells you how often the person needs incentive spirometry and how many breaths the person needs to take. Follow agency policy for cleaning and replacing disposable mouthpieces.

ASSISTING WITH OXYGEN THERAPY

Disease, injury, and surgery often interfere with breathing. The amount of oxygen in the blood may be less than normal (hypoxemia). If so, the doctor orders supplemental oxygen.

Oxygen is treated as a drug. The doctor orders the amount of oxygen to give and the device to use. The order also states if oxygen is given continuously or intermittently (periodically). *Continuous oxygen therapy* means that the oxygen is never stopped. That is, the administration of oxygen is not interrupted for any reason. *Intermittent oxygen therapy* is for symptom relief. Chest pain and exercise are common reasons for intermittent oxygen. The oxygen helps relieve chest pain. Persons with chronic respiratory diseases may have enough oxygen at rest. With mild exercise or activities of daily living, they become short of breath. Oxygen helps to relieve the shortness of breath.

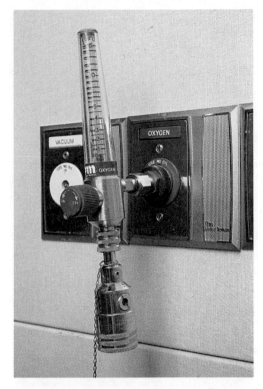

Fig. 21-11 *Wall oxygen outlet.*

You are not responsible for administering oxygen. The RN and respiratory therapist start and maintain oxygen therapy. You assist the RN in providing safe care to persons receiving oxygen.

Oxygen Sources

Oxygen is supplied through wall outlets, oxygen tanks, and oxygen concentrators. With the wall outlet (Fig. 21-11), O_2 is piped into each patient unit. Each unit is connected to a centrally located oxygen supply.

The oxygen tank is portable. It is brought to the person's unit when the doctor orders oxygen therapy. Small tanks are used during emergencies and transfers. Some ambulatory persons need continuous oxygen. Portable tanks are used when walking (Fig. 21-12, p. 512). The gauge on the tank tells how much oxygen is left in the tank (Fig. 21-13, p. 512). Tell the RN if the tank is low.

Oxygen concentrators (Fig. 21-14, p. 512) do not need an oxygen source (wall outlet or tank). The concentrator removes oxygen from the air. A power source is needed. If the concentrator is not portable, moving about is limited. The person stays close to the machine. A portable oxygen tank is needed in case of a power failure and for mobility. (See Focus on Home Care on p. 512.)

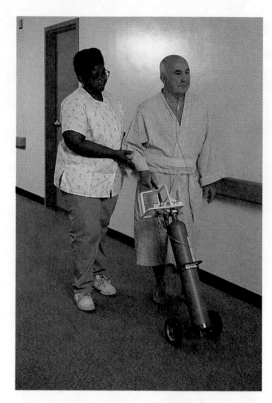

Fig. 21-12 *The person uses a portable oxygen tank during ambulation.*

HOME CARE

Oxygen tanks and oxygen concentrators are used in home care. The source ordered depends on the person's needs. The tank or concentrator is supplied by a medical supply company. Keep the company's name and phone number near the telephone.

The patient and family must practice safety measures where oxygen is used and stored. The safety measures to prevent fire are practiced (Box 21-3). Also, the oxygen tank is kept away from open flames and heat sources. These include candles, gas stoves, heating ducts, radiators, heating pipes, space heaters, and kerosene heaters and lamps. Keep a fire extinguisher in the room. If a fire occurs, turn off the oxygen. Then get the person and other family members out of the home and call the fire department.

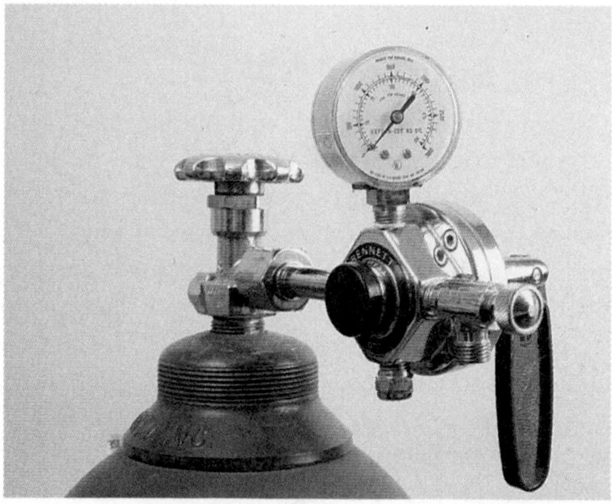

Fig. 21-13 *The gauge shows the amount of oxygen remaining in the tank.*

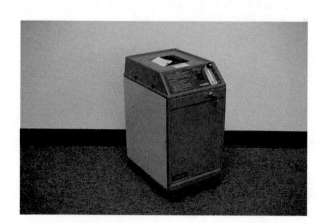

Fig. 21-14 *Oxygen concentrator.*

SAFETY RULES FOR FIRE AND USING OXYGEN

- Place "No Smoking" signs in the room and on the room door.
- Remove smoking materials from the room (cigarettes, cigars, pipes, matches, lighters).
- Remove materials from the room that ignite easily (alcohol, nail polish remover, oils, greases).
- Keep oxygen tanks away from heat sources.
- Turn off electrical items before unplugging them.
- Use electrical equipment that is in good repair (e.g., razor, radio, TV).
- Use only electrical equipment with three-prong plugs.
- Do not use materials that cause static electricity (wool and synthetic fabrics).

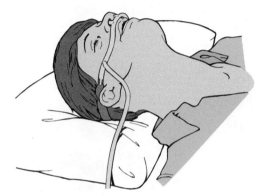

Fig. 21-15 *Nasal cannula.*

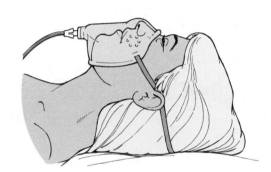

Fig. 21-16 *Simple face mask.*

Devices Used to Administer Oxygen

The doctor orders the device used to administer oxygen. These devices are common:

- **Nasal cannula** (Fig. 21-15)—two prongs project from the tubing. The prongs are inserted a short distance into the nostrils. The prongs point downward. This prevents drying of the sinuses. An elastic headband or tubing brought behind the ears keeps the cannula in place. The person can eat and talk with a cannula in place. Nasal irritation occurs with tight prongs. Pressure on the ears is possible.
- **Simple face mask** (Fig. 21-16)—covers the nose and mouth. The mask has small holes in the sides. Carbon dioxide escapes during exhalation. Room air enters during inhalation.
- **Partial-rebreathing mask** (Fig. 21-17)—a reservoir bag is added to the simple face mask. The bag is for exhaled air. With inhalation, the person inhales oxygen and some of the exhaled air. Some room air is also inhaled. The bag should not totally deflate when the person inhales.

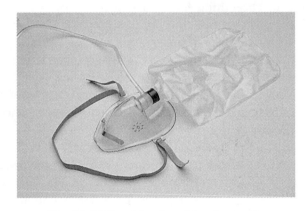

Fig. 21-17 *Partial-rebreathing face mask.*

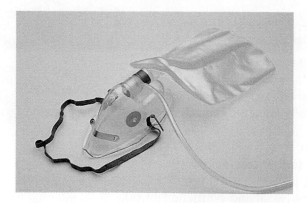

Fig. 21-18 *Nonrebreathing face mask.*

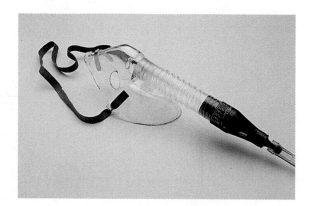

Fig. 21-19 *Venturi mask.*

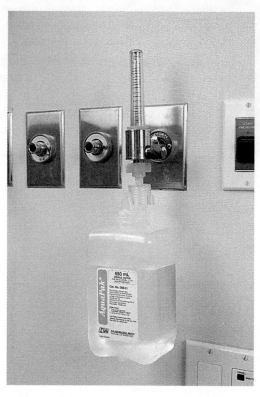

Fig. 21-20 *Oxygen administration system with humidifier.*

- **Nonrebreathing face mask** (Fig. 21-18)—prevents exhaled air from entering the reservoir bag. Exhaled air leaves through holes in the mask. When the person inhales, oxygen from the reservoir bag is inhaled. The bag must not totally collapse during exhalation.
- **Venturi mask** (Fig. 21-19)—allows precise amounts of oxygen to be given. Color-coded adaptors indicate the amount of oxygen being delivered.

Special care is needed when masks are used. Masks make talking difficult. Listen carefully to what the person is saying. Moisture can build up under masks. Keep the person's face clean and dry to help prevent irritation from the mask. Masks are removed for eating. Usually oxygen is administered by nasal cannula during meals.

Oxygen Flow Rates

The amount of oxygen given is called the *flow rate*. This is ordered by the doctor. The flow rate is measured in liters per minute (L/min). The flow rate is anywhere from 2 to 15 liters of oxygen per minute. The flowmeter (see Fig. 21-11) is set for the desired rate. This is done by the RN or respiratory therapist.

The RN tells you what the flow rate is for the person. When giving care and checking patients, always check the flow rate. Tell the RN immediately if the flow rate is too high or too low. The flow rate is adjusted by an RN or respiratory therapist. Some states and agencies let assistive personnel adjust oxygen flow rates.

✦ Preparing for Oxygen Administration

Your job description may let you set up the oxygen administration system (Fig. 21-20). The RN tells you the following:

- The person's name and room and bed number
- The oxygen administration device ordered
- If humidification was ordered

Oxygen is a dry gas. If not humidified (made moist), oxygen dries the airway's mucous membranes. Distilled water is added to the humidifier to create water vapor. Oxygen tubing is attached to the humidifier. Oxygen picks up water vapor as it flows into the system. Bubbling in the humidifier means water vapor is being produced. If humidification is not ordered, distilled water and the humidifier are not used.

◆ SETTING UP FOR OXYGEN ADMINISTRATION

PROCEDURE ALERT

- Does your state allow assistive personnel to perform the procedure?
- Is the procedure in your job description?

- Do you have the necessary training and education?
- Is an RN available to answer questions and to supervise you?

PRE-PROCEDURE

1 Review the doctor's orders with the RN.

2 Wash your hands.

3 Collect the following:

- Oxygen administration device with connecting tubing

- Flowmeter

- Humidifier (if ordered)

- Distilled water (if using a humidifier)

4 Identify the person. Check the ID bracelet with your assignment sheet.

5 Explain to the person what you are going to do.

PROCEDURE

6 Make sure the flowmeter is in the *OFF* position.

7 Attach the flowmeter to the wall outlet.

8 Fill the humidifier with distilled water.

9 Attach the humidifier to the bottom of the flowmeter.

10 Attach the oxygen administration device and connecting tubing to the humidifier. *Do not set the flowmeter or apply the oxygen administration device on the person.*

POST-PROCEDURE

11 Discard packaging.

12 Make sure the cap is securely on the distilled water. Store it according to agency policy.

13 Make sure the person is comfortable and the call bell is within reach.

14 Tell the RN that you completed the procedure. *The RN will:*

- *Turn on the oxygen and set the flow rate*

- *Apply the oxygen administration device on the person*

15 Wash your hands.

BOX 21-4

SAFETY RULES FOR OXYGEN THERAPY

- Never remove the device (cannula, mask) used to administer oxygen.
- Make sure the oxygen administration device is secure but not tight.
- Check for signs of irritation from the device. Check behind the ears, under the nose (cannula), and around the face (mask).
- Never shut off oxygen flow from the wall outlet, tank, or oxygen concentrator.
- Do not adjust the flow rate unless allowed by your state and agency.
- Notify the RN immediately if the flow rate is too high or too low.
- Make sure the humidifier is bubbling. Notify the RN immediately if the humidifier is not bubbling.
- Tape connecting tubing to the person's gown. Tubing must be secured in place.
- Make sure there are no kinks in the tubing.
- Make sure the person is not lying on any part of the tubing.
- Report signs and symptoms of hypoxia, respiratory distress, or abnormal breathing patterns to the RN immediately (see Boxes 21-1 and 21-2).
- Give oral hygiene as directed by the RN.
- Make sure the device is clean and free of mucus.
- Maintain an adequate water level in the humidifier.

Oxygen Safety

Remember, you assist the RN with oxygen therapy. You are not responsible for administering oxygen. You do not adjust the flow rate unless allowed by your state and agency. However, you must give safe care to persons receiving oxygen. Box 21-4 lists the rules for assisting with oxygen therapy. Also follow the rules in Box 21-3.

ARTIFICIAL AIRWAYS

Artificial airways keep the airway patent (open). They are used when:

- The airway is obstructed from disease, injury, secretions, or aspiration
- The person is semiconscious or unconscious
- The person is recovering from anesthesia
- The person needs mechanical ventilation (see p. 532)

Intubation is the process of inserting an artificial airway. Usually plastic, disposable airways are used. They come in adult, pediatric, and infant sizes. The following airways are common:

- **Oropharyngeal airway**—is inserted through the mouth and into the pharynx (Fig. 21-21, A). An RN can insert the airway.
- **Nasopharyngeal airway**—is inserted through a nostril and into the pharynx (Fig. 21-21, B). An RN can insert the airway.

- **Endotracheal tube**—is inserted through the mouth or nose and into the trachea (Fig. 21-21, C). A doctor or RN with special training intubates using a lighted scope. A balloon (called a *cuff*) at the end of the tube is inflated to keep the airway in place.
- **Tracheostomy tube**—is inserted through a surgical incision (*ostomy*) into the trachea (*tracheo*) (Fig. 21-21, D). Some tracheostomy tubes have cuffs. The cuff is inflated to keep the tube in place. The tracheostomy is done by a doctor.

You assist the RN in caring for persons with an artificial airway. The person's vital signs are checked often. The person is observed for hypoxia and other respiratory signs and symptoms. If an airway comes out or is dislodged, tell the RN immediately. The person needs frequent oral hygiene. The RN tells you when and how to perform oral hygiene.

Talking is hard with oropharyngeal and nasopharyngeal airways. Persons with endotracheal tubes cannot speak. Some tracheostomy tubes allow the person to speak. Paper and pencils, Magic Slates, communication boards, and hand signals are ways to communiate.

Gagging and choking sensations are common with artificial airways. Imagine something in your mouth, nose, or throat. The person needs comforting and reassurance. Remind the person that the airway helps breathing. Use touch to show you care.

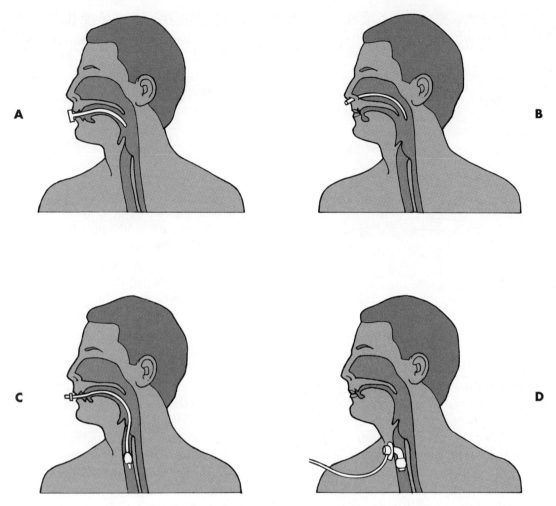

Fig. 21-21 *Artificial airways.* **A,** *Oropharyngeal airway.* **B,** *Nasopharyngeal airway.* **C,** *Endo-tracheal tube.* **D,** *Tracheostomy tube.*

Tracheostomies

Tracheostomies are temporary or permanent. They are temporary when the person requires mechanical ventilation (see p. 532). They are permanent when airway structures are surgically removed. Some cancers require removing airway structures. Sometimes a permanent tracheostomy is required when severe trauma injures the airway. (See Focus on Children.)

Tracheostomy tubes are made of plastic or metal. A tracheostomy tube has three parts (Fig. 21-22, p. 518): the outer tube, the inner tube, and the obturator. *Cannula* is another word for tube. The inner and outer tubes are often called the inner and outer cannulas.

The obturator has a rounded end. It is used to insert the outer cannula. After the outer cannula is inserted, the obturator is removed. (The obturator is placed within easy reach in case the tracheostomy tube falls out and needs to be reinserted. It is taped to the wall or bedside

focus on

CHILDREN

Some children are born with congenital defects. (*Congenitus* is a Latin word that means *to be born with.*) Therefore congenital defects are present at birth. Tracheostomies are needed for some congenital defects affecting the neck and airway. Some infections cause airway structures to swell. This obstructs airflow. Foreign body aspiration also obstructs airflow. These situations can require emergency tracheostomies.

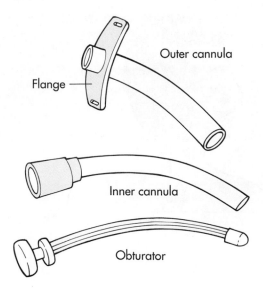

Fig. 21-22 *Parts of a tracheostomy tube.*

stand.) The inner cannula is inserted and locked in place. The outer cannula is secured in place with ties around the person's neck or a Velcro collar. The inner cannula is removed for cleaning and mucus removal. This keeps the airway patent. The outer cannula is not removed.

Some plastic tracheostomy tubes do not have inner cannulas. These are used for persons who are suctioned often. With frequent suctioning, mucus does not stick to the cannula.

The cuffed tracheostomy tube provides a seal between the cannula and the trachea (see Fig. 21-21, *D*). This type is used with mechanical ventilation. The cuff prevents air from leaking around the tube. It also prevents aspiration. The RN or respiratory therapist inflates and deflates the cuff.

Securing tracheostomy tubes in place is important. The tube must not come out (extubation). If not secured properly, the tube could come out with coughing or if pulled on. Damage to the airway is possible if the tube is loose and moves up and down in the trachea.

The tracheostomy tube must remain patent (open). Some persons can cough secretions up and out of the tracheostomy. Others require suctioning (see p. 524).

Measures are needed to prevent aspiration. Nothing can enter the stoma. Otherwise the person can aspirate. The RN teaches the person and family the following:

- Make sure dressings do not have loose gauze or lint.
- Keep the stoma or tube covered when outside. Wear a stoma cover, scarf, or shirt or blouse that buttons at the neck. The cover prevents dust, insects, and other small particles from entering the stoma.

- Take tub baths instead of showers. If showers are taken, wear a shower guard and use a hand-held nozzle. Direct water away from the stoma.
- Be careful when shampooing. Ask another person to help you.
- Cover the stoma when shaving.
- Do not swim. Water will enter the tube or stoma.
- Wear a medical alert bracelet. Also carry a medical alert ID card.

✦ *Tracheostomy care*

Tracheostomy care involves cleaning the inner cannula, cleaning the stoma, and applying clean ties or Velcro collar. Cleaning the inner cannula removes mucus. This keeps the airway patent. A clean stoma and clean ties or collar help prevent infection at the tracheostomy site. Cleaning the stoma also helps prevent skin breakdown.

Some inner cannulas are disposable. They are used once and then discarded. The inner cannula is not cleaned. A new one is inserted.

The RN tells you when to do tracheostomy care. It may be done daily or every 8 to 12 hours. Tracheostomy care is done when there are excess secretions, the ties or collar is soiled, or the dressing is soiled or moist. A co-worker assists you. When the ties are removed, your co-worker holds the outer cannula in place. *If a co-worker is not available, do not remove the old ties or Velcro collar until you secure the new ones in place.* Ties or collar must be secure but not tight. A finger should slide under the ties or collar (Fig. 21-23).

Some states let assistive personnel give tracheostomy care when the stoma is permanent and healed. Before giving tracheostomy care, make sure that:

- Your state allows assistive personnel to perform the procedure
- The procedure is in your job description
- You have the necessary training
- You are familiar with the equipment
- You review the procedure with an RN
- An RN is available to answer questions and to supervise you

Call for the RN if the person shows signs and symptoms of hypoxia or respiratory distress during the procedure. Also call the RN if the outer cannula comes out during the procedure.

(See Focus on Children and Focus on Home Care.)

Text continued on p. 524

CHILDREN

As with adults, the ties must be secure but not tight. Only a fingertip should slide under the ties (see Fig. 21-23, *B*). Ties are too loose if you can slide your whole finger under them.

The tracheostomy care procedure is done with the help of a co-worker. The co-worker holds the child still. Your co-worker also positions the child's head so that the neck is slightly extended.

HOME CARE

A family member can help you during the procedure. Explain the procedure and what you want the family member to do.

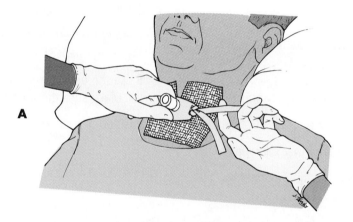

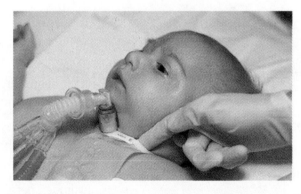

Fig. 21-23 *A, A finger is inserted under the ties.* **B,** *For children, only a fingertip is inserted under the ties.* (**B** *from Wong DL:* Whaley & Wong's nursing care of infants and children, *ed 5, St Louis, 1995, Mosby.*)

GIVING TRACHEOSTOMY CARE

PROCEDURE ALERT

- Does your state allow assistive personnel to perform the procedure?

- Is the procedure in your job description?

- Do you have the necessary training and education?

- Is an RN available to answer questions and to supervise you?

PRE-PROCEDURE

1 Review the procedure with the RN.

2 Ask a co-worker to help you. Explain what you want him or her to do.

3 Explain the procedure to the patient.

4 Wash your hands.

5 Collect the following (some may be in a tracheostomy kit):

- Tracheostomy suction supplies (see p. 529)

- Sterile tracheostomy dressing

- Three sterile 4 × 4 gauze square packages

- Hydrogen peroxide

- Sterile saline (to clean the inner cannula)

- Three sterile cotton swab packages

- Sterile basin (to clean the inner cannula)

- Sterile brush (to clean the inner cannula)

- Tracheostomy ties or Velcro collar

- Disposable inner cannula (check with the RN)

- Scissors

- Sterile gloves (two pairs)

- Cotton twill tape

- Face shield

- Towel

6 Arrange supplies on the overbed table.

7 Identify the person. Check the ID bracelet against the assignment sheet. Provide for privacy.

8 Raise the bed to a level for good body mechanics. Make sure the far bed rail is up.

9 Position the patient supine or in Fowler's position.

PROCEDURE

10 Suction the tracheostomy tube (see *Suctioning a Tracheostomy*, p. 529). Remember to wear a face shield.

11 Prepare a sterile field on the overbed table:

  a Open two sterile 4 × 4 gauze packages.

  b Open two sterile swab packages.

  c Pour sterile saline onto one sterile 4 × 4 gauze package and one sterile swab package.

  d Pour hydrogen peroxide onto one sterile 4 × 4 gauze package and one sterile swab package.

  e Open the sterile tracheostomy dressing package.

  f Open the sterile basin. Pour hydrogen peroxide into the basin. The peroxide should be about 3/4-inch deep in the basin.

  g Open the sterile brush package.

12 Put on the sterile gloves.

13 Remove the inner cannula:

  a Unlock the inner cannula with your nondominant hand. Turn the lock counterclockwise. (This hand is now contaminated.)

  b Pull the inner cannula toward you with your nondominant hand.

  c Drop the inner cannula into the basin with hydrogen peroxide. Or discard the cannula if it is disposable.

PROCEDURE—cont'd

14 Clean the inner cannula. Go to step 15 if using a disposable inner cannula.

   a Clean the inside and outside of the cannula with the sterile brush (Fig. 21-24, p. 522). Use your dominant hand to clean with the brush.

   b Check the cannula to make sure all secretions and crusts are removed.

   c Pick up the bottle of sterile saline with your nondominant hand.

   d Hold the cannula over the basin with hydrogen peroxide. (Use your dominant hand.)

   e Pour sterile saline over the inner cannula.

   f Tap the inner cannula against the inside of the sterile basin. This removes excess fluid to prevent aspiration.

15 Suction the outer cannula if secretions are present (see *Suctioning a Tracheostomy*, p. 529).

16 Replace the inner cannula with your dominant hand. Follow the direction of the tube's curve (Fig. 21-25, p. 522).

17 Lock the inner cannula in place. Turn the lock clockwise to an upright position.

18 Clean the flange of the outer cannula with your dominant hand. Use sterile swabs and sterile 4 × 4 gauze moistened with hydrogen peroxide (Fig. 21-26, p. 523). Use a new swab or gauze square for each stroke. *Make sure fluid does not enter the stoma.*

19 Remove the tracheostomy dressing with your nondominant hand.

20 Clean under the stoma. Clean in circular motions away from the stoma (see p. 675). Use sterile swabs and sterile 4 × 4 gauze moistened with hydrogen peroxide. Use one swab or gauze square for each stroke. *Make sure fluid does not enter the stoma.*

21 Rinse the flange and under the stoma. Rinse outward from the stoma using sterile swabs and sterile 4 × 4 gauze moistened with sterile saline. *Make sure fluid does not enter the stoma.*

22 Pat dry the area around the stoma and the flange. Use the dry sterile swabs and the dry sterile 4 × 4 dressing.

23 Ask your co-worker to put on sterile gloves.

24 Have your co-worker hold the tracheostomy tube in place. The tube is held in place for steps 25–27.

25 Cut the ties, or remove the Velcro collar following the manufacturer's instructions.

26 Change the ties, or apply a new Velcro collar. Follow the manufacturer's instructions for applying the collar. Change ties as follows:

   a Cut a length of twill tape about 24 to 30 inches long for the ties. Cut the tape longer if the person has a large neck.

   b Insert one end of the tie through the eyelet on the flange of the outer cannula (Fig. 21-27, p. 523).

   c Slide the ends of the tie under the person's neck.

   d Bring the ends of the ties around to the eyelet on the other side of the flange.

   e Insert one tie through the eyelet.

   f Pull the ties so they are snug but not tight. You should be able to place a finger under the tie (see Fig. 21-23).

   g Tie the ties with two square knots at the side of the person's neck.

27 Apply the sterile tracheostomy dressing under the flange and clean ties (Fig. 21-28, p. 523). Check the dressing for loose gauze and lint. Get a new dressing if necessary.

28 Ask your co-worker to let go of the outer cannula. Thank your co-worker for helping you.

29 Remove and discard the gloves and face shield.

Continued

GIVING TRACHEOSTOMY CARE—cont'd

POST-PROCEDURE

30 Make sure the person is comfortable.

31 Place the call bell within reach.

32 Lower the bed to its lowest horizontal position.

33 Raise or lower bed rails as instructed by the RN.

34 Unscreen the person.

35 Make sure that an extra tracheostomy tube is at the bedside. It must be the correct size for the person.

36 Empty the sterile basin.

37 Cap the hydrogen peroxide and saline bottles. Mark the date and time on each bottle. Store the bottle according to agency policy.

38 Discard used supplies and equipment according to agency policy.

39 Report your observations to the RN:

- The amount of secretions suctioned

- The color and consistency of secretions (see Box 21-2)

- The condition of the stoma and the skin around it

- How the person tolerated the procedure

- Any other observations

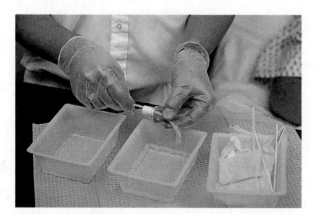

Fig. 21-24 *Clean the inner cannula with the brush. (From Elkin MK, Perry AG, Potter PA: Nursing interventions and clinical skills, St Louis, 1996, Mosby.)*

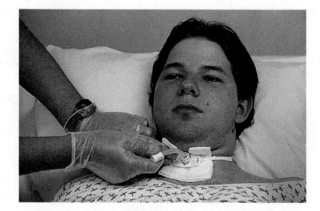

Fig. 21-25 *The inner cannula is replaced. (From Elkin MK, Perry AG, Potter PA: Nursing interventions and clinical skills, St Louis, 1996, Mosby.)*

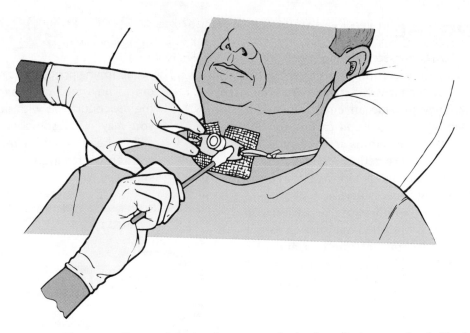

Fig. 21-26 *The outer flange of the tracheostomy tube is cleaned. A co-worker holds the tracheostomy tube in place as in step 24.*

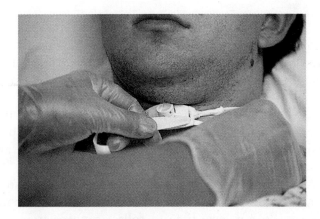

Fig. 21-27 *The tie is inserted through an eyelet on the flange. Note that the old ties are still in place when you perform the procedure by yourself. (From Elkin MK, Perry AG, Potter PA:* Nursing interventions and clinical skills, *St Louis, 1996, Mosby.)*

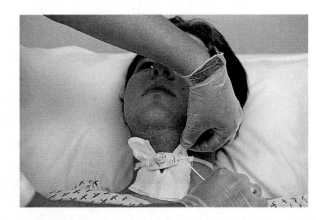

Fig. 21-28 *The tracheostomy dressing is applied under the flange and clean ties. (From Elkin MK, Perry AG, Potter PA:* Nursing interventions and clinical skills, *St Louis, 1996, Mosby.)*

SUCTIONING THE AIRWAY

Injury and illness often cause secretions to collect in the upper airway. Removing the secretions is necessary so air can flow into and out of the airway. Retained secretions obstruct the airway. They provide an environment for microbes and interfere with oxygen and carbon dioxide exchange. Hypoxia occurs if secretions are not removed. Usually coughing removes the secretions. Sometimes the person cannot cough or the cough is too weak to remove secretions. Then suctioning is necessary.

Suction is the process of withdrawing or sucking up fluid (secretions). A tube is connected to a suction source (wall outlet or suction machine) at one end and to a suction catheter at the other end. The catheter is inserted into the airway. Secretions are withdrawn through the catheter.

States and agencies vary about the role of assistive personnel in airway suctioning. Before you perform suctioning procedures, make sure that:

- Your state allows assistive personnel to perform the procedure
- The task is in your job description
- You know how to use the agency's equipment and supplies
- You review the procedure with the RN before you begin
- An RN is available to answer your questions and to supervise you

Suctioning Routes

The nose, mouth, and pharynx make up the upper airway. The trachea and bronchi are the lower parts of the airway.

The *oropharyngeal* route involves suctioning the mouth *(oral)* and pharynx *(pharyngeal)*. The suction catheter is passed through the mouth and into the pharynx. The *nasopharyngeal* route involves suctioning the nose *(nasal)* and pharynx *(pharyngeal)*. The suction catheter is passed through the nose and into the pharynx. These routes are used for persons who cannot expectorate or swallow secretions after coughing. Some states let assistive personnel do oropharyngeal suctioning.

Lower airway suctioning is done through an endotracheal tube or a tracheostomy tube (see p. 528). Some states allow assistive personnel to suction permanent tracheostomies.

Safety Measures

If not done correctly, suctioning can seriously harm the person. Suctioning removes oxygen from the airway. Therefore the person does not get a fresh supply of oxy-

focus on CHILDREN

Suctioning procedures may frighten children. They need clear explanations about the procedure. As with other procedures, you may need someone to control the child's head and arm movements. A co-worker or family member can hold the child still.

focus on HOME CARE

Agency policies differ about cleaning or changing the suction container. Some change the container every 24 hours. Others require daily cleaning of the container with hot water and soap. Follow agency policies for discarding or cleaning suction catheters, connecting tubing, and containers.

gen during suctioning. Hypoxia and life-threatening complications can arise from the respiratory, cardiovascular, and nervous systems. Cardiac arrest can occur. Infection and injury to the airway's mucous membranes also are possible. You need to understand the principles and safety measures involved in safe suctioning. These are described in Box 21-5.

Always make sure needed suction equipment and supplies are at the bedside. When the person needs suctioning you do not have time to collect supplies from the supply area. (See Focus on Children and Focus on Home Care.)

✦ Oropharyngeal Suctioning

Take no more than 10 to 15 seconds to complete a suction cycle. One complete cycle involves inserting the catheter, suctioning, and removing the catheter. (Hold your breath during the suction cycle. This helps you experience what the person feels during suctioning.)

Some patients have large amounts of thick secretions. The Yankauer suction catheter is often used for these persons (Fig. 21-29). It is larger and stiffer than other suction catheters.

Text continued on p. 528

BOX 21-5

PRINCIPLES AND SAFETY MEASURES FOR SUCTIONING

- Do not suction a person unless the RN tells you to do so. Even if oropharyngeal suctioning or tracheostomy suctioning is included in your job description, the person's condition may require the care of an RN.
- Review the procedure with the RN. Make sure the RN is available if you have questions or have problems.
- Suctioning is done as needed *(prn)*. Coughing and signs and symptoms of respiratory distress signal the need for suctioning. The RN tells you what signs to look for in each person. Suctioning is not done at scheduled intervals.
- Standard Precautions and the Bloodborne Pathogen Standard are followed. Remember, secretions can contain blood and are potentially infectious.
- The mouth is clean, not sterile. Microbes enter the mouth through breathing, eating, and drinking. Sterile technique is not required for oropharyngeal suctioning.
- Sterile technique is used when suctioning a tracheostomy (see Chapter 11).
- Use the catheter size as directed by the RN. Airway injury can occur if the catheter is too large.
- Limit the amount of suction as directed by the RN. Wall suction pressures usually are limited to 80 to 120 mm Hg in adults (80 to 100 mm Hg in children). Injury and complications are possible when suction pressure is too great.
- Do not apply suction while inserting the catheter. When suction is applied, air is sucked out of the person's airway.
- Clear the catheter with water or saline after removal.
- Insert the catheter smoothly. This helps prevent injury to the mucous membranes.
- Pass (insert) a suction catheter no more than 3 times. The risk of injury and hypoxia increases each time the suction catheter is passed.
- Check the person's pulse, respirations, and pulse oximeter before, during, and after the procedure. Also observe the person's level of consciousness. Call for the RN immediately if any of the following occur:
  - A drop in pulse rate or a pulse rate less than 60 beats per minute
  - Irregular cardiac rhythms
  - A drop or rise in blood pressure
  - Respiratory distress
  - A drop in the SpO_2 (see p. 504)

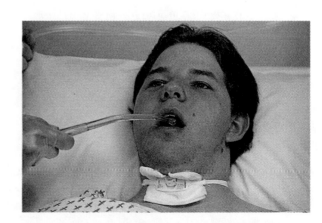

Fig. 21-29 *The Yankauer suction catheter. (From Elkin MK, Perry AG, Potter PA: Nursing interventions and clinical skills, St Louis, 1996, Mosby.)*

OROPHARYNGEAL SUCTIONING

PROCEDURE ALERT

- Does your state allow assistive personnel to perform the procedure?
- Is the procedure in your job description?
- Do you have the necessary training and education?
- Is an RN available to answer questions and to supervise you?

PRE-PROCEDURE

1 Review the procedure with the RN.

2 Wash your hands.

3 Collect the following:

   - Suction catheter (the RN tells you the kind and size)
   - Connecting tubing
   - Water (about 100 ml)
   - Clean basin
   - Suction machine (if no wall outlet suction)
   - Gloves
   - Face shield if the person is likely to cough
   - Towel

4 Identify the person. Check the ID bracelet against the assignment sheet.

5 Explain the procedure to the person.

6 Provide for privacy.

7 Raise the bed for good body mechanics. Make sure the far bed rail is raised.

PROCEDURE

8 Position the person in semi-Fowler's position. Turn his or her head toward you.

9 Place the towel under the person's chin and across the chest.

10 Wash your hands. Make sure both bed rails are raised before leaving the bedside. Lower the rail near you when you return to the person.

11 Put on the gloves. Also put on the face shield if needed.

12 Fill the basin with water.

13 Turn on the suction. The RN tells you what suction pressure to use.

14 Attach the connecting tubing to the wall suction or suction machine.

15 Attach the suction catheter to the connecting tubing (Fig. 21-30).

16 Check equipment function. Suction some water out of the basin.

17 Remove the oxygen mask if the person is using one.

18 Insert the suction catheter into the person's mouth along the gum line to the pharynx (Fig. 21-31).

19 Apply suction as you move the catheter along the gum lines and around the mouth.

20 Remove the catheter.

21 Rinse the catheter and connecting tubing. Rinse by suctioning a small amount of water from the basin.

22 Repeat steps 18–21 no more than two times.

23 Reapply the oxygen mask.

24 Clear the catheter and connecting tubing of secretions. Suction water from the basin until the tubing is clear.

25 Turn off the suction.

26 Disconnect the catheter from the connecting tubing.

27 Follow agency policy for reusing or discarding the catheter and suction container.

28 Remove the towel.

29 Remove and discard your gloves.

OROPHARYNGEAL SUCTIONING—cont'd

POST-PROCEDURE

30 Make sure the person is comfortable. Place the call bell within the person's reach.

31 Lower the bed to its lowest horizontal position. Raise or lower bed rails as instructed by the RN.

32 Unscreen the person.

33 Empty the basin. Follow agency policy for reusing or discarding the basin.

34 Discard used supplies.

35 Wash your hands.

36 Report your observations to the nurse:

- The amount of secretions suctioned

- The color and consistency of secretions (see Box 21-2)

- Signs and symptoms of hypoxia or respiratory distress

- How the person tolerated the procedure

- Any other observations

37 Collect supplies used during the procedure. Replace them at the bedside.

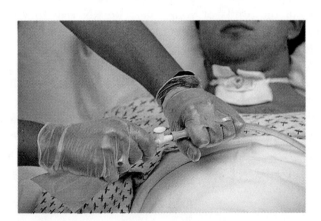

Fig. 21-30 *The suction catheter is attached to the connecting tubing.* (From Elkin MK, Perry AG, Potter PA: Nursing interventions and clinical skills, *St Louis, 1996, Mosby.*)

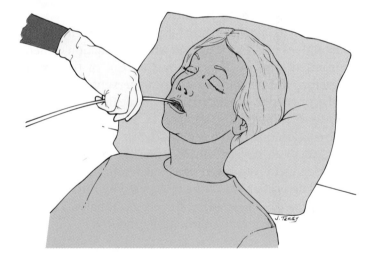

Fig. 21-31 *The suction catheter is inserted along the gum line.*

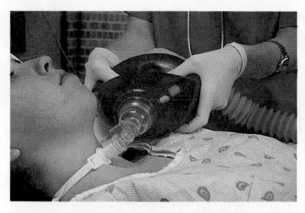

Fig. 21-32 *The Ambu bag. Two hands are used to compressed the bag.*

✦ Tracheostomy Suctioning

When the person is seriously ill or requires mechanical ventilation (see p. 532), you can assist the RN with suctioning the tracheostomy. The RN may ask you to perform the procedure when:

- The person's condition is stable and not likely to change suddenly
- The tracheostomy is healed

Hypoxia is a risk during suctioning. Remember, the person does not receive oxygen when the suction catheter is inserted. Also, suction removes air out of the airway. Therefore the person's lungs are hyperventilated before applying suction. To *hyperventilate* means to give extra (hyper) breaths (ventilate). This is done with a manual resuscitation or Ambu bag (Fig. 21-32). The Ambu bag is attached to an oxygen source. Then the oxygen delivery device is removed from the tracheostomy tube. The Ambu bag is attached to the tracheostomy tube. The bag is compressed (squeezed) as the person inhales. Three to five breaths are given as directed by the RN.

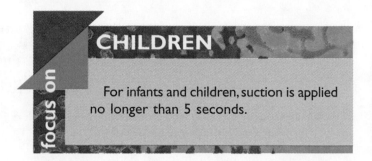

CHILDREN

focus on

For infants and children, suction is applied no longer than 5 seconds.

Both hands are used to compress the Ambu bag. You wear sterile gloves to hold and use the suction catheter. Therefore you cannot touch the Ambu bag. A co-worker is needed to help you. The co-worker uses the Ambu bag during the procedure.

Remember, an oxygen source is attached to the Ambu bag. Oxygen is treated like a drug. Assistive personnel are not allowed to administer drugs. Therefore you need to check if your state and agency allow you to use an Ambu bag attached to an oxygen source. It may be necessary for an RN or respiratory therapist to hyperventilate the lungs during the suction procedure. Remember, it takes two staff members to suction a tracheostomy. By having an RN hyperventilate the lungs, you are doing what your state and job description allow (suctioning). Because the RN administers the oxygen, you are not functioning beyond the limits of your role. The RN is with you if problems arise but is able to do other things while you tend to pre-procedure and post-procedure activities.

Ask the RN about the length of time to apply suction. Some agencies limit suctioning to 10 seconds. Others allow 10 to 15 seconds for the suction cycle (inserting the catheter, applying suction, and removing the catheter). Make sure you clearly understand the RN's directions. You must know the difference between the length time for applying suction and the length of time for the suction cycle. (See Focus on Children.)

Text continued on p. 532

SUCTIONING A TRACHEOSTOMY

PROCEDURE ALERT

- Does your state allow assistive personnel to perform the procedure?
- Is the procedure in your job description?
- Do you have the necessary training and education?
- Is an RN available to answer questions and to supervise you?

PRE-PROCEDURE

1   Review the procedure with the RN.

2   Ask an RN or respiratory therapist to perform the hyperventilation function.

3   Wash your hands.

4   Collect the following:

- Sterile suction catheter (the RN tells you the kind and size)
- Connecting tubing
- Sterile water or sterile saline (about 100 ml)
- Sterile basin
- Suction machine (if no wall outlet suction)
- Sterile gloves
- Face shield
- Sterile drape
- Ambu bag
- Leakproof bag

5   Identify the person. Check the ID bracelet against the assignment sheet.

6   Explain the procedure to the person.

7   Provide for privacy.

8   Arrange equipment on the bedside table.

9   Raise the bed for good body mechanics. Make sure the far bed rail is raised.

PROCEDURE

10   Position the person in semi-Fowler's position. Turn his or her head toward you.

11   Wash your hands. Make sure both bed rails are raised before leaving the bedside. Lower the bed rail near you when you return to the person.

12   Open the sterile towel. Place it across the person's chest.

13   Open the sterile basin.

14   Pour the sterile water or saline into the basin.

15   Turn on the suction. The RN tells you what suction pressure to use.

16   Attach the connecting tubing to the wall suction or suction machine.

17   Open the sterile suction catheter package. Do not let the suction catheter touch any nonsterile surface.

18   Attach the suction catheter to the connecting tubing. Touch only the connecting end of the catheter.

19   Put on the face shield.

20   Put on the sterile gloves.

21   Pick up the suction catheter with your dominant hand. Hold the catheter with your thumb and forefinger.

22   Check equipment function. Suction some water or saline out of the basin.

23   Ask the RN or respiratory therapist to hyperventilate the person's lungs.

24   Insert the suction catheter into the tracheostomy. Insert the catheter until the person coughs or you feel resistance (usually about 6 inches for adults). *Do not apply suction.*

Continued

SUCTIONING A TRACHEOSTOMY—cont'd

PROCEDURE—cont'd

25 Pull the catheter back about ½ inch (1 to 2 cm). *Do not apply suction.*

26 Apply suction intermittently for no more than 10 seconds (5 seconds in children). Intermittent suction means that you alternate covering and uncovering the thumb port (Fig. 21-33). Use your nondominant hand to cover and uncover the thumb port.

27 Rotate the catheter, and slowly withdraw it as you apply intermittent suction. Rotate the catheter by rolling it between your thumb and forefinger (see Fig. 21-33).

28 Remove the catheter after 10 seconds. Release the suction by uncovering the thumb port.

29 Ask the RN or respiratory therapist to hyper-ventilate the person's lungs.

30 Rinse the catheter and connecting tubing. Rinse by suctioning a small amount of water from the basin.

31 Wait 1 to 3 minutes before repeating steps 23-30. Repeat the steps no more than two times.

32 Ask the RN or respiratory therapist to connect the oxygen delivery device to the tracheostomy.

33 Clear the catheter and connecting tubing of secretions. Suction water or saline from the basin until the tubing is clear.

34 Disconnect the catheter from the connecting tubing.

35 Roll the catheter into a ball in your hand, or wrap it around your gloved hand.

36 Remove the sterile glove on the hand holding the catheter. The catheter is inside the glove as the glove is pulled off.

37 Put the glove with the catheter in your other hand.

38 Pull the glove over the glove in your hand.

39 Discard the gloves and catheter into a leak-proof bag.

40 Turn off the suction.

41 Remove the sterile towel. Discard it into the leakproof bag.

POST-PROCEDURE

42 Make sure the person is comfortable. Place the call bell within the person's reach.

43 Lower the bed to its lowest horizontal position. Raise or lower bed rails as instructed by the RN.

44 Unscreen the person.

45 Disconnect the Ambu bag from the oxygen source.

46 Empty the basin. Follow agency policy for repro-cessing or discarding the basin.

47 Remove and discard the face shield.

48 Wash your hands.

49 Report your observations to the nurse:

- The amount of secretions suctioned

- The color and consistency of secretions (see Box 21-2)

- Signs and symptoms of hypoxia or respiratory distress

- How the person tolerated the procedure

- Any other observations

50 Collect supplies used during the procedure. Re-place them at the bedside. Make sure a sterile tracheostomy tube is at the bedside. It must be the correct size for the person.

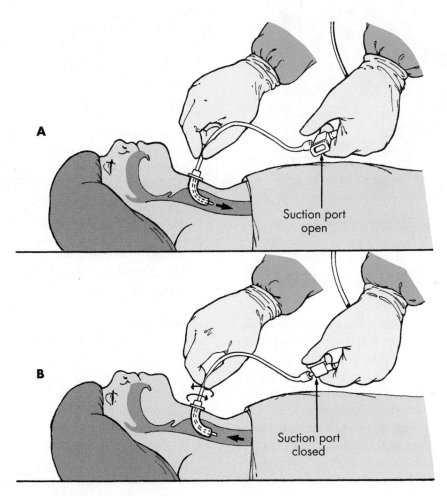

Fig. 21-33 *Intermittent suction is applied.* **A,** *The thumb port is uncovered.* **B,** *The thumb port is covered.* *(From Wong DL:* Whaley & Wong's nursing care of infants and children, *ed 5, St Louis, 1995, Mosby.)*

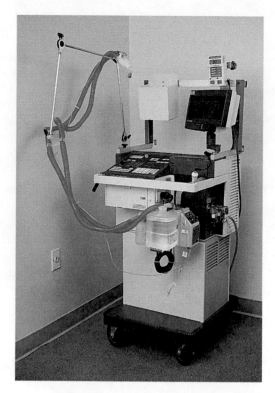

Fig. 21-34 *A mechanical ventilator.*

MECHANICAL VENTILATION

Weak muscle effort, airway obstruction, and damaged lung tissue cause hypoxia. Central nervous system diseases and injuries can affect the respiratory center in the brain. Nerve damage can interfere with messages being sent between the lungs and the brain. Drug overdose can depress the brain. These and other respiratory problems are so severe that some patients cannot breathe on their own. Or they cannot maintain enough oxygen in the blood. These persons often need mechanical ventilation. **Mechanical ventilation** is using a machine to move air into and out of the lungs (Fig. 21-34). Oxygen enters the lungs, and carbon dioxide leaves the lungs.

Persons on mechanical ventilation have artificial airways. Depending on the person's problems, an endotracheal tube or tracheostomy tube is used. You assist the RN with the person's care.

Ventilators have alarms that warn when something is wrong. One alarm is for when the person gets disconnected from the ventilator. *When any alarm sounds, first check to see if the person's endotracheal tube or tracheostomy tube is attached to the ventilator. If it is disconnected, attach the tube to the ventilator.* Then notify the RN immediately about the alarm. Do not reset alarms. Remember, the person is on a ventilator because of respiratory difficulties. The person can die if not connected to the ventilator.

Persons needing mechanical ventilation are seriously ill. They often have other problems and injuries. Their reactions to mechanical ventilation are many. Some are confused, disoriented, or unable to think clearly. Many are frightened by the machine and fear dying. Some feel relief when their bodies get enough oxygen. Many fear having to remain on the machine for life. Mechanical ventilation can be painful for those with chest injuries or chest surgery. Tubes and hoses restrict movement, adding to the person's discomfort.

The RN may ask you to assist with the person's care. The following are important aspects of the person's care:

- Keep the call bell within the person's reach.
- Make sure there is enough slack on hoses and connecting tubing. They should not pull on the endotracheal or tracheostomy tube.
- Answer call bells promptly. Remember, the person depends on others for basic needs.
- Explain who you are and what you are going to do whenever you enter the room.
- Orient the person to day, date, and time.
- Tell the RN immediately if the person shows signs of respiratory distress or discomfort.
- Do not change any settings on the ventilator or reset alarms.
- Provide a means of communication. Remember, the person on mechanical ventilation cannot talk.
- Use established hand or eye signals for "yes" and "no." All health team members (nursing staff, doctors, respiratory therapists, and others) and the family must use the same signals. Otherwise, communication does not occur.
- Ask questions that have simple answers. The person may not have the strength to write out long responses.
- Be careful what you say when within the person's hearing distance. The person may pay close attention to what is being said. Do not say anything that could upset the person.
- Watch your nonverbal communication. Although seriously ill and unable to speak, the person may be very aware of nonverbal messages. Avoid communicating worry and concern to the person.
- Take time to comfort and reassure the person. Tell the person what you are going to do and why. Also tell the person about such things as the weather, pleasant news events, and gifts and cards.
- Meet the person's basic needs for personal and oral hygiene, elimination, and activity (repositioning, range-of-motion exercises, sitting in a chair) as directed by the RN.

- Apply a moist washcloth or lubricant to the person's lips as directed by the RN. This helps prevent the lips from drying and cracking.
- Use touch to reassure and comfort the person.
- Tell the person when you are leaving the room and when you will be back.

(See Focus on Long-Term Care and Focus on Home Care.)

CHEST TUBES

When the chest is entered, air, blood, or fluid can collect in the pleural space (sac or cavity). Chest entry occurs with chest surgery or injury. **Pneumothorax** is the collection of air *(pneumo)* in the pleural space *(thorax)*. **Hemothorax** is the collection of blood *(hemo)* in the pleural space *(thorax)*. **Pleural effusion** is the collection of fluid (effusion) in the pleural space.

Pressure caused by the collection of air, blood, or fluid collapses the lung. Air cannot reach the affected aveoli. O_2 and CO_2 are not exchanged at the alveoli. Respiratory distress and hypoxia result. Sometimes there is pressure on the heart. This affects the heart's ability to pump blood and is a life-threatening problem.

The doctor inserts chest tubes to remove the air, fluid, or blood (Fig. 21-35). The sterile procedure is done in surgery, in the emergency room, or at the bedside. An RN assists with the procedure.

The chest tubes are attached to a drainage system (Fig. 21-36, p. 534). The system must be airtight so that air does not enter the pleural space. Water-seal drainage is used to keep the system airtight (Fig. 21-37, p. 534). This is done as follows:

- A chest tube is attached to connecting tubing.
- Connecting tubing is then attached to a tube in the drainage container.
- The tube in the drainage container extends under water. The water prevents air from entering the chest tube and then the pleural space.

A one-, two-, or three-bottle system or a disposable system is used (see Fig. 21-37). Disposable systems are common. Bottles are shown in Figure 21-37 to give you a clearer understanding of how the system works. Sometimes suction is applied to the drainage system.

When caring for persons with chest tubes, you need to:

- Keep the drainage system below the level of the person's chest.
- Measure the person's vital signs as directed by the RN. Report any changes in vital signs immediately.
- Report signs and symptoms of hypoxia and respiratory distress to the RN immediately. Also report patient complaints of pain or difficulty breathing.

LONG-TERM CARE

focus on

Often patients are taken off the ventilator within hours or days of needing the device. However, some persons need the ventilator for longer periods. These patients may require long-term or subacute care. Often the person needs to be weaned from the ventilator. That is, the person needs to breathe without the ventilator. It may take several weeks to get the person off the ventilator. The respiratory therapist and RN plan the weaning process.

HOME CARE

focus on

Home care is often arranged for ventilator-dependent persons. The RN teaches you how to care for each patient. You may be asked to give tracheostomy care and to suction the person. Family members also are taught how to assist with the person's care. Always make sure that an RN is available by phone when you are in the person's home. Make sure delegated tasks are allowed by your state and agency.

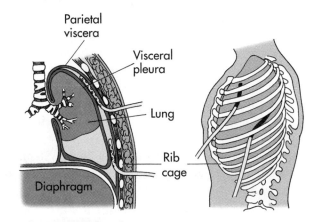

Fig. 21-35 *Chest tubes inserted into the pleural space. (From Elkin MK, Perry AG, Potter PA:* Nursing interventions and clinical skills, *St Louis, 1996, Mosby.)*

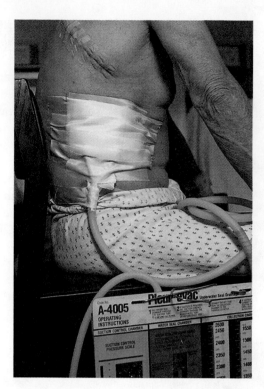

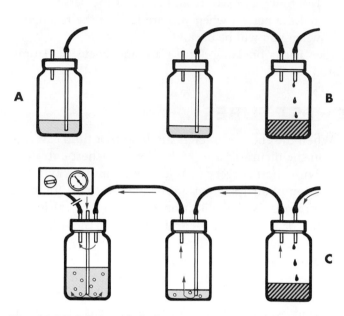

Fig. 21-36 *Chest tubes attached to a disposable water-seal drainage system.* (From Elkin MK, Perry AG, Potter PA: Nursing interventions and clinical skills, *St Louis, 1996, Mosby.*)

Fig. 21-37 *Water-seal drainage system.* **A,** *One-bottle system,* **B,** *Two-bottle system.* **C,** *Three-bottle system.* (From Potter PA, Perry AG: Fundamentals of nursing: concepts, process, and practice, ed 4, St Louis, 1997, Mosby.)

- Keep connecting tubing coiled on the bed. Allow enough slack so the chest tubes are not dislodged when the person moves. If tubing hangs in loops, drainage collects in the loop.
- Make sure the tubing is not kinked. Kinking obstructs the chest tube, causing air, blood, or fluid to collect in pleural space.
- Observe chest drainage. Immediately report to the RN any change in chest drainage. This includes increases in drainage or the appearance of bright red drainage.
- Record chest drainage according to agency policy.
- Turn and position the person as directed by the RN. The person must be turned carefully and gently to prevent the chest tubes from dislodging.
- Assist the person with coughing and deep breathing as directed by the RN. Also assist with incentive spirometry as directed.
- Note bubbling activity in the drainage system. Tell the RN immediately if the bubbling increases, decreases, or stops.

- Tell the RN immediately if any part of the system is loose or disconnected.
- Make sure petrolatum gauze is at the bedside in case a chest tube comes out.
- Call for help immediately if a chest tube comes out. Cover the insertion site with sterile petrolatum gauze. Stay with the person until an RN arrives. Follow the RN's directions.

CARDIOPULMONARY RESUSCITATION

Persons with respiratory injuries and problems are at risk for respiratory and cardiac arrest. Agency policy will require you to be certified in basic life support procedures (see Chapter 35). Such procedures include cardiopulmonary resuscitation. The American Heart Association, National Safety Council, and the American Red Cross have courses in basic life support. Your training program may include one of these courses. They also are available through many community agencies.

REVIEW QUESTIONS

Circle the best answer.

1 Alcohol and narcotics affect oxygen needs because they
   a Depress the brain
   b Are pollutants
   c Cause allergies
   d Cause a pneumothorax

2 Hypoxia is
   a A deficiency of oxygen in the blood
   b The amount of hemoglobin that contains oxygen
   c A deficiency of oxygen in the cells
   d The lack of carbon dioxide

3 One of the earliest signs of hypoxia is
   a Cyanosis
   b Increased pulse and respiratory rates
   c Restlessness
   d Dyspnea

4 A person can breathe deeply and comfortably only while sitting or standing. This is called
   a Biot's respirations
   b Orthopnea
   c Bradypnea
   d Kussmaul's respirations

5 The person will probably need to rest after
   a A chest x-ray
   b A lung scan
   c Arterial blood gases
   d Pulmonary function tests

6 A person has pulse oximetry. The person's SpO_2 is 98%. Which is *true*?
   a The machine is not accurate.
   b The person's pulse is 98 beats per minute.
   c The measurement is within normal range.
   d The person needs suctioning.

7 Which is not a site for a pulse oximetry sensor?
   a Toe   c Earlobe
   b Finger   d Upper arm

8 The best time to collect a sputum specimen is
   a On awakening
   b After meals
   c At bedtime
   d After suctioning

9 Before collecting a sputum specimen, you should
   a Ask the person to use mouthwash
   b Ask the person to rinse the mouth with clear water
   c Ask the person to brush the teeth
   d Apply lubricant to the person's lips

10 You are assisting a person with coughing and deep breathing. Which is *false*?
   a The person inhales through pursed lips.
   b The person needs to be in a comfortable sitting position.
   c The person inhales deeply through the nose.
   d The person holds a small pillow over an incision.

11 Which is useful for deep breathing?
   a Pulse oximeter
   b Incentive spirometry
   c Chest tubes
   d Partial-rebreathing mask

12 You are assisting with oxygen therapy. You can
   a Turn the oxygen on and off
   b Start the oxygen
   c Decide what device to use
   d Make sure the connecting tubing is secure and free of kinks

13 A person has a tracheostomy. Which is *false*?
   a A nondisposable inner cannula is removed for cleaning.
   b The obturator is inserted after the outer cannula.
   c The outer cannula must be secured in place.
   d The person must be protected from aspiration.

14 A person has a tracheostomy. The person can do the following *except*

a Shampoo

b Shave

c Shower with a hand-held nozzle

d Swim

15 You are giving tracheostomy care by yourself. The old ties are removed after

a Removing the inner cannula

b Cleaning the flange and stoma

c Removing the dressing

d Securing the new ties

16 These statements are about oropharyngeal suctioning. Which is *true*?

a Suction is applied while inserting the catheter.

b Suctioning is done every 2 hours.

c A suction cycle is no more than 10 to 15 seconds.

d The mouth is considered sterile.

17 Oropharyngeal suctioning requires

a Following Standard Precautions and the Blood-borne Pathogen Standard

b Sterile technique

c An artificial airway

d All of the above

18 A child has a tracheostomy. Suction is applied no longer than

a 5 seconds

b 5 to 10 seconds

c 10 seconds

d 10 to 15 seconds

19 A person's lungs are hyperventilated before suctioning the tracheostomy. Which is used to hyperventilate the lungs?

a Incentive spirometer

b Pulse oximeter

c Ambu bag

d Partial-rebreathing mask

20 When suctioning a tracheostomy, suction is applied

a Continuously

b Intermittently

c Every 10 seconds

d As directed by the RN

21 During suction procedures, you can insert the catheter no more than

a Two times

b Three times

c Four times

d Five times

22 Mr. Long requires mechanical ventilation. Which is *false*?

a He has an endotracheal tube or a tracheostomy tube.

b The call bell must always be within his reach.

c You should use touch to provide comfort and reassurance.

d You can reset alarms on the ventilator.

REVIEW QUESTIONS—cont'd

23 An alarm sounds on Mr. Long's ventilator. What should you do first?
   a Reset the alarm.
   b Check to see if his airway is attached to the ventilator.
   c Call the nurse immediately.
   d Ask him what is wrong.

24 A person has a pneumothorax. This is the collection of
   a Fluid in the pleural space
   b Blood in the pleural space
   c Air in the pleural space
   d Respiratory secretions in the pleural space

25 A person has chest tubes attached to water-seal drainage. You should do the following *except*
   a Notify the RN if bubbling increases, decreases, or stops
   b Make sure the tubing is not kinked
   c Keep the drainage system below the person's chest
   d Hang tubing in loops

Answers to these questions are on p. 852.

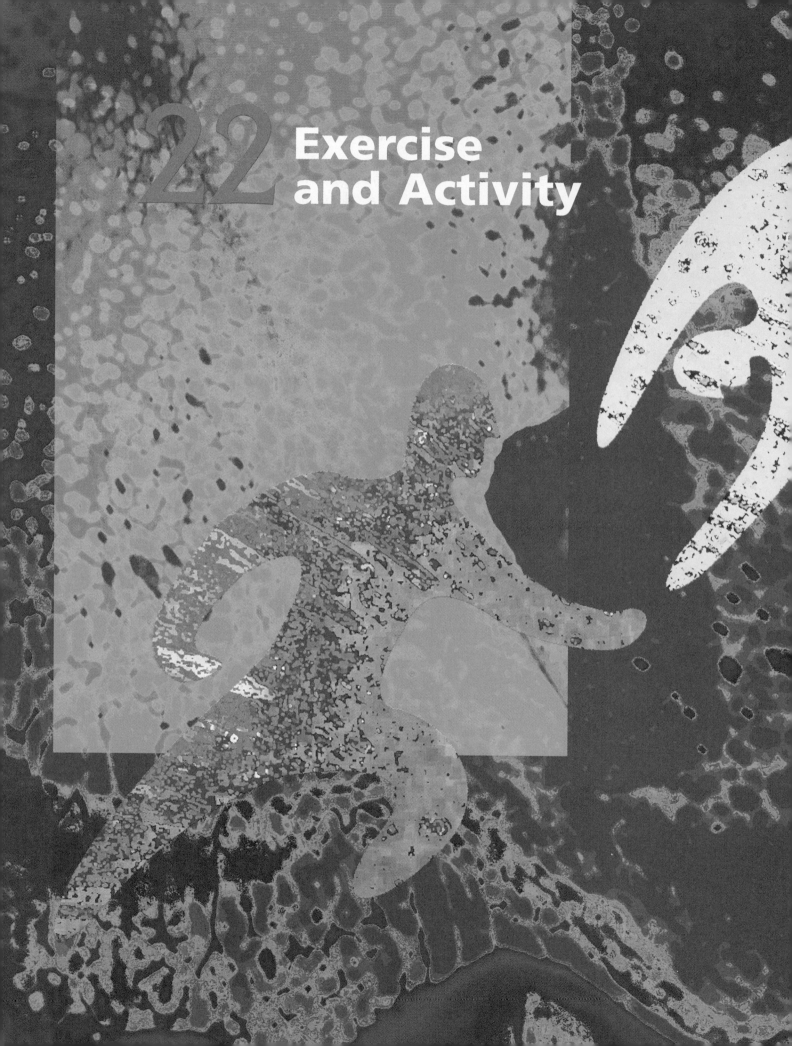

22 Exercise and Activity

- Define the key terms in this chapter
- Describe bedrest
- Describe the complications of bedrest and how to prevent them
- Describe the devices used to support and maintain body alignment
- Explain the purpose of a trapeze
- Describe range-of-motion exercises
- Explain how to help a falling person
- Describe four walking aids
- Perform the procedures described in this chapter

abduction Moving a body part away from the body

adduction Moving a body part toward the body

atrophy A decrease in size or a wasting away of tissue

contracture A condition in which a joint is flexed and fixed in position caused by the abnormal shortening of a muscle

dorsiflexion Bending backward

extension Straightening of a body part

external rotation Turning the joint outward

flexion Bending a body part

footdrop Plantar flexion

hyperextension Excessive straightening of a body part

internal rotation Turning the joint inward

orthostatic hypotension A drop in *(hypo)* blood pressure when the person stands (*ortho* and *static*); postural hypotension

plantar flexion The foot *(plantar)* is bent *(flexion);* footdrop

postural hypotension Orthostatic hypotension

pronation Turning downward

range of motion The movement of a joint to the extent possible without causing pain

supination Turning upward

syncope A brief loss of consciousness; fainting

Being active is important for physical and mental well-being. Most people move about and function without help. However, illnesses, surgery, injuries, and pain cause weakness and some activity limits. Some people are weak from chronic illnesses. Others are in bed for a long time. Some have permanent paralysis. Some disorders are progressive, causing decreases in activity. Examples include multiple sclerosis, Parkinson's disease, arthritis, and nervous system and muscular disorders (see Chapter 30). Inactivity, whether minor or severe, affects the normal function of every body system. Mental well-being is also affected.

RNs use the nursing process to promote exercise and activity in all persons to the extent possible. An RN assesses and plans for the person's need. The nursing care plan includes the person's activity level and needed exercises.

To assist in promoting exercise and activity, you need to understand:

- Bedrest
- How to prevent complications from bedrest
- How to help persons exercise

BEDREST

Bedrest is ordered by the doctor to treat a person's health problem. Generally bedrest is ordered to:

- Reduce physical activity
- Reduce pain
- Encourage rest
- Regain strength
- Promote healing

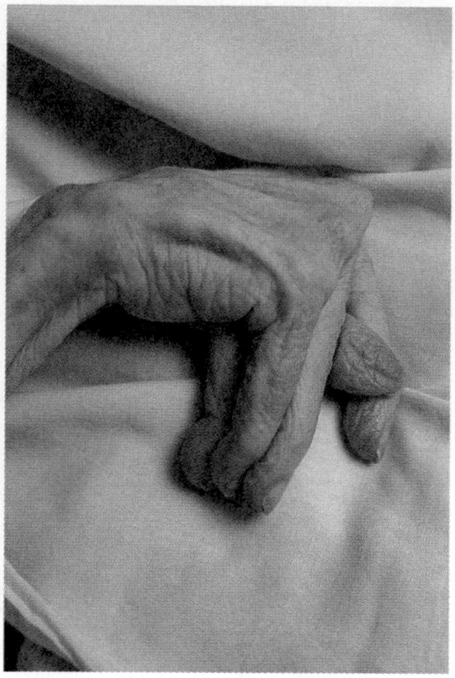

Fig. 22-1 *A contracture.*

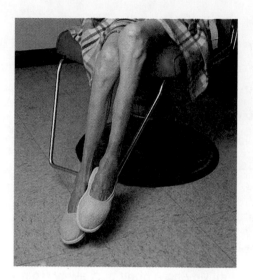

Fig. 22-2 *Muscle atrophy.*

The following types of bedrest are common. Always ask the RN what bedrest means for each patient:

- *Bedrest*—the person remains in bed but some activities of daily living (ADL) are allowed. Self-feeding, oral hygiene, bathing, shaving, and hair care are often allowed.
- *Strict bedrest*—everything is done for the person. No ADL are allowed.
- *Bedrest with commode privileges*—the person can use the bedside commode for elimination needs.
- *Bedrest with bathroom privileges (bedrest with BRP)*—the person can use the bathroom for elimination needs.

Complications of Bedrest

Bedrest and lack of exercise and activity can cause serious complications. Every body system is affected. Pressure ulcers, constipation, and fecal impaction can result. Urinary tract infections, renal calculi (renal stones), and pneumonia (infection of the lung) can occur.

Contractures and muscle atrophy occur in the musculoskeletal system. A **contracture** is a condition in which a joint is flexed and fixed in position caused by the abnormal shortening of a muscle. The contracted muscle is fixed into position, is deformed, and cannot stretch (Fig. 22-1). Common sites are the fingers, wrists, elbows, toes, ankles, knees, and hips. Contractures can occur also in the neck and spine. The person with a contracture is permanently deformed and disabled. **Atrophy** is the decrease in size or the wasting away of tissue. Muscle atrophy is a decrease in size or a wasting away of muscle (Fig. 22-2). These complications must be prevented to maintain normal body movement.

Orthostatic hypotension and blood clots occur in the cardiovascular system. **Orthostatic hypotension** is a drop in *(hypo)* blood pressure when the person stands *(ortho* and *static)*. When a person moves from lying or sitting to a standing position, the blood pressure drops. The person experiences dizziness, weakness, and spots before the eyes. Syncope can occur. **Syncope** (fainting) is a brief loss of consciousness. (Syncope comes from the Greek word *synkoptein,* which means to cut short.) Orthostatic hypotension is also called **postural hypotension.** *(Postural* relates to posture or standing.) Box 22-1 lists the measures that prevent orthostatic hypotension. Slowly changing positions is key.

Complications from bedrest are prevented by good nursing care. Positioning in good body alignment and range-of-motion exercises are important preventive measures. These are part of the person's care plan.

Positioning

Body alignment and positioning were discussed in Chapter 12. Supportive devices are often used to support and maintain the person in a certain position:

BOX 22-1

PREVENTING ORTHOSTATIC HYPOTENSION

- Measure blood pressure when the person is supine. Also count the person's pulse and respirations.
- Raise the head of the bed so the person is in Fowler's position. Raise the head of the bed slowly.
  - Ask the person about weakness, dizziness, or spots before the eyes. Lower the head of the bed if these symptoms occur.
  - Measure blood pressure, pulse, and respirations when the person is in Fowler's position.
  - Keep the person in Fowler's position for a short while. Ask the person about weakness, dizziness, or spots before the eyes.
- Assist the person to sit on the side of the bed (see Chapter 12).
  - Ask the person about weakness, dizziness, or spots before the eyes. Assist the person to Fowler's position if any of these symptoms occur.
  - Measure blood pressure, pulse, and respirations when the person is sitting on the side of the bed.
  - Have the person continue to sit on the side of the bed for a short while.
- Assist the person to stand.
  - Ask the person about weakness, dizziness, or spots before the eyes. Help the person sit on the side of the bed if any of these symptoms occur.
  - Measure blood pressure, pulse, and respirations.
- Help the person sit in a chair or walk as directed by the RN.
  - Ask the person about weakness, dizziness, or spots before the eyes. If the person is walking, help the person to sit if symptoms occur.
  - Measure blood pressure, pulse, and respirations.
- Report blood pressure, pulse, and respirations to the RN. Also report other symptoms.

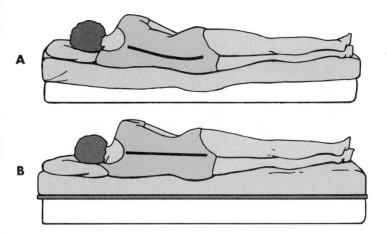
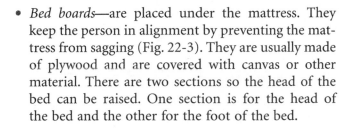

Fig. 22-3 **A,** *Mattress sagging without bed boards.* **B,** *Bed boards are placed under the mattress. No sagging occurs.*

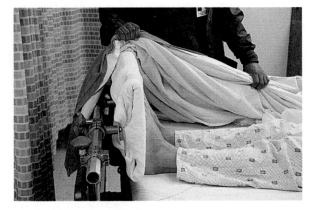

Fig. 22-4 *Footboard. Feet are flush with the board to keep them in normal alignment.*

- *Bed boards*—are placed under the mattress. They keep the person in alignment by preventing the mattress from sagging (Fig. 22-3). They are usually made of plywood and are covered with canvas or other material. There are two sections so the head of the bed can be raised. One section is for the head of the bed and the other for the foot of the bed.

- *Footboards*—are placed at the foot of mattresses (Fig. 22-4). They prevent **plantar flexion (footdrop).** In plantar flexion the foot *(plantar)* is bent *(flexion).* The footboard is placed so the soles of the feet are flush against it. The feet are in good alignment as when standing. Footboards also serve as bed cradles. They keep top linens off the feet.

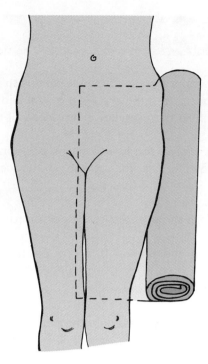

Fig. 22-5 *Trochanter roll made from a bath blanket. It extends from the hip to the knee.*

- *Trochanter rolls*—prevent the hips and legs from turning outward (external rotation) (Fig. 22-5). They are made from bath blankets. A blanket is folded to the desired length and rolled up. The loose end is placed under the person from the hip to the knee. Then the roll is tucked alongside the body. Pillows or sandbags also are used to keep the hips and knees in alignment.
- *Hip abduction wedges*—keep the hips abducted (Fig. 22-6). The wedge is positioned between the person's legs. These are common after hip replacement surgery.
- *Hand rolls or hand grips*—prevent contractures of the thumb, fingers, and wrist. Commercial hand rolls and rolled-up washcloths are common (Fig. 22-7). Foam rubber sponges, rubber balls, and finger cushions (Fig. 22-8) also are used.
- *Splints*—keep the elbows, wrists, thumbs, fingers, ankles, and knees in normal position. They are usually secured in place with Velcro. Some have foam padding (Fig. 22-9).
- *Bed cradles*—keep the weight of top linens off the feet (see Fig. 14-29, p. 327). The weight of top linens can cause footdrop and pressure ulcers.

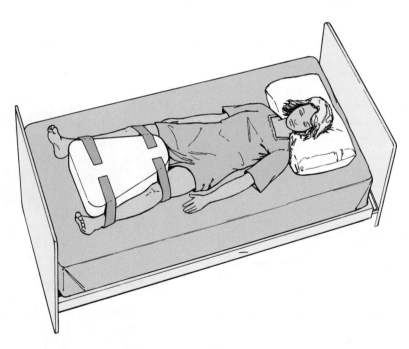

Fig. 22-6 *Hip abduction wedge.*

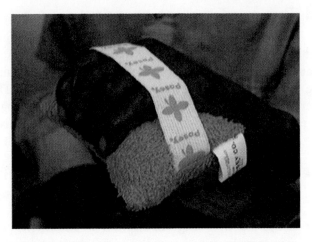

Fig. 22-7 *Hand roll. (Courtesy J. T. Posey Co, Arcadia, Calif.)*

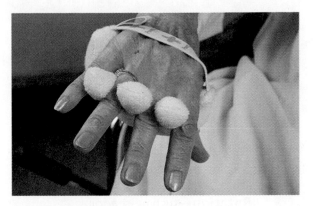

Fig. 22-8 *Finger cushion. (Courtesy J. T. Posey Co, Arcadia, Calif.)*

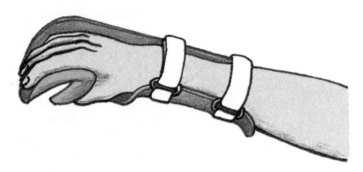

Fig. 22-9 *Splint. (From Birchenall J, Streight, E: Mosby's textbook for the home care aide, St Louis, 1997, Mosby.)*

Exercise

Exercise helps prevent contractures, muscle atrophy, and other complications of bedrest. Some exercise occurs with activities of daily living and when turning and moving in bed without assistance. Additional exercises are needed for muscles and joints.

A trapeze is used for exercises to strengthen arm muscles. The trapeze is suspended from an overbed frame (Fig. 22-10). The person grasps the bar with both hands to lift the trunk off the bed. The trapeze is used also to move up and turn in bed.

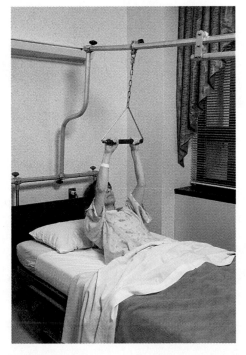

Fig. 22-10 *Trapeze is used to strengthen the arm muscles.*

BOX 22-2

JOINT MOVEMENTS

Abduction—moving a body part away from the body

Adduction—moving a body part toward the body

Extension—straightening a body part

Flexion—bending a body part

Hyperextension—excessive straightening of a body part

Dorsiflexion—bending backward

Rotation—turning the joint

Internal rotation—turning the joint inward

External rotation—turning the joint outward

Pronation—turning downward

Supination—turning upward

✦ *Range-of-motion exercises*

The movement of a joint to the extent possible without causing pain is the **range of motion (ROM)** of that joint. Range-of-motion exercises involve exercising the joints through their complete range of motion. The exercises are usually done at least twice a day. Range-of-motion exercises are active, passive, or active-assistive:

- *Active* range-of-motion exercises are done by the person.
- *Passive* range-of-motion exercises involve having another person move the joints through their range of motion.
- *Active-assistive* range of motion is when the person does the exercises with some help from another person.

Range-of-motion exercises naturally occur during activities of daily living. Bathing, hair care, eating, reaching, and walking all involve joint movements. Persons on bedrest have little activity. Therefore range-of-motion exercises are done. The RN tells you which joints to exercise and if the exercises are to be active, passive, or active-assistive. Box 22-2 describes the movements involved in range-of-motion exercises.

Range-of-motion exercises can cause injury if not done properly. Muscle strain, joint injury, and pain are possible. The rules in Box 22-3 are practiced when performing or assisting with range-of-motion exercises. (See Focus on Children and Focus on Long-Term Care.)

Text continued on p. 554

BOX 22-3

RULES FOR PERFORMING RANGE-OF-MOTION EXERCISES

- Exercise only the joints the RN tells you to exercise.
- Expose only the body part being exercised.
- Use good body mechanics.
- Support the extremity being exercised.
- Move the joint slowly, smoothly, and gently.
- Do not force a joint beyond its present range of motion or to the point of pain.
- *Perform range-of-motion exercises to the neck only if allowed by agency policy.* In some agencies neck exercises are done only by physical therapists or occupational therapists. This is because of the danger of neck injuries.

CHILDREN

Depending on the child's activity limits, almost any play activity promotes active range-of-motion exercises in children. Some examples are:

- Kicking a Mylar balloon or foam rubber ball
- Playing "pat-a-cake" and having the child clap, kick, jump, or do other motions
- Playing basketball using a wastebasket and a foam rubber ball or wadded paper
- Playing video games for finger and hand movements
- Playing with finger paints, clay, or play dough
- Having tricycle or wheelchair races
- Playing "hide and seek" by hiding a toy in the bed or room

Always check with the RN for the child's activity limits.

(Modified from Wong, DL: *Whaley and Wong's nursing care of infants and children,* ed 5, St Louis, 1995, Mosby.)

LONG-TERM CARE

The Omnibus Budget Reconciliation Act of 1987 (OBRA) requires activity programs for residents. Recreational activities are important for the physical and mental well-being of older persons. Joints and muscles are exercised, and circulation is stimulated. Recreational activities also provide social opportunities and are mentally stimulating.

The activities must meet the interests and physical, mental, and psychosocial needs of each resident. Bingo, movies, dances, exercise groups, shopping trips, museum trips, concerts, and guest speakers are often arranged. Some centers have gardening activities.

The right to personal choice is protected. The resident chooses which activities to take part in. OBRA requires that activities promote physical, intellectual, social, and emotional well-being. Well-being is promoted when the resident attends activities of personal choice. The resident must not be forced to take part in an activity that has no interest for him or her.

Residents may need help getting to an activity. Some also need help in participating. You must provide assistance as necessary.

PERFORMING RANGE-OF-MOTION EXERCISES

PRE-PROCEDURE

1 Identify the person. Check the ID bracelet against the assignment sheet.

2 Explain the procedure to the person.

3 Wash your hands.

4 Obtain a bath blanket.

5 Provide for privacy.

6 Raise the bed to the best level for good body mechanics.

PROCEDURE

7 Lower the bed rails.

8 Position the person supine and in good alignment.

9 Cover the person with a bath blanket. Fanfold top linens to the foot of the bed.

10 Exercise the neck *if allowed by your agency and if the RN instructs you to do so* (Fig. 22-11, p. 549):

  a Place your hands over the person's ears to support the head.

  b Flexion—bring the head forward so the chin touches the chest.

  c Extension—straighten the head.

  d Hyperextension—bring the head backward until the chin is pointing up.

  e Rotation—turn the head from side to side.

  f Lateral flexion—move the head to the right and to the left.

  g Repeat flexion, extension, hyperextension, rotation, and lateral flexion five times.

11 Exercise the shoulder (Fig. 22-12, p. 550):

  a Grasp the wrist with one hand and the elbow with the other.

  b Flexion—raise the arm straight in front and over the head.

  c Extension—bring the arm down to the side.

  d Hyperextension—move the arm behind the body. (This can be done if the person is standing or sitting in a straight-back chair.)

  e Abduction—move the straight arm away from the side of the body.

  f Adduction—move the straight arm to the side of the body.

  g Internal rotation—bend the elbow and place it at the same level as the shoulder. Move the forearm down toward the body.

  h External rotation—move the forearm toward the head.

  i Repeat flexion, extension, hyperextension, abduction, adduction, and internal and external rotations five times.

PERFORMING RANGE-OF-MOTION EXERCISES—cont'd

PROCEDURE—cont'd

12 Exercise the elbow (Fig. 22-13, p. 551):

  a Grasp the person's wrist with one hand and the elbow with the other.

  b Flexion—bend the arm so the same-side shoulder is touched.

  c Extension—straighten the arm.

  d Repeat flexion and extension five times.

13 Exercise the forearm (Fig. 22-14, p. 551):

  a Pronation—turn the hand so the palm is down.

  b Supination—turn the hand so the palm is up.

  c Repeat pronation and supination five times.

14 Exercise the wrist (Fig. 22-15, p. 551):

  a Hold the wrist with both of your hands.

  b Flexion—bend the hand down.

  c Extension—straighten the hand.

  d Hyperextension—bend the hand back.

  e Radial flexion—turn the hand toward the thumb.

  f Ulnar flexion—turn the hand toward the little finger.

  g Repeat flexion, extension, hyperextension, and radial and ulnar flexions five times.

15 Exercise the thumb (Fig. 22-16, p. 551):

  a Hold the person's hand with one hand and the thumb with your other hand.

  b Abduction—move the thumb out from the inner part of the index finger.

  c Adduction—move the thumb back next to the index finger.

  d Opposition—touch each fingertip with the thumb.

  e Flexion—bend the thumb into the hand.

  f Extension—move the thumb out to the side of the fingers.

  g Repeat flexion, extension, abduction, adduction, and opposition five times.

16 Exercise the fingers (Fig. 22-17, p. 552):

  a Abduction—spread the fingers and the thumb apart.

  b Adduction—bring the fingers and thumb together.

  c Extension—straighten the fingers so the fingers, hand, and arm are straight.

  d Flexion—make a fist.

  e Repeat abduction, adduction, extension, and flexion five times.

Continued

PERFORMING RANGE-OF-MOTION EXERCISES—cont'd

PROCEDURE—cont'd

17 Exercise the hip (Fig. 22-18, p. 552):

   a Place one hand under the knee and the other under the ankle to support the leg.

   b Flexion—raise the leg.

   c Extension—straighten the leg.

   d Abduction—move the leg away from the body.

   e Adduction—move the leg toward the other leg.

   f Internal rotation—turn the leg inward.

   g External rotation—turn the leg outward.

   h Repeat flexion, extension, abduction, adduction, and internal and external rotations five times.

18 Exercise the knee (Fig. 22-19, p. 553):

   a Place one hand under the knee and the other under the ankle to support the leg.

   b Flexion—bend the leg.

   c Extension—straighten the leg.

   d Repeat flexion and extension of the knee five times.

19 Exercise the ankle (Fig. 22-20, p. 553):

   a Place one hand under the foot and the other under the ankle to support the part.

   b Dorsiflexion—pull the foot forward and push down on the heel at the same time.

   c Plantar flexion—turn the foot down or point the toes.

   d Repeat dorsiflexion and plantar flexion five times.

20 Exercise the foot (Fig. 22-21, p. 553):

   a Pronation—turn the outside of the foot up and the inside down.

   b Supination—turn the inside of the foot up and the outside down.

   c Repeat pronation and supination five or six times.

21 Exercise the toes (Fig. 22-22, p. 553):

   a Flexion—curl the toes.

   b Extension—straighten the toes.

   c Abduction—spread the toes apart.

   d Adduction—pull the toes together.

   e Repeat flexion, extension, abduction, and adduction five times.

22 Cover the leg, and raise the bed rail.

23 Go to the other side. Lower the bed rail.

24 Repeat steps 11 through 21.

PERFORMING RANGE-OF-MOTION EXERCISES—cont'd

POST-PROCEDURE

25 Make sure the person is comfortable.

26 Cover the person. Remove the bath blanket.

27 Raise or lower bed rails as instructed by the RN.

28 Lower the bed to its lowest level.

29 Place the call bell within reach.

30 Unscreen the person.

31 Return the bath blanket to its proper place.

32 Wash your hands.

33 Report the following to the nurse:

- The time the exercises were performed

- The joints exercised

- The number of times the exercises were performed on each joint

- Any complaints of pain or signs of stiffness or spasm

- The degree to which the person participated in the exercises

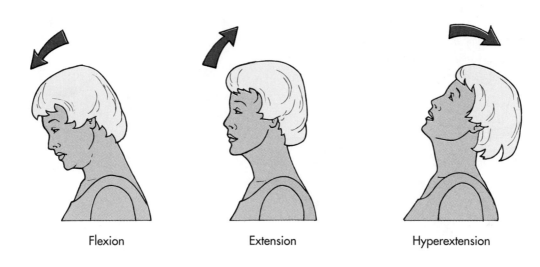

Flexion   Extension   Hyperextension

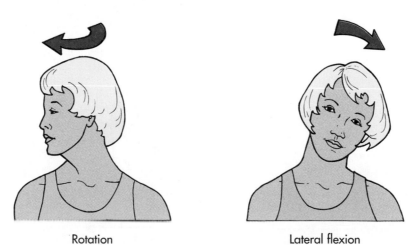

Rotation   Lateral flexion

Fig. 22-11 *Range-of-motion exercises for the neck.*

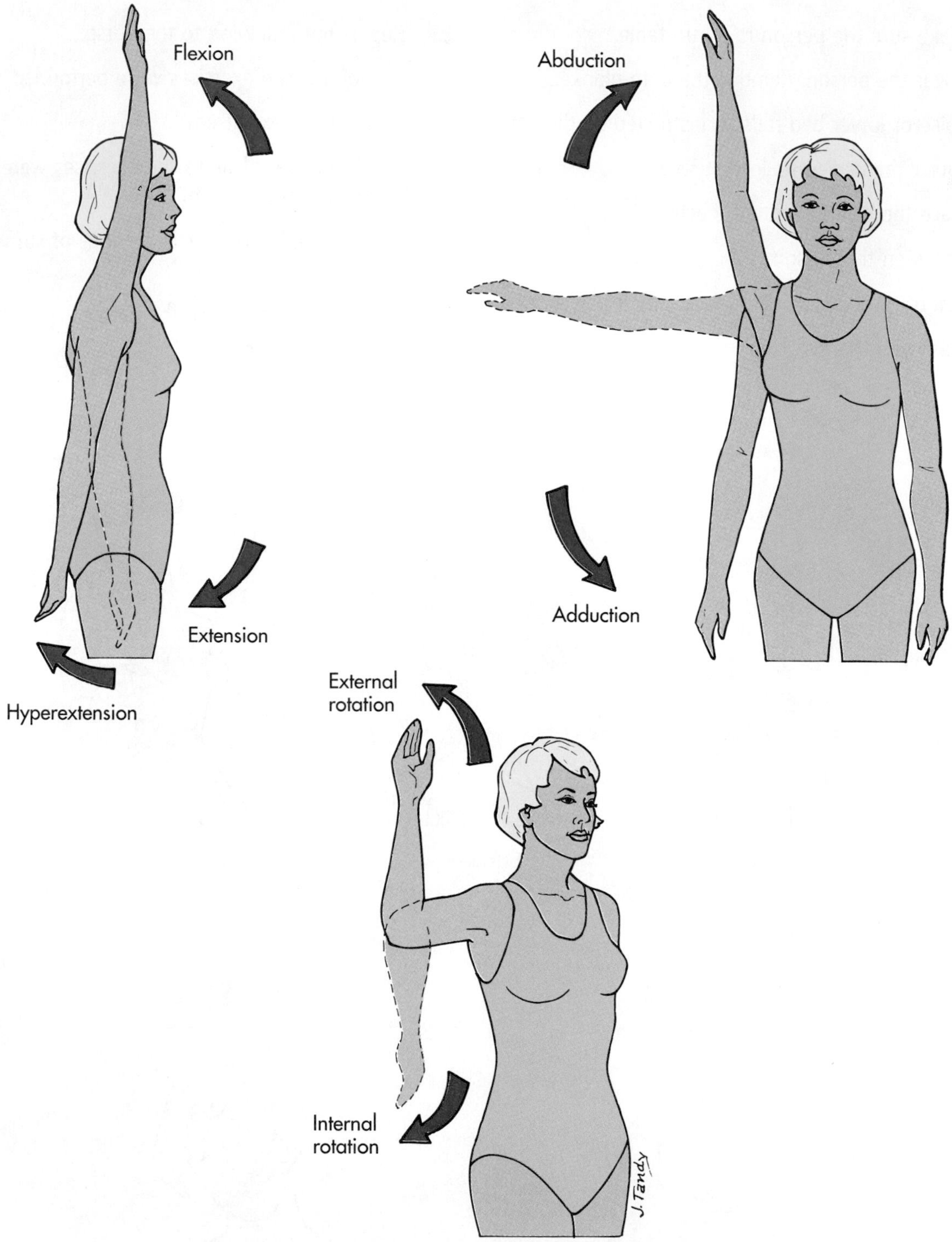

Fig. 22-12 *Range-of-motion exercises for the shoulder.*

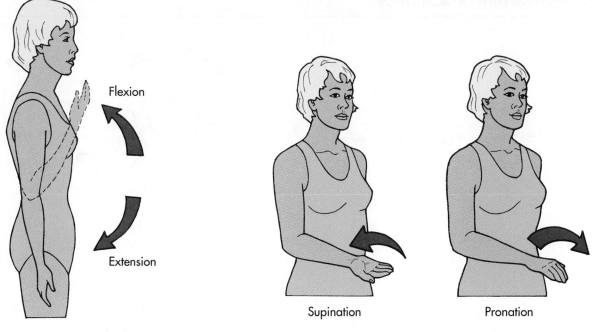

Fig. 22-13 *Range-of-motion exercises for the elbow.*

Fig. 22-14 *Range-of-motion exercises for the forearm.*

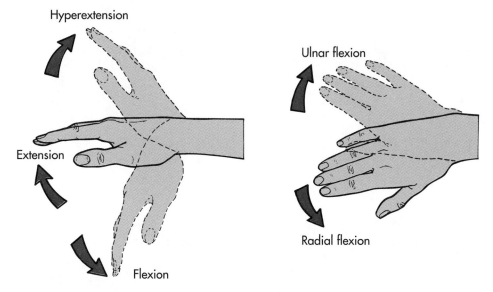

Fig. 22-15 *Range-of-motion exercises for the wrist.*

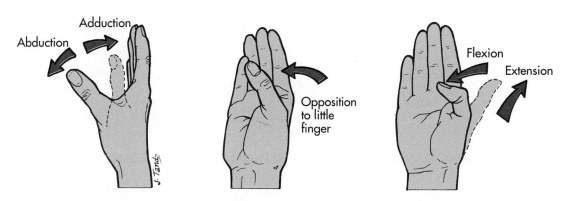

Fig. 22-16 *Range-of-motion exercises for the thumb.*

Fig. 22-17 *Range-of-motion exercises for the fingers.*

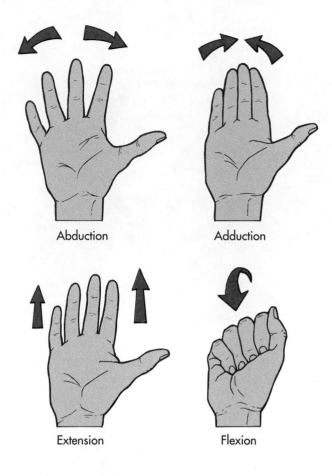

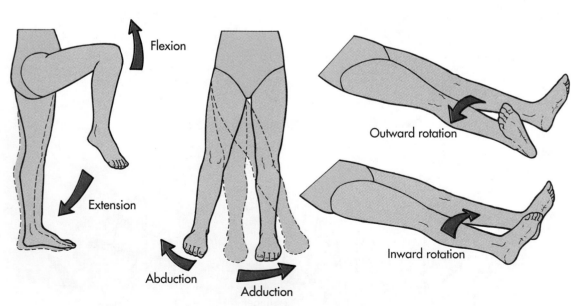

Fig. 22-18 *Range-of-motion exercises for the hip.*

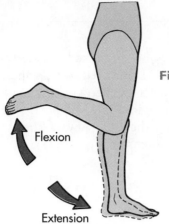

Fig. 22-19 *Range-of-motion exercises for the knee.*

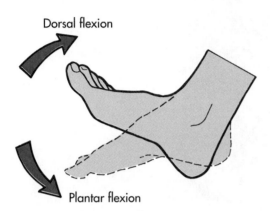

Fig. 22-20 *Range-of-motion exercises for the ankle.*

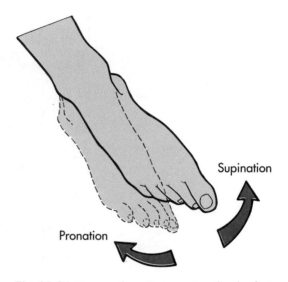

Fig. 22-21 *Range-of-motion exercises for the foot.*

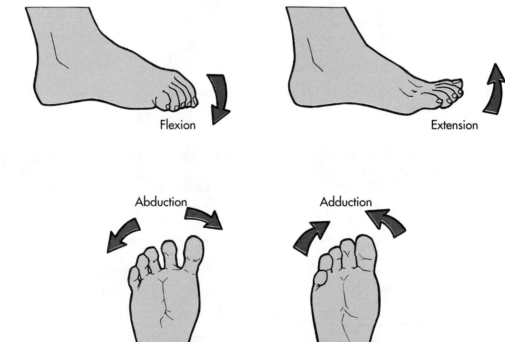

Fig. 22-22 *Range-of-motion exercises for the toes.*

✦ AMBULATION

For most persons on bedrest, activity is increased slowly and in steps. First the person dangles (sits on the side of the bed). The next step is to sit in a bedside chair. Walking about in the room and then in the hallway are the next steps. **Ambulation,** the act of walking, is not a problem if complications were prevented. Contractures and muscle atrophy are prevented by proper positioning and exercise.

Persons may be weak and unsteady from bedrest, surgery, or injury. You need to help these persons walk. Use a gait (transfer or safety) belt if the person is weak or unsteady. For additional support, the person uses handrails along the wall. Always check the person for orthostatic hypotension (see p. 541).

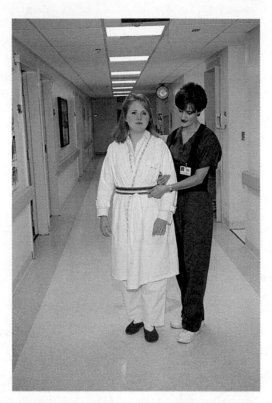

Fig. 22-23 *Assist with ambulation by walking at the person's side. Use a transfer (safety) belt for the person's safety.*

✦ HELPING THE PERSON TO WALK

PRE-PROCEDURE

1 Explain the procedure to the person.

2 Wash your hands.

3 Collect the following:

- Robe and nonskid shoes

- Paper or sheet to protect bottom linens

- Transfer (gait or safety) belt

4 Identify the person. Check the ID bracelet against the assignment sheet.

5 Provide for privacy.

HELPING THE PERSON TO WALK—cont'd

PROCEDURE

6 Move furniture if necessary for moving space for you and the person.

7 Lower the bed to its lowest position. Lock the bed wheels.

8 Fanfold top linens to the foot of the bed.

9 Place the paper or sheet under the person's feet. This protects the bottom sheet from the shoes. Put the shoes on the person.

10 Help the person to dangle. (*See Helping the Person to Sit on the Side of the Bed,* p. 253.)

11 Help the person put on the robe.

12 Apply the transfer belt. (See *Applying a Transfer [Gait] Belt,* p. 254.)

13 Help the person stand:

  a Stand facing the person.

  b Grasp the transfer belt at each side.

  c Brace your knees against the person's knees. Block his or her feet with your feet (see Fig. 12-23, p. 257).

  d Pull the person up into a standing position as you straighten your knees (see Fig. 12-24, p. 257).

14 Stand at the person's side while he or she gains balance. Do not let go of the transfer belt. Grasp the belt at the side and back.

15 Encourage the person to stand erect with the head up and back straight.

16 Assist the person to walk. Walk to the side and slightly behind the person. Provide support with the transfer belt (Fig. 22-23).

17 Encourage the person to walk normally. The heel of the foot strikes the floor first. Discourage shuffling, sliding, or walking on tiptoes.

18 Walk the required distance if the person can tolerate the activity. Do not rush the person.

19 Help the person return to bed:

  a Have the person stand at the side of the bed.

  b Pivot him or her a quarter turn. The backs of the knees should touch the bed.

  c Grasp the sides of the transfer belt.

  d Lower the person onto the bed as you bend your knees. Remove the transfer belt and robe.

  e Help the person lie down. (*See Helping the Person to Sit on the Side of the Bed,* p. 253.)

20 Lower the head of the bed. Help the person to the center of the bed.

21 Remove the shoes, and remove the paper or sheet over the bottom sheet.

POST-PROCEDURE

22 Make sure the person is comfortable. Cover the person.

23 Place the call bell within reach.

24 Raise or lower bed rails as instructed by the RN.

25 Return the robe and shoes to their proper place.

26 Return furniture to its proper location.

27 Unscreen the person.

28 Wash your hands.

29 Report the following to the RN:

- How well the person tolerated the activity

- The distance walked

✦ The Falling Person

A person may start to fall when standing or walking. The person may be weak, lightheaded, or dizzy. Fainting may occur. Falling may be caused by slipping or sliding on spills, waxed floors, throw rugs, or improper shoes (see Chapter 10).

When a person is falling, there is a tendency to try to prevent the fall. However, trying to prevent a fall could cause greater harm. You could injure yourself and the person as you twist and strain to stop the fall. Balance is lost as a person is falling. If you try to prevent the fall, you could lose your balance. Thus both you and the person could fall or cause the other person to fall. Head, hip, and knee injuries are common from falls.

If a person starts to fall, ease him or her to the floor. This lets you control the direction of the fall. You can also protect the person's head.

✦ HELPING THE FALLING PERSON

PROCEDURE

1 Stand with your feet apart. Keep your back straight.

2 Bring the person close to your body as quickly as possible. Use the gait belt if one is worn. If not, wrap your arms around the person's waist. You can also hold the person under the arms (Fig. 22-24, *A*).

3 Move your leg so the person's buttocks rest on it (Fig. 22-24, *B*). Move the leg near the person.

4 Lower the person to the floor. Let him or her slide down your leg to the floor (Fig. 22-24, *C*). Bend at your hips and knees as you lower the person.

5 Call an RN to check the person.

6 Help the RN return the person to bed. Get other staff to help if necessary.

7 Report the following to the RN:

- How the fall occurred

- How far the person walked

- How activity was tolerated before the fall

- Any complaints before the fall

- The amount of assistance needed by the person while walking

8 Complete an incident report.

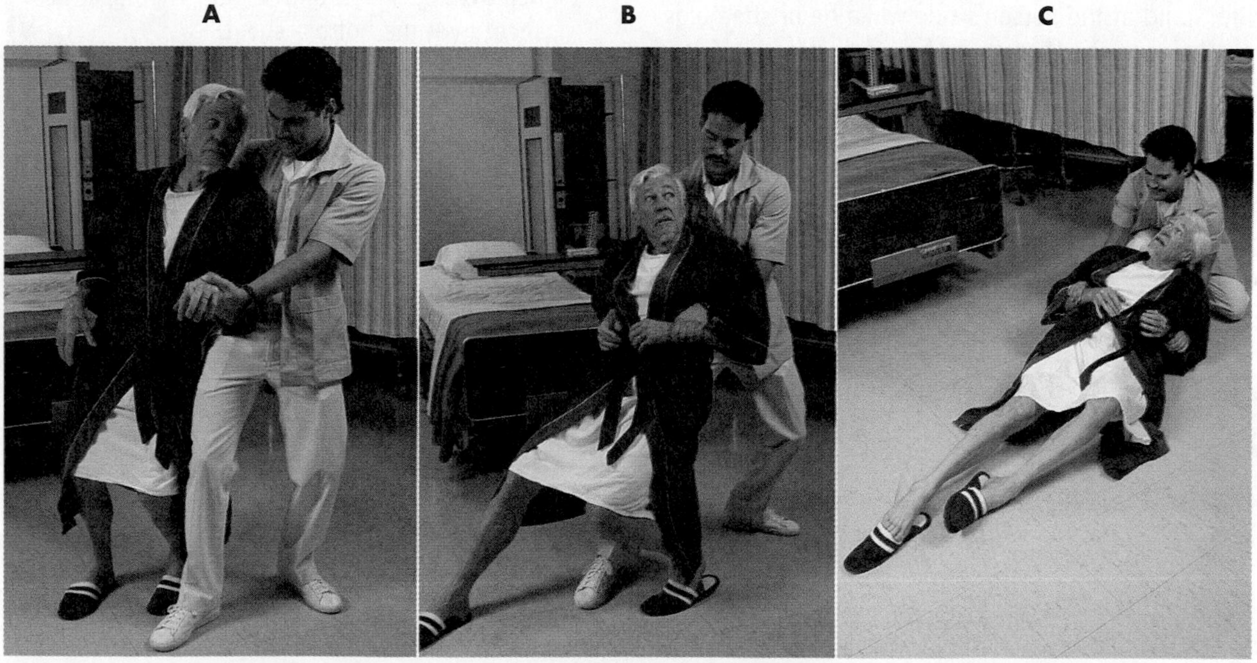

A **B** **C**

Fig. 22-24 **A,** *Support the falling person under the arms.* **B,** *The person's buttocks rest on your leg.* **C,** *Slide the person down your leg to the floor.*

Walking Aids

Walking aids support the body. They are ordered by the doctor. The type ordered depends on the person's physical condition, the amount of support needed, and the type of disability. The physical therapist or RN teaches the person to use the walking aid. Its use may be temporary or permanent.

Crutches

Crutches are used when the person cannot use one leg or when one or both legs need to gain strength. Some persons with permanent leg weakness can use crutches. They usually use Lofstrand crutches (Fig. 22-25). These crutches are made of metal. A metal band fits around the forearm. Axillary crutches extend from the underarm (axilla) to the ground (Fig. 22-26). They are made of wood or metal.

The person learns to crutch walk, climb up and down stairs, and sit and stand. Safety is important. The person on crutches is at risk of falling. The following safety measures are followed:

- The crutches must fit. An RN or physical therapist measures and fits the person with crutches. An improper fit increases the risk of falling and further injury. Back pain, nerve damage, and injuries to the underarms and palms are other risks.
- Crutch tips must be attached to the crutches. They must not be worn down, torn, or wet. Replace worn or torn crutch tips. Dry wet tips with a towel or paper towels.
- Crutches are checked for flaws. Check wooden crutches for cracks and metal crutches for bends. All bolts on both types must be tight.
- Street shoes are worn. They must be flat and have nonskid soles.
- Clothes must fit well. Loose clothing may get caught between the crutches and underarms. Loose clothing also can hang forward and block the person's view of the feet and crutch tips.

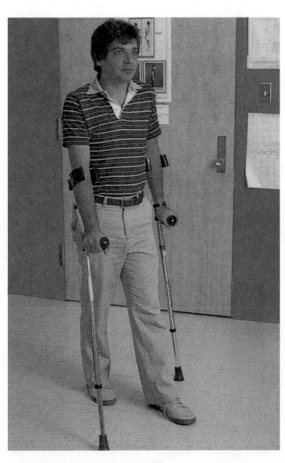

Fig. 22-25 *Lofstrand crutches.(From Elkin MK, Perry AG, Potter PA: Nursing interventions and clinical skills, St Louis, 1996, Mosby.)*

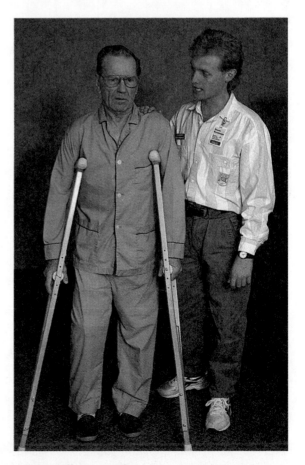

Fig. 22-26 *Axillary crutches. (From Elkin MK, Perry AG, Potter PA: Nursing interventions and clinical skills, St Louis, 1996, Mosby.)*

- Safety rules to prevent falls are followed (see Chapter 10).
- Crutches are kept where the person can reach them. Place them next to the person's chair or against a wall.
- Know which crutch gait the person uses:
  - Four-point alternating gait (Fig. 22-27)
  - Three-point alternating gait (Fig. 22-28)
  - Two-point alternating gait (Fig. 22-29)
  - Swing-to gait (Fig. 22-30)
  - Swing-through gait (Fig. 22-31)

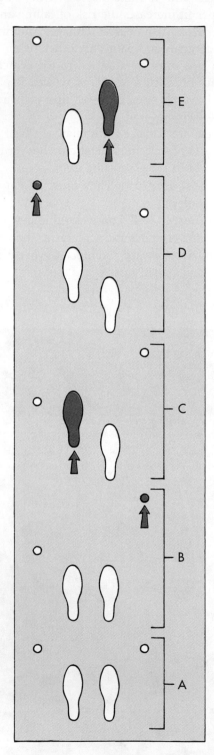

Fig. 22-27 *The four-point alternating gait. The person uses both legs. The right crutch is moved forward and then the left foot. Then the left crutch is moved forward followed by the right foot.*

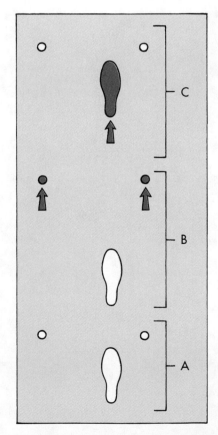

Fig. 22-28 *The three-point alternating gait. One leg is used. Both crutches are moved forward. Then the good foot is moved forward.*

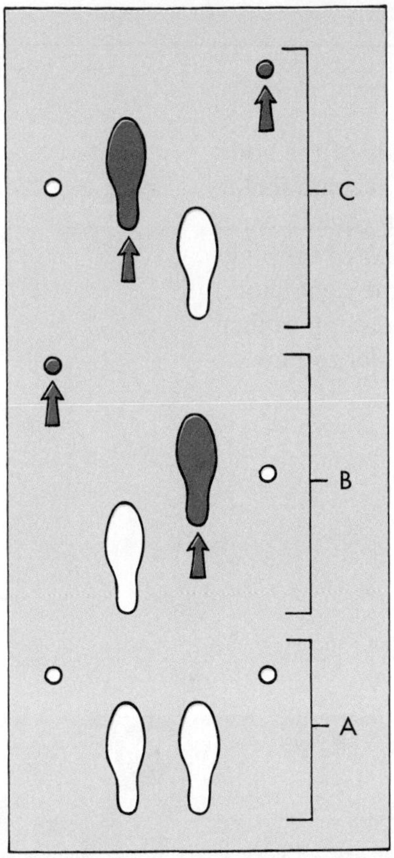

Fig. 22-29 *The two-point alternating gait. The person bears some weight on each foot. The left crutch and right foot are moved forward at the same time. Then the right crutch and left foot are moved forward.*

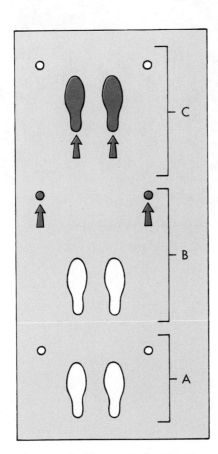

Fig. 22-30 *Swing-to gait. The person bears some weight on each leg. Both crutches are moved forward. Then the person lifts both legs and swings to the crutches.*

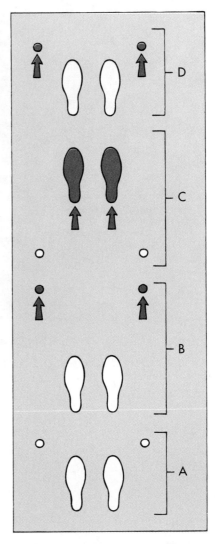

Fig. 22-31 *Swing-through gait. The person bears some weight on each leg. Both crutches are moved forward. Then the persons lifts both legs and swings through the crutches.*

Canes

Canes are used for weakness on one side of the body. They help provide balance and support. There are single-tip, three-point (tripod), and four-point (quad) canes (Fig. 22-32). A cane is held on the *strong side* of the body. (If the left leg is weak, the cane is held in the right hand.) Three-point and four-point canes give more support than single-tipped canes. However, they are harder to move.

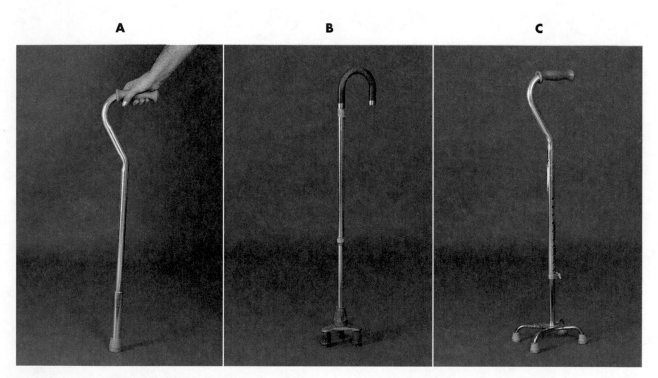

Fig. 22-32 A, *Single-tip cane.* **B,** *Three-point (tripod) cane.* **C,** *Four-point (quad) cane.*

The cane tip is about 6 to 10 inches to the side of the foot and about 6 to 10 inches in front of the foot on the strong side. The grip is level with the hip. The person walks as follows:

Step A: The cane is moved forward 6 to 10 inches (Fig. 22-33, *A*).

Step B: The weak leg (opposite the cane) is moved forward even with the cane (Fig. 22-33, *B*).

Step C: The strong leg is brought forward and ahead of the cane and the weak leg (Fig. 22-33, *C*).

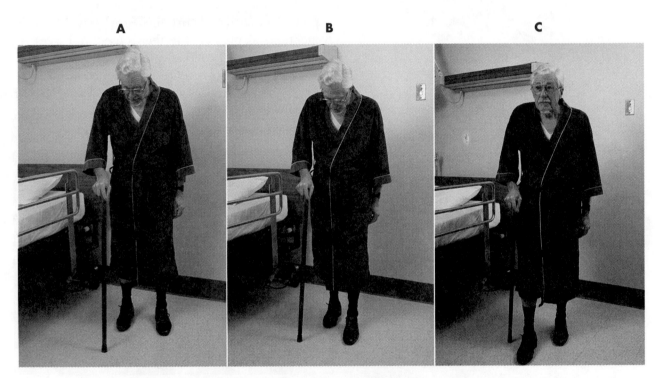

A **B** **C**

Fig. 22-33 *Walking with a cane.* **A,** *The cane is moved forward about 6 to 10 inches.* **B,** *The leg opposite the cane (weak leg) is brought forward even with the cane.* **C,** *The leg on the cane side (strong leg) is moved ahead of the cane and the weak leg.*

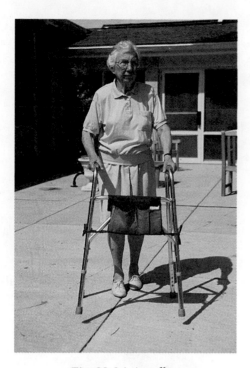

Fig. 22-34 A walker.

Walkers

A walker is a four-point walking aid (Fig. 22-34). It gives more support than a cane. Many people feel safer and more secure with a walker than with a cane. There are many kinds of walkers. The standard walker is picked up and moved about 6 to 8 inches in front of the person. The person then moves the right foot and then the left foot up to the walker (Fig. 22-35).

Baskets, pouches, and trays can be attached to walkers (see Fig. 22-34). The attachment is used to carry needed items. The person is more independent and does not have to rely on others. The attachment also keeps the hands free to grip the walker.

Braces

Braces support weak body parts. They are used also to prevent or correct deformities or to prevent joint movement. Metal, plastic, or leather is used for braces. A brace is applied over the ankle, knee, or back (Fig. 22-36). An ankle-foot orthosis (AFO) is positioned in the shoe (Fig. 22-37). Then the foot is inserted. The device is secured in place with a Velcro strap. Bony points under braces are protected. Otherwise skin breakdown can occur.

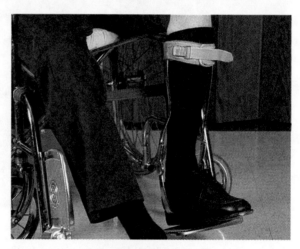

Fig. 22-36 Leg brace.

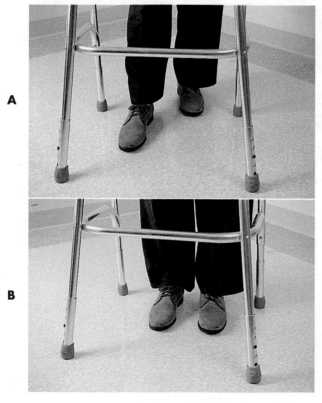

Fig. 22-35 Walking with a walker. A, The walker is moved about 6 inches in front of the person. B, The right foot and then the left foot are moved up to the walker.

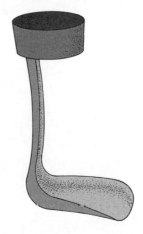

Fig. 22-37 Ankle-foot orthosis (AFO).

REVIEW QUESTIONS

Circle the best *answer.*

1 Mr. Parker is on bedrest. Which statement is *false?*
  a He has orthostatic hypotension.
  b Bedrest helps reduce pain and promote healing.
  c Complications of bedrest include pressure ulcers, constipation, and blood clots.
  d Contractures and muscle atrophy can occur.

2 Which helps to prevent plantar flexion?
  a Bed boards   c Trochanter rolls
  b A footboard   d Hand rolls

3 Which prevents the hip from turning outward?
  a Bed boards   c Trochanter roll
  b A footboard   d All of the above

4 A trapeze is used to
  a Lift the trunk off the bed
  b Move up or turn in bed
  c Strengthen arm muscles
  d All of the above

5 Passive range-of-motion exercises are performed by
  a The person
  b A health team member
  c The person with the assistance of another
  d The person with the use of a trapeze

6 ROM exercises are ordered for Mr. Parker. You should do the following *except*
  a Support the extremity being exercised
  b Move the joint slowly, smoothly, and gently
  c Force the joint through full range of motion
  d Exercise only the joints indicated by the RN

7 Flexion involves
  a Bending the body part
  b Straightening the body part
  c Moving the body part toward the body
  d Moving the body part away from the body

8 Which statement about ambulation is *false?*
  a A transfer belt is used if the person is weak or unsteady.
  b The person is allowed to shuffle or slide when beginning to walk after bedrest.
  c Walking aids may be needed permanently or temporarily.
  d Crutches, canes, walkers, and braces are common walking aids.

9 You are getting a person ready to crutch walk. You should do the following *except*
  a Check the crutch tips
  b Have the person wear street shoes
  c Get any pair of crutches from physical therapy
  d Tighten the bolts on the crutches

10 A single-tipped cane is used
  a At waist level
  b On the strong side
  c On the weak side
  d On either side

Circle T *if the statement is true or* F *if the statement is false.*

11 T F A single-tipped cane and a four-point cane give equal support.

12 T F When using a cane, the feet are moved first.

13 T F Mr. Parker uses a walker. First he moves the walker in front of him. Then he moves his right and left feet forward.

14 T F Mr. Parker starts to fall. You should try to prevent the fall.

15 T F A person has a brace. Bony areas need protection from skin breakdown.

Answers to these questions are on p. 853.

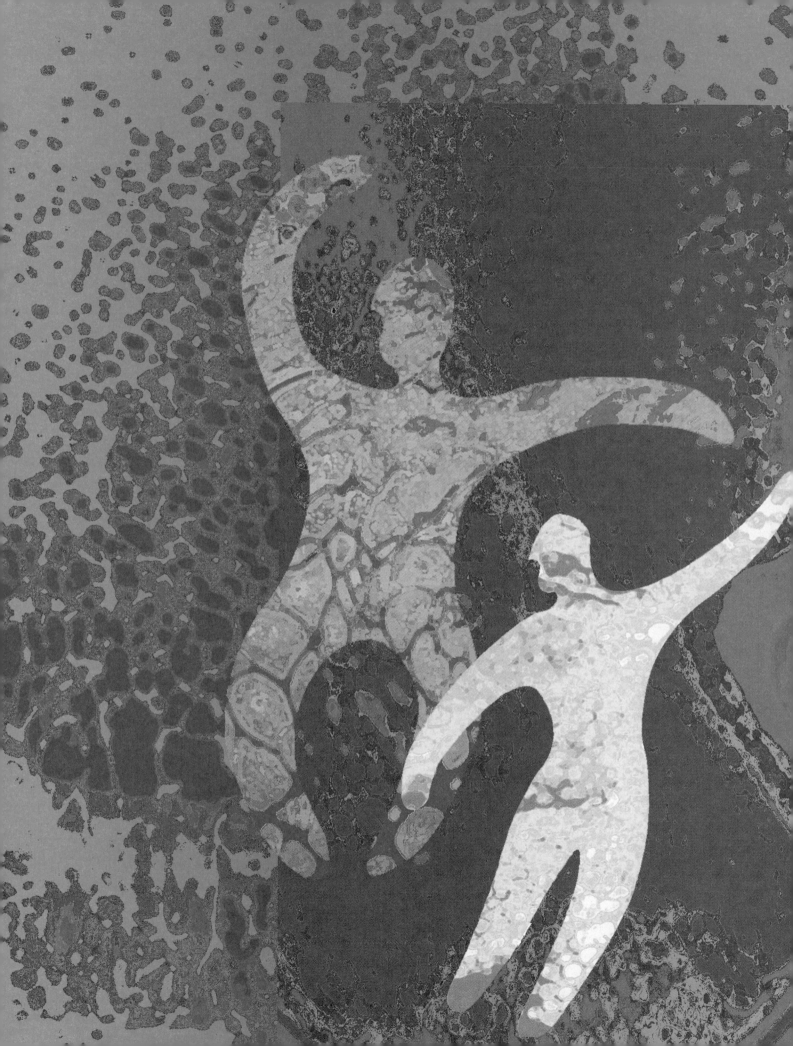

Unit VI
Assisting With Assessment

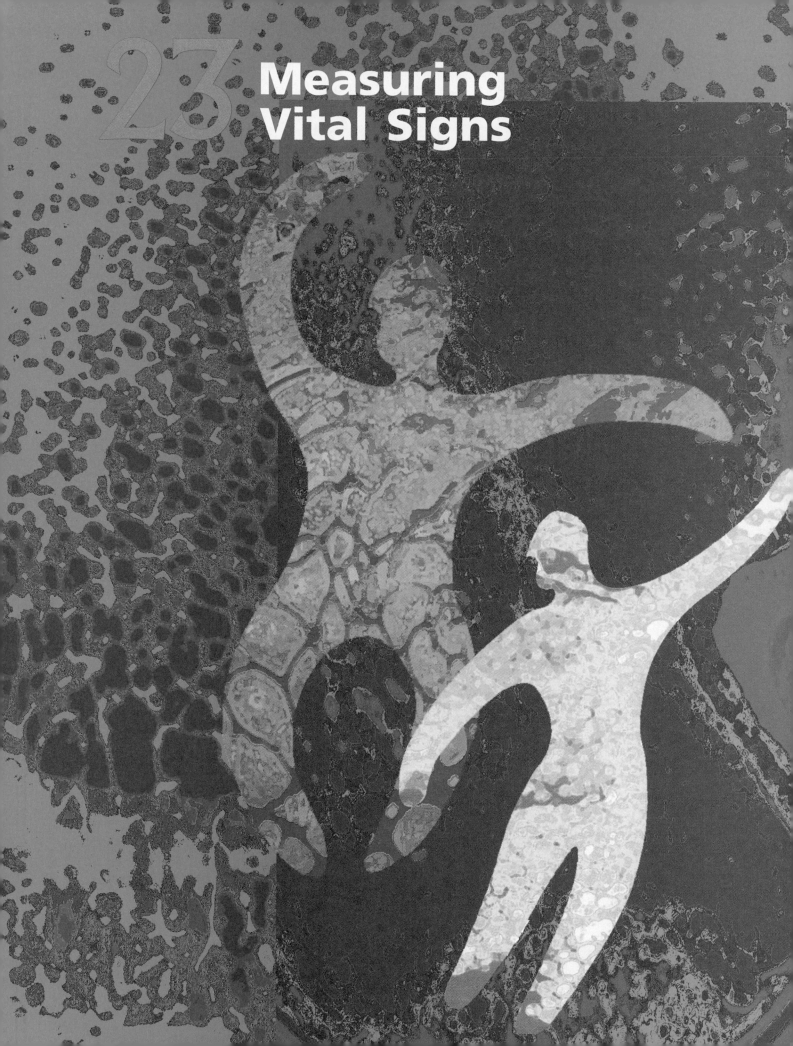

23 Measuring Vital Signs

- Define the key terms in this chapter
- Explain why vital signs are measured
- List the factors affecting vital signs
- Identify the normal ranges of oral, rectal, axillary, and tympanic membrane temperatures
- Know when to take oral, rectal, axillary, and tympanic membrane temperatures
- Identify the sites for taking a pulse
- Describe normal respirations
- Describe the factors affecting blood pressure
- Describe the practices that are followed when measuring blood pressure
- Know the normal pulse, respiration, and blood pressure ranges for different age-groups
- Perform the procedures described in this chapter

KEY TERMS

apical-radial pulse Taking the apical and radial pulses at the same time

blood pressure The amount of force exerted against the walls of an artery by the blood

body temperature The amount of heat in the body that is a balance between the amount of heat produced and the amount lost by the body

bradycardia A slow *(brady)* heart rate *(cardia)*; the rate is less than 60 beats per minute

diastole The period of heart muscle relaxation

diastolic pressure The pressure in the arteries when the heart is at rest

hypertension Persistent blood pressure measurements above the normal systolic (140 mm Hg) or diastolic (90 mm Hg) pressures

hypotension A condition in which the systolic blood pressure is below 90 mm Hg and the diastolic blood pressure is below 60 mm Hg

pulse The beat of the heart felt at an artery as a wave of blood passes through the artery

pulse deficit The difference between the apical and radial pulse rates

pulse rate The number of heartbeats or pulses felt in 1 minute

respiration The act of breathing air into (inhalation) and out of (exhalation) the lungs

sphygmomanometer The instrument used to measure blood pressure

stethoscope An instrument used to listen to the sounds produced by the heart, lungs, and other body organs

systole The period of heart muscle contraction

systolic pressure The amount of force it takes to pump blood out of the heart into the arterial circulation

tachycardia A rapid *(tachy)* heart rate *(cardia)*; the rate is more than 100 beats per minute

vital signs Temperature, pulse, respirations, and blood pressure

Vital signs reflect the function of three body processes essential for life: regulation of body temperature, breathing, and heart function. The four **vital signs** of body function are temperature, pulse, respirations, and blood pressure.

MEASURING AND REPORTING VITAL SIGNS

A person's vital signs vary within certain limits during any 24-hour period. Many factors affect vital signs. They include sleep, activity, eating, weather, noise, exercise, drugs, anger, fear, anxiety, and illness.

Vital signs are measured to detect changes in normal body function. They tell about a person's response to treatment. They often signal life-threatening events. Vital signs are part of the assessment step of the nursing process. Vital signs are always measured:

- During physical examinations
- When a person is admitted to a health care agency
- Several times a day for hospital patients
- Before and after surgery
- Before and after complex procedures or diagnostic tests
- After some nursing procedures or measures, such as ambulation
- When drugs are taken that affect the respiratory or circulatory systems
- Whenever the person complains of pain, fainting, shortness of breath, rapid heart rate, or not feeling well

Vital signs show even minor changes in a person's condition. Accuracy is essential in measuring, recording, and reporting vital signs. If unsure of your measurements, promptly ask the RN to take them again. Unless otherwise ordered, take vital signs with the person lying or sitting. The person is at rest when vital signs are measured. Immediately report to the RN:

- Any vital sign that is changed from a previous measurement
- Vital signs above the normal range
- Vital signs below the normal range

Many agencies have *temp boards* or *TPR books*. These are divided into columns. Patient names are written down the left side of the page. The other columns are for times (such as 0800, 1200, 1600, 2000). Vital signs are recorded on the line in the column appropriate for the person and time. In some agencies, changed or abnormal vital signs are circled in red. The RN or doctor compares current and previous measurements. (See Focus on Long-Term Care.)

BODY TEMPERATURE

Body temperature is the amount of heat in the body. It is a balance between the amount of heat produced and the amount lost by the body. Heat is produced as food is used for energy. It is lost through the skin, breathing, urine, and feces. Body temperature remains fairly stable. It is lower in the morning and higher in the afternoon and evening. Factors affecting body temperature include age, weather, exercise, pregnancy, the menstrual cycle, emotions, stress, and illness.

Normal Body Temperature

Temperature is measured using the Fahrenheit (F) and centigrade or Celsius (C) scales. Common sites for measuring body temperature are the mouth, rectum, axilla (underarm), and ear (tympanic membrane). Normal body temperature depends on the site and usually stays within a normal range (Table 23-1).

Thermometers are used to measure temperature. Glass and disposable thermometers are common in homes. So are tympanic thermometers. Electronic and tympanic thermometers are common in hospitals and nursing centers. Glass and disposable thermometers also are used for patients requiring isolation. (See Focus on Older Persons.)

Glass Thermometers

The glass thermometer (clinical thermometer) is a hollow glass tube with a mercury-filled bulb (Fig. 23-1). When heated, the mercury expands and rises in the tube.

23-1 TABLE	NORMAL BODY TEMPERATURES		
Site	Baseline	Normal Range	
Oral	98.6° F (37.0° C)	97.6° to 99.6° F (36.5° to 37.6° C)	
Rectal	99.6° F (37.6° C)	98.6° to 100.6° F (37.0° to 38.1° C)	
Axillary	97.6° F (36.5° C)	96.6° to 98.6° F (35.9° to 37.0° C)	
Tympanic membrane	98.6° F (37.0° C)	98.6° F (37.0° C)	

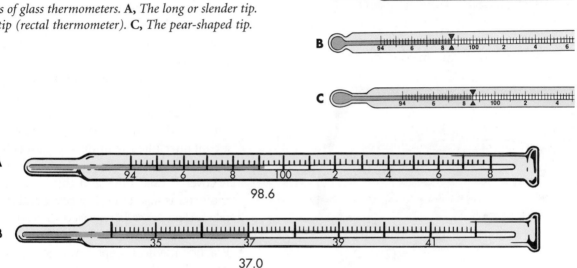

Fig. 23-1 *Types of glass thermometers.* **A,** *The long or slender tip.* **B,** *The stubby tip (rectal thermometer).* **C,** *The pear-shaped tip.*

98.6

37.0

Fig. 23-2 A, *Fahrenheit thermometer. The mercury level is at 98.6° F.* **B,** *Centigrade thermometer. The mercury level is at 37.0° C.*

The mercury contracts and moves down the tube when cooled.

Long-tip or slender-tip thermometers are used for oral and axillary temperatures. So are thermometers with stubby and pear-shaped tips. Rectal thermometers have stubby tips that are color-coded in red.

Glass thermometers are reusable. However, they have the following disadvantages:

- They take a long time to register—3 to 10 minutes depending on the site. Oral temperatures take 2 to 3 minutes, rectal temperatures take at least 2 minutes, and axillary temperatures take 5 to 10 minutes.
- They break easily. Broken rectal thermometers can injure the rectum and colon.
- The person may bite down on an oral thermometer and cause it to break. Cuts to the oral mucous membranes are risks. Any swallowed mercury can cause mercury poisoning.

How to read a glass thermometer

Fahrenheit thermometers have long and short lines. Every other long line is marked in an even degree from 94° to 108° F. The short lines indicate 0.2 (two tenths) of a degree (Fig. 23-2, *A*).

Centigrade thermometers also have long and short lines. Each long line represents 1 degree, from 34° to 42° C. Each short line represents 0.1 (one tenth) of a degree (Fig. 23-2, *B*).

Do the following to read a glass thermometer:

- Hold the thermometer at the stem (Fig. 23-3, p. 570). Bring it to eye level.
- Rotate the thermometer until you can see both the numbers and the long and short lines.
- Turn the thermometer back and forth slowly until you see the silver (or red) mercury line.
- Read the thermometer to the nearest degree (long line). Read the nearest tenth of a degree (short line)—an even number if you are using a Fahrenheit thermometer.

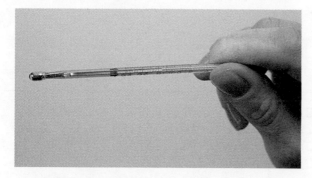

Fig. 23-3 *The thermometer is read at eye level.*

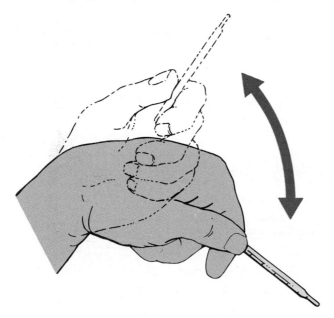

Fig. 23-4 *The wrist is snapped to shake down the thermometer.*

Using a glass thermometer

The thermometer is inserted into the mouth, rectum, or axilla. Each area has many microbes. Therefore each person has a thermometer. This prevents the spread of microbes and infection. The following measures are practiced when using a glass thermometer:

- Use only the person's thermometer.
- Rinse the thermometer under cold running water if it was soaking in a disinfectant. Use tissues to dry it from the stem to the bulb end.
- Check the thermometer for breaks and chips.
- Shake down the thermometer so the mercury is below the lines and numbers. Hold the thermometer at the stem. Stand away from walls, tables, or other hard surfaces. Flex and snap your wrist until the mercury is shaken down (Fig. 23-4).
- Clean and store the thermometer following agency policy. Wipe it with tissues first to remove mucus or feces. Do not use hot water for cleaning. It causes the mercury to expand so much that the thermometer could break. After cleaning, rinse the thermometers under cold running water. Then store it in a case or a container filled with disinfectant solution.
- Use plastic covers following agency policy (Fig. 23-5). A cover is used once and then discarded. The thermometer is inserted into a cover and the temperature taken. The cover is removed to read the thermometer. The thermometer never touches the person.
- Practice medical asepsis and Standard Precautions. Also follow the Bloodborne Pathogen Standard.

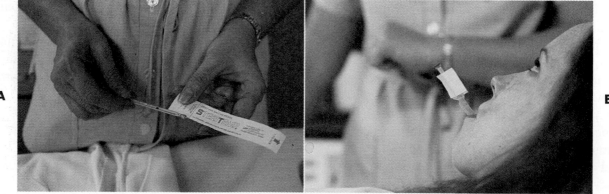

A **B**

Fig. 23-5 **A,** *The thermometer is inserted into a plastic cover.* **B,** *The patient's temperature is taken with the thermometer in the plastic cover.*

✦ *Taking oral temperatures*

Oral temperatures are usually taken on older children and adults. The glass thermometer remains in place 2 to 3 minutes or as required by agency policy. Temperatures are not taken orally if the person:

- Is an infant or a child younger than 4 or 5 years
- Is unconscious
- Has had surgery or an injury to the face, neck, nose, or mouth
- Is receiving oxygen
- Breathes through the mouth
- Has a nasogastric tube in place
- Is delirious, restless, confused, or disoriented
- Is paralyzed on one side of the body
- Has a sore mouth
- Has a history of convulsive disorders

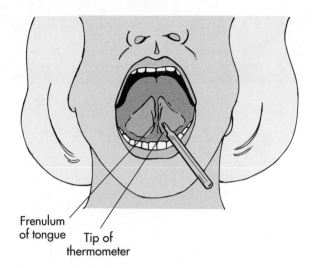

Frenulum of tongue   Tip of thermometer

Fig. 23-6 *The thermometer is positioned at the base of the tongue next to the frenulum.*

TAKING AN ORAL TEMPERATURE WITH A GLASS THERMOMETER

PRE-PROCEDURE

1 Explain the procedure to the person. Ask him or her not to eat, drink, smoke, or chew gum for at least 15 minutes.

2 Collect the following:

- Oral thermometer and holder
- Tissues
- Plastic covers if used
- Gloves

3 Wash your hands.

4 Identify the person. Check the ID bracelet, and call the person by name.

5 Provide for privacy.

PROCEDURE

6 Put on the gloves.

7 Rinse the thermometer in cold water if it was soaking in a disinfectant solution. Dry it with tissues.

8 Check the thermometer for breaks or chips.

9 Shake down the thermometer.

10 Place a plastic cover on the thermometer if used.

11 Ask the person to moisten his or her lips.

12 Place the bulb end of the thermometer under the person's tongue (Fig. 23-6).

13 Ask the person to close his or her lips around the thermometer to hold it in place. Ask the person not to talk while the thermometer is in place.

14 Leave the thermometer in place for 2 to 3 minutes or as required by agency policy.

15 Remove the thermometer by grasping the stem.

16 Use tissues to remove the plastic cover. Wipe the thermometer with a tissue from the stem to the bulb end if no cover was used.

17 Read the thermometer.

18 Record the person's name and temperature on your notepad.

19 Shake down the thermometer.

20 Clean the thermometer according to agency policy.

Continued

TAKING AN ORAL TEMPERATURE WITH A GLASS THERMOMETER—cont'd

POST-PROCEDURE

21 Make sure the person is comfortable and the call bell is within reach.

22 Unscreen the person.

23 Remove the gloves, and wash your hands.

24 Report any abnormal temperature to the nurse. Record the measurement in the proper place.

✦ Taking rectal temperatures

Rectal temperatures are taken when the oral route cannot be used. Rectal temperatures are not taken if the person has diarrhea or a rectal disorder or injury or has had rectal surgery. Rectal temperatures are dangerous also for persons with heart disease. The thermometer can stimulate the vagus nerve in the rectum. This nerve also affects the heart. Stimulation of the vagus nerve slows the heart rate. The heart rate can slow to dangerous levels in some persons.

The rectal thermometer is lubricated for easy insertion and to prevent tissue injury. The thermometer is held in place so it is not lost into the rectum or broken. A glass thermometer remains in the rectum for 2 minutes or as required by agency policy.

Privacy is important when taking rectal temperatures. The buttocks and anus are exposed. Many people are embarrassed by the procedure.

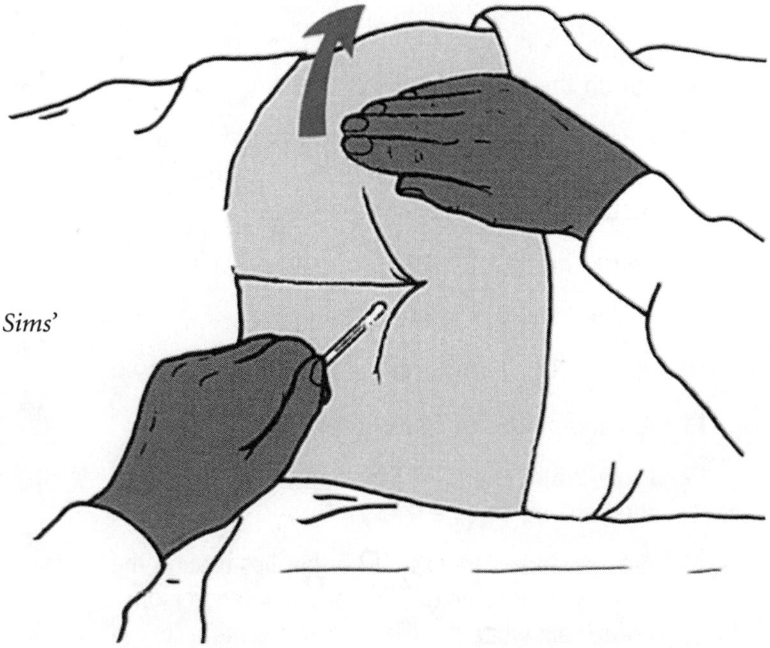

Fig. 23-7 *The rectal temperature is taken with the patient in Sims' position. The buttock is raised to expose the anus.*

TAKING A RECTAL TEMPERATURE WITH A GLASS THERMOMETER

PRE-PROCEDURE

1 Explain the procedure to the person.

2 Collect the following:

- Rectal thermometer and holder
- Toilet tissue
- Plastic covers if used
- Gloves
- Water-soluble lubricant

3 Wash your hands.

4 Identify the person. Check the ID bracelet, and call the person by name.

5 Provide for privacy.

PROCEDURE

6 Rinse the thermometer in cold water if it was soaking in a disinfectant solution. Dry it with tissues.

7 Check the thermometer for breaks or chips.

8 Shake down the thermometer.

9 Place a plastic cover on the thermometer if used.

10 Position the person in Sims' position.

11 Put on the gloves.

12 Put a small amount of lubricant on a tissue. Lubricate the bulb end of the thermometer.

13 Fold back top linens to expose the anal area.

14 Raise the upper buttock to expose the anus (Fig. 23-7).

15 Insert the thermometer 1 inch into the rectum.

16 Hold it in place for 2 minutes or as required by the agency.

17 Remove the thermometer.

18 Remove the plastic cover. Wipe the thermometer with tissues from the stem to the bulb end if no cover was used.

19 Place the used toilet tissue on a paper towel or on several thicknesses of toilet tissue. Place the thermometer on clean toilet tissue.

20 Wipe the anal area to remove excess lubricant and any feces. Cover the person.

21 Make sure the person is comfortable and the call bell is within reach.

22 Dispose of tissue.

23 Read the thermometer. Record the person's name and temperature on your notepad. Write *R* to indicate a rectal temperature.

24 Shake down the thermometer.

25 Clean the thermometer according to agency policy.

26 Remove the gloves, and wash your hands.

POST-PROCEDURE

27 Unscreen the person.

28 Report any abnormal temperature. Record the measurement with an *R* in the proper place.

✦ *Taking axillary temperatures*

Axillary temperatures are less reliable than oral, rectal, or tympanic membrane temperatures. They are used when the other routes cannot be used. The axilla must be dry for the measurement. This site is not used right after bathing. The thermometer is held in place to maintain proper position. A glass thermometer is held in place for 5 to 10 minutes or as required by agency policy.

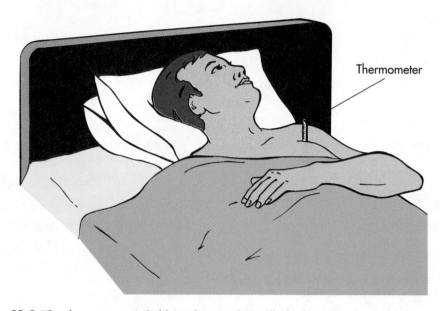

Thermometer

Fig. 23-8 *The thermometer is held in place in the axilla by bringing the patient's arm over the chest.*

TAKING AN AXILLARY TEMPERATURE WITH A GLASS THERMOMETER

PRE-PROCEDURE

1 Explain the procedure to the person.

2 Collect the following:

- Oral glass thermometer and holder

- Plastic covers if used

- Tissues

- Towel

3 Wash your hands.

4 Identify the person. Check the ID bracelet, and call the person by name.

5 Provide for privacy.

PROCEDURE

6 Rinse the thermometer in cold water if it was soaking in a disinfectant solution. Dry it with tissues.

7 Check the thermometer for breaks or chips.

8 Shake down the thermometer.

9 Place a plastic cover on the thermometer if used.

10 Help the person remove an arm from the gown. Do not expose the person.

11 Dry the axilla with the towel.

12 Place the bulb end of the thermometer in the center of the axilla.

13 Ask the person to place the arm over the chest to hold the thermometer in place (Fig. 23-8). Hold it and the arm in place if he or she cannot help or if the person is an infant or child.

14 Leave the thermometer in place for 5 to 10 minutes or as required by agency policy.

15 Remove the thermometer from the plastic cover. Wipe the thermometer with tissues from the stem to the bulb end if no cover was used.

16 Read the thermometer.

17 Record the person's name and temperature with an *A* (for axillary temperature) on your notepad.

18 Help the person put the gown back on.

19 Make sure the person is comfortable and the call bell is within reach.

20 Shake down the thermometer.

21 Rinse and wash the thermometer. Place it in the holder with disinfectant or in a plastic cover.

POST-PROCEDURE

22 Unscreen the person.

23 Follow agency policy for soiled linen.

24 Wash your hands.

25 Report any abnormal temperature. Record the measurement with an *A* in the proper place.

✦ Electronic Thermometers

Electronic thermometers are battery operated. They measure temperature in a few seconds. The temperature is displayed on the front of the instrument. Some models have a battery charger. The hand-held unit is kept in a battery charger when not in use.

Electronic thermometers have oral and rectal probes. A disposable cover (sheath) covers the probe. Disposable probe covers are used once and then discarded. This helps prevent the spread of infection. Medical asepsis, Standard Precautions, and the Bloodborne Pathogen Standard also help prevent the spread of infection.

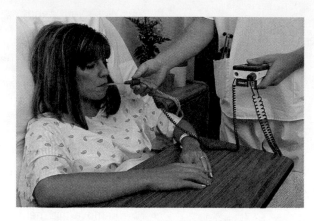

Fig. 23-9 *The covered probe of the electronic thermometer is inserted under the tongue.*

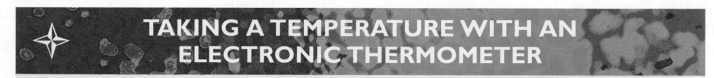

TAKING A TEMPERATURE WITH AN ELECTRONIC THERMOMETER

PRE-PROCEDURE

1 Explain the procedure to the person. Ask him or her not to eat, drink, smoke, or chew gum for at least 15 minutes if you will take an oral temperature.

2 Collect the following:

- Electronic thermometer

- Probe (blue for an oral or axillary temperature; red for a rectal temperature)

- Disposable probe covers

- Toilet tissue (for a rectal temperature)

- Water-soluble lubricant (for a rectal temperature)

- Gloves

3 Plug the probe into the thermometer.

4 Wash your hands.

5 Identify the person. Check the ID bracelet, and call the person by name.

TAKING A TEMPERATURE WITH AN ELECTRONIC THERMOMETER—cont'd

PROCEDURE

6 Provide for privacy. Position the person for an oral, rectal, or axillary temperature.

7 Put on gloves if contact with body fluid or body substances is likely.

8 Insert the probe into a probe cover.

9 For an *oral temperature:*

   a Ask the person to open the mouth and raise the tongue.

   b Place the covered probe at the base of the tongue on either side (Fig. 23-9).

   c Ask the person to lower the tongue and close the mouth.

   For a rectal temperature:

   a Lubricate the end of the covered probe using the lubricant on the toilet tissue.

   b Fold back top linens to expose the anal area.

   c Raise the upper buttock to expose the anus.

   d Insert the probe ½ inch into the rectum.

   For an axillary temperature:

   a Help the person remove an arm from the gown. Do not expose the person.

   b Dry the axilla with the towel.

   c Place the covered probe in the axilla. Place the person's arm over the chest.

10 Hold the probe in place until you hear a tone or see a flashing or steady light.

11 Read the temperature on the display. A tone or a flashing or steady light means the temperature was measured.

12 Remove the probe. Press the eject button to discard the cover.

13 Record the person's name and temperature on your notepad.

14 Return the probe to the holder.

15 Make sure the person is comfortable. Help the person put the gown back on if an axillary temperature was taken. For a *rectal temperature:*

   a Wipe the anal area with tissue to remove lubricant.

   b Cover the person.

   c Discard used toilet tissue.

   d Remove the gloves.

POST-PROCEDURE

16 Place the call bell within the person's reach.

17 Unscreen the person.

18 Remove the gloves, and wash your hands.

19 Return the thermometer to the charging unit.

20 Wash your hands.

21 Report any abnormal temperature. Record the measurement in the proper place. Note if an oral, rectal, or axillary temperature was taken.

✦ Tympanic Membrane Thermometers

Tympanic membrane thermometers measure temperature at the tympanic membrane in the ear (Fig. 23-10). The covered probe is gently inserted into the ear. The temperature is measured in 1 to 3 seconds. These thermometers are battery operated and use disposable probe covers. They must be kept charged.

Tympanic membrane thermometers are comfortable for the person. They are not invasive like rectal thermometers. They are useful for children because of their speed and comfort. There are fewer microbes in the ear than in the mouth or rectum. Therefore the risk of spreading infection is reduced. These thermometers are not used if there is drainage from the ear.

✦ TAKING A TYMPANIC MEMBRANE TEMPERATURE

PRE-PROCEDURE

1 Explain the procedure to the person.

2 Get the tympanic membrane thermometer and a probe cover.

3 Wash your hands.

4 Identify the person. Check the ID bracelet, and call the person by name.

5 Provide for privacy.

PROCEDURE

6 Ask the person to turn his or her head so the ear is in front of you.

7 Insert the probe gently. Pull back on the ear to straighten the ear canal (Fig. 23-11).

8 Start the thermometer.

9 Read the measurement when you hear a tone or see a flashing light.

10 Remove the probe from the ear.

11 Record the person's name and temperature on your notepad. Note that a tympanic temperature was taken.

12 Press the eject button, and discard the probe.

POST-PROCEDURE

13 Make sure the person is comfortable and the call bell is within reach.

14 Unscreen the person.

15 Return the thermometer to the charging unit.

16 Wash your hands.

17 Report any abnormal temperature. Record the measurement in the proper place. Note that a tympanic membrane temperature was taken.

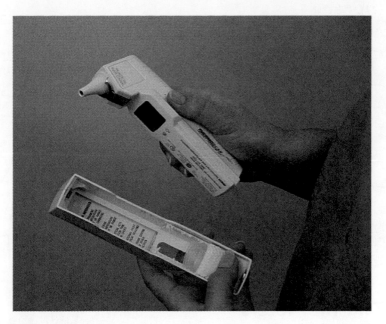

Fig. 23-10 *Tympanic membrane thermometer.* *(Courtesy Braun Thermoscan, Inc, Boston, Mass.)*

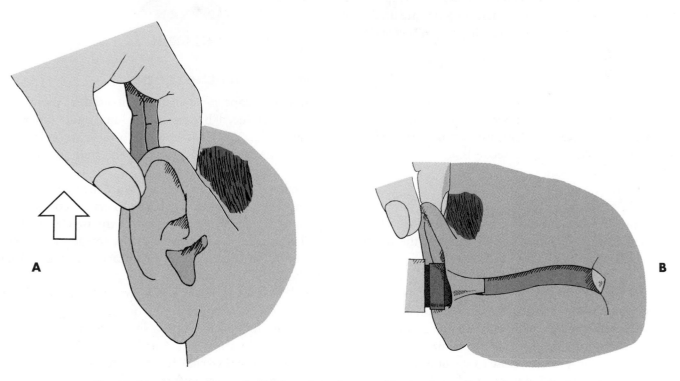

Fig. 23-11 **A,** *The ear is pulled back and,* **B,** *the tympanic membrane thermometer probe is inserted into the ear canal.*

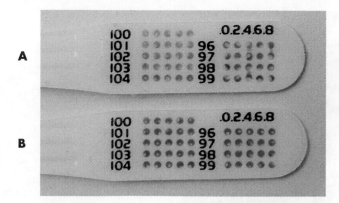

Fig. 23-12 A, *Disposable oral thermometer with chemical dots.* **B,** *The dots change color when the temperature is taken.*

Disposable Oral Thermometers

Disposable oral thermometers have small chemical dots (Fig. 23-12). The dots change color when heated by the body. Each dot must be heated to a certain temperature before it changes color. These thermometers are used only once. They measure temperature in 45 to 60 seconds.

Temperature-Sensitive Tape

Temperature-sensitive tape changes color in response to body heat. The tape is applied to the forehead or abdomen. It shows if the temperature is normal or above normal. Exact body temperature is not measured. The color change takes about 15 seconds.

PULSE

The **pulse** is defined as the beat of the heart felt at an artery as a wave of blood passes through the artery. A pulse can be felt every time the heart beats.

Sites for Taking a Pulse

The temporal, carotid, brachial, radial, femoral, popliteal, and dorsalis pedis (pedal) pulses are on both sides of the body (Fig. 23-13). Pulses are easy to feel at these sites. The arteries are close to the body's surface and lie over a bone. The radial site is used most often because it is easy to reach and find. You can take a radial pulse without disturbing or exposing the person. The carotid pulse is taken during cardiopulmonary resuscitation (CPR) and other emergencies (see Chapter 35).

The apical pulse is felt over the apex (top) of the heart. It is taken with a stethoscope.

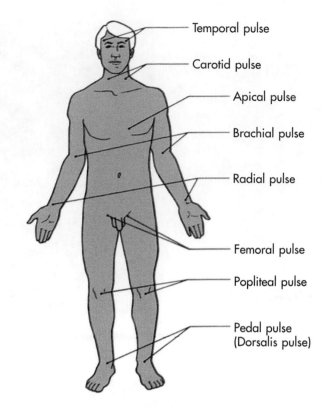

Fig. 23-13 *The pulse sites.*

Using a Stethoscope

A **stethoscope** is an instrument used to listen to the sounds produced by the heart, lungs, and other body organs (Fig. 23-14). It is used to take the apical pulse and to measure blood pressure. The stethoscope amplifies the sounds for easy hearing.

Stethoscopes are in contact with many persons and health team members. Therefore infection control is important. The earpieces and diaphragm are cleaned before and after use. Cleaning prevents the spread of microbes.

The following measures are practiced when using a stethoscope:
- Wipe the earpieces and diaphragm with alcohol wipes.
- Warm the diaphragm in your hand (Fig. 23-15).
- Place the earpiece tips in your ears so the bend of the tips points forward. Earpieces should fit snugly to block out external noises. They should not cause pain or ear discomfort.
- Place the diaphragm over the artery. Hold it in place as in Figure 23-16.
- Prevent noise. Do not let anything touch the tubing. Ask the person to be silent during the procedure.
- Wipe the earpiece tips and diaphragm with alcohol wipes after the procedure.

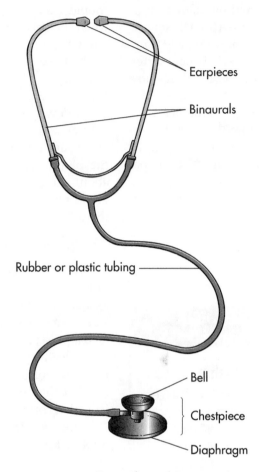

Earpieces

Binaurals

Rubber or plastic tubing

Bell

Chestpiece

Diaphragm

Fig. 23-14 *Parts of a stethoscope.*

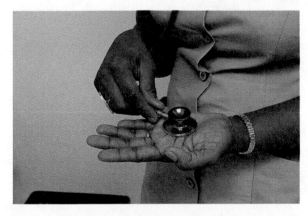

Fig. 23-15 *The diaphragm of the stethoscope is warmed in the palm of the hand.*

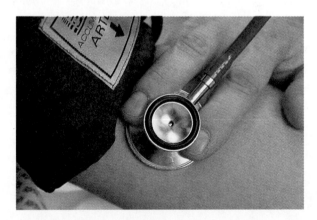

Fig. 23-16 *The stethoscope is held in place with the fingertips of the index and middle fingers.*

Pulse Rate

The **pulse rate** is the number of heartbeats or pulses felt in 1 minute. The rate varies for different age-groups (Table 23-2). The pulse rate is affected by many factors. They include elevated body temperature (fever), exercise, fear, anger, anxiety, excitement, heat, position, and pain. These and other factors cause the heart to beat faster. Some drugs also increase the pulse rate. Other drugs slow down the pulse.

The adult pulse rate is between 60 and 100 beats per minute. A rate of less than 60 or more than 100 is considered abnormal. **Tachycardia** is a rapid *(tachy)* heart rate *(cardia)*. The heart rate is more than 100 beats per minute. **Bradycardia** is a slow *(brady)* heart rate *(cardia)*. The rate is less than 60 beats per minute. Report abnormal rates to the RN immediately.

TABLE 23-2 PULSE RANGES FOR DIFFERENT AGES	
Age	Pulse Rates per Minute
Birth to 4 weeks	80-180
4 weeks to 1 year	80-160
1 to 2 years	80-130
2 to 6 years	80-120
6 to 12 years	70-110
12 years and older	60-100

Rhythm and Force of the Pulse

The rhythm of the pulse should be regular. That is, a pulse should be felt in a pattern. The same time interval should occur between beats. An irregular pulse occurs when the beats are unevenly spaced or beats are skipped (see Chapter 24).

The force of the pulse relates to its strength. A forceful pulse is easy to feel and is described as *strong, full,* or *bounding.* Pulses that are hard to feel are described as *weak, thready,* or *feeble.*

Electronic blood pressure equipment (see p. 588) can also count pulses. The pulse rate is displayed along with the blood pressure. However, no information is given about the rhythm and force of the pulse. If electronic blood pressure equipment is used, you still need to feel the pulse to determine rhythm and force.

✦ Taking a Radial Pulse

The radial pulse is used for routine vital signs. The pulse is felt by placing the first three fingers of one hand against the radial artery. The radial artery is on the thumb side of the wrist (Fig. 23-17). Do not use your thumb to take a pulse; it has a pulse of its own. You could mistake the pulse in your thumb for the person's pulse. Count the pulse for 30 seconds. Then multiply the number by 2 to get the number of beats per minute. If the pulse is irregular, count the pulse for 1 full minute.

Some agencies require that all radial pulses be taken for 1 full minute. Follow your agency's policy.

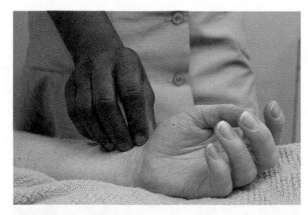

Fig. 23-17 *The middle three fingers are used to locate the radial pulse on the thumb side of the wrist.*

TAKING A RADIAL PULSE

PRE-PROCEDURE

1 Wash your hands.

2 Identify the person. Check the ID bracelet, and call the person by name.

3 Explain the procedure to the person.

4 Provide for privacy.

PROCEDURE

5 Have the person sit or lie down.

6 Locate the radial pulse with your 3 middle fingers (see Fig. 23-17).

7 Note if the pulse is strong or weak, and regular or irregular.

8 Count the pulse for 30 seconds. Multiply the number of beats by 2. Or count the pulse for 1 full minute if required by agency policy.

9 Count the pulse for 1 full minute if it is irregular.

10 Record the person's name and pulse on your notepad. Make a note about the strength of the pulse and if it was regular or irregular.

POST-PROCEDURE

11 Make sure the person is comfortable and the call bell is within reach.

12 Unscreen the person.

13 Wash your hands.

14 Report the following to the RN:

- A pulse rate of less than 60 or more than 100 beats per minute is reported immediately

- Whether the pulse is regular or irregular

- The pulse rate

- The strength of the pulse (strong, full, or bounding; or weak, thready, or feeble)

15 Record the pulse rate in the proper place.

✦ Taking an Apical Pulse

The apical pulse is taken with a stethoscope. This method is used on infants and children up to about 3 years of age. Apical pulses are also taken on adults who have heart disease or who take drugs that affect the heart. The apical pulse is on the left side of the chest slightly below the nipple (Fig. 23-18). The apical pulse is counted for 1 full minute.

The heartbeat normally sounds like a *lub-dub*. Each *lub-dub* is counted as 1 beat. Do not count the *lub* as 1 beat and the *dub* as another.

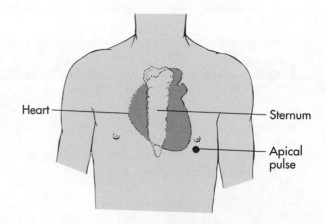

Fig. 23-18 *The apical pulse is located 2 to 3 inches to the left of the sternum (breastbone) and below the left nipple.*

TAKING AN APICAL PULSE

PRE-PROCEDURE

1 Collect the following:

   • Stethoscope with diaphragm

   • Alcohol wipes

2 Wash your hands.

3 Identify the person. Check the ID bracelet, and call the person by name.

4 Explain the procedure to the person.

5 Provide for privacy.

PROCEDURE

6 Wipe the earpieces and diaphragm with alcohol wipes.

7 Have the person sit or lie down.

8 Warm the diaphragm in your palm.

9 Expose the nipple area of the left chest.

10 Place the earpieces in your ears.

11 Locate the apical pulse. Place the diaphragm 2 to 3 inches to the left of the breastbone and below the left nipple (see Fig. 23-18).

12 Count the pulse for 1 full minute. Note if it is regular or irregular.

13 Cover the person. Remove the earpieces.

14 Record the person's name and pulse on your notepad. Note whether the pulse was regular or irregular.

15 Make sure the person is comfortable and the call bell is within reach.

16 Unscreen the person.

17 Clean the earpieces and diaphragm of the stethoscope with alcohol wipes.

18 Return the stethoscope to its proper place.

POST-PROCEDURE

19 Wash your hands.

20 Report the following to the nurse:

   • A pulse rate of less than 60 or more than 100 beats per minute is reported immediately

   • Whether the pulse was regular or irregular

   • The pulse rate

21 Record the pulse rate in the proper place with an *Ap* for an apical pulse.

⚜ Taking an Apical-Radial Pulse

The apical and radial pulse rates should be equal. Sometimes heart contractions are not strong enough to create pulses in the radial artery. This may occur in people with heart disease. The radial pulse may be less than the apical pulse. To see if there is a difference between the apical and radial rates, the pulses are taken at the same time by two staff members. This is called an **apical-radial pulse.** The **pulse deficit** is the difference between the apical and radial pulse rates. To obtain the pulse deficit, subtract the radial rate from the apical rate. The apical pulse rate is never less than the radial pulse rate.

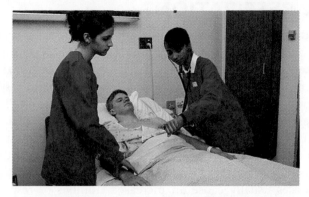

Fig. 23-19 *Two workers take an apical-radial pulse. One worker takes the apical pulse, and the other takes the radial pulse.*

✦ TAKING AN APICAL-RADIAL PULSE

PRE-PROCEDURE

1 Ask a nurse or another assistive person to help you.

2 Collect a stethoscope and alcohol wipes.

3 Wash your hands.

4 Identify the person. Check the ID bracelet, and call the person by name.

5 Explain the procedure to the person.

6 Provide for privacy.

PROCEDURE

7 Wipe the earpieces and diaphragm with the alcohol wipes.

8 Have the person sit or lie down.

9 Warm the diaphragm in your palm.

10 Expose the left nipple area of the chest.

11 Place the earpieces in your ears.

12 Find the apical pulse. Have your co-worker find the radial pulse (Fig. 23-19).

13 Give the signal to begin counting.

14 Count the pulse for 1 full minute.

15 Give the signal to stop counting.

16 Cover the person. Remove the earpieces.

17 Record the person's name and the apical and radial pulses on your notepad. Subtract the radial pulse from the apical pulse for the pulse deficit. Note whether the pulse was regular or irregular.

18 Make sure the person is comfortable and the call bell is within reach.

19 Unscreen the person.

20 Clean the earpieces and diaphragm with alcohol wipes.

21 Return the stethoscope to its proper place.

POST-PROCEDURE

22 Wash your hands.

23 Report the following to the nurse:

- An apical pulse rate of less than 60 or more than 100 beats per minute is reported immediately

- The apical and radial pulse rates

- The pulse deficit

- Whether the pulse was regular or irregular

24 Record the pulses in the proper place. Indicate that an apical-radial pulse was taken.

✦ RESPIRATIONS

Respiration is the act of breathing air into the lungs (inhalation) and out of the lungs (exhalation). Oxygen is taken into the lungs during inhalation. Carbon dioxide is moved out of the lungs during exhalation. Each respiration involves one inhalation and one exhalation. The chest rises during inhalation and falls during exhalation.

The healthy adult has 10 to 20 respirations per minute. The respiratory rate is affected by many of the factors that affect body temperature and pulse. Heart and respiratory diseases usually cause an increased number of respirations per minute.

Respirations are normally quiet, effortless, and regular. Both sides of the chest rise and fall equally. See Chapter 21 for abnormal respiratory patterns.

Respirations are counted when the person is at rest. The person is positioned so you can see the chest rise and fall. The depth and rate of breathing can be voluntarily controlled to a certain extent. People tend to change breathing patterns when they know their respirations are being

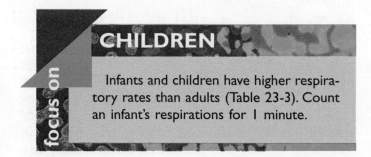

CHILDREN

focus on

Infants and children have higher respiratory rates than adults (Table 23-3). Count an infant's respirations for 1 minute.

counted. Therefore the person should be unaware that you are counting respirations.

Respirations are counted right after taking a pulse. Keep your fingers or stethoscope over the pulse site. (The person assumes you are still taking the pulse.) Count respirations by watching the rise and fall of the chest. Count them for 30 seconds. Then multiply the number by 2 for the total number of respirations in 1 minute. If an abnormal pattern is noted, count the respirations for 1 full minute. (See Focus on Children.)

✦ COUNTING RESPIRATIONS

PROCEDURE

1. Continue to hold the wrist after taking the radial pulse. Keep the stethoscope in place if you took an apical pulse.

2. Do not tell the person you are counting respirations.

3. Begin counting when the chest rises. Count each rise and fall of the chest as 1 respiration.

4. Observe if respirations are regular and if both sides of the chest rise equally. Also note the

depth of respirations and if the person has any pain or difficulty in breathing.

5. Count respirations for 30 seconds. Multiply the number by 2.

6. Count an adult's respirations for 1 full minute if they are abnormal or irregular.

7. Record the person's name, respiratory rate, and other observations on your notepad.

POST-PROCEDURE

8. Make sure the person is comfortable and the call bell is within reach.

9. Wash your hands.

10. Report the following to the RN:

    • The respiratory rate

    • Equality and depth of respirations

    • If the respirations were regular or irregular

    • If the person experienced pain or difficulty in breathing

    • Any respiratory noises

    • Any abnormal respiratory patterns (see Chapter 21)

11. Record the respiratory rate in the proper place.

TABLE 23-3 NORMAL RESPIRATORY RATES FOR CHILDREN

Age	Respirations per Minute
Newborn	35
1 to 11 months	30
2 years	25
4 years	23
6 years	21
8 years	20
10 years	19
12 years	19
14 years	18
16 years	17
18 years	16-18

(From Wong DL: *Whaley & Wong's nursing care of infants and children,* ed 5, St Louis, 1995, Mosby.)

focus on CHILDREN

As with the other vital signs, infants and children have lower blood pressures than adults. A newborn's blood pressure is usually about 70/55 mm Hg. At 1 year the blood pressure increases to 90/55 mm Hg. Blood pressure continues to increase as the child grows older. Adult levels are reached between 14 and 18 years of age.

Blood pressures are not measured routinely in infants and young children. The RN tells you when to measure their blood pressures.

focus on OLDER PERSONS

Arteries narrow and lose their elasticity. The heart has to work harder to pump blood through the vessels. Therefore both the systolic and diastolic pressures are higher in older persons. A blood pressure of 160/90 mm Hg is normal for many older persons.

Older persons also are at risk for orthostatic hypotension (see Chapter 22).

BLOOD PRESSURE

Blood pressure is the amount of force exerted against the walls of an artery by the blood. Blood pressure is controlled by:

- The force of heart contractions
- The amount of blood pumped with each heartbeat
- How easily the blood flows through the blood vessels

The period of heart muscle contraction is called **systole.** The period of heart muscle relaxation is called **diastole.**

Both the systolic and diastolic pressures are measured. The **systolic pressure** is the higher pressure. It represents the amount of force needed to pump blood out of the heart into the arterial circulation. The **diastolic pressure** is the lower pressure. It reflects the pressure in the arteries when the heart is at rest. Blood pressure is measured in millimeters (mm) of mercury (Hg). The systolic pressure is recorded over the diastolic pressure. The average adult has a systolic pressure of 120 mm Hg and a diastolic pressure of 80 mm Hg. This is written as 120/80 mm Hg.

Factors Affecting Blood Pressure

Blood pressure can change from minute to minute. Such changes are related to the factors described in Box 23-1 on p. 588.

Because it can vary so easily, blood pressure has normal ranges. Systolic pressures between 100 and 140 mm Hg are considered normal. Normal diastolic pressures are between 60 and 90 mm Hg.

Persistent measurements above the normal systolic and diastolic pressures are abnormal. This condition is known as **hypertension.** Report any systolic pressure above 140 mm Hg to the RN immediately. A diastolic pressure above 90 mm Hg also is reported immediately. Likewise, systolic pressures below 90 mm Hg and diastolic pressures below 60 mm Hg are reported. This is called **hypotension.** Some people normally have low blood pressures. However, hypotension may be a sign of a serious condition that can lead to death if it is not corrected. (See Focus on Children and Focus on Older Persons.)

BOX 23-1

FACTORS AFFECTING BLOOD PRESSURE

- **Age**—blood pressure increases as a person grows older. It is lowest in infancy and childhood and highest in adulthood. Blood pressure continues to increase with aging.
- **Gender** (male or female)—women usually have lower blood pressures than men. Blood pressures rise in women after menopause.
- **Blood volume**—is the amount of blood in the system. Severe bleeding lowers the blood volume. Therefore the blood pressure lowers. The rapid administration of IV fluids increases the blood volume. The blood pressure rises.
- **Stress**—includes anxiety, fear, and emotions. Heart rate and blood pressure increase as part of the body's response to stress.
- **Pain**—generally increases blood pressure. However, severe pain can cause shock. Blood pressure is seriously low in the state of shock (see Chapter 35).
- **Exercise**—increases heart rate and blood pressure. Blood pressure should not be measured right after exercise.
- **Weight**—blood pressure is higher in overweight persons. The blood pressure lowers with weight loss.
- **Race**—black persons generally have higher blood pressures than white persons.
- **Diet**—a high-sodium diet increases the amount of water in the body. The extra fluid volume increases blood pressure.
- **Medications**—drugs can be given to raise or lower blood pressure. Other drugs have the side effects of high or low blood pressure.
- **Position**—blood pressure is generally lower when lying down and higher in the standing position. Sudden changes in position can cause sudden changes in blood pressure (orthostatic hypotension). A person who stands suddenly may have a sudden drop in blood pressure. Dizziness and fainting can occur. (See Chapter 22).
- **Smoking**—increases blood pressure. Nicotine in cigarettes causes blood vessels to narrow. The heart must work harder to pump blood through narrowed vessels.
- **Alcohol**—excessive alcohol intake can raise blood pressure.

Equipment

A stethoscope and a sphygmomanometer are used to measure blood pressure. The **sphygmomanometer** consists of a cuff and a measuring device. There are three types of sphygmomanometers: aneroid, mercury, and electronic. The aneroid type has a round dial and a needle that points to the calibrations (Fig. 23-20, *A*). The aneroid manometer is small and easy to carry. The mercury manometer is more accurate than the aneroid type. The mercury type has a column of mercury within a calibrated tube (Fig. 23-20, *B*). Many agencies have wall-mounted mercury sphygmomanometers in patient rooms.

Electronic sphygmomanometers display the systolic and diastolic blood pressures on the front of the instrument (Fig. 23-21). The pulse is usually displayed also. The cuff automatically inflates and deflates on some models. Others have automatic deflation only. If electronic blood pressure equipment is used where you work, you need to learn how to use the equipment. Follow the manufacturer's instructions. Electronic devices are available also for home use.

The blood pressure cuff is wrapped around the upper arm. Tubing connects the cuff to the manometer. Another tube connects the cuff to a small hand-held bulb. A valve on the bulb is turned so the cuff inflates as the bulb is squeezed. The inflated cuff causes pressure over the brachial artery. The valve is turned in the other way for cuff deflation. Blood pressure is measured as the cuff is deflated.

Sounds are produced as blood flows through the arteries. The stethoscope is used to listen to the sounds in the brachial artery as the cuff is deflated. Stethoscopes are not needed with electronic sphygmomanometers. (See Focus on Children on p. 589.)

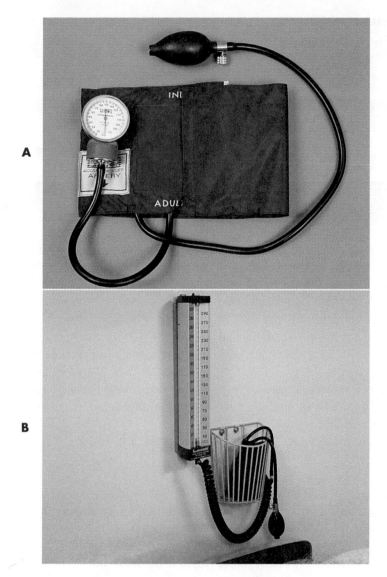

Fig. 23-20 **A,** *Aneroid manometer and cuff.* **B,** *Mercury manometer and cuff.*

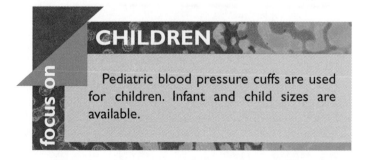

CHILDREN

focus on

Pediatric blood pressure cuffs are used for children. Infant and child sizes are available.

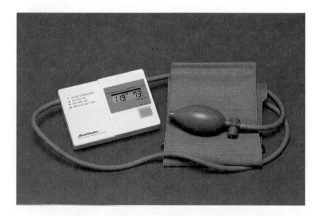

Fig. 23-21 *Electronic sphygmomanometer.*

Measuring Blood Pressure

Blood pressure normally is measured in the brachial artery. Box 23-2 lists the guidelines for measuring blood pressure.

BOX 23-2

GUIDELINES FOR MEASURING BLOOD PRESSURE

- Do not take blood pressure on an arm with an IV infusion, a cast, or a dialysis access site. If a person has had breast surgery, blood pressure is not taken on that side. Also avoid taking blood pressure on an injured arm.
- Let the person rest for 10 to 20 minutes before measuring the blood pressure.
- Measure blood pressure with the person sitting or lying. Sometimes the doctor orders measurement of blood pressure in the standing position.
- Apply the cuff to the bare upper arm. Clothing can affect the measurement. Do not apply the cuff over clothing.
- Make sure the cuff is snug. Loose cuffs can cause inaccurate readings.
- Place the diaphragm of the stethoscope firmly over the artery. The entire diaphragm must be in contact with the skin.
- Make sure the room is quiet. Talking, television, radio, and sounds from the hallway can affect an accurate measurement.
- Have the sphygmomanometer clearly visible.
- Locate the radial artery, and then inflate the cuff. When you no longer feel the radial pulse, inflate the cuff another 30 mm Hg. This prevents cuff inflation to an unnecessarily high pressure, which is painful to the person.
- Measure the systolic and diastolic pressures. Expect to hear the first blood pressure sound at the point where you last felt the radial pulse. The first sound is the systolic pressure. The point where the sound disappears is the diastolic pressure.
- Take the blood pressure again if you are not sure of an accurate measurement. Wait 30 to 60 seconds before repeating the measurement.
- Notify the RN immediately if you cannot hear the blood pressure.

✦ MEASURING BLOOD PRESSURE

PRE-PROCEDURE

1 Collect the following:

- Sphygmomanometer (blood pressure cuff)
- Stethoscope
- Alcohol wipes

2 Wash your hands.

3 Identify the person. Check the ID bracelet, and call the person by name.

4 Explain the procedure to the person.

5 Provide for privacy.

PROCEDURE

6 Wipe the stethoscope earpieces and diaphragm with alcohol wipes.

7 Have the person sit or lie down.

8 Position the person's arm so it is level with the heart. The palm should be up.

9 Stand no more than 3 feet away from the sphygmomanometer. A mercury model should be vertical, on a flat surface, and at eye level. The aneroid type should be directly in front of you.

10 Expose the upper arm.

11 Squeeze the cuff to expel any remaining air. Close the valve on the bulb.

12 Find the brachial artery at the inner aspect of the elbow.

13 Place the arrow on the cuff over the brachial artery (Fig. 23-22, A, p. 592). Wrap the cuff around the upper arm at least 1 inch above the elbow. It should be even and snug.

14 Place the stethoscope earpieces in your ears.

15 Locate the radial artery. Inflate the cuff until you can no longer feel the pulse. Inflate the cuff 30 mm Hg beyond the point where you last felt the pulse.

16 Position the diaphragm over the brachial artery (Fig. 23-22, B, p. 592).

17 Deflate the cuff at an even rate of 2 to 4 millimeters per second. Turn the valve counterclockwise to deflate the cuff.

18 Note the point on the scale where you hear the first sound. This is the systolic reading. It should be near the point where the radial pulse disappeared.

19 Continue to deflate the cuff. Note the point where the sound disappears for the diastolic reading.

20 Deflate the cuff completely. Remove it from the person's arm. Remove the stethoscope.

21 Record the person's name and blood pressure on your notepad.

22 Return the cuff to the case or wall holder.

POST-PROCEDURE

23 Make sure the person is comfortable and the call bell is within reach.

24 Unscreen the person.

25 Clean the earpieces and diaphragm with alcohol wipes.

26 Return the equipment to its proper place.

27 Wash your hands.

28 Report the blood pressure. Record it in the proper place.

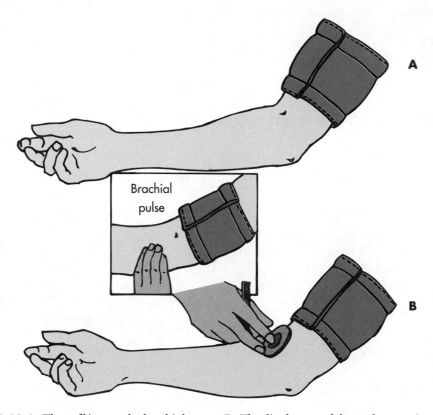

Fig. 23-22 A, *The cuff is over the brachial artery.* **B,** *The diaphragm of the stethoscope is over the brachial artery.*

REVIEW QUESTIONS

Circle the best answer.

1 Which statement is *false?*
- a The vital signs are temperature, pulse, respirations, and blood pressure.
- b Vital signs detect changes in body function.
- c Vital signs change only during illness.
- d Sleep, exercise, drugs, emotions, and noise affect vital signs.

2 Which temperature should you report immediately?
- a An oral temperature of 98.4° F
- b A rectal temperature of 101.6° F
- c An axillary temperature of 97.6° F
- d An oral temperature of 99.0° F

3 A rectal temperature is *not* taken when the person
- a Is unconscious
- b Is an infant
- c Has a nasogastric tube
- d Has had rectal surgery

4 Which gives the least accurate measurement of body temperature?
- a Oral temperature
- b Rectal temperature
- c Axillary temperature
- d Tympanic temperature

5 Which is usually used to take a pulse?
- a The radial pulse
- b The apical-radial pulse
- c The apical pulse
- d The brachial pulse

6 Which is reported to the RN immediately?
- a An adult has a pulse of 120 beats per minute
- b An infant has a pulse of 130 beats per minute
- c An adult has a pulse of 80 beats per minute
- d All of the above

7 Which statement about apical-radial pulses is *true?*
- a The pulse can be taken by one person.
- b The radial pulse can be more than the apical pulse.
- c The apical pulse can be more than the radial pulse.
- d The apical and radial pulses are always equal.

8 Normal respirations are
- a Between 10 and 20 per minute
- b Quiet and effortless
- c Regular with both sides of the chest rising and falling equally
- d All of the above

9 Respirations are usually counted
- a After taking the temperature
- b After taking the pulse
- c Before taking the pulse
- d After taking the blood pressure

10 Which blood pressure is normal for an adult?
- a 88/54 mm Hg
- b 210/100 mm Hg
- c 130/82 mm Hg
- d 152/90 mm Hg

11 When taking a blood pressure, you should do the following *except*
- a Take the blood pressure in the arm with an IV infusion
- b Apply the cuff to a bare upper arm
- c Turn off the television and radio
- d Locate the brachial artery

12 Which is the systolic blood pressure?
- a The point at which the pulse is no longer felt
- b The point where the first sound is heard
- c The point where the last sound is heard
- d The point 30 mm Hg above where the pulse was felt

Answers to these questions are on p. 853.

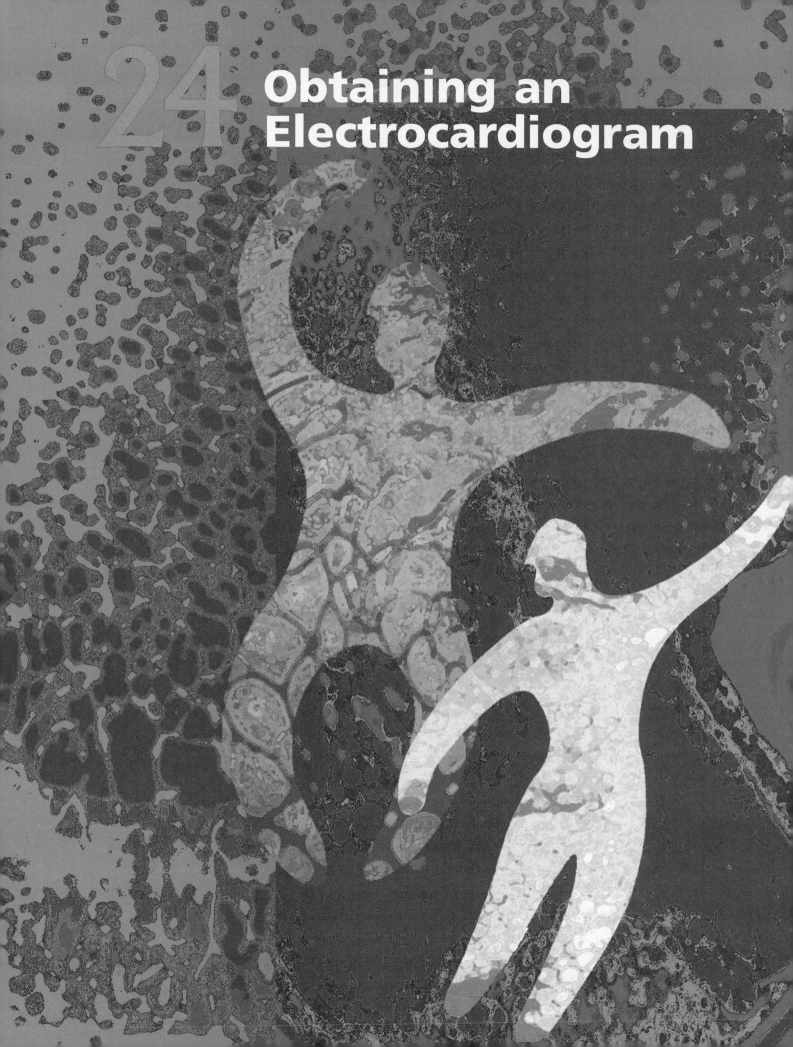

24

Obtaining an Electrocardiogram

OBJECTIVES

- **Define the key terms in this chapter**
- **Explain why electrocardiograms are obtained**
- **Describe the structures and function of the heart**
- **Explain the conduction system of the heart**
- **Identify the normal waves of an electrocardiogram**
- **Locate the sites for limb leads and chest leads**
- **Identify the functions of the electrocardiograph**
- **Describe electrocardiograph paper**
- **Calculate the heart rate using a 6-second strip**
- **Explain how to prepare the person for an electrocardiogram**
- **Obtain an electrocardiogram**
- **Know the dysrhythmias that are life threatening**

KEY TERMS

arrhythmia Without *(a)* a rhythm

artifact Interference on the electrocardiogram

dysrhythmia An abnormal *(dys)* rhythm

electrocardiogram A recording *(gram)* of the electrical activity *(electro)* of the heart *(cardio)*; ECG or EKG

electrocardiograph An instrument *(graph)* that records the electrical activity *(electro)* of the heart *(cardio)*

lead A pair of electrodes; electrical activity is recorded between the electrodes

An **electrocardiogram** (ECG or EKG) is a recording *(gram)* of the electrical activity *(electro)* of the heart *(cardio)*. Changes occur in the ECG when the heart muscle is damaged. The doctor can locate the area of heart damage by studying the ECG. An irregular heart rhythm is detected by taking a pulse. However, an ECG is required to identify the type of irregular rhythm.

Therefore doctors order ECGs for persons with chest pain, pain in the upper arms, and irregular heart rhythms. Persons with abnormal blood pressures also require ECGs. These signs and symptoms may signal heart disease.

ECGs also are done before surgery. This is to make sure that the person does not go to surgery with a heart problem. Fitness tests and health physical examinations often include ECGs. By detecting heart problems early, life-threatening heart diseases can be prevented.

Obtaining ECGs is commonly done by assistive personnel. As with other procedures, make sure that:

- Your state allows you to perform the procedure
- The procedure is in your job description
- You have the necessary education and training
- You know how to use the facility's equipment
- An RN is available to answer questions and supervise you

THE HEART

The heart is a muscle. It pumps blood through the blood vessels to the tissues and cells. The heart lies in the middle to lower part of the chest cavity toward the left side (Fig. 24-1 on p. 596). The heart is hollow and has three layers (Fig. 24-2 on p. 596):

- The *pericardium* is the outer layer. It is a thin sac covering the heart.
- The *myocardium* is the second layer. This layer is the thick, muscular portion of the heart.
- The *endocardium* is the inner layer. It is the membrane lining the inner surface of the heart.

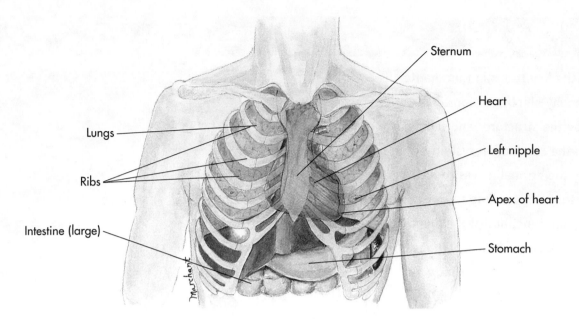

Fig. 24-1 *Location of the heart in the chest cavity.*

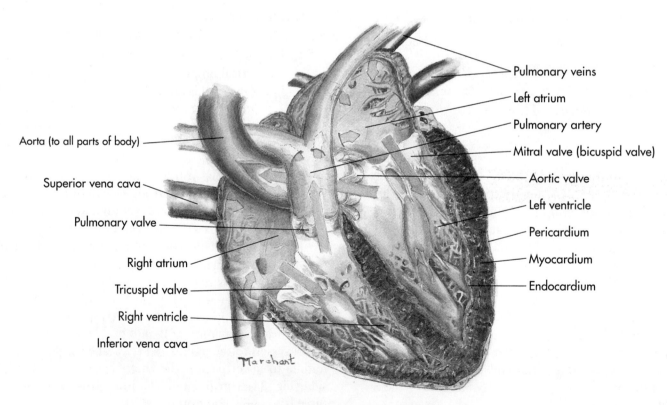

Fig. 24-2 *Structures of the heart.*

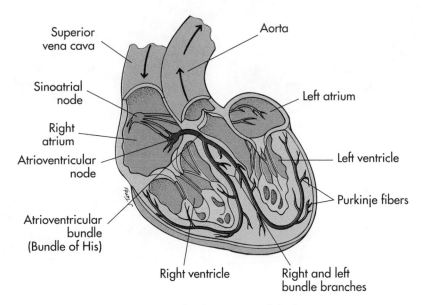

Fig. 24-3 *Conduction system of the heart.*

The heart has four chambers (see Fig. 24-2). Upper chambers receive blood and are called the *atria*. The *right atrium* receives blood from body tissues. The *left atrium* receives blood from the lungs. Lower chambers are called ventricles. Ventricles pump blood. The *right ventricle* pumps blood to the lungs for oxygen. The *left ventricle* pumps blood to all parts of the body.

There are two phases of heart action. During *diastole*, the resting phase, heart chambers fill with blood. The heart relaxes during this phase. During *systole*, the working phase, the heart contracts. Blood is pumped through the blood vessels when the heart contracts. Systole and diastole make up the *cardiac cycle*.

Conduction System

The conduction system controls the cardiac cycle. The heart muscle must relax (fill with blood) and contract (pump) blood in a coordinated fashion. Otherwise cells do not get enough blood and oxygen.

To coordinate the cardiac cycle, the heart's muscle fibers are linked together. An electrical impulse starts in the wall of the right atrium. It passes through (is conducted or transmitted to) muscle fibers in the right and left atria, causing the atria to contract. Then the impulse moves to the ventricles, causing the ventricles to contract. For every heartbeat, an electrical impulse is conducted through the heart.

Four structures in the heart wall make up the conduction system (Fig. 24-3). They are the sinoatrial node, atrioventricular node, atrioventricular bundle, and the Purkinje fibers.

- *Sinoatrial node (SA node)* starts the impulse in the right atrium. The SA node is also called the *pacemaker*. It sets the pace (beat) of the heart.
- The electrical impulse travels from SA node to the right and left atria.
- The right and left atria contract as the impulse travels through them. Blood is pumped to the ventricles.
- The electrical impulse reaches the *atrioventricular node (AV node)*. It is located at the bottom of the right atrium *(atrio)* near the right ventricle *(ventricular)*.
- The impulse travels through the AV node to the *atrioventricular bundle (AV bundle)* in the wall separating the right and left ventricles. (The AV bundle is also called the *bundle of His*.)
- The AV bundle has right and left branches that extend to all parts of the ventricular wall. The *right bundle branch* conducts the impulse to the right ventricle. The *left bundle branch* conducts the impulse to the left ventricle.
- *Purkinje fibers* branch into the myocardium (heart muscle) from the right and left bundle branches. When the impulse reaches the ventricular muscle, the ventricles contract.
- After contracting, the ventricles relax.

Areas outside the SA node can act as a pacemaker. That is, they can start an impulse. This causes an irregular heartbeat. Some rhythms are life threatening.

Blocks can occur in the conduction system. A block prevents the impulse from traveling through the conduction system in a normal manner. Blocks also can be life threatening.

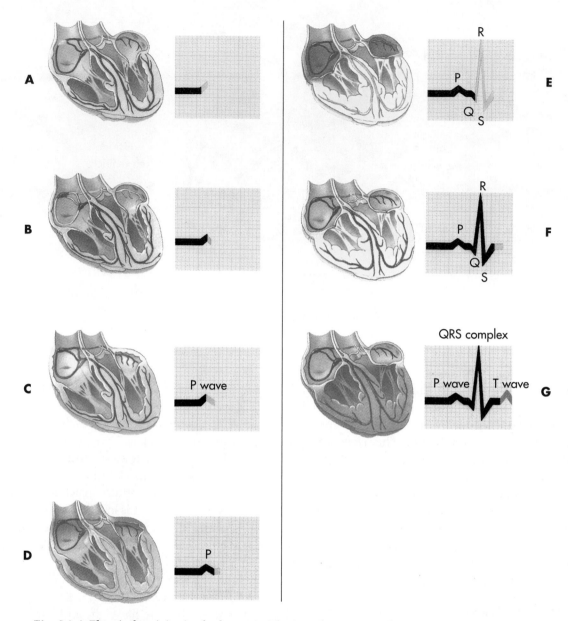

Fig. 24-4 *Electrical activity in the heart.* **A,** *The impulse starts in the SA node.* **B,** *The impulse spreads to the right and left atria.* **C,** *The atria contract. The P wave is formed.* **D,** *The impulse reaches the AV node and the AV bundle. The atria relax.* **E,** *The ventricles contract. The QRS complex forms.* **F,** *The ventricles start to relax.* **G,** *The ventricles relax. The T wave forms.* (From Thibodeau GA, Patton KT: Structure and function of the body, *ed 10, St Louis, 1997, Mosby.)*

THE ELECTROCARDIOGRAM

ECGs record the electrical activity of the conduction system. The electrical activity is recorded in waves. The waves give the cardiac cycle a distinct appearance. Each wave represents electrical activity in a certain part of the heart. The *P wave, QRS complex,* and *T wave* are the major parts of the cardiac cycle. Figure 24-4 shows the electrical activity in the cardiac cycle.

If a problem occurs in a part of the conduction system, the wave representing that part appears abnormal. Problems can occur in any part of the conduction system. ECG changes also occur if the heart muscle is damaged. By studying the ECG, the doctor determines the site of the problem in the conduction system or the area of heart muscle damage.

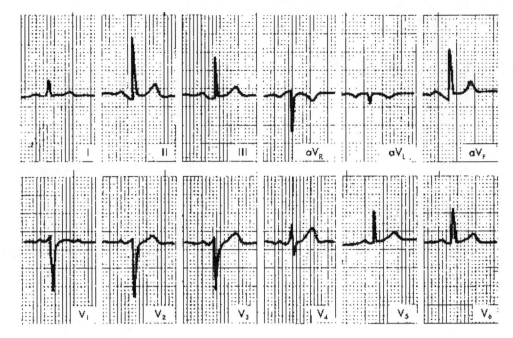

Fig. 24-5 *Twelve leads of the electrocardiogram.* *(From Kinney M, Packa D, Andreoli K, Zipes D: Comprehensive cardiac care, ed 8, St Louis, 1996, Mosby.)*

ECG Leads

The cardiac cycle involves electrical currents passing through the heart. The currents travel in many directions. These currents also are conducted to the body's surface. The currents can be detected with electrodes placed on the body's surface. Electrical activity is recorded between two electrodes. Each pair of electrodes is called a **lead.**

The standard ECG involves 12 leads. It is called a *12-lead ECG.* The heart's electrical activity is recorded from different directions. The cardiac cycle (P wave, QRS complex, and T wave) appears different from each of the 12 directions (Fig. 24-5).

Limb leads

Electrical current from the heart travels to the arms and legs—the limbs. Electrodes are attached to each limb. The six limb leads involve three standard limb leads and three augmented limb leads.

The *standard limb leads* are numbered with Roman numerals. They also are called *bipolar limb leads.* They measure electrical activity between two *(bi)* points *(poles)* (Fig. 24-6).

- Lead I—records electrical activity between the right arm (RA) and left arm (LA).
- Lead II—records electrical activity between the right arm (RA) and left leg (LL).
- Lead III—records electrical activity between the left arm (LA) and left leg (LL).

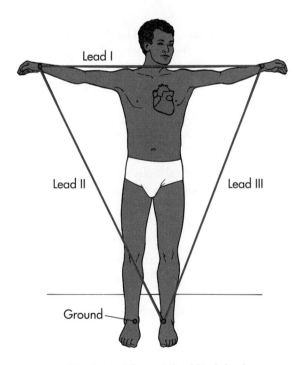

Fig. 24-6 *The standard limb leads.*

The *augmented unipolar limb leads* produce larger wave forms that are easier to read. (To *augment* means to increase or enlarge.) They record the heart's electrical activity from one *(uni)* limb lead *(pole)* to the midpoint of the two other leads (Fig. 24-7, p. 600). These three leads

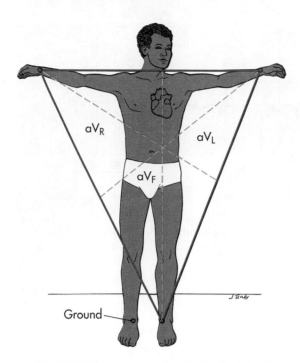

Fig. 24-7 *The augmented unipolar limb leads.*

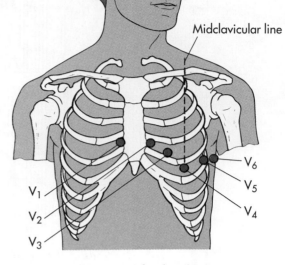

Fig. 24-8 *The chest leads.*

are called aV$_R$, aV$_L$, and aV$_F$. (The letter *a* means *augmented*. The letter *V* stands for unipolar.)

- aV$_R$—records electrical activity from the right arm (R) to the midpoint between the electrodes on the left arm and left leg.
- aV$_L$—records electrical activity from the left arm (L) to the midpoint between the electrodes on the right arm and left leg.
- aV$_F$—records electrical activity from the left leg (F) to the midpoint between the electrodes on the right arm and left arm.

Chest leads

Chest leads also are called precordial leads. Precordial means in front of *(pre)* the heart *(cor)*. These leads are placed at six different sites on the chest (Fig. 24-8). The sites are over the heart. The six chest leads are numbered V$_1$ through V$_6$. (The V stands for *unipolar.*)

The chest leads are placed as follows:

- V$_1$—is at the fourth intercostal space on the right side of the sternum. *Intercostal* means between *(inter)* the ribs *(costal)*. The fourth intercostal space is between the third and fourth ribs.
- V$_2$—is at the fourth intercostal space on the left side of the sternum.
- V$_3$—is halfway between V$_2$ and V$_4$.

- V$_4$—is at the fifth intercostal space at the midclavicular line. The fifth intercostal space is between the fifth and sixth ribs. *Midclavicular* means in the middle *(mid)* of the *(clavicle)*. To find the midclavicular line, find the clavicle. Then find the middle of the clavicle. Draw an imaginary line down to the fifth intercostal space. (This is usually below the left nipple.)
- V$_5$—is at the level of V$_4$ and the anterior axillary line. The *anterior axillary* line is in front of *(anterior)* the underarm *(axillary)*.
- V$_6$—is at the level of V$_4$ and the midaxillary line. *Midaxillary* means the middle *(mid)* of the underarm *(axillary)*.

The Electrocardiograph

The **electrocardiograph** is an instrument *(graph)* that records the electrical activity *(electro)* of the heart *(cardio)*. The machine is portable and is brought to the person's bedside when an ECG is ordered (Fig. 24-9).

The ECG machine senses the heart's electrical activity from the electrodes. Cables attach the electrodes on the person's body to the machine. The machine processes electrical activity. Then it displays the activity in the form of a graph (Fig. 24-10).

All ECG machines sense, process, and display the heart's electrical activity. You will learn how to use the ECG machines in your agency. Always follow the manufacturer's instructions.

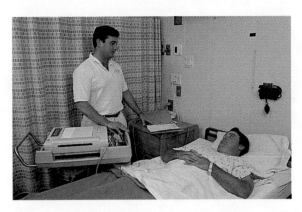

Fig. 24-9 *The electrocardiograph is brought to the person's bedside.*

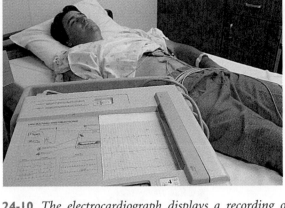

Fig. 24-10 *The electrocardiograph displays a recording of the heart's electrical activity.*

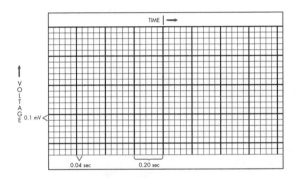

Fig. 24-11 *Electrocardiograph paper.* (*From Phipps WJ, Sands J, Lehman MK, Cassmeyer V:* Medical-surgical nursing: concepts and clinical practice, *ed 5, St Louis, 1995, Mosby.*)

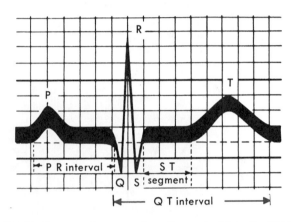

Fig. 24-12 *Pattern of a normal cardiac cycle. Note the PR interval and the ST segment.* (*From Kinney M, Packa D, Andreoli K, Zipes D:* Comprehensive cardiac care, *ed 8, St Louis, 1996, Mosby.*)

Electrocardiograph paper

Electrocardiograph paper is divided into squares (Fig. 24-11). The larger squares (heavy black lines) are divided into smaller squares (light black lines).

Moving vertically (from bottom to top), the squares represent *voltage*. Voltage is a measure of electrical force. The greater the force coming from the heart muscle, the higher the wave formed on the ECG. When studying the ECG, the doctor looks at the height of the waves in each lead. Depending on the lead, the wave may be above the baseline or below it.

Moving horizontally (from left to right), the squares represent *time*. Each small square represents 0.04 second. Note that each large square has five small squares. Therefore each large square represents 0.20 second (0.04 second × 5 = 0.20 second).

The P wave, QRS complex, and T wave of the cardiac cycle normally occur in a certain pattern (Fig. 24-12). Normal time intervals occur between the P wave and QRS complex (PR interval) and between the QRS complex and the T wave (QT interval). Abnormal patterns and time intervals signal heart problems.

The ECG paper is marked also along the top white margin (Fig. 24-13, p. 602). The notches occur in 1-second intervals. The indicator lines are longer or darker every 3 seconds. Note that there are 5 large boxes between two notches. Remember, each large box represents 0.20 second. Therefore 5 large boxes represent 1 second (0.20 second × 5 = 1 second). These notches are useful for estimating the person's heart rate. Simply count the number of R waves within a 6-second strip. Multiply that number by 10. In Figure 24-14 on p. 602, the heart rate is 70.

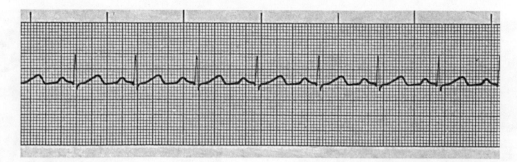

Fig. 24-13 *Indicator lines on ECG paper. Each small line represents 1 second. The longer lines represent 3 seconds. (From Atwood S, Stanton C, Storey J:* Introduction to basic cardiac dysrhythmias, *ed 2, St Louis, 1996, Mosby.)*

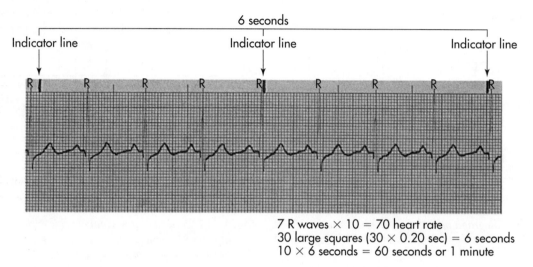

7 R waves × 10 = 70 heart rate
30 large squares (30 × 0.20 sec) = 6 seconds
10 × 6 seconds = 60 seconds or 1 minute

Fig. 24-14 *Estimating the heart rate with a 6-second strip. Seven R waves × 10 = 70 beats per minute. (From Atwood S, Stanton C, Storey J:* Introduction to basic cardiac dysrhythmias, *ed 2, St Louis, 1996, Mosby.)*

Artifact

Sometimes interference occurs on the ECG. This is called **artifact.** P waves, QRS complexes, and T waves are not clear and distinct (Fig. 24-15, *A* and *B*). Sometimes the baseline looks fuzzy (Fig. 24-15, *C*). Poorly connected or loose electrodes can cause artifact. Excess chest hair and·sweating can interfere with electrode contact with the skin. Broken cable wires also cause artifact. So can patient movements such as shivering and rapid breathing. Do not confuse artifact with abnormal rhythms (see pp. 606-612). If in doubt, call for the RN.

◆ **Obtaining an ECG**

The person must be mentally and physically prepared for an ECG. Often ECGs are done when the person is experiencing chest pain. The person may be having a heart attack. The person is frightened and in pain and may have difficulty breathing. This life-threatening situation requires prompt action and a calm manner.

The RN tells you when to obtain an ECG. Sometimes ECGs are ordered *stat*. Stat is an abbreviation for the Latin word *statim*, which means immediately.

The RN explains the procedure to the person and why it is necessary. As you perform the procedure, you also explain what you are going to do. This helps calm the person.

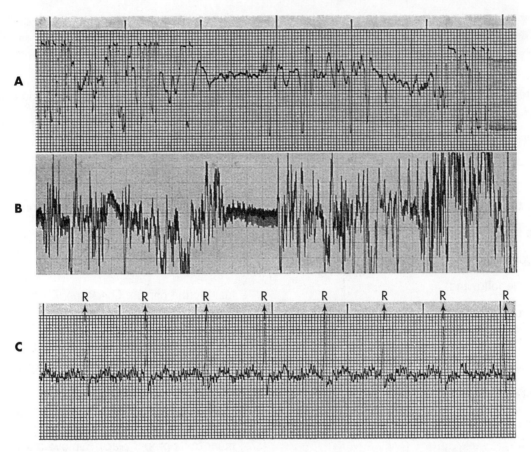

Fig. 24-15 *Artifact. (From Atwood S, Stanton C, Storey J:* Introduction to basic cardiac dysrhythmias, *ed 2, St Louis, 1996, Mosby.)*

The supine position is preferred for the ECG. However, persons with severe chest pain and difficulty breathing may find the supine position uncomfortable. Ask the RN how you should position the person.

The electrodes must have good contact with the skin for a clear recording. Skin preparation is important. Electrode sites are wiped with alcohol. This removes skin oils and perspiration. Allow the sites to dry before applying the electrodes.

Excessive chest and body hair can prevent good skin–electrode contact. Shaving electrode sites often is necessary. Explain to the person why you need to shave these sites. Be careful not to nick or cut the skin. Wear gloves when shaving to avoid possible contact with blood. Standard Precautions and the Bloodborne Pathogen Standard are followed.

You must call for the RN immediately if the person develops problems during the ECG. Stay with the person until the RN arrives. Then follow the RN's instructions. Call for the RN immediately if the person has any of the following:

- Chest pain
- Pain in the jaw or down the arms
- Dyspnea or shortness of breath
- Changes in mental function
- Tachycardia (calculate a 6-second strip)
- Bradycardia (calculate a 6-second strip)
- Abnormal beats (see pp. 606-612)
- An abnormal rhythm (see pp. 606-612)

OBTAINING AN ECG

PROCEDURE ALERT

- Does your state allow assistive personnel to perform the procedure?
- Is the procedure in your job description?
- Do you have the necessary training and education?
- Is an RN available to answer questions and to supervise you?

PRE-PROCEDURE

1   Review the procedure with the RN.

2   Explain the procedure to the person.

3   Wash your hands.

4   Collect the following:

- Electrocardiograph
- Electrodes
- Alcohol wipes
- Razor
- Towel
- Gloves
- Requisition slip

5   Review the manufacturer's instructions for the ECG machine.

6   Arrange equipment in a convenient location in the person's room.

7   Identify the person. Check the ID bracelet against the requisition slip.

8   Provide for privacy.

9   Raise the bed to the best level for good body mechanics.

10 Assist the person with elimination needs. This helps the person relax. Clean and return equipment to its proper place. Remove gloves, and wash your hands. (The person may be seriously ill. The person's condition may not allow time for this step.)

PROCEDURE

11 Measure the person's vital signs. Make a note of them.

12 Position the person supine.

13 Expose only the person's chest, arms, and legs.

14 Determine if you will need to shave any electrode sites.

15 Shave electrode sites as needed:

a   Place a towel under the site.

b   Put on the gloves.

c   Shave the site.

d   Move the towel to the next site. Avoid getting hair on bed linens.

e   Shave that site.

f   Repeat steps 15 d and e as necessary.

g   Remove and discard the gloves.

16 Clean the electrode sites with the alcohol wipes.

17 Allow electrode sites to dry.

18 Apply the electrodes to the chest, arms, and legs (see Figs. 24-6 and 24-8).

19 Connect the cables from the machine to the electrodes (Fig. 24-16).

20 Plug the ECG machine into a wall outlet.

21 Ask the person to lie still. Remind the person not to talk or to cross his or her legs.

22 Obtain an 8- to 12-inch tracing of each lead. Call for the RN if you see any abnormal patterns (see pp. 606-612).

23 Turn off the ECG machine.

24 Tear the tracing off the machine.

OBTAINING AN ECG—cont'd

PROCEDURE—cont'd

25 Label the tracing with the person's identifying information: full name, ID number, room and bed number, and age. Also note the date and time.

26 Disconnect the cables.

27 Remove the electrodes.

28 Cover the person.

POST-PROCEDURE

29 Make sure the person is comfortable.

30 Place the call bell within reach.

31 Raise or lower bed rails as instructed by the RN.

32 Lower the bed to its lowest horizontal position.

33 Unscreen the person.

34 Discard used supplies. Follow agency policy for soiled linen.

35 Unplug and return the ECG machine to its proper location.

36 Show the ECG to the RN. Report any observations or patient complaints.

37 Take or send the ECG and requisition slip to the appropriate department.

38 Wash your hands.

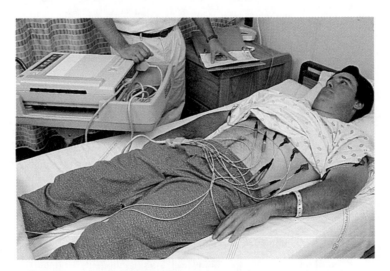

Fig. 24-16 *Cables are connected from the machine to the electrodes.*

DYSRHYTHMIAS

A **dysrhythmia** is an abnormal *(dys)* rhythm. The term *arrhythmia* often is used. **Arrhythmia** means without *(a)* a rhythm. The doctor or RN studies the ECG for dysrhythmias. Treatment depends on the cause and type of dysrhythmia.

Some dysrhythmias are life threatening. Immediate action must be taken. If you see anything abnormal on a tracing, you must call for the RN immediately. Figures 24-13 and 24-14 show normal rhythms. The QRS complexes occur at regular intervals. The P waves and T waves appear normal. These are normal sinus rhythms. That is, the rhythm starts in the sinoatrial node (SA node) and passes through the conduction system normally. Figures 24-17 through 24-32 show some dysrhythmias that must be reported to the RN immediately:

- *Sinus tachycardia*—the heart rate is rapid (Fig. 24-17). Impulses start in the SA node.

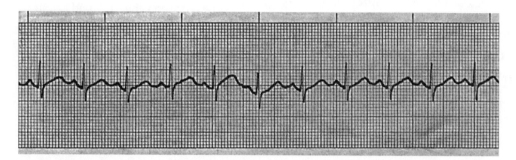

Fig. 24-17 *Sinus tachycardia. The heart rate is 110. (From Atwood S, Stanton C, Storey J:* Introduction to basic cardiac dysrhythmias, *ed 2, St Louis, 1996, Mosby.)*

- *Sinus bradycardia*—the heart rate is slow (Fig. 24-18). Impulses start in the SA node.

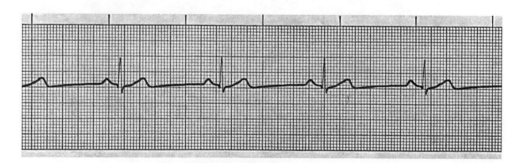

Fig. 24-18 *Sinus bradycardia. The heart rate is 40. (From Atwood S, Stanton C, Storey J:* Introduction to basic cardiac dysrhythmias, *ed 2, St Louis, 1996, Mosby.)*

- *Premature atrial contraction (PAC)*—the SA node sends out an impulse early (Fig. 24-19).

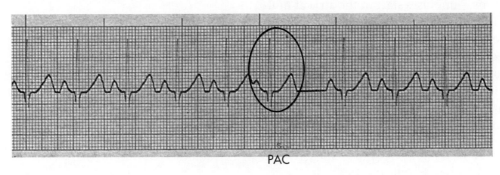

PAC

Fig. 24-19 *Premature atrial contraction (PAC).* *(From Atwood S, Stanton C, Storey J:* Introduction to basic cardiac dysrhythmias, *ed 2, St Louis, 1996, Mosby.)*

- *Paroxysmal atrial tachycardia (PAT)*—a normal rhythm suddenly turns into tachycardia. Bursts (paroxysms) of tachycardia occur. The tachycardia stops suddenly (Fig. 24-20).

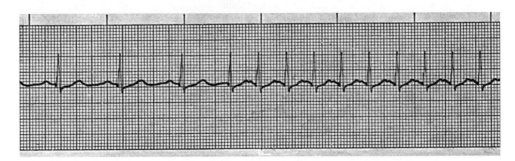

Fig. 24-20 *Paroxysmal atrial tachycardia (PAT).* *(From Atwood S, Stanton C, Storey J:* Introduction to basic cardiac dysrhythmias, *ed 2, St Louis, 1996, Mosby.)*

- *Atrial flutter*—impulses start in the atria at a rapid rate. The ventricles do not respond to every impulse (Fig. 24-21). There are more P waves (flutter or F waves) than QRS complexes. QRS complexes occur at regular intervals. The person's pulse is regular.

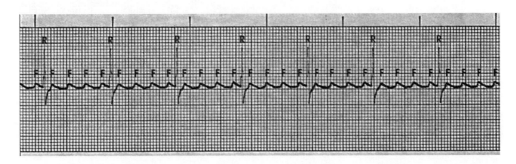

Fig. 24-21 *Atrial flutter. Note the F waves.* *(From Atwood S, Stanton C, Storey J:* Introduction to basic cardiac dysrhythmias, *ed 2, St Louis, 1996, Mosby.)*

- *Atrial fibrillation*—impulses start in the atria at multiple sites. There are no P waves. Impulses are conducted to the ventricles at irregular intervals (Fig. 24-22). QRS complexes occur at irregular intervals. Therefore the pulse is irregular. The atria quiver, not contract. Blood is not pumped from the atria to the ventricles in normal amounts. Therefore the ventricles pump inadequate amounts of blood to the rest of the body.

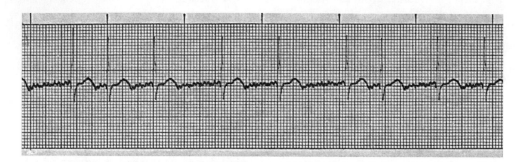

Fig. 24-22 *Atrial fibrillation. No P waves occur and the rhythm is irregular. (From Atwood S, Stanton C, Storey J:* Introduction to basic cardiac dysrhythmias, *ed 2, St Louis, 1996, Mosby.)*

- *Junctional rhythms*—impulses start in the AV node. There are no P waves (Fig. 24-23). Junctional rhythms can occur at normal or slow rates.

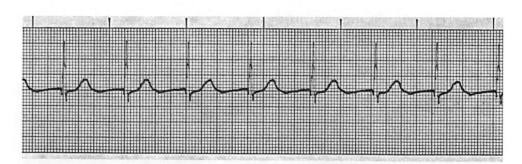

Fig. 24-23 *Junctional rhythm. No P waves. (From Atwood S, Stanton C, Storey J:* Introduction to basic cardiac dysrhythmias, *ed 2, St Louis, 1996, Mosby.)*

- *Third-degree heart block*—the impulse is blocked between the atria and ventricles (Fig. 24-24). The impulse cannot reach the ventricles. The ventricles must create their own impulses. P waves appear but are not related to the QRS complexes. The QRS complexes are wider than normal. The heart rate is very slow. ***This is a life-threatening dysrhythmia.***

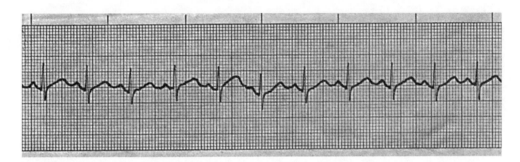

Fig. 24-24 *Third-degree heart block. The atrial rate (P waves) is faster than the ventricular rate.* (From Atwood S, Stanton C, Storey J: Introduction to basic cardiac dysrhythmias, *ed 2, St Louis, 1996, Mosby.*)

- *Premature ventricular contraction (PVC)*—the impulse is created in the ventricles. It occurs earlier than the next regular beat. The QRS complex is wide and bizarre (Fig. 24-25). *Unifocal PVCs* come from one *(uni)* site *(focal)*. They all look the same. *Multifocal PVCs* are created in many *(multi)* sites *(focal)* as in Figure 24-26 on p. 610. Bigeminy *is when every second* (bi) *complex is a PVC* (Fig. 24-27, p. 610). With trigeminy, *every third* (tri) *complex is a PVC.* (Geminus *means twin.*) Two PVCs can occur in a row (Fig. 24-28, p. 610). They can be unifocal or multifocal and are called *coupled PVCs*. A *run of ventricular tachycardia* is several PVCs in a row (Fig. 24-29, p. 611). The rhythm returns to normal. PVCs mean that the heart muscle is irritable. ***PVCs are life threatening.***

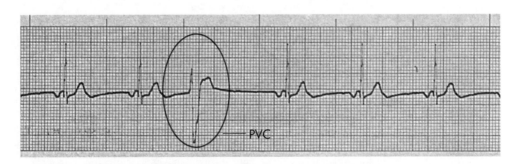

PVC

Fig 24-25 *Premature ventricular contraction (PVC).* (From Atwood S, Stanton C, Storey J: Introduction to basic cardiac dysrhythmias, *ed 2, St Louis, 1996, Mosby.*)

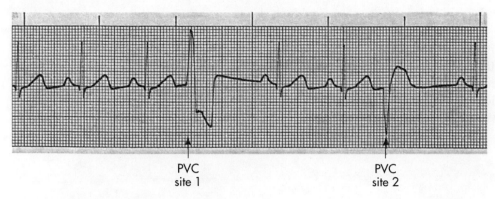

Fig. 24-26 *Multifocal PVCs. (From Atwood S, Stanton C, Storey J:* Introduction to basic cardiac dysrhythmias, *ed 2, St Louis, 1996, Mosby.)*

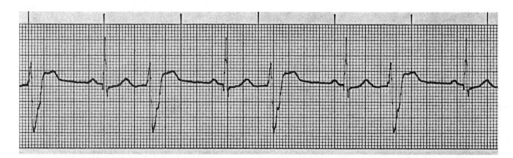

Fig. 24-27 *Bigeminy. (From Atwood S, Stanton C, Storey J:* Introduction to basic cardiac dysrhythmias, *ed 2, St Louis, 1996, Mosby.)*

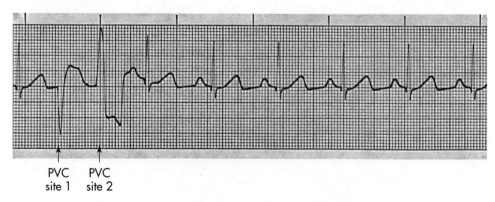

Fig. 24-28 *Coupled PVCs. Two PVCs occur in a row. The PVCs are multifocal. (From Atwood S, Stanton C, Storey J:* Introduction to basic cardiac dysrhythmias, *ed 2, St Louis, 1996, Mosby.)*

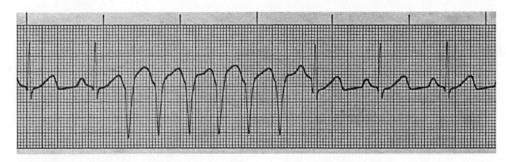

Fig. 24-29 *Run of ventricular tachycardia. (From Atwood S, Stanton C, Storey J:* Introduction to basic cardiac dysrhythmias, *ed 2, St Louis, 1996, Mosby.)*

- *Ventricular tachycardia (VT)*—impulses start in the ventricles. The heart rate can range from 40 to 250 beats per minute. QRS complexes are wide and bizarre. The rhythm looks like a series of PVCs (Fig. 24-30). **Ventricular tachycardia is life threatening. If not corrected, it progresses to ventricular fibrillation.**

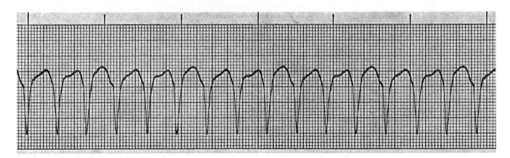

Fig. 24-30 *Ventricular tachycardia (VT). The rate is 160. (From Atwood S, Stanton C, Storey J:* Introduction to basic cardiac dysrhythmias, *ed 2, St Louis, 1996, Mosby.)*

- *Ventricular fibrillation (V Fib)*—impulses start from multiple sites in the ventricles. P waves and QRS complexes are not present (Fig. 24-31). The ventricles quiver, not contract. **Ventricular fibrillation is deadly. The person is in cardiac arrest.**

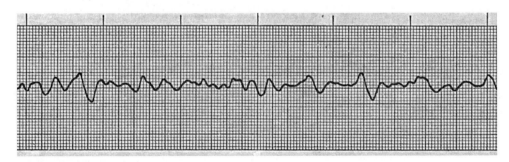

Fig. 24-31 *Ventricular fibrillation—no P waves or QRS complexes. (From Atwood S, Stanton C, Storey J:* Introduction to basic cardiac dysrhythmias, *ed 2, St Louis, 1996, Mosby.)*

- *Asystole*—means no *(a)* contraction *(systole)*. No electrical activity occurs in the heart (Fig. 24-32). **Asystole is deadly. The person is in cardiac arrest.**

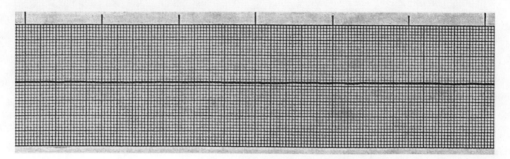

Fig. 24-32 *Asystole. (From Atwood S, Stanton C, Storey J:* Introduction to basic cardiac dysrhythmias, *ed 2, St Louis, 1996, Mosby.)*

Always look at the person when you see ECG patterns similar to ventricular tachycardia (see Fig. 24-30), ventricular fibrillation (see Fig. 24-31), and asystole (see Fig. 24-32). Check to see if the person is moving and breathing. Disconnected cables, improper electrode placement, and patient movements can cause similar patterns (see p. 603). Initiate your facility's life-support procedures if the person:

- Is unresponsive
- Is not breathing
- Has no pulse

REVIEW QUESTIONS

Circle the best answer.

1 The recording of the electrical activity of the heart is an
   a Electrocardiograph
   b Electrocardiogram
   c Arrhythmia
   d Electrode

2 The muscular portion of the heart is called the
   a Pericardium
   b Myocardium
   c Endocardium
   d Dyscardium

3 The heart muscle contracts during
   a Systole
   b Diastole
   c Fibrillation
   d Conduction

4 In normal rhythms, the impulse is created in the
   a SA node
   b AV node
   c Bundle of His
   d Purkinje fibers

5 The normal ECG has the following waves *except*
   a P waves
   b QRS complexes
   c T waves
   d F waves

6 The standard ECG involves
   a 3 leads
   b 6 leads
   c 12 leads
   d Unipolar leads

7 The chest leads also are called
   a Precordial leads   c Augmented limb leads
   b Limb leads   d Bipolar leads

8 To estimate the heart rate with an ECG tracing, you need a
   a 3-second strip
   b 6-second strip
   c 3-inch strip
   d 6-inch strip

9 Before applying electrodes to the skin, electrode sites are cleaned
   a By shaving
   b With soap and water
   c With alcohol wipes
   d With water

10 A person develops chest pain during an ECG. What should you do?
    a Take the person's vital signs.
    b Ask about other symptoms.
    c Continue taking the ECG.
    d Call for the RN.

11 Which dysrhythmia is not life threatening?
    a Atrial flutter
    b Ventricular tachycardia
    c Ventricular fibrillation
    d Third-degree heart block

12 The ECG tracing appears to show asystole. What should you do?
    a Call for the RN.
    b Start life-support procedures.
    c Continue taking the ECG.
    d Check to see if the person is moving and breathing.

Answers to these questions are on p. 853.

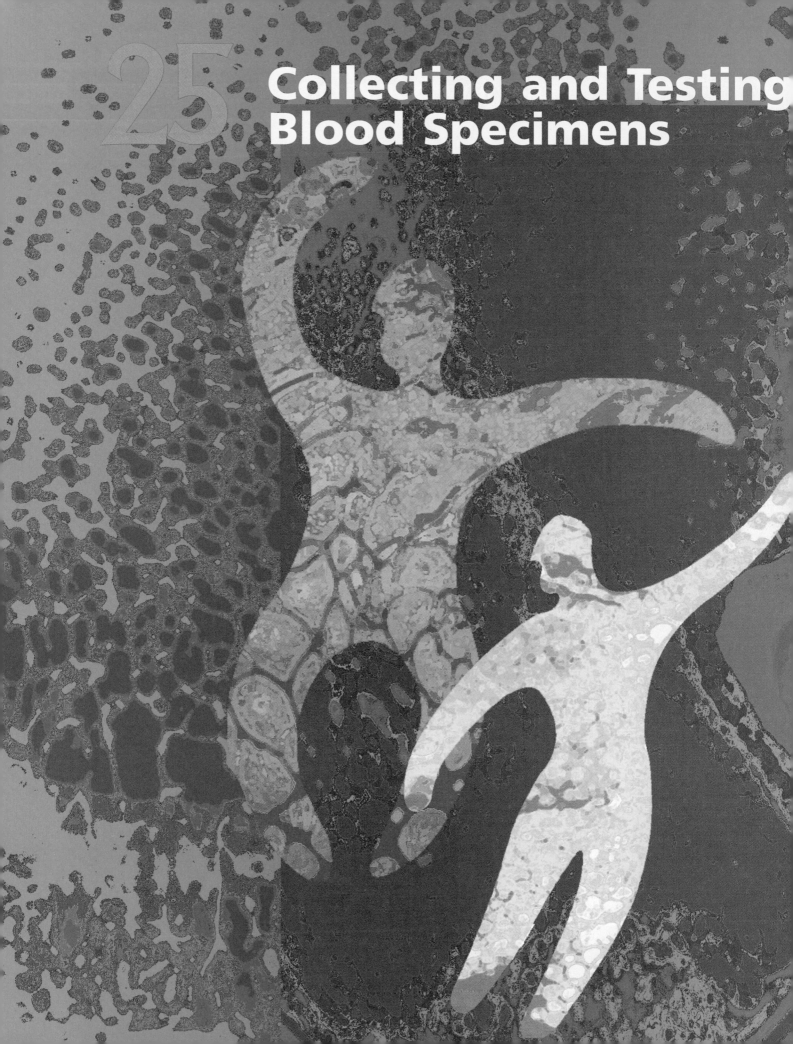

25 Collecting and Testing Blood Specimens

OBJECTIVES

- Define the key terms in this chapter
- Identify the sources of blood specimens
- Identify the sites for a skin puncture
- Describe three venipuncture methods
- Explain how to select tubes for blood specimens
- Identify the information required for labeling blood specimens
- Identify the common venipuncture sites for collecting blood specimens
- Explain how to select a venipuncture site
- Explain the importance of blood glucose testing
- Describe two methods of blood glucose testing
- Explain the rules for blood glucose testing
- Perform the procedures described in this chapter

KEY TERMS

callus A thick, hardened area on the skin

hematology The study *(ology)* of blood *(hemat)*

hematoma A swelling *(oma)* that contains blood *(hemat)*

lancet A short, pointed, disposable blade

palpate To feel or touch using your hands or fingers

tourniquet A constricting device applied to a limb to control bleeding

venipuncture A technique in which a vein *(veni)* is punctured

Hematology is the study of *(ology)* blood *(hemat)*. Blood tests are very common in health care. They play a role in preventing disease and in detecting and treating disease. Blood tests are ordered by doctors. Most tests are done in the laboratory. Some are done at the bedside or in home settings by nurses and assistive personnel.

Blood specimens are drawn by laboratory personnel and nurses. Many states and agencies allow assistive personnel to obtain blood specimens. Before collecting and testing blood specimens, make sure:

- Your state allows assistive personnel to perform the procedures
- The procedures are in your job description
- You have the necessary training
- You know how to use the agency's equipment
- You review the procedures with an RN
- The RN is available to answer questions and to supervise you

Standard Precautions and the Bloodborne Pathogen Standard are followed when collecting and testing blood specimens. Contact with blood is likely.

SOURCES OF BLOOD SPECIMENS

Most blood tests require blood obtained from skin punctures or venipunctures. Sometimes arterial blood is needed. Persons with respiratory diseases and those on mechanical ventilation often require blood gas analysis. The tests measure the amount of oxygen and carbon dioxide in the arterial blood. The specimen is collected by making an arterial stick. Laboratory technicians, RNs, and respiratory therapists with special training do arterial sticks.

✦ Skin Punctures

With skin punctures, a few drops of capillary blood are obtained. A fingertip is the most common site for skin punctures. The earlobe also is a site. These sites provide easy access and do not require clothing removal. The patient feels a sharp pinch. Discomfort is brief.

Inspect the site carefully. Look for signs of trauma. Avoid sites that are swollen, bruised, cyanotic (bluish color), scarred, or calloused. Blood flow to these areas is poor. A **callus** is a thick, hardened area on the skin. Calluses often form over areas that are used frequently, such as the tips of the thumbs and index fingers. Therefore the thumbs and index fingers are not good sites for skin punctures. Also avoid sites that have skin breaks.

Avoid using the center, fleshy part of the fingertip. The site has many nerve endings. A puncture at the site is painful. Use the side or top of the fingertip (Fig. 25-1).

A sterile lancet is used to puncture the skin (Fig. 25-2). A **lancet** is a short, pointed blade. Because the blade is short, it punctures but does not cut the skin. The lancet is enclosed in a protective cover. You do not touch the actual blade. Different types of lancets are available. All are disposable. A lancet is used once and discarded into the sharps container. (See Focus on Children, Focus on Older Persons, and Focus on Home Care.)

focus on CHILDREN

The heel is used for skin punctures in infants. Finger and earlobe sites are used for children. Give the child a choice of sites. Then let the child choose the site for the skin puncture. This gives the child a sense of control.

focus on OLDER PERSONS

Older persons often have poor circulation in their fingers. Applying a warm washcloth or washing the hands in warm water helps increase blood flow.

focus on HOME CARE

An RN teaches patients and family members to do skin punctures in the home setting.

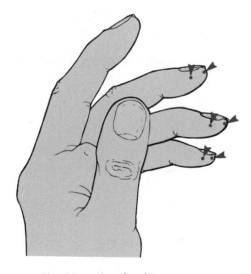

Fig. 25-1 *Sites for skin punctures.*

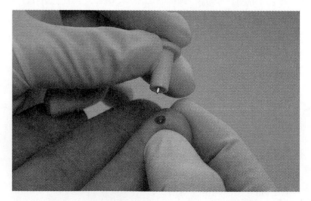

Fig. 25-2 *A lancet. (From Zakus SM: Clinical procedures for medical assistants, ed 3, St Louis, 1995, Mosby.)*

PERFORMING A SKIN PUNCTURE

PROCEDURE ALERT

- Does your state allow assistive personnel to perform the procedure?
- Is the procedure in your job description?
- Do you have the necessary training and education?
- Is an RN available to answer questions and to supervise you?

PRE-PROCEDURE

1 Review the procedure with the RN.

2 Explain the procedure to the person.

3 Wash your hands.

4 Collect the following:

   - Sterile lancet
   - Alcohol wipes
   - Gloves
   - Cotton balls
   - Washcloth
   - Soap, towel, and wash basin

5 Read the manufacturer's instructions for the lancet.

6 Arrange supplies in a convenient location.

7 Identify the person. Check the ID bracelet against the assignment sheet or laboratory requisition form.

8 Provide for privacy.

PROCEDURE

9 Help the person assume a comfortable position.

10 Ask the person to wash his or her hands. Provide necessary supplies and equipment.

11 Open the lancet and alcohol wipes.

12 Put on the gloves.

13 Inspect the person's fingers. Select a skin puncture site.

14 Warm the finger or earlobe if it is cold. To warm the part, gently rub it or apply a warm washcloth.

15 Massage the hand and finger toward the puncture site. This brings more blood to the site.

16 Lower the finger so the hand is below the person's waist. This increases blood flow to the site.

17 Hold the finger with your thumb and forefinger (see Fig. 25-2). Use your nondominant hand. Hold the finger until step 23.

18 Clean the site with alcohol. *Do not touch the site after cleaning.*

19 Allow the site to dry.

20 Pick up the sterile lancet.

21 Place the lancet against the side of the finger or the top of the fingertip (Fig. 25-3, p. 618).

22 Puncture the skin by pushing the button on the lancet. (Follow the manufacturer's instructions.)

23 Wipe away the first blood drop. Use a cotton ball.

24 Apply gentle pressure below the puncture site.

25 Allow a large drop of blood to form (Fig. 25-4, p. 618).

26 Collect and test the specimen (see p. 628).

27 Apply pressure to the puncture site until bleeding stops. Use a cotton ball. If the person is able, let the person continue to apply pressure to the site.

28 Discard the lancet into the sharps container.

29 Discard the cotton balls following agency policy. Remember, they contain blood.

30 Remove and discard the gloves.

Continued

PERFORMING A SKIN PUNCTURE—cont'd

POST-PROCEDURE

31 Help the person to a comfortable position.

32 Make sure the call bell is within reach.

33 Raise or lower bed rails as instructed by the RN.

34 Lower the bed to its lowest horizontal position.

35 Unscreen the person.

36 Discard used supplies. Clean and return the bath basin to its proper place.

37 Follow agency policy for soiled linen.

38 Wash your hands.

39 Report the following to the RN:

- The time the specimen was collected

- The test results (see p. 628)

- The site used

- How the person tolerated the procedure

- Other observations or patient complaints

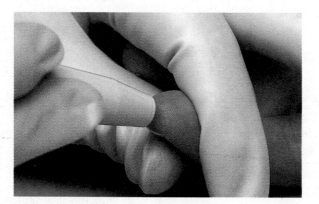

Fig. 25-3 *Puncturing the skin with a lancet.* (*From Elkin MK, Perry AG, Potter PA:* Nursing interventions and clinical skills, *St Louis, 1996, Mosby.*)

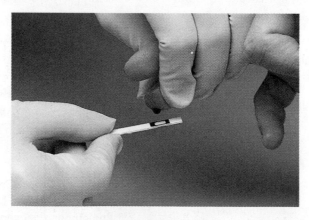

Fig. 25-4 *A large drop of blood forms.* (*From Elkin MK, Perry AG, Potter PA:* Nursing interventions and clinical skills, *St Louis, 1996, Mosby.*)

✦ Venipunctures

Venipunctures are done when large amounts of blood are needed. **Venipuncture** is a technique in which a vein *(veni)* is punctured with a needle.

The needle is attached to a syringe or a Vacutainer. With the syringe method, you pull back on the plunger to withdraw blood into the barrel (Fig. 25-5). (Review parts of a syringe on p. 405.) After the blood is collected, it is transferred to a test tube.

With a Vacutainer, blood flows into the tube (Fig. 25-6). The Vacutainer system has a needle, needle and tube holder, and evacuated tube with rubber stopper (Fig. 25-7). In evacuated tubes, air is removed, creating a vacuum. When a vein is punctured, blood flows into the tube. The Vacutainer system allows the collection of many blood specimens with one venipuncture. After a tube fills, it is removed and a new one is attached to the holder.

Selecting collection tubes

Blood collection tubes come in different sizes. The blood test ordered determines the amount of blood needed. Also, some tests require additives. Additives are chemicals that are added to the collection tube. The chemicals preserve the blood until testing.

In the Vacutainer system, the tubes contain the necessary additives. The rubber stoppers are color-coded. Red, lavender, blue, green, gray, and yellow are common colors. The color-coding signals the type of additive, the amount of blood to collect, and the recommended blood tests. Color-coding may vary with agencies. Always follow your agency's procedures. Check the Vacutainer tube guide (Fig. 25-8) when selecting tubes for blood tests.

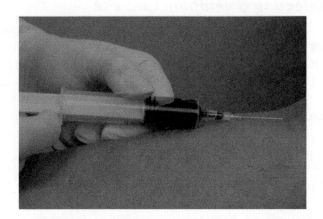

Fig. 25-5 *Needle and syringe method. Blood collects in the barrel as the plunger is pulled back. (From Zakus SM:* Clinical procedures for medical assistants, *ed 3, St Louis, 1995, Mosby.)*

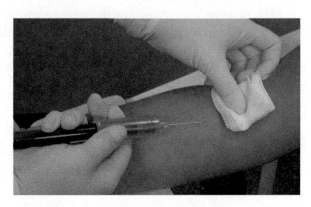

Fig. 25-6 *Blood collects in a Vacutainer tube. (From Zakus SM:* Clinical procedures for medical assistants, *ed 3, St Louis, 1995, Mosby.)*

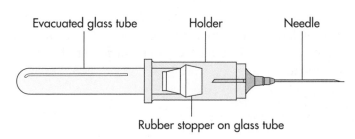

Evacuated glass tube · Holder · Needle · Rubber stopper on glass tube

Fig. 25-7 *Parts of the Vacutainer. (From Zakus SM:* Clinical procedures for medical assistants, *ed 3, St Louis, 1995, Mosby.)*

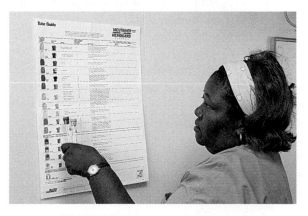

Fig. 25-8 *Checking the Vacutainer guide.*

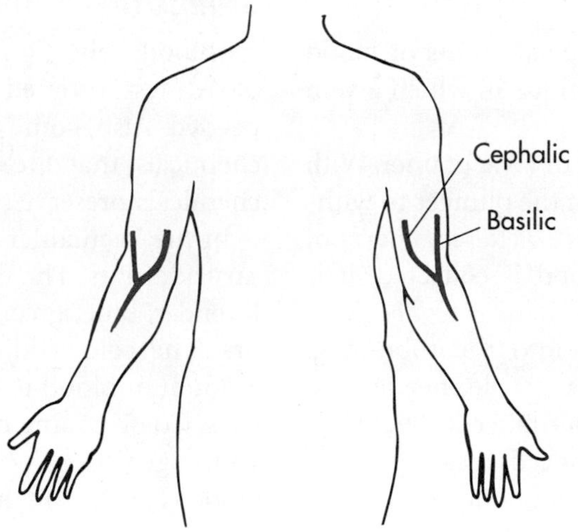

Fig. 25-9 *Veins in the antecubital space. (From Cooper MG, Cooper DE, Burrows NJ:* The medical assistant, *ed 6, St Louis, 1993, Mosby.)*

After selecting the collection tubes, place them in order of use. The order is important to prevent tube contamination. Different tubes have different additives. The additives must not be transferred from one tube to another. Follow agency procedures for the order in which to collect blood specimens.

Labeling collection tubes

Before blood specimens are sent to the laboratory, the collection tube must be labeled with the person's identifying information. Labeling is done at the bedside after the specimens are collected. Labeling is necessary to make sure that the right tests are done for the right person. Otherwise, wrong test results are reported for the person. This leads to the wrong treatment. The person can suffer serious harm.

Follow your agency's procedure for labeling blood specimens. Labeling includes:
- The person's full name—last name, first name, and middle name or initial
- The person's ID number
- The person's bed and room number
- The person's age
- The person's gender (male or female)
- Doctor's name
- Date and time the specimen was collected
- Your name or initials
- Blood test ordered

Selecting a venipuncture site

The basilic and cephalic veins in the antecubital space are the most common venipuncture sites (Fig. 25-9). These veins are large and near the skin surface. Hand veins offer alternative sites.

Before selecting a vein, select the arm that you will use. Avoid the arm on the side of a mastectomy (removal of a breast) or on the side of hemiplegia. If a person has an IV infusion, do not use that arm. Do not use the arm with an access site for hemodialysis. Always discuss site selection with the RN. The RN tells you what side to avoid.

Inspect the arm you will use. Look for skin breaks and hematomas. A **hematoma** is a swelling *(oma)* that contains blood *(hemat)*. Do not use sites with skin breaks or hematomas.

To select a vein, apply a tourniquet (Fig. 25-10). A **tourniquet** is a constricting device applied to a limb to control bleeding. The device is applied above the bleeding site. It prevents arterial blood flow to the part below the tourniquet. Likewise, it prevents venous blood from returning to the heart. Therefore tourniquets are useful for venipunctures. The veins fill with blood and distend (enlarge). They are firmer and easier to see and feel. The tourniquet is removed after collecting the blood specimen.

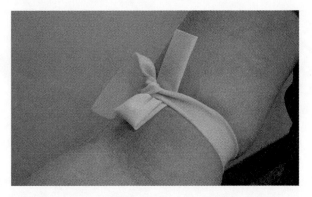

Fig. 25-10 *A tourniquet is applied to select a venipuncture site.* (*From Zakus SM:* Clinical procedures for medical assistants, *ed 3, St Louis, 1995, Mosby.*)

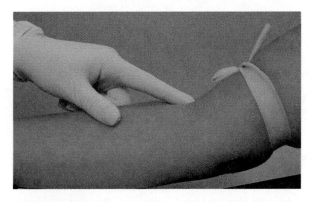

Fig. 25-11 *Palpating a vein.* (*From Zakus SM:* Clinical procedures for medical assistants, *ed 3, St Louis, 1995, Mosby.*)

focus on CHILDREN

Children are often afraid of needles. Explain what you are going to do. Ask a parent or another staff member to hold and comfort the child. Use toys or books to distract the child. Also keep the needle out of the child's sight for as long as possible. Perform the venipuncture and collect the blood quickly.

Children fear the loss of blood. Explain that they have a lot of blood and that their bodies constantly make blood. Placing an adhesive bandage over the site is comforting. It reassures the child that blood will not leak from the body.

focus on OLDER PERSONS

Older persons often have fragile or sclerosed veins. Ask the RN to assist you with site selection.

When used for venipunctures, tourniquets serve to prevent venous blood flow—not arterial blood flow. The tourniquet must be tight so that the veins distend. However, you should feel the radial pulse. If you do not feel a radial pulse, the arm is not getting arterial blood. Release and reapply the tourniquet. Feel for the radial pulse again. A tourniquet is applied no longer than 1 minute.

To select a vein in the antecubital space, apply a tourniquet 3 to 4 inches above the elbow. Then ask the person to open and close a fist. With the fist closed, look and feel for a vein. Look for a straight vein. The vein should feel full and firm. It should be elastic and rebound (spring back) after you palpate it. To **palpate** means to feel or touch using your hands or fingers. You use your fingers to palpate veins (Fig. 25-11). Avoid veins that are:

- Small and narrow—they are usually fragile
- Weak—weak veins are soft and do not rebound
- Sclerosed—*sclero* means hardened; sclerosed veins are hard and rigid
- Easy to roll—the vein rolls when palpated

(See Focus on Children and Focus on Older Persons.)

Text continued on p. 628

COLLECTING BLOOD SPECIMENS WITH A NEEDLE AND SYRINGE

PROCEDURE ALERT

- Does your state allow assistive personnel to perform the procedure?

- Is the procedure in your job description?

- Do you have the necessary training and education?

- Is an RN available to answer questions and to supervise you?

PRE-PROCEDURE

1 Review the procedure with the RN. Discuss site selection.

2 Explain the procedure to the person.

3 Wash your hands.

4 Collect the following:

   - Alcohol swabs

   - Tourniquet

   - Sterile 2 × 2 gauze dressings

   - Tape or adhesive bandage

   - Sterile needle

   - Sterile syringe

   - Color-coded vacuum test tubes (check the expiration date)

   - Laboratory requisition forms

   - Labels for the blood specimens

   - Towel

   - Gloves

   - Leakproof plastic bag

   - Portable sharps container (optional)

5 Complete the labels for the blood specimens.

6 Arrange equipment on the overbed table. If using a blood collection tray, place it on the bedside table or the chair. (The tray is used for many patients. It can contaminate the overbed table that is used for eating and other nursing procedures.)

7 Identify the person. Check the ID bracelet against the laboratory requisition forms.

8 Provide for privacy.

9 Raise the bed to the best level for good body mechanics.

PROCEDURE

10 Help the person assume a comfortable position. The person should be supine, sitting, or in semi-Fowler's position.

11 Inspect both arms for skin breaks and hematomas. Ask the person if he or she prefers the right or left arm for the venipuncture.

12 Choose the side you will use. Position the overbed table so you can reach supplies easily.

13 Place a rolled towel under the arm.

14 Position the arm. Extend the arm with the palm side up.

15 Prepare the supplies:

   a Open the alcohol swabs.

   b Open the sterile gauze squares.

   c Open the adhesive bandage.

   d Open the needle and syringe package.

   e Attach the needle to the syringe.

16 Put on the gloves.

COLLECTING BLOOD SPECIMENS WITH A NEEDLE AND SYRINGE—cont'd

PROCEDURE—cont'd

17 Apply the tourniquet 3 or 4 inches above the elbow:

a Cross one end tightly over the other.

b Tuck the upper end under the band to form a half bow (see Fig. 25-10).

18 Palpate the radial pulse. Release and reapply the tourniquet if you do not feel a pulse.

19 Ask the person to open and close the fist a few times.

20 Look and palpate for a vein in the antecubital space (see Fig. 25-11).

21 Select a vein. Avoid veins that are narrow, weak, sclerosed, or rolling.

22 Release the tourniquet if it has been on longer than 1 minute.

23 Wait 1 minute before reapplying the tourniquet.

24 Reapply the tourniquet.

25 Palpate the vein again.

26 Clean the site with an alcohol swab. Clean in a circular motion from the site outward about 2 inches. *Do not touch the site after cleaning.*

27 Let the site dry.

28 Pick up the needle and attached syringe.

29 Remove the needle cover. Pull it straight off. *Do not touch the needle.*

30 Pull the skin over the site taut. Use the thumb or first two fingers of your nondominant hand (Fig. 25-12, p. 625). Hold the site taut until step 33.

31 Hold the needle and syringe so that the needle bevel is up. (The bevel is the pointed end.)

32 Position the needle at a 15- to 30-degree angle to the person's arm.

33 Insert the needle into the vein gently and smoothly (Fig. 25-13, p. 625).

34 Pull back on the plunger slowly to withdraw blood (Fig. 25-14, p. 625). Use your nondominant hand.

35 Release the tourniquet. Pull on the half bow.

36 Continue to pull back on the plunger until you have withdrawn the necessary amount of blood. Keep the needle stable so it does not move.

37 Hold a gauze square over the puncture site. Do not apply pressure.

38 Pull the needle straight out.

39 Apply pressure to the venipuncture site with the gauze square. Ask the person to apply pressure to the arm. Bleeding stops in 1 to 3 minutes.

40 Transfer blood from the syringe into the vacuum tube. Be very careful not to stick yourself with the needle. Follow agency policy for tube order (see p. 619).

a Method 1:

• Insert the needle through the rubber stopper on the tube.

• Let the vacuum tube fill (Fig. 25-15, p. 625).

• Discard the needle and syringe into the sharps container. *Do not recap the needle.*

b *Method 2:*

• Remove the needle from the syringe. Discard it into the sharps container. *Do not recap the needle.*

• Remove the rubber stopper from the tube.

• Inject blood directly into the tube by pushing down on the plunger.

• Insert the rubber stopper.

• Check the outside of the tube for blood. Remove any blood with alcohol swabs.

Continued

COLLECTING BLOOD SPECIMENS WITH A NEEDLE AND SYRINGE—cont'd

PROCEDURE—cont'd

41 Identify the tubes with additives. Mix the blood and additives by gently inverting each tube back and forth. Follow the manufacturer's instructions for the number of times to invert the tube (usually 8 to 10 times). Do not shake the tube.

42 Check the venipuncture site for bleeding.

43 Remove the gauze square.

44 Apply a new gauze square or adhesive bandage. Secure the gauze square with tape.

45 Discard the syringe into the sharps container if you have not yet done so.

46 Apply labels to the blood specimens.

47 Put the specimens into the plastic bag (if this is your agency's policy).

48 Remove the towel under the person's arm. Follow agency policy for soiled linen. The towel may contain blood.

49 Discard cotton balls, gauze, and alcohol swabs following agency policy. These supplies may contain blood.

50 Remove and discard the gloves.

POST-PROCEDURE

51 Assist the person to a comfortable position.

52 Place the call bell within reach.

53 Raise or lower bed rails as instructed by the RN.

54 Lower the bed to its lowest horizontal position.

55 Discard any other used supplies.

56 Unscreen the person.

57 Take the blood specimens to the nurses' station.

58 Report the following to the RN:

   • The time the specimens were collected

   • The site used

   • The amount of bleeding at the site

   • Any signs of hematoma

   • How the person tolerated the procedure

   • Patient complaints of pain at the site

   • Any other observations or patient complaints

   • What you did with the specimens

59 Take or send the specimens to the laboratory as directed by the RN.

60 Wash your hands.

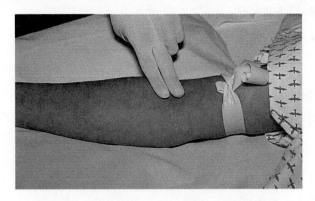

Fig. 25-12 *Pulling the skin taut over the venipuncture site. (From Potter PA, Perry AG:* Fundamentals of nursing: concepts, process, and practice, *ed 4, St Louis, 1997, Mosby.)*

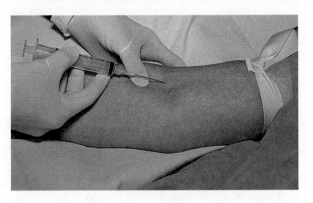

Fig. 25-13 *Inserting the needle into the vein. (From Potter PA, Perry AG:* Fundamentals of nursing: concepts, process, and practice, *ed 4, St Louis, 1997, Mosby.)*

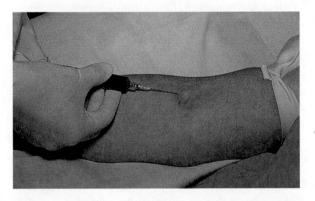

Fig. 25-14 *Pulling back on the plunger to withdraw blood. (From Potter PA, Perry AG:* Fundamentals of nursing: concepts, process, and practice, *ed 4, St Louis, 1997, Mosby.)*

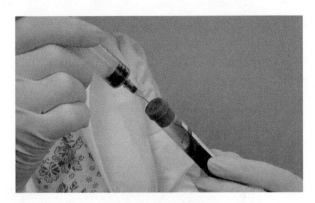

Fig. 25-15 *Transferring blood from the syringe into the vacuum tube. (From Zakus SM:* Clinical procedures for medical assistants, *ed 3, St Louis, 1995, Mosby.)*

COLLECTING BLOOD SPECIMENS USING THE VACUTAINER SYSTEM

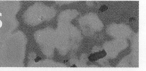

PROCEDURE ALERT

- Does your state allow assistive personnel to perform the procedure?

- Is the procedure in your job description?

- Do you have the necessary training and education?

- Is an RN available to answer questions and to supervise you?

PRE-PROCEDURE

1 Review the procedure with the RN. Discuss site selection.

2 Explain the procedure to the person.

3 Wash your hands.

4 Collect the following:

- Alcohol swabs

- Tourniquet

- Sterile 2 × 2 gauze dressings

- Tape or adhesive bandage

- Vacutainer tube holder

- Sterile double-ended Vacutainer needle

- Vacutainer tubes (check the expiration date)

- Laboratory requisition forms

- Labels for the blood specimens

- Towel

- Gloves

- Leakproof plastic bag

5 Complete the labels for the blood specimens.

6 Arrange equipment on the overbed table.

7 Identify the person. Check the ID bracelet against the laboratory requisition forms.

8 Provide for privacy.

9 Raise the bed to the best level for good body mechanics.

PROCEDURE

10 Follow steps 10 through 14 in *Collecting Blood Specimens With a Needle and Syringe.*

11 Prepare the supplies:

a Open the alcohol swabs.

b Open the sterile gauze squares.

c Open the adhesive bandage.

d Open the double-ended needle.

e Attach the needle to the Vacutainer tube holder (Fig. 25-16).

f Place the first tube to be used inside the holder. Do not attach it to the needle.

g Arrange tubes in order of use. Follow agency policy.

12 Follow steps 16 through 27 in *Collecting Blood Specimens With a Needle and Syringe.*

13 Pick up the Vacutainer needle and tube holder.

14 Remove the needle cover. Pull it straight off. *Do not touch the needle.*

15 Pull the skin over the site taut. Use the thumb or first two fingers of your nondominant hand. Hold the site taut until step 19.

16 Hold the needle so that the needle bevel is up. (The bevel is the pointed end.)

17 Position the needle at a 15- to 30-degree angle to the person's arm.

18 Insert the needle into the vein gently and slowly (Fig. 25-17).

COLLECTING BLOOD SPECIMENS USING THE VACUTAINER SYSTEM—cont'd

PROCEDURE—cont'd

19 Push the tube forward onto the end of the needle in the holder. Push gently.

20 Let the tube fill with blood (Fig. 25-18, p. 628).

21 Remove the filled tube from the holder. Grasp it firmly.

22 Insert the next tube. Repeat steps 19 through 22 for the other tubes.

23 Release the tourniquet after the last tube fills.

24 Hold a gauze square over the puncture site. Do not apply pressure.

25 Pull the needle straight out.

26 Apply pressure to the venipuncture site with the gauze square. Ask the person to apply pressure to the arm. Bleeding stops in 1 to 3 minutes.

27 Remove the last tube from the tube holder. *Do not recap the needle.*

28 Discard the needle and tube holder into the sharps container.

29 Identify the tubes with additives. Mix the blood and additives by gently inverting each tube back and forth. Follow the manufacturer's instructions for the number of times to invert the tube (usually 8 to 10 times). Do not shake the tube.

30 Check the venipuncture site for bleeding.

31 Remove the gauze square.

32 Apply a new gauze square or adhesive bandage. Secure the gauze square with tape.

33 Apply labels to the blood specimens.

34 Put the specimens into the plastic bag (if this is your agency's policy).

35 Remove the towel under the person's arm. Follow agency policy for soiled linen. The towel may contain blood.

36 Discard cotton balls, gauze, and alcohol swabs following agency policy. These supplies may contain blood.

37 Remove and discard the gloves.

POST-PROCEDURE

38 Follow steps 51 through 60 in *Collecting Blood Specimens With a Needle and Syringe.*

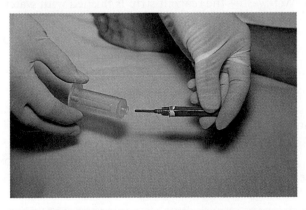

Fig. 25-16 *Attaching the double-ended needle to the Vacutainer needle and tube holder. (From Potter PA, Perry AG: Fundamentals of nursing: concepts, process, and practice, ed 4, St Louis, 1997, Mosby.)*

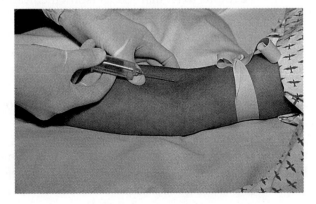

Fig. 25-17 *Inserting the needle into the vein. (From Potter PA, Perry AG: Fundamentals of nursing: concepts, process, and practice, ed 4, St Louis, 1997, Mosby.)*

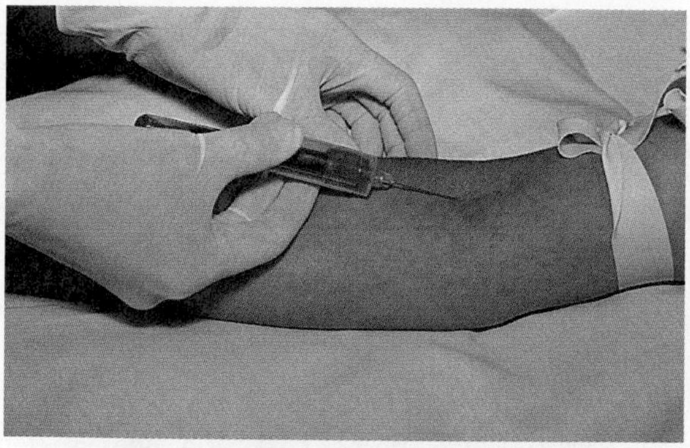

Fig. 25-18 *The Vacutainer tube fills with blood.* (From Potter PA, Perry AG: Fundamentals of nursing: concepts, process, and practice, ed 4, St Louis, 1997, Mosby.)

Butterfly Method

Some people have small or weak hand veins. Other sites may be bruised from frequent venipunctures. The butterfly method is useful for such persons. The method involves using a butterfly needle (see Fig. 20-9, *B* on p. 482), a vacuum tube needle and tube holder, and vacuum tubes.

The vacuum tube needle and tube holder attach to the butterfly needle tubing. The butterfly needle is used for the venipuncture. Blood flows into the butterfly needle, into the vacuum tube needle, and into the vacuum tube. The method also allows the collection of many specimens.

BLOOD GLUCOSE TESTING

Diabetes mellitus is a chronic disease in which the pancreas fails to secrete enough insulin. Insufficient amounts of insulin prevent the body from using sugar for energy. Sugar builds up in the blood if it cannot be used. Blood glucose testing is done to measure blood sugar levels. The doctor uses the results to regulate the person's medication and diet. Inaccurate results are harmful to the person.

Complex tests are done in the laboratory. Two simple blood glucose tests are done at the bedside or in home settings. Both involve reagent strips. The blood reacts with the test area on the reagent strip. The reaction causes the test area to change color. Capillary blood is used for both tests. A skin puncture is done to obtain the specimen.

One method involves exposing the reagent strip to blood. After waiting the recommended amount of time, the blood is wiped or rinsed off the reagent strip. Then the reagent strip is compared with a color chart. The results are read and reported to the RN. You record them following agency policy. As always, follow the manufacturer's instructions for using the reagent strips.

focus on HOME CARE

Patients and families monitor blood glucose in the home setting. The person may have a routine for testing blood glucose. Ask the person how he or she does the test. Report the routine to the RN. The RN lets you follow the routine if it is safe for the person. If it is unsafe, the RN plans for patient and family teaching.

The patient keeps a record of the test results. Share the results with the person, and report them to the RN. Also record the results following agency policy.

The other method involves using a glucose meter (glucometer). A drop of blood is applied to the reagent strip. The strip is inserted into the glucose meter. The blood glucose level is displayed on the monitor. The speed with which results are displayed varies with the manufacturer. Some take as long as 2 minutes. Others take 15 seconds. Many different glucose meters are available. Always read and follow the manufacturer's instructions. Make sure you know how to use the equipment before testing blood. Also check the manufacturer's instructions for the reagent strip to use. Use only the type of reagent strip specified by the manufacturer. Otherwise you will get inaccurate results.

Also check the manufacturer's instructions about how to treat a strip before inserting it into the glucose meter. The manufacturer requires one of the following:

- Dry-wipe—blood is wiped off the reagent strip with a cotton ball.
- Wet-wash—the reagent strip is flushed with water to rinse off blood.
- No-wipe—no wiping or rinsing; the reagent strip is inserted directly into the glucose meter.

In agencies, glucose meters are tested daily for accuracy. Inaccurate results can harm the person. The manufacturer has specific instructions for testing the meter. Specially trained staff members perform the tests.

Accurate results are important. The rules in Box 25-1 are followed when testing blood specimens for glucose. (See Focus on Home Care.)

BOX 25-1

RULES FOR BLOOD GLUCOSE TESTING

- Read the manufacturer's instructions. Make sure you understand them.
- Make sure you know how to use the equipment. Request any necessary training.
- Make sure the glucose meter was tested for accuracy. Check the testing log.
- Check the color of reagent strips. Do not use them if they are discolored.
- Check the expiration date of the reagent strips. Do not use them if the date has passed.
- Use a watch with a sweep hand to time the test. Follow the manufacturer's instructions for test times.
- Report the results immediately to the RN.
- Record the result following agency policy.
- Practice Standard Precautions.
- Follow the Bloodborne Pathogen Standard.

MEASURING BLOOD GLUCOSE

PROCEDURE ALERT

- Does your state allow assistive personnel to perform the procedure?
- Is the procedure in your job description?
- Do you have the necessary training and education?
- Is an RN available to answer questions and to supervise you?

PRE-PROCEDURE

1 Review the procedure with the RN.

2 Explain the procedure to the person.

3 Wash your hands.

4 Collect the following:

- Sterile lancet
- Alcohol swab
- Cotton balls
- Glucose testing meter
- Reagent strips (Make sure they are the correct ones for the meter. Check the expiration date.)
- Gloves
- Paper towel
- Soap, towel, and wash basin

5 Arrange supplies on the overbed table.

6 Identify the person. Check the ID bracelet against the assignment sheet.

7 Raise the bed to a good level for body mechanics.

Continued

MEASURING BLOOD GLUCOSE—cont'd

PROCEDURE

8   Ask the person to wash his or her hands. Provide necessary supplies and equipment.

9   Help the person assume a comfortable position.

10 Prepare the supplies:

    a   Open the alcohol swabs.

    b   Remove a reagent strip from the bottle. Place it on the paper towel. Place the cap securely on the bottle.

    c   Prepare the lancet.

    d   Turn on the glucose meter.

11 Put on the gloves.

12 Perform a skin puncture to obtain a drop of blood (see *Performing a Skin Puncture* on p. 617).

13 Wipe off the first drop of blood with a cotton ball.

14 Apply gentle pressure below the puncture site.

15 Allow a large drop of blood to form (see Fig. 25-4).

16 Hold the test area of the reagent strip close to the drop of blood.

17 Lightly touch the reagent strip to the blood drop. Do not smear the blood.

18 Set the timer on the glucose meter.

19 Set the reagent strip on the paper towel. Or follow the manufacturer's instructions.

20 Wait the length of time required by the manufacturer.

21 Apply pressure to the puncture site until bleeding stops. Use a cotton ball. If the person is able, let the person continue to apply pressure to the site.

22 Treat the reagent strip according to the manufacturer's instructions. Use the dry-wipe, wet-wash, or no-wipe method (see p. 628).

23 Insert the reagent strip into the glucose meter (Fig. 25-19). Follow the manufacturer's instructions.

24 Read the result on the display (Fig. 25-20). Write down the result, and tell the person the result.

25 Turn off the glucose meter.

26 Discard the lancet into the sharps container.

27 Discard the cotton balls following agency policy. (The cotton balls contain blood.)

28 Remove and discard the gloves.

POST-PROCEDURE

29 Help the person to a comfortable position.

30 Make sure the call bell is within reach.

31 Raise or lower bed rails as instructed by the RN.

32 Lower the bed to its lowest horizontal position.

33 Unscreen the person.

34 Discard used supplies. Clean and return the bath basin to its proper place.

35 Follow agency policy for soiled linen.

36 Wash your hands.

37 Report the following to the RN immediately:

- The time the specimen was collected

- The test results

- The site used

- How the person tolerated the procedure

- Other observations or patient complaints

38 Record the result following agency policy.

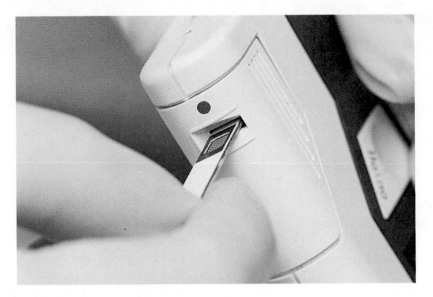

Fig. 25-19 *Inserting the reagent strip into the glucose meter. (From Elkin MK, Perry AG, Potter PA:* Nursing interventions and clinical skills, *St Louis, 1996, Mosby.)*

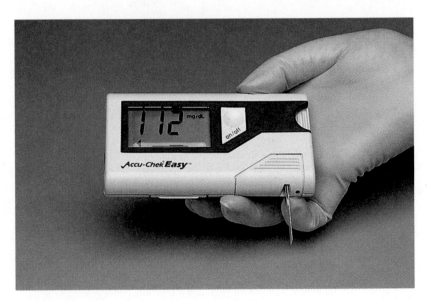

Fig. 25-20 *Reading the result on the glucose meter display. (From Elkin MK, Perry AG, Potter PA:* Nursing interventions and clinical skills, *St Louis, 1996, Mosby.)*

REVIEW QUESTIONS

Circle the best answer.

1 A tourniquet is
   a A swelling that contains blood
   b A blood test
   c A device to control bleeding
   d A short, pointed, disposable blade

2 The most common site for a skin puncture is
   a The earlobe
   b The heel
   c The thumb
   d A fingertip

3 You inspect a skin puncture site. You avoid the site if it is
   a Calloused
   b Swollen or bruised
   c Scarred
   d All of the above

4 To avoid painful skin punctures, puncture the fingertip
   a At the side of the fingertip
   b In the center of the fingertip
   c In the fleshy part of the fingertip
   d All of the above

5 You perform a skin puncture. The first drop of blood is
   a Saved
   b Wiped off with a cotton ball
   c Tested in case you cannot get another drop
   d Rinsed off with water

6 After puncturing the skin, the lancet is
   a Discarded into the sharps container
   b Sterilized for reuse
   c Discarded with other supplies
   d Capped

7 Blood specimens are labeled at the nurses' station.
   a True
   b False

8 You are to perform a venipuncture. What veins should you use?
   a Hand veins
   b Foot veins
   c Veins in the antecubital space
   d All of the above

9 You are selecting a vein for a venipucture. The vein should
   a Rebound after palpating it
   b Be narrow
   c Be sclerosed
   d Roll easily

REVIEW QUESTIONS—cont'd

10 The needle and syringe method is used to obtain a blood specimen. Which is *true*?

a The needle is capped. The needle and syringe are sent to the laboratory.

b The needle is discarded. The syringe is capped and sent to the laboratory.

c The blood is transferred from the syringe to a test tube.

d Blood is collected in Vacutainers.

11 You are going to test blood glucose with a glucose meter. Which is *false*?

a The blood specimen is obtained by venipuncture.

b The manufacturer's instructions must be followed.

c The expiration date on the reagent strips is checked.

d The results are immediately reported to the RN.

12 The manufacturer requires the dry-wipe method for reagent strips. This means that

a Blood is rinsed off before inserting the reagent strip into the glucose meter.

b The first drop of blood from the skin puncture is wiped off with a cotton ball.

c Blood is wiped off with a cotton ball before inserting the reagent strip into the glucose meter.

d The reagent strip is inserted directly into the glucose meter.

Answers to these questions are on p. 853.

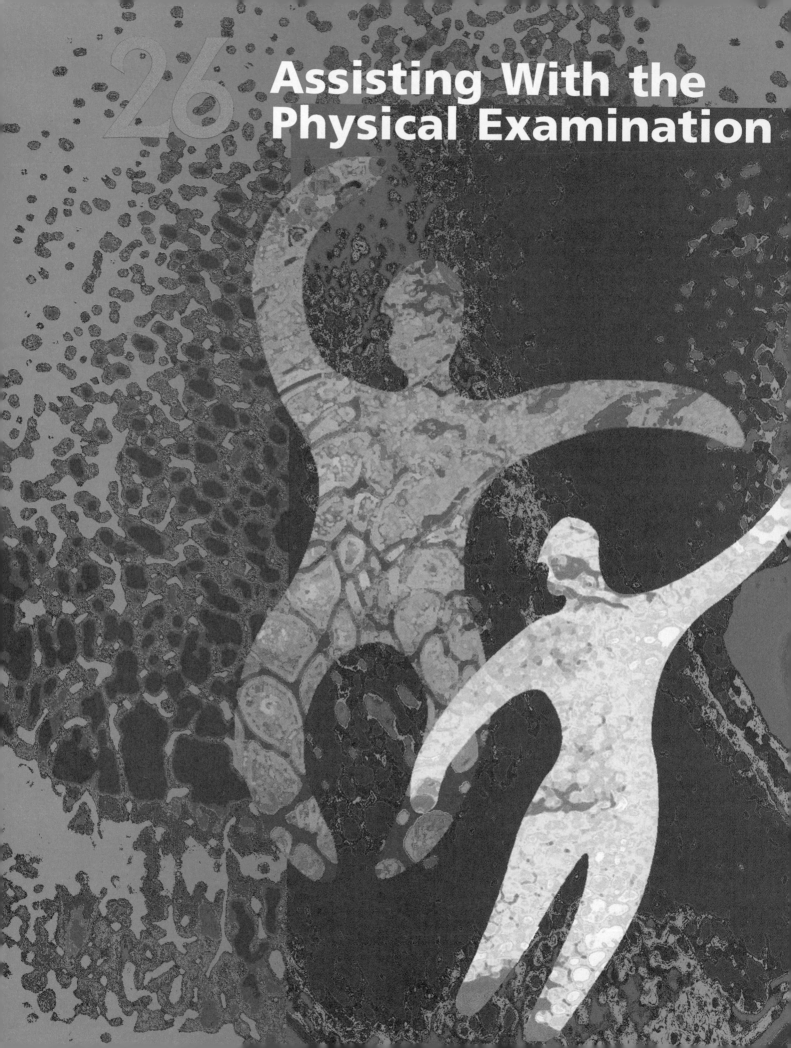

26 Assisting With the Physical Examination

- Define the key terms in this chapter
- Explain your responsibilities before, after, and during a physical examination
- Identify the equipment used during a physical examination
- Describe how to prepare a person for an examination
- Describe four examination positions and how to drape the person for each position
- Prepare a person for an examination
- Explain the rules for assisting with a physical examination
- Perform the procedures described in this chapter

KEY TERMS

dorsal recumbent position The supine or back-lying examination position; the legs are together

horizontal recumbent position The dorsal recumbent position

knee-chest position The person kneels and rests the body on the knees and chest; the head is turned to one side, the arms are above the head or flexed at the elbows, the back is straight, and the body is flexed about 90 degrees at the hips

laryngeal mirror An instrument used to examine the mouth, teeth, and throat

lithotomy position The person is in a back-lying position, the hips are brought down to the edge of the examination table, the knees are flexed, the hips are externally rotated, and the feet are supported in stirrups

nasal speculum An instrument used to examine the inside of the nose

ophthalmoscope A lighted instrument used to examine the internal structures of the eye

otoscope A lighted instrument used to examine the external ear and the eardrum (tympanic membrane)

percussion hammer An instrument used to tap body parts to test reflexes; reflex hammer

Sims' position A side-lying position in which the upper leg is sharply flexed so that it is not on the lower leg and the lower arm is behind the person

tuning fork An instrument used to test hearing

vaginal speculum An instrument used to open the vagina so that it and the cervix can be examined

Physical examinations are usually done by doctors. Many RNs also perform them. They are done for many reasons. Routine health examinations are done to promote health. Preemployment physicals are done to determine fitness for work. Physical examinations are used also to diagnose and treat disease. You may be asked to assist a doctor or RN with a physical examination.

RESPONSIBILITIES OF ASSISTIVE PERSONNEL

Your responsibilities depend on the agency's policies and procedures. The examiner's preferences also affect what you are expected to do. You may do some or all of the following:

- Collect linens for draping the person and for the procedure.
- Collect equipment and supplies used for the examination.
- Prepare the room for the examination.
- Provide enough lighting.
- Measure vital signs, height, and weight.
- Position and drape the person for the examination.
- Hand equipment and instruments to the examiner.
- Label specimen containers.
- Dispose of soiled linen, and discard used disposable supplies.
- Clean reusable equipment after the examination.
- Help the person dress or assume a comfortable position after the examination.

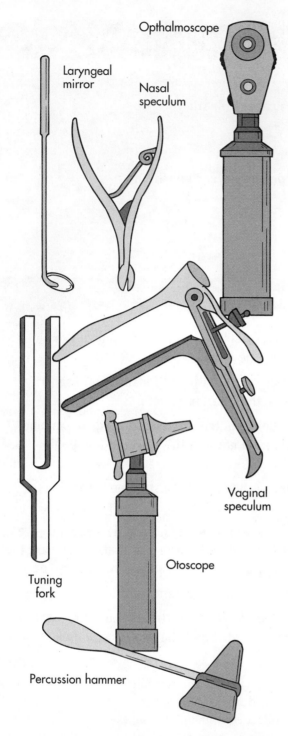

Fig. 26-1 *Instruments used for a physical examination.*

EQUIPMENT

Some equipment and supplies used in a physical examination are used for nursing care. You may recognize some of the instruments. You need to know the instruments in Figure 26-1:

- **Ophthalmoscope**—is a lighted instrument used to examine the internal structures of the eye.
- **Otoscope**—is used to examine the external ear and the eardrum (tympanic membrane). The otoscope is a lighted instrument. Some scopes have interchangeable parts. They are changed into an ophthalmoscope or otoscope.
- **Percussion hammer**—is used to tap body parts to test reflexes. It is also called a *reflex hammer*.
- **Vaginal speculum**—is used to open the vagina so it and the cervix can be examined.
- **Nasal speculum**—is used to examine the inside of the nose.
- **Tuning fork**—is vibrated to test hearing.
- **Laryngeal mirror**—is used to examine the mouth, teeth, and throat.

Many agencies have examination trays in the central supply department. If not, collect needed items. Items listed in *Preparing the Person for an Examination* on p. 638 usually are used for an examination. They are arranged on a tray or table for the examiner.

✦ PREPARING THE PERSON

The physical examination causes anxiety for many people. They are concerned about possible findings. Other factors can add to their anxiety. These include discomfort, embarrassment, the fear of exposure, and unfamiliarity with the procedure. You need to be sensitive to the person's feelings and concerns. The person is prepared physically and psychologically for the examination. The RN explains the purpose of the examination and what to expect. This could be your responsibility, depending on the situation and the agency.

Usually all clothes are removed for a complete physical examination. The person is covered with a drape. It may be a disposable paper drape, a bath blanket, a sheet, or a drawsheet. Usually a hospital gown is worn. It reduces the feeling of nakedness and the fear of exposure. Explain to the person that there is little exposure during the examination. The person needs to understand that some exposure is necessary to examine the body. However, only the body part being examined is exposed. You must screen the person and close the door to the room. This further protects the person's right to privacy. (See Focus on Children and Focus on Long-Term Care.)

The person urinates before the examination. An empty bladder is necessary for the examiner to feel the abdominal organs. A full bladder can change the normal position and shape of organs. It also can cause discomfort, especially when the abdominal organs are felt. If a urine specimen is needed, obtain it at this time. Explain how to collect the specimen, and label the container properly (see Chapter 17).

Warmth is a major concern during the examination. The person is protected from chilling, especially if ill, an older person, or a child. An extra bath blanket should be nearby. Also take measures to prevent drafts.

The examiner may want height, weight, and vital signs measured. These are obtained before the examination starts. They are recorded on the examination form. The person is then positioned and draped for the examination.

focus on

CHILDREN

Toddlers, preschool children, and school-age children are allowed to wear underpants during the examination. The underpants are lowered or removed as necessary during the procedure.

focus on

LONG-TERM CARE

The resident's quality of life must be promoted. The resident has the right to personal choice. The doctor or RN is responsible for informing the resident about the examination. Reasons for the examination are given. The resident is told who will do the examination and when it will be done. The procedure is explained. The resident must give consent. The resident may want a different examiner. Or the resident may want a family member present. Some residents may want the examination results explained with a family member present. All of these are part of the resident's right to personal choice.

✦ PREPARING THE PERSON FOR AN EXAMINATION

PROCEDURE

1 Explain the procedure to the person.

2 Wash your hands.

3 Assemble the following items on a tray at the bedside or in the examination room:

- Flashlight
- Sphygmomanometer
- Stethoscope
- Thermometer
- Tongue depressors (blades)
- Laryngeal mirror
- Ophthalmoscope
- Otoscope
- Nasal speculum
- Percussion (reflex) hammer
- Tuning fork
- Tape measure
- Gloves
- Water-soluble lubricant
- Vaginal speculum
- Cotton-tipped applicators
- Specimen containers and labels
- Disposable bag
- Emesis basin
- Towel
- Bath blanket
- Tissues
- Drape (sheet, bath blanket, drawsheet, or disposable drape)
- Paper towels
- Cotton balls
- Waterproof bed protector
- Eye chart (Snellen chart)
- Slides
- Gown
- Alcohol wipes
- Wastebasket
- Container for soiled instruments
- Marking pencils or pens

4 Identify the person. Check the ID bracelet, and call the person by name.

5 Provide for privacy.

6 Ask the person to put on the gown. Instruct him or her to remove all clothes. Assist as necessary.

7 Ask the person to urinate. If the person is not ambulatory, offer the bedpan or urinal. Provide for privacy.

8 Transport the person to the examination room.

9 Weigh and measure the person (see p. 639).

10 Help the person get on the examination table. Have him or her use a stool if necessary. Omit this step if the examination will be done in the person's room.

11 Position the person as directed (see p. 641). Raise the bed to its highest level. Raise the bed rails if the person is in bed.

12 Drape the person.

13 Place a bed protector under the buttocks.

14 Arrange for adequate lighting.

15 Put the call bell on for the RN or examiner. Do not leave the person unattended.

⚡ MEASURING HEIGHT AND WEIGHT

The person wears only a gown (or pajamas if not part of the physical examination). Clothes add weight. Shoes or slippers also add weight and add to the height measurement. The person urinates before being weighed. A full bladder affects the weight measurement. If a urine specimen is needed, collect it at this time.

Standing, chair, and lift scales are used (Fig. 26-2). Chair and lift scales are used for persons who cannot stand. Follow the manufacturer's instructions when using a chair or lift scale. (See Focus on Children.)

focus on CHILDREN

Birth weight serves as the baseline for measuring an infant's growth. The RN also uses the weight measurements for the nursing process. Weighing infants is described on p. 803.

Length, not height, is measured in children under 2 years of age. The child lies on a measuring board or on a paper. Two people hold the child still. One holds the head still, and the other extends and holds the legs still. The measurement is taken from the top of the head to the heels. If using paper, mark the paper at the head and heels. Measure the distance between the two points.

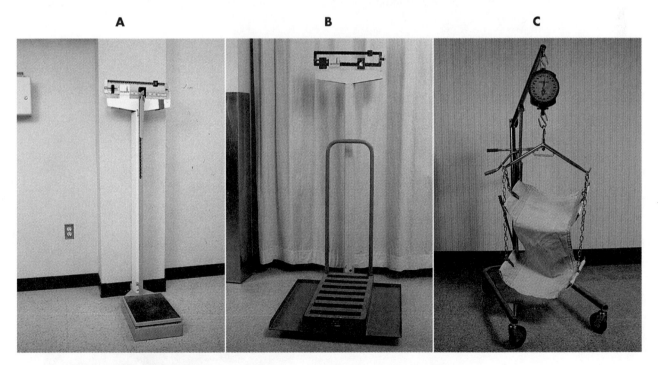

Fig. 26-2 A, *Standing scale.* **B,** *Chair scale.* **C,** *Lift scale*

MEASURING HEIGHT AND WEIGHT

PRE-PROCEDURE

1 Explain the procedure to the person.

2 Ask the person to urinate.

3 Wash your hands.

4 Collect the following:

- Portable balance scale

- Paper towels

5 Identify the person. Check the ID bracelet, and call the person by name.

6 Provide for privacy.

PROCEDURE

7 Place the paper towels on the scale platform.

8 Raise the height rod.

9 Help the person stand on the scale platform. Arms are at the sides.

10 Move the weights until the balance pointer is in the middle (Fig. 26-3).

11 Record the weight on the examination form.

12 Ask the person to stand very straight.

13 Lower the height rod until it rests on the person's head (Fig. 26-4).

14 Record the height on the examination form.

POST-PROCEDURE

15 Assist the person onto the examination table or back to bed. Make sure he or she is comfortable.

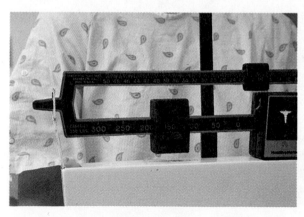

Fig. 26-3 *The weight is read when the balance pointer is in the middle.*

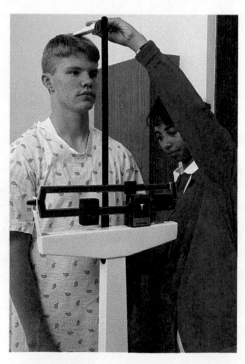

Fig. 26-4 *Height is measured.*

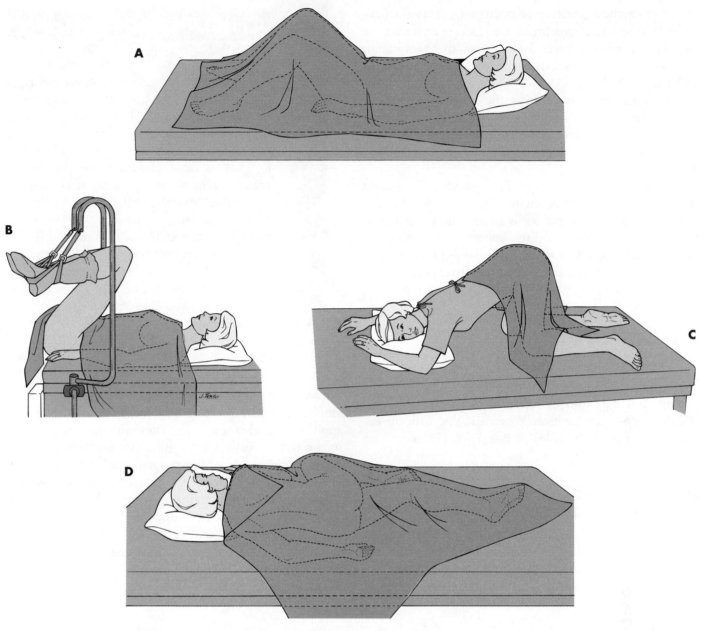

Fig. 26-5 *Positioning and draping for the physical examination.* **A,** *Dorsal recumbent position.* **B,** *Lithotomy position.* **C,** *Knee-chest position.* **D,** *Sims' position.*

POSITIONING AND DRAPING

The person may have to assume a special position for the examination. Some examination positions (Fig. 26-5) are uncomfortable and embarrassing. The examiner tells you how to position the person. Help the person assume and maintain the position. But first explain the following to the person:

- The need for the position
- How the position is assumed
- How the body is draped
- How long the person can expect to stay in the position

The **dorsal recumbent (horizontal recumbent)** or supine position is used to examine the abdomen, anterior chest, and breasts. The person is supine with the legs together. If the perineal area is to be examined, the knees are flexed and hips externally rotated (see Fig. 26-5, *A*). The person is draped as for perineal care (see *Female Perineal Care,* p. 318).

The **lithotomy position** (Fig. 26-5, *B*) is used to examine the vagina. The person lies on her back, and her hips are brought to the edge of the examination table. The knees are flexed, and the hips are externally rotated. The feet are supported in stirrups. The person is draped as for the dorsal recumbent position. Some agencies provide socks to cover the feet and calves.

The **knee-chest position** (Fig. 26-5, *C*) is used to examine the rectum. Sometimes it is used to examine the vagina. The person kneels on the bed or examination table. Then the person rests his or her body on the knees and chest. The head is turned to one side, and the arms are above the head or flexed at the elbows. The back is straight, and the body is flexed about 90 degrees at the hips. The person wears a gown and sometimes socks. The drape is applied in a diamond shape to cover the back, buttocks, and thighs.

The **Sims' position** (Fig. 26-5, *D*) is sometimes used to examine the rectum or vagina. This is a side-lying position in which the upper leg is sharply flexed so that it is not on the lower leg and the lower arm is behind the person. The drape is applied in a diamond shape. The corner near the examiner is folded back to expose the rectum or vagina.

ASSISTING WITH THE EXAMINATION

You may be asked to prepare, position, and drape the person. You may also be asked to assist the doctor or RN during the examination. When assisting with the examination, follow the rules in Box 26-1. (See Focus on Children.)

After the Examination

After the examination the person is taken back to the room. In a clinic, the person dresses in the examination room. Assist as needed. Lubricant is used for the vaginal or rectal examination. The area is wiped or cleaned before the person dresses or returns to the room.

focus on CHILDREN

The examination of an infant or child is like an adult examination. However, a parent is present. The parent may need to hold the infant or child still during some parts of the procedure if the infant or child is uncooperative. Being held still may frighten an infant. The child may also fear separation from the parent. Some children fear being physically harmed during the examination. A calm, comforting manner helps both the child and the parent. Remember, the parent may be anxious too.

The equipment needed is like that used for the adult examination. Toys are used to assess development. Vaginal speculums are not used.

Used disposable items are put in a waste container. Examples are bed protectors, paper drapes, tongue blades, applicators, and cotton balls. These supplies are replaced so the tray is ready for the next examination. Reusable items are cleaned according to agency policy and returned to the tray. This includes the otoscope and ophthalmoscope tips, speculum, and stethoscope. The examination table is covered with a clean drawsheet or paper. All specimens are labeled and sent to the laboratory with a requisition slip. The person's unit or examination room should be neat and orderly after the examination. Follow agency policy for soiled linens.

BOX 26-1   RULES FOR ASSISTING WITH THE PHYSICAL EXAMINATION

- Wash your hands before and after the examination.
- Provide for privacy. This is done by screening, closing doors, and draping. Expose only the body part being examined.
- Assist the person in assuming positions as directed by the examiner.
- Place instruments and equipment in a handy location for the examiner.
- Stay in the room when a female is examined (unless you are a male). When a woman is examined by a man, another female is in the room. This is for the legal protection of the woman and the male examiner. A female attendant also adds to the psychological comfort of the woman.
- Protect the person from falling.
- Anticipate the examiner's need for equipment.
- Place paper or paper towels on the floor if the person is asked to stand.
- Practice medical asepsis and Standard Precautions. Also follow the Bloodborne Pathogen Standard.

REVIEW QUESTIONS

Circle the best answer.

1 The otoscope is used to
   a Examine the internal structures of the eye
   b Examine the external ear and the eardrum
   c Test reflexes
   d Open the vagina

2 You are preparing Mrs. Porter for an examination. You should do the following *except*
   a Have her urinate
   b Ask her to undress
   c Drape her
   d Go tell the nurse when Mrs. Porter is ready

3 Which part of Mrs. Porter's examination can you do?
   a Examine her eyes and ears
   b Inspect her mouth, teeth, and throat
   c Measure her height, weight, and vital signs
   d Observe her perineum and rectum

4 Before being weighed, Mrs. Porter needs to
   a Urinate
   b Put on shoes or slippers
   c Have vital signs measured
   d All of the above

5 Mrs. Porter is supine. Her hips are flexed and externally rotated. Her feet are supported in stirrups. She is in the
   a Dorsal recumbent position
   b Lithotomy position
   c Knee-chest position
   d Sims' position

6 You will assist with Mrs. Porter's examination. Which is *false*?
   a Handwashing is done before and after the examination.
   b Instruments are placed near the examiner.
   c You leave the room when Mrs. Porter is examined.
   d Provide for privacy by screening, closing the door, and proper draping.

Answers to these questions are on p. 853.

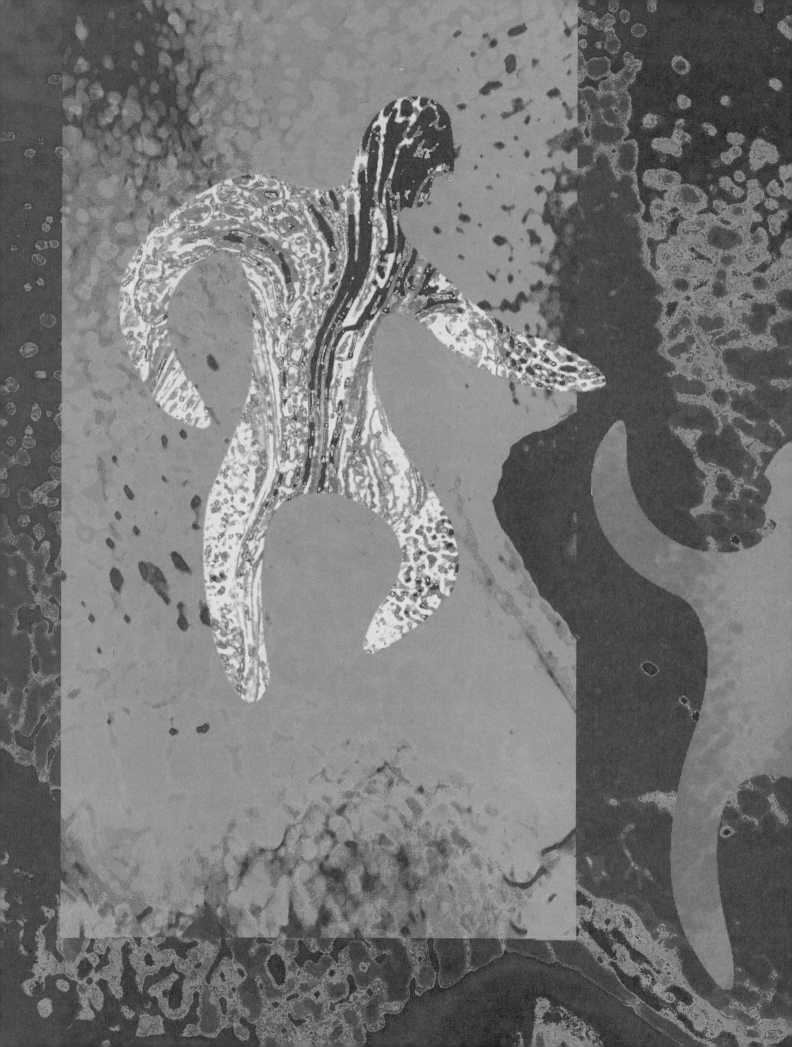

Unit VII
Assisting With the Healing Process

27 The Surgical Patient

- Define the key terms in this chapter
- Describe the common fears and concerns of surgical patients
- Explain how persons are physically and psychologically prepared for surgery
- Describe how to prepare a room for the postoperative patient
- List the signs and symptoms that are reported to the RN postoperatively
- Explain how circulation is stimulated after surgery
- Describe how to meet personal hygiene, nutrition, fluids, and elimination needs after surgery
- Perform the procedures described in this chapter

anesthesia The loss of feeling or sensation produced by a drug

elective surgery Scheduled surgery a person chooses to have at a certain time

embolus A blood clot that travels through the vascular system until it lodges in a distant blood vessel

emergency surgery Unscheduled surgery done immediately to save the person's life or limb

general anesthesia Unconsciousness and the loss of feeling or sensation produced by a drug

local anesthesia The loss of sensation in a small area

postoperative After surgery

preoperative Before surgery

regional anesthesia The loss of sensation or feeling in a part of the body produced by the injection of a drug; the person does not lose consciousness

thrombus A blood clot

urgent surgery Surgery necessary for the person's health; it must be done soon to prevent further damage or disease

Surgery is done for many reasons. Common reasons include removing a diseased organ or body part, removing a tumor, or repairing injured tissue. Surgery is done also to diagnose a disease, improve appearance, and relieve symptoms.

Many surgeries require hospital stays. The person is admitted 1 or 2 days before the surgery and stays for a few or several days after the surgery. However, ambulatory surgery (outpatient surgery, one-day surgery, and same-day surgery) is quite common. It does not require an overnight hospital stay. The person is in the hospital less than 23 hours. Many outpatient surgeries are done in clinics or surgical centers that are part of doctors' offices.

Surgeries are elective, urgent, or emergency:

- **Elective surgery** is done for the person's well-being. It is not lifesaving and may not be necessary for the person's health. The surgery is scheduled anywhere from 1 day to months in advance. Cosmetic surgery—surgery to improve appearance—is often elective surgery.
- **Urgent surgery** is needed for the person's health. It must be done soon to prevent further damage or disease. Cancer surgery and coronary artery bypass surgery are examples.
- **Emergency surgery** is done immediately to save a person's life or limb. The need is sudden and unexpected. Accidents, stabbings, and bullet wounds often require emergency surgery.

The person is prepared for what happens before, during, and after surgery. This involves physical and psychological preparation. RNs and doctors prepare the person for the surgical experience.

In hospitals you will have contact with persons before and after surgery. In nursing centers many residents are recovering from surgery. Many postoperative patients need home care.

PSYCHOLOGICAL CARE

Illness or injury causes many fears and concerns (Box 27-1, p. 648). Surgery increases these fears. The person's deepest and worst fears are often felt. How would you feel if you needed surgery tomorrow? Would you fear cancer

COMMON FEARS AND CONCERNS OF SURGICAL PATIENTS

The fear of . . .
- Cancer
- Disfigurement and scarring
- Disability
- Pain during surgery
- Dying during surgery
- Anesthesia and its effects
- Going to sleep or not waking up after surgery
- Exposure
- Severe pain or discomfort after surgery
- Tubes, needles, and other equipment used for care

- Complications
- Prolonged recovery
- More surgery or treatments
- Separation from family and friends

Concern about . . .
- Caring for children and other family members
- Pets or plants
- The house, lawn, and garden
- Monthly bills, loan payments, mortgages, or rent
- Insurance coverage for hospital and doctor bills

or the loss of an organ or body part? Would you have fears about pain or death? Who will care for your children and your home? Who will earn money while you are in the hospital? Imagine you are in an accident. You wake up hours later. You are told that your right leg was amputated during surgery.

Feelings are affected by past experiences. Some persons have had surgery before. Others have not. Family and friends usually share their surgical experiences with the patient. Their experiences also can affect the patient. Most people know about tragic surgical events—surgery on the wrong person, surgery on the wrong body part, instruments left in the body, death during surgery. Some people do not talk about their fears and concerns. They may cry, be quiet and withdrawn, or constantly talk about other things. Some pace or are very cheerful.

Psychological preparation is important. You must respect the person's fears and concerns. The health team must show the person warmth, sensitivity, and caring.

Patient Information

The doctor explains the need for surgery to the patient and family. They are told about the surgical procedure, risks, and possible complications. Risks from not having surgery also are explained. Information is given about who will do the surgery, when it is scheduled, and how long it will take. The person and family may have questions about the surgery and what to expect. Questions and misunderstandings are cleared up. Instructions about care also are given. All information before surgery is given by the doctor or RN.

After surgery the doctor tells the patient and the family about the results. The doctor decides what and when to tell them. Often the health team knows before the person does. Patients and families are usually anxious to know the results. They often ask nurses, assistive personnel, and other health workers. Often they ask if reports are back from the laboratory or what the reports say. Knowing what the person was told is very important. You do not tell of any diagnosis. Nor do you give incomplete or inaccurate information. The RN tells you what and when the person and family were told.

Your Role

You can assist in the psychological care of the surgical patient. Do the following if you are involved in preoperative and postoperative care:
- Listen to the person who voices fears or concerns about surgery
- Refer any questions about the surgery or its results to the RN
- Explain procedures you will perform to the person and why they are being done
- Follow the rules of communication (see Chapter 4)
- Use verbal and nonverbal communication (see Chapter 6)
- Perform procedures and tasks with skill and ease
- Report verbal and nonverbal signs of patient fear or anxiety to the RN
- Report a person's request to see a member of the clergy to the RN

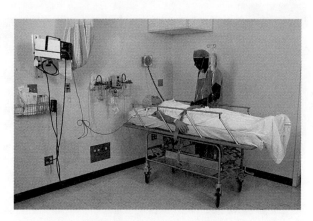

Fig. 27-1 *Recovery room.*

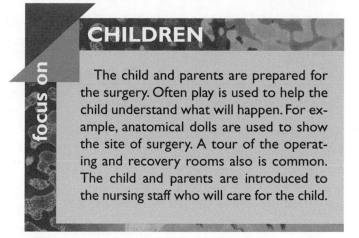

THE PREOPERATIVE PERIOD

The **preoperative** (before surgery) period may be many days or just a few minutes. If time permits, the person is prepared psychologically and physically for the effects of anesthesia and surgery. Good preoperative preparation prevents complications after surgery.

Preoperative Teaching

An RN does the preoperative teaching. The RN explains what to expect before and after surgery. Teaching includes the following:

- *Preoperative activities*—This includes tests and their purpose, skin preparation, personal care, and the purpose and effects of preoperative medications.
- *Deep breathing, coughing, and leg exercises*—These are taught and practiced. After surgery they are done every 1 or 2 hours when the person is awake.
- *The recovery room*—This is where the patient wakes up (Fig. 27-1). Care in the recovery room is explained.
- *Vital signs*—These are taken frequently until stable.
- *Food and fluids*—The patient is NPO and has an intravenous (IV) infusion after surgery. The doctor orders food and oral fluids when the person's condition is stable.
- *Turning and repositioning*—The patient is usually turned and repositioned every 2 hours after surgery.
- *Early ambulation*—Usually the patient walks a short distance the evening of surgery.
- *Pain*—The person is told about the type and amount of pain to expect and about pain medications.
- *Needed treatments and equipment*—The person also may need a urinary catheter, nasogastric (NG) tube, oxygen, wound suction, a cast, or traction.
- *Position restrictions*—Some surgeries require certain positions. For example, the hip is abducted following hip replacement surgery (see Chapter 30).

(See Focus on Children.)

Special Tests

Before surgery the doctor orders tests to evaluate the person's circulatory, respiratory, and urinary systems. These tests include a chest x-ray examination, a complete blood count (CBC), and urinalysis. An electrocardiogram (ECG or EKG) detects any cardiac (heart) problems (see Chapter 24). If blood loss is expected, type and cross-matching are done for blood replacement (see Chapter 20). Other tests are done depending on the person's condition and the surgery. The person is prepared for the tests as needed. The results must be on the chart by the time of surgery.

Nutrition and Fluids

A light meal is usually allowed. Then the person is NPO 6 to 8 hours before the surgery. These measures reduce the risk of vomiting and aspiration during anesthesia and after surgery. An NPO sign is placed in the person's room. Remember, the water pitcher and glass are removed when the person is NPO.

Elimination

Abdominal surgeries usually require a preoperative enema. Cleansing enemas are common before intestinal surgeries. Remember, feces contain microbes. When the intestine is opened, feces can spill into the sterile abdominal cavity. This contamination is prevented by cleansing enemas that clear the colon of feces.

Enemas are given also when straining or a bowel movement could cause postoperative problems. Such problems include pain, severe bleeding (hemorrhage), or stress on the operative area. The doctor orders what enema to give and when.

Some surgeries require catheters. For pelvic and abdominal surgeries, the bladder must be empty. A full bladder is easily injured during surgery. Catheters also allow accurate output measurements during and after surgery.

Personal Care

Personal care before surgery usually involves the following:

- A complete bed bath, shower, or tub bath is taken. A special soap or cleanser may be ordered. A shampoo is included. The bath and shampoo reduce the number of microbes on the body at the time of surgery.
- Makeup and nail polish are removed. The skin, lips, and nail beds are observed for color and circulation during and after surgery.
- Long hair is braided. All hairpins, clips, combs, and similar items are removed. So are wigs and hairpieces. Some agencies have both men and women wear surgical caps. A cap keeps hair out of the face and the operative area.
- Oral hygiene is performed to promote comfort. Being NPO causes thirst and a dry mouth. The person must not swallow any water during oral hygiene.
- Dentures are removed. They are removed before preoperative medications are given. They are cleaned and kept moist in a denture cup. They are kept in a safe place. Some persons do not like being seen without their dentures. Let them wear their dentures as long as possible. This promotes the person's sense of dignity and esteem.

(See Focus on Children.)

Valuables

Valuables are removed for safekeeping. These include dentures, glasses, contact lenses, hearing aids, and jewelry. Artificial eyes and limbs also are removed. These items are easily lost or broken during surgery. Transfers to the

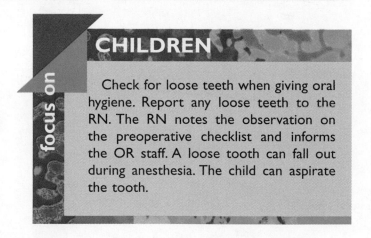

focus on CHILDREN

Check for loose teeth when giving oral hygiene. Report any loose teeth to the RN. The RN notes the observation on the preoperative checklist and informs the OR staff. A loose tooth can fall out during anesthesia. The child can aspirate the tooth.

operating room (OR), recovery room, and back to the person's room also present safety risks. A note is made on the person's chart about the valuables removed and where they are kept. The person may want to wear a wedding band or religious medal. The item is secured in place with gauze or tape according to agency policy.

✦ Skin Preparation

The skin and hair shafts contain microbes that could enter the body through the surgical incision. A serious infection could result. The skin cannot be sterilized. However, a *skin prep* (preparation) can reduce the number of microbes.

Agency policy and the surgeon's preferences determine the area to be prepared for a specific surgery (Fig. 27-2). The incision site and a large area around the area are *prepped*.

Text continued on p. 654

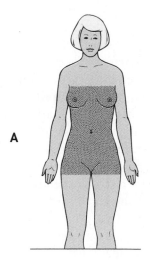
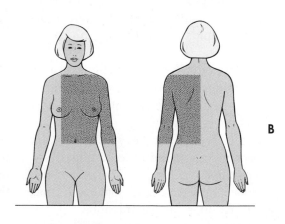

Fig. 27-2 *Skin preparation sites for surgeries on various body areas. The shaded area indicates the area to shave.* **A,** *Abdominal surgery.* **B,** *Chest or thoracic surgery.*

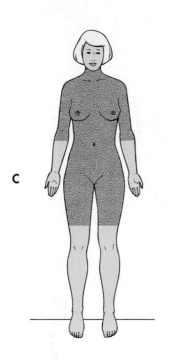

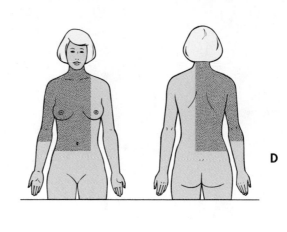

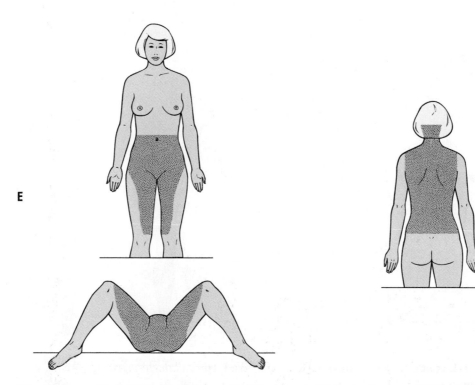

Fig. 27-2, cont'd **C**, *Open-heart surgery.* **D**, *Breast surgery.* **E**, *Perineal surgery.* **F**, *Cervical spine surgery.*

Continued

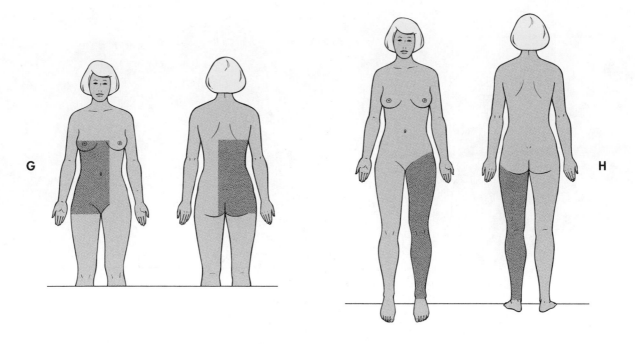

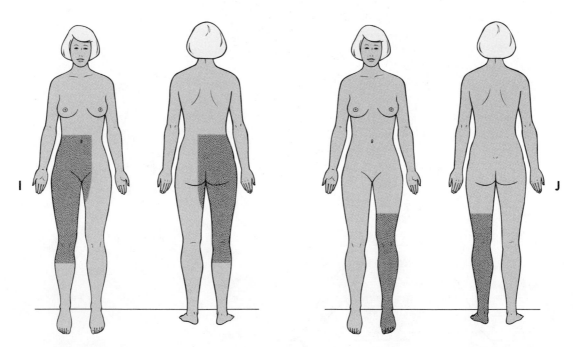

Fig. 27-2, cont'd *G, Kidney surgery.* **H,** *Knee surgery.* **I,** *Hip and thigh surgery.* **J,** *Lower leg and foot surgery.*

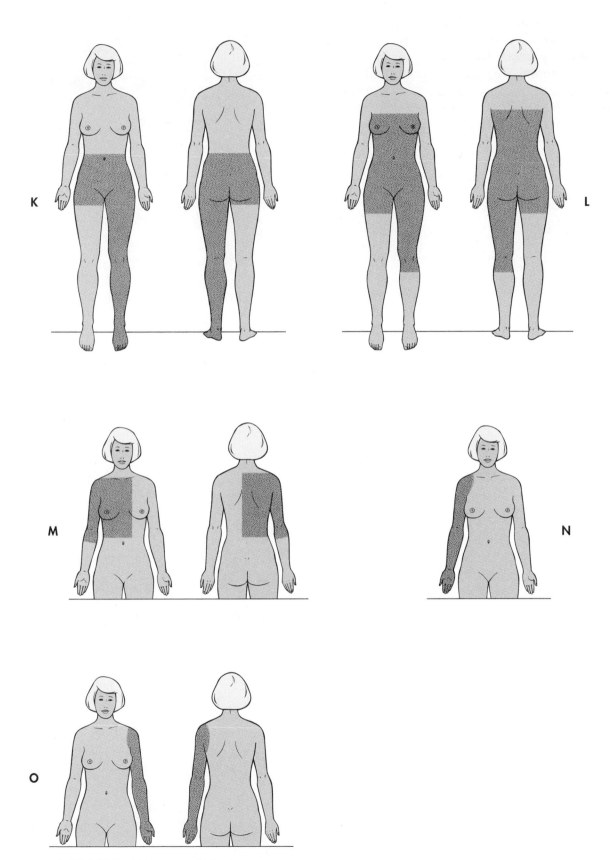

Fig. 27-2, cont'd K, *Complete lower extremity surgery.* **L,** *Abdominal and leg surgery.* **M,** *Upper arm surgery.* **N,** *Lower arm surgery.* **O,** *Elbow surgery.*

The skin prep is done right before the surgery. It is done in the person's room or in the OR. Hair is removed by applying a depilatory (cream hair remover) or by shaving.

Disposable prep kits are used for shaving. A kit has a razor, a sponge filled with soap, a basin, and a drape and towel (Fig. 27-3). The skin is lathered with soap. Then the skin is shaved in the direction of hair growth (Fig. 27-4). Any skin break is a possible infection site. If you do a skin prep, be very careful not to cut, scratch, or nick the skin. Standard Precautions and the Bloodborne Pathogen Standard are followed.

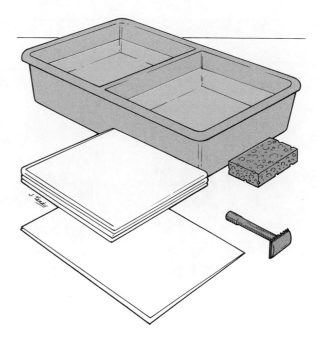

Fig. 27-3 *Skin prep kit.*

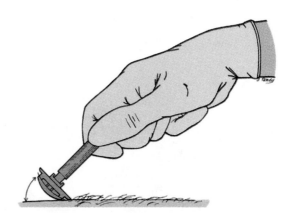

Fig. 27-4 *The skin is held taut. Shaving is done in the direction of hair growth.*

THE SURGICAL SKIN PREP

PRE-PROCEDURE

1 Explain the procedure to the person.

2 Wash your hands.

3 Collect the following:

- Disposable skin prep kit
- Bath blanket
- Warm water
- Gloves
- Waterproof pad
- Bath towel

4 Identify the person. Check the ID bracelet against the assignment sheet.

5 Provide for privacy.

PROCEDURE

6 Make sure you have good lighting. There should be no glares or shadows.

7 Raise the bed to the best level for good body mechanics. Lower the bed rail.

8 Cover the person with a bath blanket. Fanfold top linens to the foot of the bed.

9 Place the waterproof pad under the area to be shaved.

10 Open the skin prep kit.

11 Position the person for the skin prep. Drape him or her with the disposable drape.

12 Add warm water to the basin. Put on the gloves.

13 Apply soap to the skin with the sponge. Work up a good lather.

14 Hold the skin taut. Shave in the direction of hair growth (see Fig. 27-4).

15 Shave outward from the center using short strokes.

16 Rinse the razor often.

17 Check to see that the entire area is free of hair. Also check for cuts, scratches, or nicks.

18 Rinse the skin thoroughly. Pat dry.

19 Remove the drape and waterproof pad. Remove the gloves.

20 Return top linens. Remove the bath blanket.

POST-PROCEDURE

21 Make sure the person is comfortable.

22 Lower the bed to its lowest position. Place the call bell within reach. Unscreen the person.

23 Return equipment to its proper place.

24 Discard supplies and soiled linen following agency policy.

25 Wash your hands.

26 Report the following to the RN:

- The time the procedure was completed
- The area prepared
- Any cuts, nicks, or scratches
- Any other observations

The Consent for Surgery

Before surgery is done, the person must give permission. The person signs an *operative permit* or *surgical consent.* The consent is signed when the person understands the information given by the doctor. Sometimes the person's spouse or nearest relative is also required to sign the consent. A parent or legal guardian signs for a minor child. The legal guardian signs for a person who is mentally incompetent. The doctor is responsible for securing the person's written consent. However, this responsibility is often delegated to the RN. *You are never responsible for obtaining the person's written consent for surgery.*

The Preoperative Checklist

A preoperative checklist (Fig. 27-5) is placed on the front of the person's chart. The RN makes sure the checklist is completed. The person is ready for surgery when the list is complete. The RN may ask you to do some things on the list. Promptly report when you complete each task. Also report any observations. Except for raising the bed rails, everything on the checklist is completed before preoperative medications are given.

Preoperative Medication

About 45 minutes to 1 hour before surgery, the preoperative medications are given. One medication helps the person relax and feel drowsy. The other dries up respiratory secretions to prevent aspiration. Drowsiness, lightheadedness, thirst, and dry mouth are normal and expected.

Falls and accidents are prevented after the drugs are given. Bed rails are raised and the person is not allowed out of bed. Therefore the person voids before the drugs are given. After the drugs are given, the patient uses the bedpan or urinal for voiding. Smoking is not allowed. The person can fall asleep while smoking.

The bed is kept in the lowest position or raised to the highest position, following agency policy. Move furniture out of the way to make room for the stretcher. Also clean off the overbed table and the bedside stand. This prevents damage to equipment and valuables. Raise the bed to the highest position for transferring the patient from the bed to a stretcher.

Transport to the Operating Room

An RN or OR attendant brings a stretcher to the room. The patient is transferred onto the stretcher and covered with a bath blanket. The blanket provides warmth and prevents exposure. Falling is prevented. Safety straps are secured, and the side rails are raised. A small pillow is sometimes placed under the person's head for comfort.

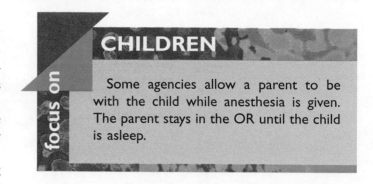

CHILDREN

focus on

Some agencies allow a parent to be with the child while anesthesia is given. The parent stays in the OR until the child is asleep.

Identification checks are made. Then the person's chart is given to the OR staff member.

The RN responsible for preoperative care may go with the person to the OR entrance. Often the family also is allowed to go this far. (See Focus on Children.)

ANESTHESIA

Anesthesia is the loss of feeling or sensation produced by a drug. There are three types of anesthesia general, regional, and local:

- **General anesthesia** produces unconsciousness and the loss of feeling or sensation. A drug is given intravenously, or a gas is inhaled (breathed in).
- **Regional anesthesia** produces loss of sensation or feeling in a large area of the body. The person does not lose consciousness. A drug is injected into a body part.
- **Local anesthesia** produces loss of sensation in a small area. A drug is injected at the specific site.

Anesthetics are given by specially educated doctors and nurses. An *anesthesiologist* is a doctor who specializes in the administration of anesthetics. An *anesthetist* is an RN who has had advanced study in the administration of anesthetics.

THE POSTOPERATIVE PERIOD

After surgery (**postoperative**) the person is taken to the recovery room (RR), or postanesthesia room (PAR). The recovery room is near the OR. There the person recovers from the anesthetic. This can take 1 to 2 hours. The person is watched very closely. Vital signs are taken and observations are made often. The person leaves the recovery room when:

- Vital signs are stable.
- The person has good respiratory function.
- The person can respond and call for help when it is needed.

The doctor gives the transfer order when appropriate.

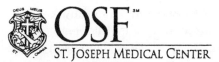

ST. JOSEPH MEDICAL CENTER

2200 E. Washington Street, Bloomington, Illinois 61701
Phone (309) 662-3311

PRE-OPERATIVE CHECKLIST

DATE OF SURGERY: _____

CHART PREPARATION	ADEQUATE INITIAL HERE	NOT ADEQUATE INITIAL HERE AND EXPLAIN
1. HISTORY AND PHYSICAL ON CHART HT. _____ WT. _____		
2. SURGICAL CONSENT ON CHART, SIGNED		
3. CONSENT FOR ADM BLOOD/BLOOD PROD.		
4. PREGNANCY TEST OBTAINED WHEN INDICATED		
5 URINALYSIS REPORT ON CHART		
6. BLOOD WORK TYPE _____		
7. TYPE AND CROSSMATCH		
8. CHEST X-RAY REPORT ON CHART		
9. EKG REPORT ON CHART READ _____		
10. KNOWN ALLERGIES AND SENSITIVITIES NOTED ON CHART		
11. KNOWN EXPOSURE AND/OR ALLERGY TO **LATEX** NOTED ON CHART		

PATIENT PREPARATION	ADEQUATE INITIAL HERE	NOT ADEQUATE INITIAL HERE AND EXPLAIN
12. FAMILY NOTIFIED OF SURGERY NAME _____ DATE/TIME _____		
13. PATIENT IDENTIFICATION ON WRIST		
14. ALL PROSTHESIS REMOVED (INCLUDING DENTURES, WIGS, HAIRPINS, CONTACT LENSES, COSMETICS, NAIL POLISH, ARTIFICIAL EYES, LIMBS, ETC)		
15. ALL JEWELRY REMOVED		
16. CLOTHING REMOVED EXCEPT HOSPITAL GOWN WITH TIES		
17. SURGICAL PREP DONE		
18. TIME OF LAST MEAL OR FLUIDS _____ TIME		
19. PRE-OP TPR AND BP: T_____ P_____ R _____ BP_____		
20. VOIDED TIME _____ OR FOLEY		
21. PRE-OP IV AND/OR ANTIBIOTIC: TIME:		

	DRUG	DOSAGE	ROUTE
PREOPERATIVE MEDICATION GIVEN,			

TIME _____ GIVEN BY _____

☐ SIDE RAILS UP

READY FOR O.R.   DATE _____ TIME _____ SIGNATURE _____

PATIENT IDENTIFIED BY TRANSPORTER AND STAFF NURSE   TIME _____

FLOOR NURSE SIGNATURE _____   OR TRANSPORTER SIGNATURE _____   OR NURSE SIGNATURE _____

IDENTIFICATION OF INITIALS			
INITIALS	SIGNATURE	INITIALS	SIGNATURE

Fig. 27-5 *Preoperative checklist. (Courtesy OSF, St. Joseph Medical Center, Bloomington, Ill.)*

Preparing the Person's Room

The room must be ready for the person's return from the recovery room. A surgical bed is made (see Chapter 13). Equipment and supplies needed for the person's care are brought to the room. The RN tells you if special measures and equipment are needed. The room is prepared after the person is taken to the OR. Preparations include:

- Making a surgical bed
- Placing equipment and supplies in the room:
  - Thermometer
  - Stethoscope
  - Sphygmomanometer
  - Kidney basin
  - Tissues
  - Waterproof bed protector
  - Vital signs flow sheet
  - I&O record
  - IV pole
  - Other items as directed by the RN
- Raising the bed to its highest position
- Lowering bed rails
- Moving furniture out of the way for the stretcher

The Person's Return From the Recovery Room

The recovery room nurse calls the nursing unit when the person is ready for transfer. The person is transported by the recovery room nurses. An RN meets the person on the nursing unit, and the person is transferred from the stretcher to bed. Assist as needed in the transfer. Also help position the person.

Vital signs are taken, and observations are made. They are compared with those reported by the recovery room nurse. The RN checks dressings for bleeding. Catheters, IV infusions, and other tube placement and function are checked. Bed rails are raised, and the call bell is placed within the person's reach. Necessary care and treatments are given. Then the family is allowed to see the person.

Measurements and Observations

The person's condition affects your role in postoperative care. Often you will measure vital signs and observe the person's condition. Vital signs are usually measured:

- Every 15 minutes the first hour
- Every 30 minutes for 1 to 2 hours
- Every hour for 4 hours
- Every 4 hours

The RN tells you how often to check the person. This is an important function. Always be alert for the signs and symptoms listed in Box 27-2. Report them to the RN immediately.

focus on OLDER PERSONS

Many older persons have stiff and painful joints. Sore muscles, bones, and joints occur from positioning on the operating room table. Remember to turn and reposition older persons slowly and gently.

Positioning

Proper positioning promotes comfort and prevents complications. The type of surgery affects positioning. Position restrictions may be ordered. The person is usually positioned for easy and comfortable breathing. Also, stress on the incision is prevented. When the person is supine, the head of the bed is usually raised slightly. The person's head may be turned to the side. These positions prevent aspiration if vomiting occurs.

Repositioning every 1 to 2 hours helps prevent respiratory and circulatory complications. It may be painful to turn. Provide support, and turn the person with smooth, gentle motions. Pillows and other positioning devices are often used (see Chapters 12 and 22).

The RN tells you when to reposition the person and the positions allowed. Usually you assist the nurse. Sometimes you will turn and reposition the person yourself. This occurs when the person's condition is stable and care is simple. (See Focus on Older Persons.)

Coughing and Deep Breathing

Respiratory complications are prevented. There are two major complications. One is *pneumonia*, an inflammation and infection in the lung. The other is *atelectasis*, the collapse of a portion of the lung. Coughing and deep breathing exercises and incentive spirometry help prevent these complications (see Chapter 21). (See Focus on Older Persons on p. 659.)

Stimulating Circulation

After surgery, circulation must be stimulated. This is especially true for blood flow in the legs. If blood flow is sluggish, blood clots may form. Blood clots (thrombi) can form in the deep leg veins (Fig. 27-6, *A*). A blood clot (**thrombus**) can break loose and travel through the bloodstream. It then becomes an embolus. An **embolus** is a blood clot that travels through the vascular system until it lodges in a distant vessel (Fig. 27-6, *B*). An embolus from a vein eventually lodges in the lungs (pulmonary embolus). A pulmonary embolus can cause severe respiratory problems and death. (See Focus on Older Persons on p. 660.)

BOX 27-2

POSTOPERATIVE OBSERVATIONS

- Choking
- A drop or rise in blood pressure
- Bright red blood from the incision, drainage tubes, or suction tubes
- A pulse rate of more than 100 or less than 60 beats per minute
- A weak or irregular pulse
- A rise or drop in body temperature
- Hypoxia (see Chapter 21)
- The need for upper airway suctioning (tachypnea, dyspnea, moist-sounding respirations or gurgling, restlessness, cyanosis)
- Shallow, slow breathing
- Rapid, gasping, or difficult respirations
- Weak cough
- Complaints of thirst
- Restlessness
- Cold, moist, clammy, or pale skin
- Cyanosis of the lips or nails
- Increased drainage on or under dressings or on bed linens (including drawsheets, bottom sheets, and pillowcases)
- Complaints of pain or nausea
- Vomiting
- Confusion or disorientation
- Additional measurements and observations:
- The amount, character, and time of the first voiding after surgery
- Intake and output
- IV flow rate
- The appearance of drainage from a urinary catheter, NG tube, or wound suction
- Any other observation that can mean a change in the person's condition

focus on OLDER PERSONS

The changes of aging increase the older person's risk for respiratory complications. Respiratory muscles are weaker. Lung tissue is less elastic. The person has less strength for coughing. Coughing, deep breathing, and incentive spirometry are very important.

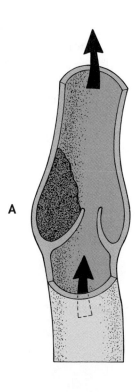
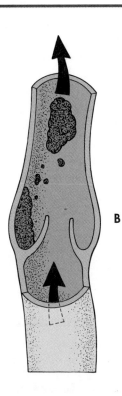

A
B

Fig. 27-6 **A,** *A blood clot is attached to the wall of a vein. The arrows show the direction of blood flow.* **B,** *Part of the thrombus has broken off and has become an embolus. The embolus will travel in the bloodstream until it lodges in a distant vessel.*

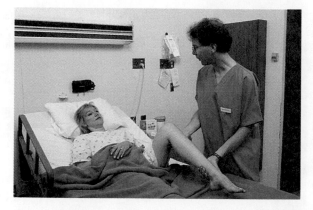

Fig. 27-7 *The knee is flexed and then extended during postoperative leg exercises.*

Leg exercises

Leg exercises increase venous blood flow. Therefore they help prevent thrombi. Leg exercises are easy to do. You assist if the person is weak. If the person had leg surgery, a doctor's order is needed for the exercises. The RN tells you when to do the exercises. They are done with the person supine. They are done at least every 1 or 2 hours while the person is awake. The following exercises are done five times:

- Ask the person to make circles with the toes. This rotates the ankles.
- Have the person dorsiflex and plantar flex the feet (see Chapter 22).
- Have the person flex and extend one knee and then the other (Fig. 27-7).
- Ask the person to raise and lower one leg off the bed (Fig. 27-8). Repeat this exercise with the other leg.

✦ Elastic stockings

Elastic stockings help prevent thrombi. The elastic exerts pressure on the veins, promoting venous blood flow to the heart.

Elastic stockings are often ordered for postoperative patients and for those with heart disease and circulatory disorders. Bedrest and pregnancy also are reasons for using elastic stockings. Affected persons can develop blood clots (thrombi).

The stockings come in many sizes. Thigh-high or knee-high lengths are available. The RN measures the person to determine the correct size. The stockings are removed at least twice each day. They are applied before the person gets out of bed.

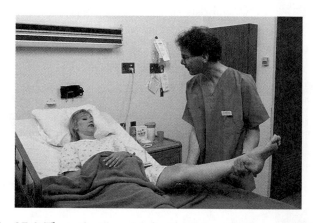

Fig. 27-8 *The patient is assisted with raising and lowering the leg.*

APPLYING ELASTIC STOCKINGS

PRE-PROCEDURE

1 Explain the procedure to the person.

2 Wash your hands.

3 Obtain elastic stockings in the correct size.

4 Identify the person. Check the ID bracelet against the assignment sheet.

5 Provide for privacy.

PROCEDURE

6 Raise the bed to the best level for good body mechanics.

7 Lower the bed rail.

8 Position the person supine.

9 Expose the legs. Fanfold top linens back toward the person.

10 Hold the foot and heel of the stocking. Gather the rest of the stocking in your hands.

11 Support the person's foot at the heel.

12 Slip the foot of the stocking over the toes, foot, and heel (Fig. 27-9, A).

13 Pull the stocking up over the leg. It should be even and snug (Fig. 27-9, B).

14 Make sure the stocking is not twisted and has no creases or wrinkles.

15 Repeat steps 10 through 14 for the other leg.

16 Return top linens to their proper position.

POST-PROCEDURE

17 Help the person to a comfortable position.

18 Lower the bed to its lowest position. Place the call bell within reach.

19 Raise or lower bed rails as instructed by the RN.

20 Unscreen the person.

21 Wash your hands.

22 Report that you applied the stockings. Report the time of application.

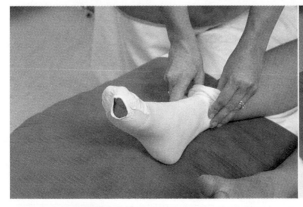 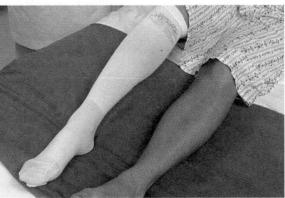

Fig. 27-9 A, *The stocking is slipped over the toes, foot, and heel.* **B,** *The stocking is pulled up over the leg.*

✦ *Elastic bandages*

Bandages are applied to an extremity. They are used for the same purposes as elastic stockings. They also provide support and reduce swelling from musculoskeletal injuries. The bandage is applied from the lower (distal) part of the extremity to the top (proximal) part. The RN gives you directions about the area to bandage. When applying bandages:

- Use the correct size. Use the proper length and width to bandage the extremity.
- Position the extremity in good alignment.
- Face the person during the procedure.
- Expose fingers or toes if possible. This allows circulation checks.
- Apply the bandage with firm, even pressure.
- Check the color and temperature of the extremity every hour.
- Reapply a loose or wrinkled bandage.

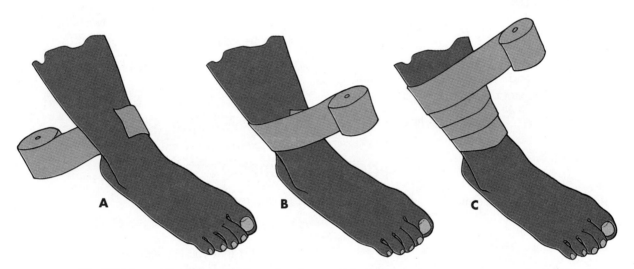

Fig. 27-10 **A,** *The roll of the elastic bandage is up. The loose end is at the bottom.* **B,** *The bandage is applied to the smallest part with two circular turns.* **C,** *The bandage is applied with spiral turns in an upward direction.*

APPLYING ELASTIC BANDAGES

PRE-PROCEDURE

1 Explain the procedure to the person.

2 Wash your hands.

3 Collect the following:

- Elastic bandage (the RN tells you what size)
- Tape or metal clips

4 Identify the person. Check the ID bracelet against the assignment sheet.

5 Provide for privacy.

6 Raise the bed to the best level for good body mechanics.

PROCEDURE

7 Help the person to a comfortable position. Expose the part to be bandaged.

8 Make sure the area is clean and dry.

9 Hold the bandage so the roll is up and the loose end is on the bottom (Fig. 27-10, *A*).

10 Apply the bandage to the smallest part of the wrist, ankle, or knee.

11 Make two circular turns around the part (Fig. 27-10, *B*).

12 Make overlapping spiral turns in an upward direction. Each turn should overlap about two-thirds of the previous turn (Fig. 27-10, *C*).

13 Apply the bandage smoothly with firm, even pressure. It should not be tight.

14 Tape or clip the end of the bandage to hold it in place. The clip must not be under the part.

15 Check the fingers or toes for cold or cyanosis. Also check for complaints of pain, numbness, or tingling. Remove the bandage if any are noted. Report your observations to the RN.

POST-PROCEDURE

16 Make sure the person is comfortable and the call bell is within reach.

17 Lower the bed.

18 Raise or lower bed rails as instructed by the RN.

19 Unscreen the person.

20 Wash your hands.

21 Report the following to the RN:

- The time the bandage was applied
- The site of the application
- Any other observations

Sequential compression devices (SCD)

A sequential compression device is a sleeve that is wrapped around the leg. Made of cloth or plastic, it is secured in place with Velcro. The device is attached to a pump. The pump inflates the device with air. This promotes venous blood flow to the heart by causing pressure on the veins. Then the pump deflates the device. After deflation, the device is inflated again. The inflation and deflation sequence is repeated as ordered by the doctor.

Early Ambulation

Early ambulation prevents postoperative circulatory complications such as thrombi. It also prevents pneumonia, atelectasis, constipation, and urinary tract infections. The person usually ambulates the evening of surgery or the next day. The person dangles first. Blood pressure and pulse are measured. If the blood pressure and pulse are stable, the person is assisted out of bed. Usually the person does not walk very far, just a few feet in the room. Distance increases as the person gains strength.

The RN tells you when to ambulate the person. Usually you assist the RN the first time.

Wound Healing

The incision needs protection. Healing is promoted, and infection is prevented. Sterile dressing changes are done by the doctor or nurse. Some states let assistive personnel do simple dressing changes. Wound healing is discussed in Chapter 28.

Nutrition and Fluids

The person has an IV infusion on return from the OR. Continued IV therapy depends on the type of surgery and the person's condition. Anesthesia can cause nausea and vomiting. The person's diet progresses from NPO to clear liquids, to full liquids, to a light diet, and then to a regular diet.

The diet is ordered by the doctor. Frequent oral hygiene is important when the person is NPO.

Some patients have a nasogastric (NG) tube (see Chapter 19). Often the NG tube is attached to suction to keep the stomach empty. The person is NPO and receives IV therapy.

Elimination

Anesthesia, the surgery, and being NPO affect normal bowel and urinary elimination. Many pain medications can cause constipation. The measures to promote elimination are practiced as directed by the RN (see Chapters 17 and 18).

Intake and output are measured postoperatively. The person must urinate within 8 hours after surgery. Report the time and amount of the person's first voiding. If the person does not void within 8 hours, a catheterization is usually ordered. Some patients have catheters after surgery. See Chapter 17 for care of the person with a catheter.

Fluid intake and return to a regular diet are needed for bowel elimination. Suppositories or enemas may be ordered for constipation. Rectal tubes may be ordered for flatulence.

Comfort and Rest

Pain is common after surgery. The degree of pain depends on the extent of surgery, incision site, and the presence of drainage tubes, casts, or other devices. Positioning during surgery can cause muscle strains and discomfort. The doctor orders pain medications for the person. The RN uses the nursing process to promote comfort and rest. Many of the measures listed in Chapter 16 are part of the person's care plan.

Personal Hygiene

Personal hygiene is important for the person's physical and mental well-being. Wound drainage and skin prep solutions can irritate the skin and cause discomfort. NPO causes a dry mouth and breath odors. Moist, clammy skin from blood pressure changes or elevated body temperatures also cause discomfort. Frequent oral hygiene, hair care, and a complete bed bath the day after surgery help refresh and renew the person physically and psychologically. The gown is changed whenever it becomes wet or soiled.

REVIEW QUESTIONS

Circle the best answer.

1 Which is true of elective surgery?
   a   The surgery is done immediately.
   b   The need for surgery is sudden and unexpected.
   c   Surgery is scheduled for a later date.
   d   General anesthesia is always used.

2 Mr. Moore said he was afraid of surgery. He might show his fear by
   a   Being quiet and withdrawn
   b   Crying
   c   Pacing or being unusually cheerful
   d   All of the above

3 You can assist in Mr. Moore's psychological preparation by explaining
   a   The reason for the surgery
   b   The procedures you are doing
   c   The risks and possible complications of surgery
   d   What to expect during the preoperative and postoperative periods

4 Preoperatively, Mr. Moore is
   a   NPO
   b   Allowed only water
   c   Given a regular breakfast
   d   Given a tube feeding

5 Cleansing enemas are ordered for Mr. Moore pre-operatively. The enemas are given

   a To clean the colon of feces
   b To prevent bleeding
   c To relieve flatus
   d To prevent pain

6 Mr. Moore's skin prep is done preoperatively to

   a Completely bathe the body
   b Sterilize the skin
   c Reduce the number of microbes on the skin
   d Destroy nonpathogens and pathogens

7 When shaving the skin before surgery

   a Shave in the direction opposite of hair growth
   b Shave toward the center of the specific area
   c Be careful not to cut, scratch, or nick the skin
   d All of the above

8 Mr. Moore's preoperative medication was given. He

   a Must remain in bed
   b Is allowed to smoke with supervision
   c Can use the commode to void
   d Is allowed only sips of water

9 General anesthesia

   a Is a specially educated nurse
   b Produces unconsciousness and the loss of feeling or sensation
   c Is a specially educated doctor
   d Produces loss of sensation or feeling in a body part

10 Mr. Moore must cough and deep breathe after surgery to prevent

   a Bleeding
   b A pulmonary embolus
   c Respiratory complications
   d Pain and discomfort

11 Leg exercises are ordered for Mr. Moore. Which is *false*?

   a Leg exercises stimulate circulation.
   b Leg exercises prevent thrombi.
   c Leg exercises are done five times every 1 or 2 hours.
   d Leg exercises are done only for leg surgery.

12 Postoperatively, Mr. Moore's position is changed

   a Every 2 hours   c Every 4 hours
   b Every 3 hours   d Every shift

13 Mr. Moore wears elastic stockings to

   a Prevent blood clots
   b Hold dressings in place
   c Reduce swelling after musculoskeletal injury
   d All of the above

14 When applying an elastic bandage

   a The extremity is in good alignment
   b The fingers or toes are covered if possible
   c It is applied from the largest to smallest part of the extremity
   d It is applied from the upper to the lower part of the extremity

Circle T if the statement is true or F if the statement is false.

15 T F Hair is kept out of the face for surgery by using pins, clips, or combs.

16 T F Nail polish is removed before surgery.

17 T F Women can wear makeup to surgery.

18 T F Pajamas are worn to the operating room.

19 T F Contact lenses are removed before surgery.

20 T F A surgical bed is made for the person's return from the recovery room.

21 T F A drop in a person's blood pressure is reported to the RN immediately.

22 T F The patient never ambulates until the day after surgery.

23 T F Intake and output are measured after surgery.

24 T F A surgical patient should urinate within 8 hours after surgery.

Answers to these questions are on p. 853.

28 Wound Care

OBJECTIVES

- Define the key terms in this chapter
- Describe the different types of wounds
- Describe the process, types, and complications of wound healing
- Describe the observations to make about a wound
- Describe the different types of wound drainage
- Explain how to measure wound drainage
- Explain how to secure dressings
- Explain the rules for applying dressings
- Explain the rules for cleaning wounds and drain sites
- Explain the purpose of binders and how to apply them
- Describe how to meet the basic needs of persons with wounds
- Perform the procedures described in this chapter

KEY TERMS

abrasion A partial-thickness wound caused by the scraping away or rubbing of the skin

chronic wound A wound that does not heal easily

clean-contaminated wound A wound occurring from the surgical entry of the urinary, reproductive, respiratory, or gastrointestinal system

clean wound A wound that is not infected; microbes have not entered the wound

closed wound A wound in which tissues are injured but the skin is not broken

contaminated wound A wound with a high risk of infection

contusion A closed wound caused by a blow to the body

dehiscence The separation of wound layers

dirty wound An infected wound

evisceration The separation of the wound along with the protrusion of abdominal organs

full-thickness wound The dermis, epidermis, and subcutaneous tissue are penetrated; muscle and bone may be involved

hematoma The collection of blood under the skin and tissues

hemorrhage The excessive loss of blood in a short period of time

incision An open wound with clean, straight edges; usually intentionally produced with a sharp instrument

infected wound A wound that contains large amounts of bacteria and that shows signs of infection; a dirty wound

intentional wound A wound created for therapy

laceration An open wound with torn tissues and jagged edges

open wound The skin or mucous membrane is broken

partial-thickness wound A wound in which the dermis and epidermis of the skin are broken

penetrating wound An open wound in which the skin and underlying tissues are pierced

puncture wound An open wound made by a sharp object; entry of the skin and underlying tissues may be intentional or unintentional

purulent drainage Thick green, yellow, or brown drainage

sanguineous drainage Bloody drainage *(sanguis)*

Key Terms continued on p. 668

---

serosanguineous drainage Thin, watery drainage *(sero)* that is blood-tinged *(sanguineous)*

serous drainage Clear, watery fluid *(serum)*

shock The condition that results when there is not enough blood supply to organs and tissues

trauma An accident or violent act that injures the skin, mucous membranes, bones, and internal organs

unintentional wound A wound resulting from trauma

wound A break in the skin or mucous membrane

A **wound** is a break in the skin or mucous membrane. Wounds result from many causes. A surgical incision leaves a wound. Often wounds result from **trauma**—an accident or violent act that injures the skin, mucous membranes, bones, and internal organs. Falls, vehicle accidents, gun shots, stabbings, and other violent acts are sources of trauma. Human and animal bites, burns, and frostbite are other types of trauma. Pressure ulcers (pressure sores) are wounds that occur from poor skin care and immobility.

The wound is a portal of entry for microorganisms. Thus infection is a major threat. Wound care involves preventing infection and preventing further injury to the wound and surrounding tissues. Preventing blood loss and pain also are important.

Your role in wound care depends on state law, your job description, and the person's condition. Whatever your role, you need to know the types of wounds, how wounds heal, and the measures that promote wound healing. A review of surgical asepsis is useful before studying this chapter (see Chapter 11).

TYPES OF WOUNDS

Wounds are described in many ways. They are intentional or unintentional, open or closed, clean or dirty, and partial-thickness or full-thickness. **Intentional wounds** are created for therapy. Surgical incisions and venipunctures for starting IV therapy or for collecting blood specimens are examples. **Unintentional wounds** result from trauma. Falls, vehicle accidents, gun shots, stabbings, and other violent acts are sources of unintentional wounds.

A wound is open or closed. An **open wound** is when the skin or mucous membrane is broken. Intentional and most unintentional wounds are open. In a **closed wound**, tissues are injured but the skin is not broken. Bruises, twists, and sprains are examples of closed wounds.

Contamination is another factor in describing wounds. A **clean wound** is not infected, and microbes have not entered the wound. Closed wounds are usually clean. So are intentional wounds created under surgically aseptic conditions. In addition, the urinary, respiratory, and gastrointestinal systems are not entered. A **clean-contaminated wound** occurs from the surgical entry of the urinary, reproductive, respiratory, or gastrointestinal system. These systems are not sterile and contain normal flora. A **contaminated wound** has a high risk of infection. Unintentional wounds generally are contaminated. Wound contamination occurs also from breaks in surgical asepsis and spillage of intestinal contents. Tissues may show signs of inflammation. An **infected wound (dirty wound)** contains large amounts of bacteria and shows signs of infection. Examples include old wounds, surgical incisions into infected areas, and traumatic injuries that rupture the bowel. A **chronic wound** is one that does not heal easily. Pressure ulcers and ulcers in persons with circulatory disorders are examples. (See Chapter 14 for a review of pressure uclers.)

Partial or full thickness describes a wound's depth. In a **partial-thickness wound** the dermis and epidermis of the skin are broken. The dermis, epidermis, and subcutaneous tissue are penetrated in a **full-thickness wound**. Muscle and bone may be involved.

Wounds also are described by their cause:

- **Abrasion**—a partial-thickness wound caused by the scraping away or rubbing of the skin
- **Contusion**—a closed wound caused by a blow to the body
- **Incision**—an open wound with clean, straight edges; usually intentionally produced with a sharp instrument
- **Laceration**—an open wound with torn tissues and jagged edges
- **Penetrating wound**—an open wound in which the skin and underlying tissues are pierced
- **Puncture wound**—an open wound made by a sharp object; entry of the skin and underlying tissues may be intentional or unintentional

WOUND HEALING

The healing process has three phases:

- *Inflammatory phase* (3 days). Bleeding stops, and a scab forms over the wound. The scab protects microorganisms from entering the wound. Blood supply to the wound increases. The blood brings nutrients and healing substances. Because of the increased blood supply, signs and symptoms of inflammation appear: redness, swelling, heat or warmth, and pain. Loss of function may occur.

- *Proliferative phase* (day 3 to day 21). Proliferate means to multiply rapidly. During this phase, tissue cells multiply to repair the wound.
- *Maturation phase* (day 21 to 1 or 2 years). The scar gains strength. The red, raised scar eventually becomes thin and pale.

Types of Wound Healing

The healing process occurs through primary intention, secondary intention, or tertiary intention. With *primary intention (first intention, primary closure)*, the wound edges are brought together. This closes the wound. Sutures (stitches), staples, clips, or adhesive strips hold the wound edges together. Special glues are now available to doctors for wound closings.

Secondary intention (second intention) is used for contaminated and infected wounds. Wounds are cleaned and dead tissue removed. Wound edges are not brought together, and the wound gaps. Healing occurs naturally. However, healing takes longer and leaves a larger scar. The threat of infection is great.

Tertiary intention (third intention, delayed intention) involves leaving a wound open and then closing it later. Thus tertiary intention combines secondary and primary intention. Infection and poor circulation are common reasons for tertiary intention.

Complications of Wound Healing

Many factors affect the healing process and increase the risk of complications. The type of wound is one factor. Other factors include the person's age, general health, nutrition, and life-style. Good circulation is important. Age, smoking, circulatory disease, and diabetes all affect circulation. Certain medications (Coumadin and heparin) can prolong bleeding. Tissue growth and repair require adequate protein in the diet. Infection is a risk for persons with immune system changes and for those taking antibiotics. Antibiotics kill pathogens. Specific antibiotics kills specific pathogens. In doing so, an environment may be created that allows other pathogens to grow and multiply.

Hemorrhage

Hemorrhage is the excessive loss of blood in a short period of time. If the bleeding is not stopped, death results. Hemorrhage may be internal or external. Internal hemorrhage cannot be seen. Bleeding occurs inside the body into tissues and body cavities. A hematoma may form. A **hematoma** is a collection of blood under the skin and tissues. The area appears swollen and has a reddish-blue color. Shock, vomiting blood, coughing up blood, and loss of consciousness are signs of internal hemorrhage.

You can see external bleeding. Bloody drainage and dressings soaked with blood are common signs. Remember, gravity causes fluid to flow down. Therefore blood can flow down and collect under the part. Always check under the body part for the pooling of blood. As with internal hemorrhage, shock can occur.

Shock results when there is not enough blood supply to organs and tissues. Signs and symptoms include low or falling blood pressure, a rapid and weak pulse, and rapid respirations. The skin is cold, moist, and pale. The person is restless and may complain of thirst. Confusion and loss of consciousness occur as shock worsens.

Hemorrhage and shock are emergencies. Immediately notify the RN, and assist as requested. Remember to practice Standard Precautions and follow the Bloodborne Pathogen Standard when in contact with blood. Gloves are always worn. Gowns, masks, and eye protection are necessary when blood splashes and splatters are likely.

Infection

Wound contamination can occur during or after the injury. Trauma is a common source of contaminated wounds. Surgical wounds can be contaminated during or after surgery. An infected wound appears inflamed (reddened) and has drainage (p. 670). The wound is painful and tender. The person has a fever.

Dehiscence

Dehiscence is the separation of the wound layers (Fig. 28-1). Separation may involve the skin layer or underlying tissues. Abdominal wounds are most commonly

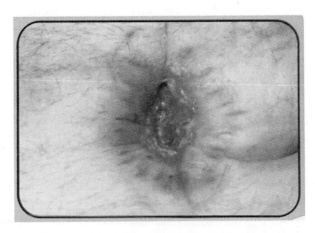

Fig. 28-1 *Wound dehiscence.* (*Courtesy Morison M et al: A colour guide to the nursing management of chronic wounds,* ed 2, London, 1997, Mosby.)

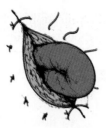

Fig. 28-2 *Wound evisceration. (From* Mosby's medical, nursing & allied health dictionary, *ed 4, St Louis, 1994, Mosby.)*

affected. Coughing, vomiting, and abdominal distention place stress on the wound. The person often describes the sensation of the wound popping open.

Evisceration

Evisceration is the separation of the wound along with the protrusion of abdominal organs (Fig. 28-2). Causes are the same as for dehiscence.

Dehiscence and evisceration are surgical emergencies. The wound is covered with large sterile dressings saturated with sterile saline. You must notify the RN immediately and assist in preparing the person for surgery.

Wound Appearance

During the healing process, doctors and nurses routinely observe the wound and its drainage. They observe for healing and complications. You need to make certain observations when assisting with wound care. You report your observations to the RN and record them according to agency policy. Box 28-1 lists the wound observations that you need to make. (See Focus on Home Care.)

Wound Drainage

During injury and the inflammatory phase of wound healing, fluid and cells escape from the tissues. The amount of drainage may be small or large depending on wound size and location. Bleeding and infection also affect the amount and kind of drainage. Wound drainage is observed and measured.

Major types of wound drainage are as follows:
* **Serous drainage**—clear, watery fluid (Fig. 28-3, *A*). The fluid in a blister is serous. *Serous* comes from the word *serum,* which is the clean, thin, fluid portion of the blood. Serum does not contain blood cells or platelets.
* **Sanguineous drainage**—bloody drainage (Fig. 28-3, *B*). Sanguineous comes from the Latin word *sanguis,* which means blood. The amount and color of sanguineous drainage is important. Hemorrhage is suspected when large amounts are present. Bright drainage indicates fresh bleeding. Older bleeding is darker.

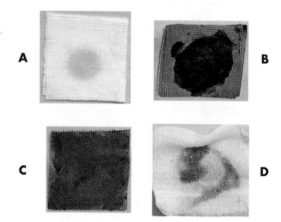

Fig. 28-3 *Wound drainage.* **A,** *Serous drainage.* **B,** *Sanguineous drainage.* **C,** *Serosanguineous drainage.* **D,** *Purulent drainage.* *(From Potter PA, Perry AG:* Fundamentals of nursing: concepts, process, and practice, *ed 4, St Louis, 1997, Mosby.)*

* **Serosanguineous drainage**—thin, watery drainage *(sero)* that is blood-tinged *(sanguineous)* (Fig. 28-3, *C*).
* **Purulent drainage**—thick drainage that is green, yellow, or brown (Fig. 28-3, *D*).

Drainage must leave the wound for healing to occur. If drainage is trapped inside the wound, underlying tissues swell. The wound may heal at the skin level, but underlying tissues do not close. This can lead to infection and other complications.

When large amounts of drainage are expected, the doctor inserts a drain. A *Penrose drain* is a rubber tube that drains onto a dressing (Fig. 28-4). Because the Penrose drain opens onto the dressing, it is an open drain and a portal of entry for microbes.

BOX 28-1

WOUND OBSERVATIONS

Wound Location
- Multiple wounds may exist from surgery or trauma.

Wound Size and Depth (measure in centimeters)
- Size: measure from top to bottom and side to side.
- Depth: (a) insert a sterile swab inside the deepest part of the wound; (b) remove the swab and measure the distance on the swab. *Only measure depth when the wound is open and with the RN's supervision.*
- Use the same ruler when measuring the wound.

Wound Appearance
- Is the wound red and swollen?
- Is the area around the wound warm to touch?
- Are sutures, staples, or clips intact or broken?
- Are wound edges closed or separated? Did the wound break open?

Drainage (see p. 670)
- Is the drainage serous, sanguineous, serosanguineous, or purulent?
- What is the amount of drainage?

Odor
- Does the wound or drainage have an odor?

Surrounding Skin
- Is surrounding skin intact?
- What is the color of surrounding skin?
- Are surrounding tissues swollen?

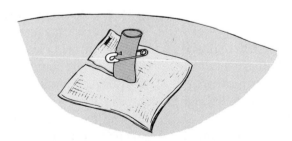

Fig. 28-4 *A Penrose drain. The safety pin prevents the drain from slipping into the wound.*
(*From Potter PA, Perry AG:* Fundamentals of nursing: concepts, process, and practice, *ed 4, St Louis, 1997, Mosby.*)

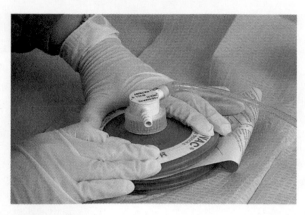

Fig. 28-5 *A Hemovac. Drains are sutured to the wound and connected to the reservoir.* (From Elkin MK, Perry AG, Potter PA: Nursing interventions and clinical skills, *St Louis, 1996, Mosby.*)

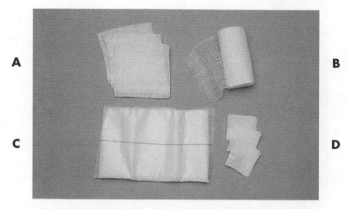

Fig. 28-7 *Gauze dressings.* **A,** *A 4 × 4 dressing.* **B,** *Gauze roll.* **C,** *Abdominal pad (ABD).* **D,** *2 × 2 dressing.*

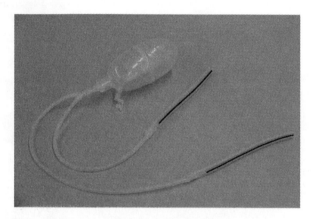

Fig. 28-6 *The Jackson-Pratt drainage system.* (From Elkin MK, Perry AG, Potter PA: Nursing interventions and clinical skills, *St Louis, 1996, Mosby.*)

Closed drainage systems prevent microbes from entering the wound. A drainage tube is placed in the wound and attached to suction. The Hemovac (Fig. 28-5) and Jackson-Pratt (Fig. 28-6) systems are examples. Other systems are used depending on the type of wound, its size, and location.

Drainage is measured in three ways:
- Note the number and size of dressings with drainage. Describe the amount and kind of drainage on them. Are dressings saturated? Is drainage on just part of the dressing? If so, which part? Is drainage through some or all layers of the dressing?
- Weigh dressings before applying them to the wound. Note the weight of each dressing. Note the weight of each dressing after removal. Subtract the weight of the dry dressing from the wet dressing.
- Measure the amount of drainage in the collecting receptacle if closed drainage is used.

DRESSINGS

Wound dressings have many functions. They protect wounds from injury and microbes. Drainage is absorbed and removed along with dead tissue. Dressings can promote comfort and cover unsightly wounds. They also provide a moist environment for wound healing. When bleeding is a problem, pressure dressings help control bleeding.

The type and size of dressing used depend on many factors. These include the type of wound, its size, and location; amount of drainage; and the presence or absence of infection. The dressing's function and the frequency of dressing changes are other factors. The RN tells you what dressing to use.

Types of Dressings

Dressings are described by the material used and application method. Many products are available for dressing wounds. You need to be familiar with the following materials:
- Gauze—comes in squares, rectangles, pads, and rolls (Fig. 28-7). Gauze dressings absorb moisture.
- Nonadherent gauze—is a gauze dressing with a nonstick surface. The dressing does not stick to the wound and removes easily without injuring tissue.
- Transparent adhesive film—prevents fluids and bacteria from reaching the wound but air can. The wound is kept moist. Drainage is not absorbed. The transparent film allows wound observation.

Some dressings contain special agents to promote wound healing. The RN is likely to change such dressings. If you assist with the dressing change, the RN explains its use to you.

Dressing application methods involve dry and wet dressings:

- *Dry-to-dry dressing*—usually called a *dry dressing.* A dry gauze dressing is placed over the wound. Additional dressings are placed on top of the first dressing as needed. Drainage is absorbed by the dressing and is removed with the dressing. A dry dressing can stick to the wound. The dressing must be removed carefully to prevent tissue injury and discomfort.
- *Wet-to-dry dressing*—a gauze dressing saturated with a solution is applied over the wound. Additional dressings are applied as needed. These dressings are also moistened with solution. The solution softens dead tissue in the wound. The dead tissue is absorbed by the dressing and is removed with the dressing. The dressings are removed when dry.
- *Wet-to-wet dressing*—a gauze dressing saturated with solution is placed in the wound. The dressing is kept moist.

Securing Dressings

Dressings must be secure over wounds. Bacteria can enter the wound, and drainage can escape if the dressing is dislodged. Tape and Montgomery ties are commonly used to secure dressings. Binders (p. 678) also hold dressings in place.

Tape

Adhesive, paper, plastic, and elastic tapes are available. Adhesive tape sticks well to the skin. However, the adhesive part can remain on the skin and is hard to remove. The adhesive can irritate the skin. Sometimes skin is removed with the tape, causing an abrasion. Many people are allergic to adhesive tape. Paper and plastic tapes are nonallergenic. This means that they do not cause allergic reactions. Elastic tape allows movement of the body part. The RN tells you what type of tape to use for the person.

Tape is available in $\frac{1}{2}$-inch, 1-inch, 2-inch, and 3-inch widths. The size used depends on the size of the dressing. The RN tells you what size to use. Tape is applied to secure the top, middle, and bottom of the dressing (Fig. 28-8). The tape should extend beyond each side of the dressing. *The tape should not encircle the entire body part. If swelling occurs, circulation to the part is impaired.*

Montgomery ties

Montgomery ties (Fig. 28-9) are used for large dressings and when frequent dressing changes are needed. A Montgomery tie consists of an adhesive strip and a cloth tie. When the dressing is in place, the adhesive strips are placed on both sides of the dressing. Then the cloth ties are secured over the dressing. Two or three Montgomery ties may be needed on each side. The cloth ties are undone for the dressing change. The adhesive strips are not removed unless soiled. (See Focus on Children at right, Focus on Older Persons and Focus on Home Care on p. 674.)

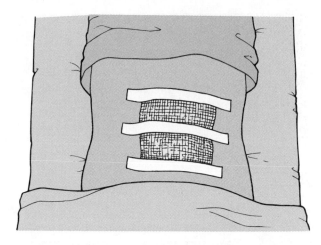

Fig. 28-8 *Tape is applied at the top, middle, and bottom of the dressing. Note that the tape extends beyond both sides of the dressing.*

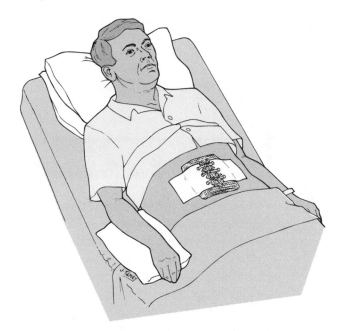

Fig. 28-9 *Montgomery ties.*

CHILDREN

focus on

Children are often afraid of dressing changes. Tape removal is often painful for them. The wound's appearance can be frightening. A calm, cooperative child is important to prevent contamination of the sterile field. Let the parent or caregiver hold the child if you can reach the wound with ease. Letting the child hold or play with a favorite toy is often comforting.

OLDER PERSONS

Older persons have thin, fragile skin. You must prevent skin tears. Extreme care is necessary when removing tape.

HOME CARE

Make sure you have the necessary supplies before leaving the agency. The RN may ask you to telephone him or her after removing the old dressings. During this telephone call, you report your observations to the RN. Then the RN gives you instructions about how to proceed.

✦ Applying Dressings

The doctor usually does the first dressing change after surgery. The RN follows the doctor's order for dressing changes. The RN tells you when to change a dressing and what supplies to use. A dressing change usually involves cleaning the wound and drain site. Box 28-2 lists the rules for applying dressings. Box 28-3 lists the rules for cleaning wounds and drain sites.

Remember, assistive personnel do not administer medications. The doctor's orders may include applying a medicated powder or ointment to the wound. The RN is responsible for applying the medication. Also, some wounds and dressings are more complex than others. An RN observes such wounds and changes the dressings. Your job description may allow you to apply simple dressings to uncomplicated wounds and to assist the RN with complex wounds.

Text continued on p. 678

BOX 28-2

RULES FOR APPLYING DRESSINGS

- Make sure your state allows assistive personnel to perform the procedure.
- Make sure the procedure is in your job description.
- Apply dressings only under the RN's direction and supervision.
- Review the procedure with the RN. A patient may require special measures.
- Allow pain medications time to take effect. The person may experience discomfort during the dressing change. The RN gives the medication and tells you how long to wait.
- Provide for the person's fluid and elimination needs before starting the procedure.
- Collect all needed equipment and supplies before you begin.
- Control your nonverbal communication. Wound odors, appearance, and drainage may be unpleasant. Do not communicate your thoughts and reactions to the person.
- Remove soiled dressings so that the underside of the dressing is away from the person's sight. The drainage and its odor may upset the person.
- Do not force the person to look at the wound. A wound can affect the person's body image and esteem. The RN helps the person deal with the wound.
- Practice Standard Precautions and follow the Bloodborne Pathogen Standard. Wear personal protective equipment as necessary.
- Wear clean, disposable gloves to remove old dressings.
- Remove tape by pulling the tape toward the wound.
- Remove dressings gently to prevent pain and discomfort. The dressing may stick to the wound and surrounding skin.
- Follow the rules of surgical asepsis to apply a sterile dressing (see p. 221).
- Set up your sterile field after removing and discarding old dressings.
- Wear sterile gloves to apply new dressings.
- Follow the rules for cleaning wounds and drain sites (see Box 28-3).

BOX 28-3

RULES FOR CLEANING WOUNDS AND DRAIN SITES

- Ask the RN about what solution to use.
- Use sterile gauze dressings to apply the solution.
- Use sterile forceps to hold the sterile gauze for cleaning.
- Clean away from the wound. Clean from the wound to the surrounding skin (Fig. 28-10).
- Use circular motions when cleaning drain sites (Fig. 28-11).
- Use a different gauze dressing for each stroke.

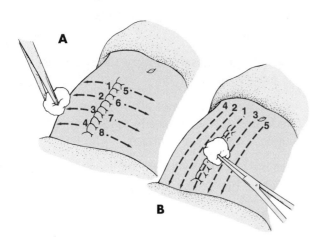

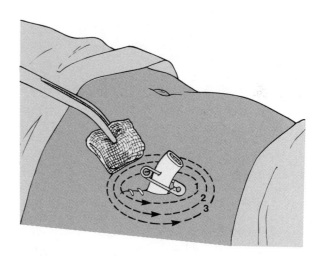

Fig. 28-10 *Cleaning a wound.* **A,** *Clean starting at the wound and stroking out to surrounding skin.* **B,** *Clean the wound from top to bottom. Start at the wound. Then clean surrounding tissues. Remember to use a new swab for each stroke.* (From Potter PA, Perry AG: Fundamentals of nursing: concepts, process, and practice, *ed 4, St Louis, 1997, Mosby.)*

Fig. 28-11 *Cleaning a drain site. Clean in circular motions starting at the drain site. Use a new swab for each stroke.*

APPLYING A DRY STERILE DRESSING

PROCEDURE ALERT

- Does your state allow assistive personnel to perform the procedure?

- Is the procedure in your job description?

- Do you have the necessary training and education?

- Is an RN available to answer questions and to supervise you?

PRE-PROCEDURE

1 Review the procedure with the RN.

2 Explain to the person what you are going to do.

3 Allow time for pain medication to take effect.

4 Provide for the person's fluid and elimination needs.

5 Wash your hands.

6 Collect needed equipment:

- Disposable gloves

- Sterile gloves

- Personal protective equipment as needed (mask, gown, eye shield)

- Sterile cleaning solution

- Sterile dressing set with sterile scissors and sterile forceps

- Sterile basin

- Sterile drape

- Tape and Montgomery ties as directed by the RN

- Sterile dressings as directed by the RN

- Sterile gauze swabs for wound cleaning

- Adhesive remover

- Leakproof plastic bag

- Bath blanket

7 Identify the person. Check the ID bracelet against the assignment sheet.

8 Provide for the person's privacy. Close the door and privacy curtain.

9 Arrange furniture for your work surface. Make sure that you will not have to reach over or turn your back on the work surface.

10 Raise the bed to a level for good body mechanics. Make sure the far bed rail is raised.

PROCEDURE

11 Help the person to a comfortable position.

12 Cover the person with a bath blanket. Fanfold top linens to the foot of the bed.

13 Expose the affected body part.

14 Remind the person not to touch supplies or the wound.

15 Make a cuff on the plastic bag. Place the bag within easy reach.

16 Put on the clean gown and mask if needed.

17 Put on the disposable gloves.

18 Undo Montgomery ties or remove tape:

a Montgomery ties: fold ties away from the wound.

b Tape: Hold the skin down, and gently pull the tape toward the wound.

19 Remove adhesive from the skin if necessary. Wet a 4 × 4 gauze dressing with the adhesive remover. Clean away from the wound.

20 Remove gauze dressings starting with the top dressing. Keep the soiled side of the dressing away from the person's sight. Place dressings in the plastic bag. Do not let the dressings touch the outside of the bag.

APPLYING A DRY STERILE DRESSING—cont'd

PROCEDURE—cont'd

21 Remove the dressing directly over the wound very gently. The dressing may stick to the wound or drain.

22 Observe the wound, drain site, and wound drainage (see Box 28-1).

23 Remove the disposable gloves. Discard them into the plastic bag.

24 Make sure the plastic bag is away from where you will set up your sterile field.

25 Wash your hands. Raise the bed rail when you leave the bedside, and lower it upon your return.

26 Set up your sterile field (see Chapter 11).

   a Place the sterile drape over your work surface.

   b Open the sterile dressing set. Drop the contents onto the sterile field.

   c Open the sterile dressings. Drop them onto the sterile field.

   d Open the sterile bowl. Place it on the sterile field.

   e Open the sterile swabs for cleaning the wound. Drop them into the sterile bowl.

   f Open the sterile cleaning solution. Pour the solution into the bowl with the sterile swabs. Place the cap and bottle outside the sterile field.

27 Put on the sterile gloves.

28 Pick up the sterile swabs with the sterile forceps. Place them in the cleaning solution. Save some swabs for drying the skin around the wound and drain site.

29 Clean the wound (see Fig. 28-10). Clean from the wound outward. Use a new swab for each stroke. Drop used swabs into the plastic bag. Do not let the forceps touch the bag.

30 Clean the area around the drain site (see Fig. 28-11). Clean from the wound outward. Use a new swab for each circular motion. Do not let the forceps touch the bag.

31 Dry the skin around the wound and drain site. Use dry swabs.

32 Apply a 4 × 4 gauze dressing to the drain site (see Fig. 28-4). Use a precut 4 × 4 dressing, or cut half-way through a 4 × 4 dressing using the sterile scissors.

33 Apply dressings over the wound and drain site as directed by the RN.

34 Secure the dressings in place. Use tape (see Fig. 28-8) or Montgomery ties (see Fig. 28-9).

35 Remove your gloves. Discard them in the plastic bag.

POST-PROCEDURE

36 Help the person to assume a comfortable position. Cover the person with the top linens, and remove the bath blanket.

37 Make sure the call bell is within the person's reach.

38 Lower the bed to its lowest position. Raise or lower bed rails as instructed by the RN.

39 Unscreen the person.

40 Discard supplies into the plastic bag. Discard the plastic bag according to agency policy.

41 Clean your work surface following the Bloodborne Pathogen Standard. Return furniture to its proper place.

42 Wash your hands.

43 Report your observations to the RN.

BOX 28-4

RULES FOR APPLYING BINDERS

- Apply the binder so that firm, even pressure is exerted over the area.
- Apply the binder so it is snug but does not interfere with breathing or circulation.
- Position the person in good alignment when the binder is applied.
- Reapply the binder if it becomes loose, wrinkled, or out of position or causes discomfort.
- Secure pins so they point away from incisional areas.
- Change binders that are moist or soiled to prevent the growth of microorganisms.

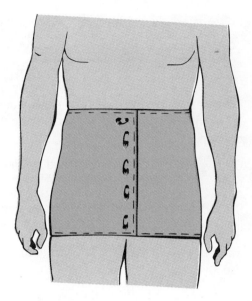

Fig. 28-12 *Straight abdominal binder.*

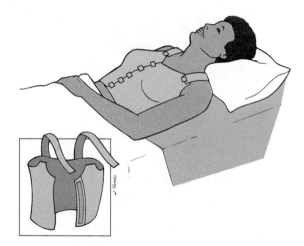

Fig. 28-13 *Breast binder.*

BINDERS

Binders are applied to the abdomen, chest, or perineal areas. Binders promote healing because they:

- Support wounds and hold dressings in place
- Reduce or prevent swelling by promoting circulation
- Promote comfort
- Prevent injury

They must be applied properly. Incorrect application can cause severe discomfort, skin irritation, and circulatory and respiratory complications. The binder's effectiveness and the person's safety depend on correct application. Box 28-4 lists the rules for applying these binders:

- *Straight abdominal binders*—provide abdominal support and hold dressings in place (Fig. 28-12). The binder is a rectangle. The binder is applied with the person supine. The top part is positioned at the person's waist. The lower part is over the hips. The binder is secured in place with pins, hooks, or Velcro.
- *Breast binders*—support the breasts after breast surgery (Fig. 28-13). They also apply pressure to the breasts after childbirth. If the mother does not breast-feed, pressure from the binder helps dry up the milk in the breasts. The binder also promotes comfort and provides support to swollen breasts after childbirth. The woman is supine when the breast binder is applied. The binder is pulled snugly across the chest and secured in place.
- T *binders*—are used to secure dressings in place after rectal and perineal surgeries. The single T binder is used for women (Fig. 28-14, *A*). The double T binder is used for men (Fig. 28-14, *B*). If perineal dressings are large, women may need double T binders. To apply a T binder, the waist bands are brought around the waist and pinned at the front. The tails are brought between the person's legs and up to the waistband. They are pinned in place at the waistband.

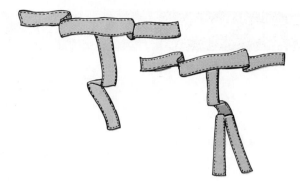

Fig. 28-14 A, *Single* T *binder.* **B,** *Double* T *binder.*

HEAT AND COLD APPLICATIONS

Heat and cold applications are often ordered for wound care. Heat and cold applications are ordered by doctors to promote healing, promote comfort, and reduce tissue swelling. Heat and cold applications are discussed in Chapter 29.

WOUND CARE AND THE PERSON'S BASIC NEEDS

This chapter focuses on wounds. However, you must remember that it is the *person* who has the wound. The wound, which can affect the person's basic needs, is only one aspect of the person's care.

You must remember that the person is recovering from surgery or trauma. The wound is a source of pain and discomfort. The wound and the pain may interfere with breathing and moving. Turning, repositioning, and ambulating may be painful. You must handle the person gently and allow pain medications to take effect before giving care.

Good nutrition is needed for healing. However, pain and discomfort can affect the person's appetite. So can odors from wound drainage. Remove soiled dressings promptly from the room, use room deodorizers, and keep drainage containers out of the person's sight. If the person has a taste for certain foods or beverages, report this information to the RN.

Infection is always a threat. You must practice Standard Precautions and follow the Bloodborne Pathogen Standard. Dressing changes require sterile technique. Also, observe the wound and the person carefully for signs and symptoms of infection.

Delayed healing is a risk for persons who are elderly or obese or have poor nutrition. Poor circulation and diabetes also affect healing. These conditions are risk factors for infection.

Many fears affect the person's sense of safety and security. The person fears scarring, disfigurement, delayed healing, and infection. Fears about the wound "popping" open are common. Costly medical bills are other concerns. Continued hospital care, home care, or long-term care may be needed.

Victims of violence have many other concerns. Future attacks, finding and convicting the attacker, and fear for family members is common. Victims of domestic violence, child abuse, and elderly abuse often hide the true source of their injuries.

The person's wound may be large or small. It may be visible to others—on the face, arms, or legs—or hidden by clothing. Wound drainage may have unpleasant odors. The wound may be extensive and disfiguring. It may affect the person's ability to perform sexually or the person's sense of being sexually attractive. The amputation of a finger, hand, arm, toe, foot, or leg can affect the person's function, everyday activities, and job. Eye injuries can affect vision. Abdominal trauma and surgery can affect eating and elimination.

Whatever the location or size of the wound, physical function and body image are affected. The person's sense of love and belonging and self-esteem are affected. You must be sensitive to the person's feelings. The person may be sad and tearful or angry and hostile. Adjustment may be difficult and rehabilitation necessary. You must be gentle and kind, give thoughtful care, and practice good communication techniques. Other health team members—social workers, psychiatrists, and the clergy—may be involved in the person's care.

REVIEW QUESTIONS

Circle the best answer.

1 Sally Jones fell off her bike. She has a laceration on her right leg. Which is *false?*

a She has an open wound.

b She has an infected wound.

c She has a contaminated wound.

d She has an unintentional wound.

2 A person had rectal surgery. What type of wound does the person have?

a A clean wound

b A dirty wound

c A clean-contaminated wound

d A contaminated wound

3 The skin and underlying tissues are pierced. This is

a A penetrating wound

b An incision

c A contusion

d An abrasion

4 A wound appears red and swollen. The area around the wound is warm to touch. These signs are characteristics of

a The inflammatory phase of wound healing

b The proliferative phase of wound healing

c Healing by primary intention

d Healing by secondary intention

5 A wound is healing by primary intention. During a dressing change you note that the wound is separating. This is called

a Dehiscence

b Tertiary intention

c Evisceration

d Hematoma

6 You note a clear, watery drainage from a wound. This drainage is called

a Purulent drainage

b Serous drainage

c Sero-purulent drainage

d Serosanguineous drainage

7 You note large amounts of sanguineous drainage in a Hemovac. Which is *true?*

a The person is bleeding.

b You need to notify the doctor.

c The person has an infection.

d The person has a Penrose drain.

8 A dressing does the following *except*

a Protect the wound from injury

b Absorb drainage

c Provide a moist environment for wound healing

d Support the wound and reduce swelling

9 Which dressing is likely to stick to a wound?

a A wet-to-wet dressing

b Nonadherent gauze

c A dry-to-dry dressing

d Montgomery ties

10 You are securing a dressing with tape. Tape is applied

a Around the entire part

b To the top and bottom of the dressing

c To the top, middle, and bottom of the dressing

d As the person prefers

11 You are going to apply a sterile dressing. You put on sterile gloves

a At the beginning of the procedure

b To remove the old dressings

c To open sterile dressings

d After setting up the sterile field

REVIEW QUESTIONS—cont'd

12 When cleaning a wound, you clean
   a   Outward from the wound
   b   Toward the wound
   c   In circular motions away from the wound
   d   In circular motions toward the wound

13 The wound is cleaned
   a   After setting up the sterile field
   b   While wearing clean disposable gloves
   c   With soap and water
   d   Daily

14 Mr. Moore has an abdominal binder. The binder is used to
   a   Prevent blood clots
   b   Prevent wound infection
   c   Provide support and hold dressings in place
   d   Decrease circulation and swelling

Answers to these questions are on p. 853.

29 Heat and Cold Applications

- Define the key terms in this chapter
- Identify the purposes, effects, and complications of heat and cold applications
- Identify the persons at risk for complications from heat and cold applications
- Explain the differences between moist and dry heat and cold applications
- Describe the rules for the application of heat and cold
- Explain how cooling and warming blankets are used
- Perform the procedures described in this chapter

KEY TERMS

constrict To narrow

cyanosis Bluish discoloration of the skin

dilate To expand or open wider

hyperthermia A body temperature *(thermia)* that is much higher *(hyper)* than normal

hypothermia A very low *(hypo)* body temperature *(thermia)*

Doctors order heat and cold applications to promote healing and comfort. They also reduce tissue swelling. Heat and cold have opposite effects on body function. Severe injuries and changes in body function can occur. The risks are great. You must thoroughly understand the purposes, effects, and complications of heat and cold applications.

In some agencies, only nurses apply heat and cold. Other agencies let assistive personnel apply heat and cold. Before you perform these procedures, make sure that:

- Your state allows you to perform the procedure
- The procedure is in your job description
- You have the necessary training
- You are familiar with the equipment
- You review the procedure with an RN
- An RN is available to answer questions and to supervise you

HEAT APPLICATIONS

Heat applications can be applied to almost any body part. They are often used for musculoskeletal injuries or problems (sprains, arthritis). Heat applications are used to:

- Relieve pain
- Relax muscles
- Promote healing
- Reduce tissue swelling
- Decrease joint stiffness

Effects

When heat is applied to the skin, blood vessels in the area dilate. **Dilate** means to expand or open wider (Fig. 29-1, p. 684). More blood flows through the vessels. The tissues have more oxygen and nutrients for healing. Excess fluid is removed from the area faster. The skin is reddened and feels warm.

Complications

High temperatures can cause burns. Pain, excessive redness, and blisters are danger signs. Report these signs immediately. Also observe for pale skin. When heat is applied too long, blood vessels **constrict** (narrow) (see Fig. 29-1, *C*). Blood flow decreases when vessels constrict. This reduces the amount of blood for the tissues. Tissue damage occurs, and the skin is pale.

Fair-skinned people are at great risk for complications. Their delicate and fragile skin is easily burned. Persons with difficulty sensing heat or pain also are at risk. Nervous system damage, loss of consciousness, and circulatory disorders interfere with sensation. So does confusion and strong pain medications.

Persons with metal implants are at risk. Metal conducts heat. Deep tissues can be burned. Pacemakers and joint replacements are made of metal. Heat is not applied in the area of the implant.

Heat is not applied to a pregnant woman's abdomen. The heat can affect fetal growth.

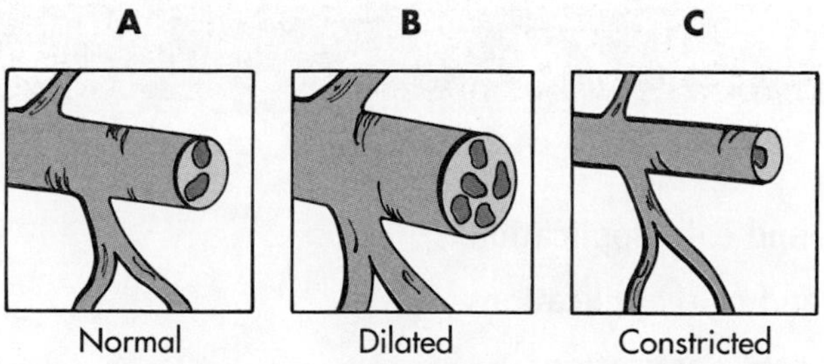

Fig. 29-1 **A,** *Blood vessel under normal conditions.* **B,** *Dilated blood vessel.* **C,** *Constricted blood vessel.*

Moist and Dry Applications

A *moist heat application* means that water is in contact with the skin. Water conducts heat. The effects from moist heat are greater and occur faster than from dry heat applications. Heat penetrates deeper with a moist application. To prevent injury, moist heat applications have lower (cooler) temperatures than dry heat applications.

Water is not in contact with the skin with *dry heat applications.* Dry heat has advantages:

- The application stays at the desired temperature longer.
- Dry heat does not penetrate as deeply as moist heat.

Because water is not used, dry heat needs higher (hotter) temperatures to achieve the desired effect. Therefore burns are still a risk.

The person must be protected from injury during local heat applications. Practice the rules in Box 29-1 to prevent burns and other complications. (See Focus on Children and Focus on Older Persons.)

focus on

CHILDREN

Infants and young children have fragile skin. They are at risk for burns. They need careful observation. Always respond to infants and young children who are crying. Crying is a way of communicating pain.

focus on

OLDER PERSONS

Older persons have thin and fragile skin. They also are at risk for burns. Other changes from aging and health problems increase the risk for burns. They include circulatory and nervous system changes. Some drugs also affect the older person's ability to sense pain. Confused persons and those with dementia may not recognize pain. Look for changes in the person's behavior. Behavior changes can signal pain.

BOX 29-1

RULES FOR APPLYING HEAT AND COLD

- Know how to operate equipment used in the procedure.
- Measure the temperature of moist applications. Use a bath thermometer.
- Follow agency policies for safe temperature ranges. See Table 29-1 for guidelines.
- Do not apply *very hot* (above 106° to 115° F, or 41.1° to 46.1° C) applications. Tissue damage can occur. A nurse applies *very hot* applications.
- Ask the RN what the temperature of the application should be:
  - Heat—cooler temperatures are used for persons at risk.
  - Cold—warmer temperatures are used for persons at risk.
- Know the precise site of the heat application. Ask the RN to show you the site.
- Cover dry heat or cold applications before applying them. Use a flannel cover, towel, or pillowcase according to agency policy.
- Observe the skin for signs of complications. Immediately report the following to the RN:
  - Complaints of pain, numbness, or burning
  - Excessive redness
  - Blisters
  - Pale, white, or gray skin
  - Cyanosis
  - Shivering
- Do not let the person change the temperature of the application.
- Ask the RN how long to leave the application in place. Carefully watch the time. Heat and cold are applied for no longer than 20 minutes.
- Follow the rules of electrical safety when using electrical appliances to apply heat.
- Expose only the body part where you will apply heat or cold. Provide for privacy through proper draping and screening.
- Place the call bell within the person's reach.

TABLE 29-1

HEAT AND COLD TEMPERATURE RANGES

Temperature	Fahrenheit Range	Centigrade Range
Very hot	106° to 115° F	41.1° to 46.1° C
Hot	98° to 106° F	36.6° to 41.1° C
Warm	93° to 98° F	33.8° to 36.6° C
Tepid	80° to 93° F	26.6° to 33.8° C
Cool	65° to 80° F	18.3° to 26.6° C
Cold	50° to 65° F	10.0° to 18.3° C

(Modified from Perry AG, Potter PA: *Clinical nursing skills and techniques,* ed 4, St Louis, 1998, Mosby.)

✦ Hot Compresses and Packs

Hot compresses and packs are moist heat applications. They consist of a washcloth, small towel, or gauze dressing. A compress is applied to a small area. Packs are applied to large areas.

The application is left in place for 20 minutes. Sometimes an aquathermia pad (p. 691) is applied over the compress or pack. This maintains the temperature of the compress or pack.

APPLYING HOT COMPRESSES

PROCEDURE ALERT

- Does your state allow assistive personnel to perform the procedure?

- Is the procedure in your job description?

- Do you have the necessary training and education?

- Is an RN available to answer questions and to supervise you?

PRE-PROCEDURE

1 Explain the procedure to the person.

2 Wash your hands.

3 Collect the following:

- Basin

- Bath thermometer

- Small towel, washcloth, or gauze squares

- Plastic wrap or aquathermia pad

- Ties, tape, or rolled gauze

- Bath towel

- Waterproof bed protector

4 Identify the person. Check the ID bracelet against the assignment sheet.

5 Provide for privacy.

PROCEDURE

6 Place the protector under the body part.

7 Fill the basin one-half to two-thirds full with hot water as directed by the RN.

8 Place the compress in the water.

9 Wring out the compress.

10 Apply the compress to the area. Note the time.

11 Cover the compress quickly. Do one of the following as directed by the RN:

  a Cover the compress with plastic wrap and then with a bath towel (Fig. 29-2). Secure the towel in place with ties, tape, or rolled gauze.

  b Cover the compress with an aquathermia pad (see p. 691).

12 Place the call bell within reach. Raise or lower bed rails as instructed by the RN.

13 Check the area every 5 minutes. Check for redness and complaints of pain, discomfort, or numbness. Remove the compress if any occur. Tell the RN immediately.

14 Change the compress if cooling occurs.

15 Remove the compress after 20 minutes or as directed by the RN. Pat the area dry with a towel. (Lower the bed rail for this step.)

POST-PROCEDURE

16 Make sure the person is comfortable and unscreened.

17 Raise or lower bed rails as instructed by the RN.

18 Place the call bell within reach.

19 Clean equipment. Discard disposable items.

20 Follow agency policy for soiled linen.

21 Wash your hands.

22 Report the following to the RN:

- Time, site, and length of the application

- Observations of the skin

- The person's response

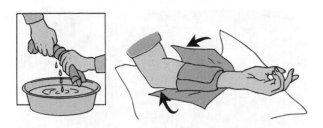

Fig. 29-2 *A hot compress is covered with plastic and a bath towel. These keep the compress warm.*

✦ *Commercial compresses*

Commercial compresses are premoistened and packaged in foil. An infrared lamp is used to heat the wrapped compress as instructed by the manufacturer. The lamp is kept in the clean utility room, treatment room, medication room, or the person's room.

Commercial compresses are sterile. Sometimes doctors order them for nonsterile compresses. RNs may decide they are needed in certain situations. Commercial compresses are costly and are used only when necessary.

✦ APPLYING A COMMERCIAL COMPRESS

PROCEDURE ALERT

- Does your state allow assistive personnel to perform the procedure?

- Is the procedure in your job description?

- Do you have the necessary training and education?

- Is an RN available to answer questions and to supervise you?

PRE-PROCEDURE

1 Explain the procedure to the person.

2 Wash your hands.

3 Collect the following:

- Commercial compress

- Infrared lamp

- Towel

- Ties, tape, or rolled gauze

- Waterproof bed protector

- Aquathermia pad (if ordered)

4 Heat the compress following the manufacturer's instructions.

5 Identify the person. Check the ID bracelet against the assignment sheet.

6 Provide for privacy.

PROCEDURE

7 Place the bed protector under the body part.

8 Open the foil-wrapped compress.

9 Apply the compress quickly. Use the outside of the foil to pick up and apply the compress.

10 Cover the compress with a towel.

11 Secure the towel in place with ties, tape, or rolled gauze.

12 Apply the aquathermia pad (if ordered). See *Applying an Aquathermia Pad*, p. 691.

13 Place the call bell within reach. Raise or lower bed rails as instructed by the RN.

14 Check the area every 5 minutes. Check for redness and complaints of pain, discomfort, or numbness. Remove the compress if any occur. Tell the RN immediately.

15 Change the compress if cooling occurs.

16 Remove the compress after 20 minutes or as directed by the RN. Pat the area dry with the towel. (Lower the bed rail for this step.)

POST-PROCEDURE

17 Follow steps 16 through 22 in *Applying Hot Compresses*.

✦ Hot Soaks

A hot soak involves putting the body part into water. This usually is used for smaller parts, such as a hand, lower arm, foot, or lower leg (Fig. 29-3). Sometimes larger areas are soaked (arm, leg, or torso). Then a tub is used. The soak lasts 15 to 20 minutes. The person's comfort and body alignment are maintained during the hot soak.

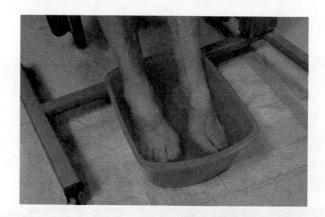

Fig. 29-3 *The hot soak.*

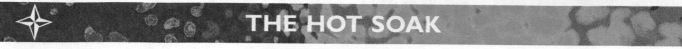

THE HOT SOAK

PROCEDURE ALERT

- Does your state allow assistive personnel to perform the procedure?
- Is the procedure in your job description?
- Do you have the necessary training and education?
- Is an RN available to answer questions and to supervise you?

PRE-PROCEDURE

1 Explain the procedure to the person.

2 Wash your hands.

3 Collect the following:

- Water basin or an arm or foot bath
- Bath thermometer
- Bath blanket
- Waterproof pads

4 Identify the person. Check the ID bracelet against the assignment sheet.

5 Provide for privacy.

PROCEDURE

6 Position the person for the treatment. Place the call bell within reach.

7 Place a waterproof pad under the area.

8 Fill the container one-half full with hot water as directed by the RN. Measure water temperature.

9 Expose the area. Avoid unnecessary exposure.

10 Place the part into the water. Pad the edge of the container with a towel. Note the time.

11 Cover the person with a bath blanket for extra warmth.

12 Check the area every 5 minutes. Check for redness and complaints of pain, numbness, or discomfort. Remove the part from the soak if any of these complications occur. Wrap the part in a towel, and tell the RN immediately.

13 Check water temperature every 5 minutes. Change water as necessary. Wrap the part in a towel while changing the water.

14 Remove the part from the water in 15 to 20 minutes. Pat dry with a towel.

POST-PROCEDURE

15 Follow steps 16 through 22 in *Applying Hot Compresses.*

✦ The Sitz Bath

The sitz bath involves immersing the pelvic area in warm or hot water for 20 minutes. (*Sitz* means *seat* in German.) Sitz baths are used to clean perineal or anal wounds. They are used also to promote healing, relieve pain and soreness, increase circulation, or stimulate voiding. They are common after rectal or female pelvic surgery, for hemorrhoids, and after childbirth.

The disposable plastic sitz bath fits onto the toilet seat (Fig. 29-4). A sitz tub is a built-in fixture with a deep seat. The person sits in a seat filled with water (Fig. 29-5).

Blood flow to the pelvic area increases. Therefore less blood flows to other body parts. The person may become weak or feel faint. Drowsiness can occur from the treatment's relaxing effect. Observe the person for signs of weakness, faintness, or fatigue. Also protect the person from injury. Check the person often, keep the call bell within reach, and prevent chills and burns.

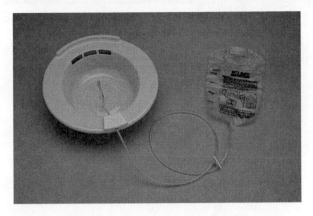

Fig. 29-4 *The disposable sitz bath.*

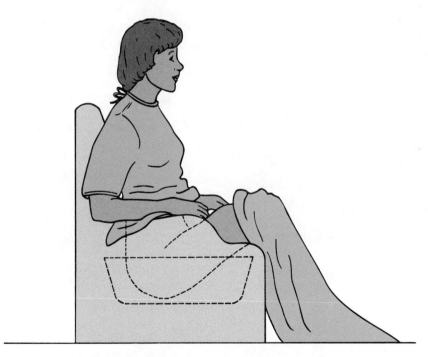

Fig. 29-5 *The built-in sitz bath.*

ASSISTING THE PERSON TO TAKE A SITZ BATH

PROCEDURE ALERT

- Does your state allow assistive personnel to perform the procedure?

- Is the procedure in your job description?

- Do you have the necessary training and education?

- Is an RN available to answer questions and to supervise you?

PRE-PROCEDURE

1 Explain the procedure to the person.

2 Wash your hands.

3 Collect the following:

- Disposable sitz bath or wheelchair if the built-in sitz bath is used

- Bath thermometer

- Large water container

- Two bath blankets, bath towels, and a clean gown

- Footstool if the person is short

- Disinfectant solution

- Utility gloves

4 Identify the person. Check the ID bracelet against the assignment sheet.

5 Provide for privacy.

PROCEDURE

6 Do one of the following:

a Place the disposable sitz bath on the toilet seat.

b Transport the person by wheelchair to the sitz bath room.

7 Fill the sitz bath two-thirds full with water as directed by the RN. Measure water temperature.

8 Use bath towels to pad the metal parts that will be in contact with the person.

9 Raise the gown, and secure it above the waist.

10 Help the person sit in the sitz bath.

11 Place a bath blanket around the shoulders. Place another over the legs for warmth.

12 Provide a footstool if the edge of the sitz bath causes pressure under the knees.

13 Make sure the call bell is within reach and the person is comfortable.

14 Stay with a person who is weak or unsteady.

15 Check the person every 5 minutes for complaints of weakness, faintness, and drowsiness. Check for a rapid pulse. If any occur, get assistance to help the person back to bed.

16 Help the person out of the sitz bath after 20 minutes or as directed by the RN.

17 Assist the person with drying and dressing.

18 Assist the person back to bed.

POST-PROCEDURE

19 Make sure the person is comfortable and unscreened.

20 Place the call bell within reach.

21 Raise or lower bed rails as instructed by the RN.

22 Clean the sitz bath with disinfectant solution. Wear utility gloves for this step.

23 Return reusable items to their proper place. Follow agency policy for soiled linen.

24 Wash your hands.

25 Report your observations to the nurse.

✦ The Aquathermia Pad

The aquathermia pad (Aqua-K, K-Pad) is an electric device used for dry heat. Tubes inside the pad are filled with distilled water. A bedside heating unit is also filled with distilled water. The heated water flows to the pad through a connecting hose (Fig. 29-6). Another hose returns water to the heating unit. The water is reheated and circulated back into the pad.

The heating unit is kept level with the pad and connecting hoses. Water must flow freely. Hoses must be free of kinks and air bubbles. The temperature is set at 105° F (40.5° C) with a key. Then the key is removed. This prevents anyone from changing the temperature. The temperature is often set in the central supply department. The key is kept in that department.

The following safety measures are practiced:

- Follow electrical safety precautions (see Chapter 10).
- Place the heating unit on an even, uncluttered surface. This prevents it from being knocked over or knocked off of the surface.
- Use a flannel cover to insulate the pad. It also absorbs perspiration at the application site. (Some agencies use a towel or pillowcase.)
- Secure the pad in place with ties, tape, or rolled gauze. Do not use pins. They can puncture the pad and cause leaking.
- Do not place the pad under the person or under a body part. This prevents the escape of heat. Burns can result if heat cannot escape.

(See Focus on Home Care.)

focus on HOME CARE

Many people have heating pads with electric coils made of wire. These coils present fire hazards if they break. Burns are a great risk because the temperature is easily adjusted. Always make sure the heating pad is in good repair. Check the temperature often to make sure the patient has not changed it.

Another type of pad serves as a heating pad or a cold application. This pad is filled with a special fluid. The pad is kept in the freezer until needed. If used as a heating pad, the pad is heated in a microwave oven following the manufacturer's instructions. The pad, whether used for heat or cold, is secured in place with attached Velcro straps.

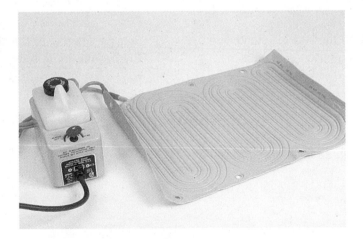

Fig. 29-6 *The aquathermia pad and heating unit.*

APPLYING AN AQUATHERMIA PAD

PROCEDURE ALERT

- Does your state allow assistive personnel to perform the procedure?

- Is the procedure in your job description?

- Do you have the necessary training and education?

- Is an RN available to answer questions and to supervise you?

PRE-PROCEDURE

1   Explain the procedure to the person.

2   Wash your hands.

3   Collect the following:

- Aquathermia pad and heating unit

- Distilled water

- Flannel cover, pillowcase, or towel

- Ties, tape, or rolled gauze

4   Identify the person. Check the ID bracelet against the assignment sheet.

5   Provide for privacy.

PROCEDURE

6   Fill the heating unit two-thirds full with distilled water.

7   Remove air bubbles. Place the pad and tubing below the heating unit. Tilt the unit from side to side.

8   Set the temperature as instructed by the RN (usually 105° F, or 40.5° C). Remove the key (give it to the RN when you complete the procedure).

9   Place the pad in the cover.

10   Plug in the unit. Let water warm to the desired temperature.

11   Set the heating unit on the bedside stand. Keep the pad and connecting hoses level with the unit. Hoses must be free of kinks.

12   Apply the pad to the part. Note the time.

13   Secure the pad in place with ties, tape, or rolled gauze. Do not use pins.

14   Unscreen the person. Place the call bell within reach.

15   Raise or lower bed rails as instructed by the RN.

16   Check the area every 5 minutes. Check the skin for redness, swelling, and blisters. Ask about pain, discomfort, or decreased sensation. Remove the pad if any occur. Tell the RN immediately.

17   Remove the pad at the specified time. (Lower the bed rail for this step.)

POST-PROCEDURE

18   Follow steps 16 through 22 in *Applying Hot Compresses.*

COLD APPLICATIONS

Cold applications are often used to treat sprains and fractures. They reduce pain, prevent swelling, and decrease circulation and bleeding. Cold cools the body when fever is present.

Effects

Cold has the opposite effect of heat. When cold is applied to the skin, blood vessels constrict (see Fig. 29-1, C). Decreased blood flow results. Less oxygen and nutrients are carried to the tissues. Cold applications are useful right after injury. The decreased circulation reduces the amount of bleeding. The amount of fluid collecting in tissues is reduced also. Cold has a numbing effect on the skin. This helps reduce or relieve pain in the part.

Complications

Complications include pain, burns and blisters, and **cyanosis** (bluish discoloration of the skin). Burns and blisters tend to occur from intense cold. They occur also when dry cold applications are in direct contact with the skin. When cold is applied for a long time, blood vessels dilate. Blood flow increases. The prolonged application of cold has the same effects as local heat applications.

Fair-skinned persons have fragile skin. They are at great risk for complications. So are persons with mental or sensory impairments. (See Focus on Children and Focus on Older Persons.)

Moist and Dry Applications

Cold applications are moist or dry. The ice bag and ice collar are dry cold applications. The cold compress is a moist application. Moist cold applications penetrate deeper than dry ones. Therefore temperatures of moist applications are not as cold as dry applications.

Injuries from cold applications are prevented. See the rules listed in Box 29-1.

✦ Ice Bags, Ice Collars, and Disposable Cold Packs

An ice bag and ice collar are dry cold applications. Ice collars are applied to the neck. The bag or collar is filled with crushed ice. Then it is placed in a cover. If the cover becomes moist, it is removed and a dry one applied.

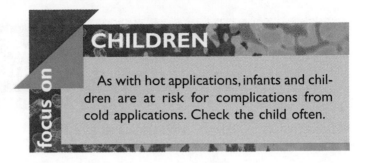

focus on CHILDREN

As with hot applications, infants and children are at risk for complications from cold applications. Check the child often.

focus on OLDER PERSONS

As with hot applications, older persons are at risk for complications from cold applications. Check the person often.

focus on HOME CARE

Disposable ice packs are common in home settings. They are kept in the freezer until needed. Plastic bags also can serve as ice bags. After filling the bag with ice, close the bag securely to prevent leaks. Then wrap the pack or bag in a towel, dishcloth, or pillowcase.

Commercial ice bags are kept frozen until needed. They can be refrozen for reuse. Covers are also needed with ice collars or commercial ice bags.

Disposable cold packs are used once and discarded. They come in many sizes. Some have an outer covering allowing direct application to the skin. Otherwise a cover is used. (See Focus on Home Care.)

APPLYING AN ICE BAG, ICE COLLAR, OR DISPOSABLE COLD PACK

PROCEDURE ALERT

- Does your state allow assistive personnel to perform the procedure?

- Is the procedure in your job description?

- Do you have the necessary training and education?

- Is an RN available to answer questions and to supervise you?

PRE-PROCEDURE

1 Explain the procedure to the person.

2 Wash your hands.

3 Collect a disposable cold pack or the following:

- Ice bag or collar

- Crushed ice

- Flannel cover, towel, or pillowcase

- Paper towels

PROCEDURE

4 Apply an ice bag or collar:

a Fill the ice bag with water. Put in the stopper. Turn the bag upside down to check for leaks.

b Empty the bag.

c Fill the bag one-half to two-thirds full with crushed ice or ice chips (Fig. 29-7).

d Remove excess air. Bend, twist, or squeeze the bag; or press it against a firm surface.

e Place the cap or stopper on securely.

f Dry the bag with the paper towels.

g Place the bag in the cover.

5 Apply a disposable cold pack:

a Squeeze, knead, or strike the cold pack as directed by the manufacturer. This releases cold.

b Place the bag in the cover.

6 Identify the person. Check the ID bracelet against the assignment sheet.

7 Provide for privacy.

8 Apply the ice bag. Secure it in place with ties, tape, or rolled gauze. Note the time.

9 Place the call bell within reach. Raise or lower bed rails as instructed by the RN.

10 Check the skin every 10 minutes. Check for blisters; pale, white, or gray skin; cyanosis; and shivering. Ask about numbness, pain, or burning. Remove the bag if any occur. Tell the RN immediately.

11 Remove the bag after 20 minutes or as directed by the RN.

POST-PROCEDURE

12 Follow steps 16 through 22 in *Applying Hot Compresses.*

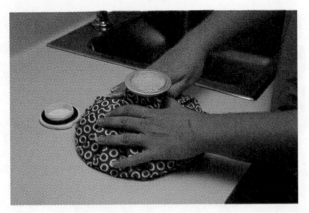

Fig. 29-7 *The ice bag is filled one-half to two-thirds full with ice.*

✦ Cold Compresses

Applying a cold compress is like applying a hot compress. The cold compress is a moist application. Moist cold compresses are left in place no longer than 20 minutes.

✦ APPLYING COLD COMPRESSES

PROCEDURE ALERT

- Does your state allow assistive personnel to perform the procedure?
- Is the procedure in your job description?
- Do you have the necessary training and education?
- Is an RN available to answer questions and to supervise you?

PRE-PROCEDURE

1 Explain the procedure to the person.

2 Wash your hands.

3 Collect the following:

- Large basin with ice
- Small basin with cold water
- Gauze squares, washcloths, or small towels
- Waterproof pad
- Bath towel

4 Identify the person. Check the ID bracelet against the assignment sheet.

5 Provide for privacy.

PROCEDURE

6 Place the small basin with cold water into the large basin with ice.

7 Place the compresses into the cold water.

8 Place a bed protector under the affected body part. Expose the area.

9 Wring out a compress so water is not dripping.

10 Apply the compress to the part. Note the time.

11 Check the area every 5 minutes. Check for blisters; pale, white, or gray skin; cyanosis; or shivering. Ask about numbness, pain, or burning. Remove the compress if any occur. Tell the RN immediately.

12 Change the compress when it warms. Usually compresses are changed every 5 minutes.

13 Remove the compress after 20 minutes or as directed by the RN.

14 Pat dry the area with the bath towel.

POST-PROCEDURE

15 Follow steps 16 through 22 in *Applying Hot Compresses.*

COOLING AND WARMING BLANKETS

Hyperthermia is a body temperature *(thermia)* that is much higher *(hyper)* than normal. Body temperature is greater than 103° F (39.4° C). It is often called *heat stroke* when caused by hot weather temperatures. Other causes include illness, dehydration, and not being able to perspire. Lowering the person's body temperature is necessary. Otherwise death can occur. The doctor orders ice packs applied to the person's head, neck, underarms, and groin. Sometimes cooling blankets are used alone or with ice packs.

A cooling blanket is an electric device. Made of rubber or plastic, the device has tubes filled with distilled water or other fluid. The fluid circulates through the tubes. The blanket is placed on the person's bed and covered with a sheet. The blanket is turned on to the cool setting and allowed to cool. The person lies on the blanket. The person's vital signs are measured often. Rapid and excess cooling are prevented.

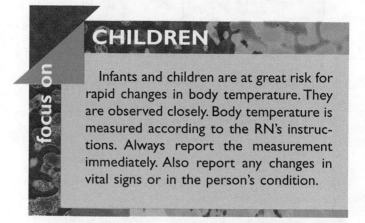

focus on

CHILDREN

Infants and children are at great risk for rapid changes in body temperature. They are observed closely. Body temperature is measured according to the RN's instructions. Always report the measurement immediately. Also report any changes in vital signs or in the person's condition.

Hypothermia is a very low *(hypo)* body temperature *(thermia)*. Body temperature is less than 95° F (35° C). Cold weather temperatures is a common cause. The person must be warmed to prevent death. The person's treatment may include a warming blanket. A warming blanket is the same as a cooling blanket except that the temperature is turned to warm. Vital signs are checked often to prevent rapid or excess warming.

When used to cool the body, the device is called a *hypothermia blanket*. When used to warm the body, it is called a *hyperthermia blanket*. The device has warm and cool settings. (See Focus on Children.)

REVIEW QUESTIONS

Circle the best answer.

1 Local heat has the following effects *except*
a Pain relief
b Muscle relaxation
c Healing
d Decreased blood flow

2 Which is the greatest threat from heat applications?
a Infection
b Burns
c Chilling
d Pressure sores

3 Who has the greatest risk of complications from local heat applications?
a A 10-year-old boy
b A teenager
c A 40-year-old woman
d An older person

4 These statements are about moist heat applications. Which is *false?*
a Water is in contact with the skin.
b The effects of moist heat are less than the effects of dry heat application.
c Moist heat penetrates deeper than dry heat.
d The temperature of a moist heat application is lower than a dry heat application.

5 The temperature of a hot application is usually between
a 80° and 93° F
b 93° and 98° F
c 98° and 106° F
d 106° and 115° F

6 These statements are about sitz baths. Which is *false?*
a The pelvic area is immersed in warm or hot water for 20 minutes.
b The sitz bath lasts 25 to 30 minutes.
c They clean the perineum, relieve pain, increase circulation, or stimulate voiding.
d Weakness and fainting can occur.

7 Mrs. Parks is using an aquathermia pad. Which is *false?*
a The aquathermia pad is a dry heat application.
b The temperature of an aquathermia pad is usually set at 105° F.
c Electrical safety precautions are practiced.
d Pins secure the pad in place.

8 Local cold applications
a Reduce pain, prevent swelling, and decrease circulation
b Dilate blood vessels
c Prevent the spread of microbes
d All of the above

9 Which is *not* a complication of local cold applications?
a Pain
b Burns and blisters
c Cyanosis
d Infection

10 Before applying an ice bag
a Place the bag in a freezer
b Measure the temperature of the bag
c Place the bag in a cover
d Ask the person to void

11 Moist cold compresses are left in place no longer than
a 20 minutes
b 30 minutes
c 45 minutes
d 60 minutes

12 A cooling blanket is used for
a Hypothermia
b Hyperthermia
c Cyanosis
d Shivering

Answers to these questions are on p. 853.

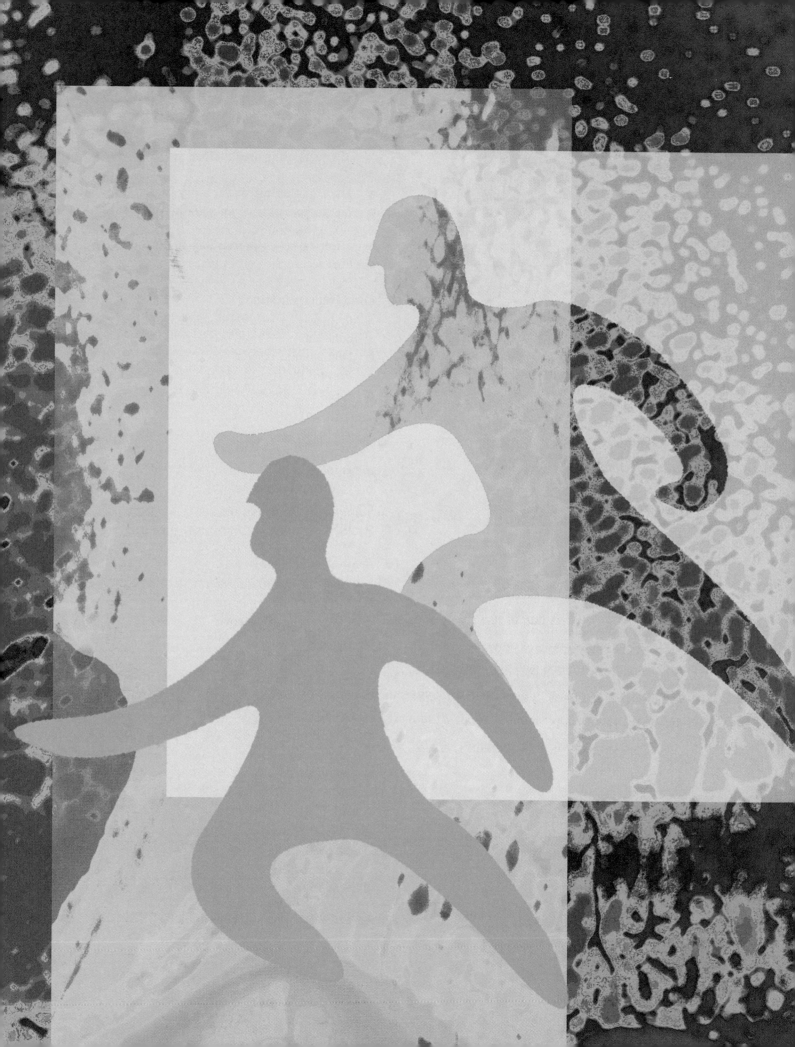

Unit VIII
Assisting With Clinical Situations

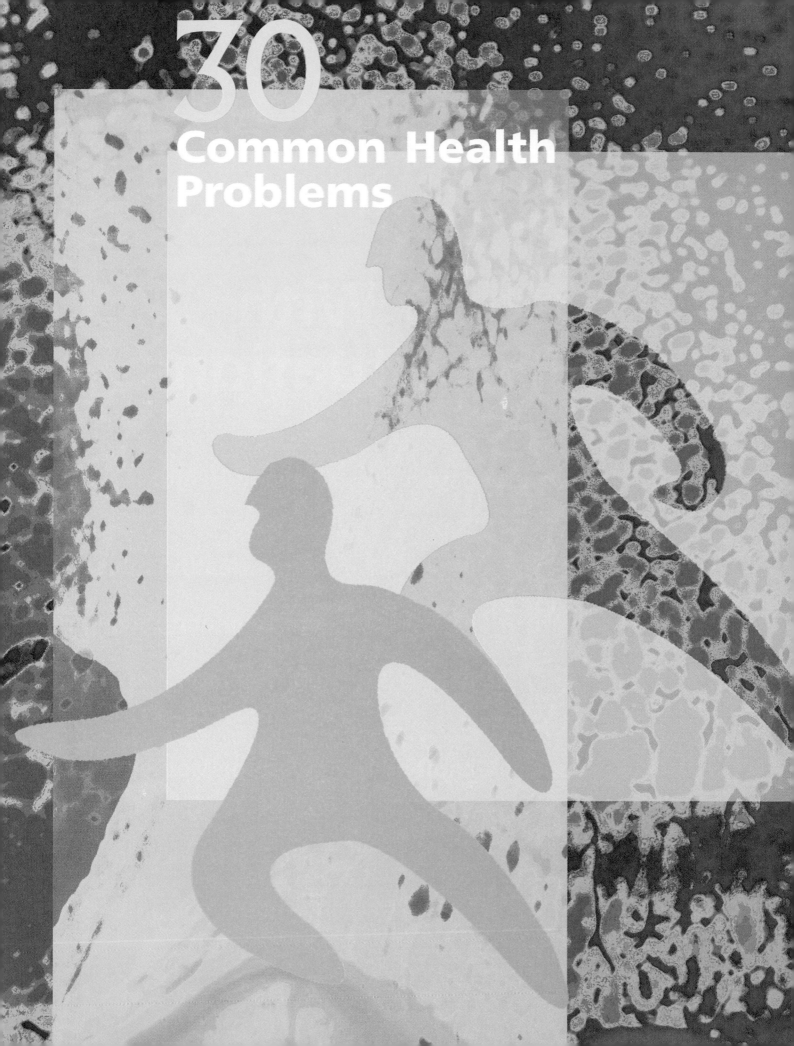

30
Common Health Problems

- Define the key terms in this chapter
- Describe cancer and its treatment
- Explain how to maintain joint function in persons with arthritis
- Explain how to care for persons in casts, in traction, and with hip pinnings
- Describe osteoporosis and the care required
- Describe the effects of amputation
- Describe stroke, its signs and symptoms, and the care required
- Describe Parkinson's disease and multiple sclerosis
- Explain how to care for persons with hearing and vision impairments
- Identify the causes and effects of head and spinal cord injuries and the care required
- Describe common respiratory disorders and the care required
- Identify the signs, symptoms, and treatment of hypertension
- List the risk factors for coronary artery disease
- Describe angina pectoris, myocardial infarction, heart failure, and the care required
- Describe the care required by persons with urinary system disorders
- Identify the signs, symptoms, and complications of diabetes
- Explain how to help the person who is vomiting
- Describe hepatitis and AIDS, their signs and symptoms, and necessary precautions
- Identify the communicable diseases common in children
- Identify sexually transmitted diseases

KEY TERMS

alopecia Loss of hair

amputation The removal of all or part of an extremity

aphasia The inability *(a)* to speak *(phasia)*

arthritis Joint *(arthr)* inflammation *(itis)*

arthroplasty Surgical replacement *(plasty)* of a joint *(arthro)*

benign tumor A tumor that grows slowly and within a localized area

braille A method of writing that uses raised dots; raised dots are arranged to represent each letter of the alphabet; the first ten letters represent the numbers 0 through 9

cancer Malignant tumor

closed fracture The bone is broken but the skin is intact; simple fracture

compound fracture The bone is broken and has come through the skin; open fracture

dialysis Process of removing waste products from the blood

dysphagia Difficulty *(dys)* swallowing *(phagia)*

expressive aphasia Difficulty expressing or sending out thoughts

expressive-receptive aphasia Difficulty expressing or sending out thoughts and difficulty receiving information

fracture A broken bone

Key Terms continued on p. 702

gangrene A condition in which there is death of tissue; tissues become black, cold, and shriveled

hemiplegia Paralysis on one side of the body

hyperglycemia High *(hyper)* sugar *(glyc)* in the blood *(emia)*

hypoglycemia Low *(hypo)* sugar *(glyc)* in the blood *(emia)*

malignant tumor A tumor that grows rapidly and invades other tissues; cancer

metastasis The spread of cancer to other parts of the body

open fracture Compound fracture

paraplegia Paralysis of the legs

quadriplegia Paralysis of the arms, legs, and trunk

receptive aphasia Difficulty receiving information

simple fracture Closed fracture

stomatitis Inflammation *(itis)* of the mouth *(stomat)*

tinnitus Ringing in the ears

tumor A new growth of cells; tumors are benign or malignant

vertigo Dizziness

This chapter gives basic information about common health problems. The RN uses the nursing process to meet the needs of persons with these and other health problems. Understanding a disorder makes the required care meaningful. An RN gives you more information as needed.

A review of Chapter 7 ("Body Structure and Function") will help you study this chapter.

CANCER

A **tumor** is a new growth of abnormal cells. Tumors are benign or malignant (Fig. 30-1). **Benign** tumors grow slowly and within a localized area. They do not usually cause death. A malignant tumor is cancerous. A **malignant** tumor (**cancer**) grows rapidly and invades healthy tissues (Fig. 30-2). Death occurs if the cancer is not treated and controlled. **Metastasis** is the spread of cancer to other body parts (Fig. 30-3). It occurs if the cancer is not treated and controlled. Cancer can occur in almost any body part. The most common sites are the lung, colon and rectum, breast, prostate, uterus, and urinary tract. Cancer is the second leading cause of death in the United States. It occurs in people of all ages.

The exact causes of cancer are unknown. However, certain factors contribute to its development. They include:

- A family history of cancer
- Exposure to radiation (including the sun)
- Exposure to certain chemicals
- Smoking
- Alcohol
- High-fat, high-calorie diet
- Food additives
- Viruses
- Hormones

BOX 30-1

SEVEN WARNING SIGNS OF CANCER

- **C**hange in bowel or bladder habits
- **A** sore that does not heal
- **U**nusual bleeding or discharge from a body opening
- **T**hickening or lump in the breast or elsewhere in the body
- **I**ndigestion or difficulty swallowing
- **O**bvious change in a wart or mole
- **N**agging cough or hoarseness

Cancer can be treated and controlled with early detection. The seven warning signs identified by the American Cancer Society (ACS) are listed in Box 30-1.

Treatment depends on the type of tumor, its site and size, and if it has spread. One or a combination of treatments is used. The three major cancer treatments are surgery, radiation therapy, and chemotherapy.

Surgery involves removing malignant tissue. Surgery is done to cure or control cancer. It is also done to relieve pain from advanced cancer. Some surgeries are very disfiguring. The person's self-esteem and body image are affected.

Radiation therapy destroys living cells. X-rays are directed at the tumor. Cancer cells and normal cells are exposed to radiation. Both are destroyed. Radiation therapy is used to cure certain cancers or to control the growth of cancer cells. Pain is relieved or prevented by controlling cell growth. Radiation therapy has side effects. Discomfort, nausea and vomiting, fatigue (tiredness),

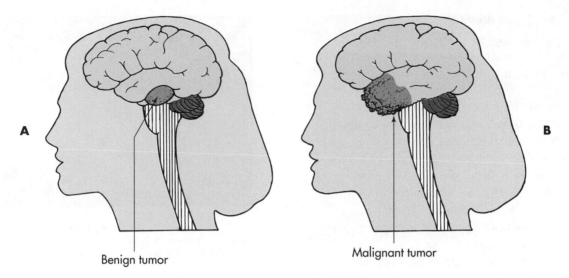

Fig. 30-1 A, *Benign tumors grow within a localized area.* **B,** *Malignant tumors invade other tissues.*

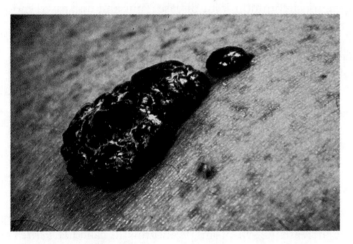

Fig. 30-2 *A malignant tumor on the skin.* (*From Belcher AE:* Cancer nursing, *St Louis, 1992, Mosby.*)

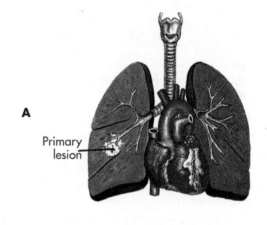

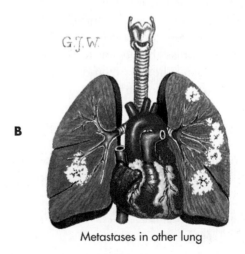

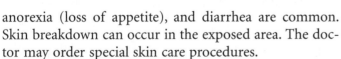

anorexia (loss of appetite), and diarrhea are common. Skin breakdown can occur in the exposed area. The doctor may order special skin care procedures.

Chemotherapy involves drugs that kill cells. Like radiation, chemotherapy affects normal cells and cancer cells. It is used to cure cancer or control the growth rate of cancer cells. Side effects can be severe. They are caused by the destruction of normal cells. The gastrointestinal tract is irritated. Nausea, vomiting, and diarrhea result. **Stomatitis,** an inflammation (*itis*) of the mouth (*stomat*), may develop also. Hair loss (**alopecia**) may occur. Decreased production of blood cells occurs. As a result, the person is at risk for bleeding and infection.

Fig. 30-3 A, *A tumor in the lung.* **B,** *The tumor has metastasized to the other lung.* (*From Belcher AE:* Cancer nursing, *St Louis, 1992, Mosby*).

CHILDREN

focus on

Leukemia is the most common type of cancer in children. Leukemia means an increased number of white blood cells *(leuk)* in the blood *(emia)*. According to the ACS, other common sites are the bones, lymph nodes, brain, nervous system, and kidneys. The ACS has identified the following warning signs of cancer in children:

- An unusual mass or swelling
- Unexplained paleness and loss of energy
- Sudden tendency to bruise
- Persistent, localized pain or limping
- Prolonged, unexplained fever or illness
- Frequent headaches, often with vomiting
- Sudden eye or vision changes
- Excessive, rapid weight loss

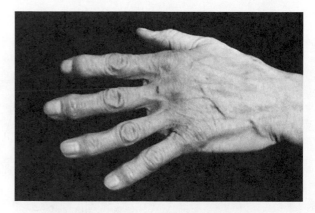

Fig. 30-4 *Heberden's nodes occur in the finger joints. (From Lewis SM, Collier IC, Heitkemper MM:* Medical-surgical nursing: assessment and management of clinical problems, *ed 4, St Louis, 1996, Mosby.)*

Persons with cancer have many needs. They include:
- Pain relief or control
- Adequate rest and exercise
- Fluids and nutrition
- Preventing skin breakdown
- Preventing bowel elimination problems (constipation occurs from pain medications; diarrhea occurs from chemotherapy)
- Dealing with the side effects of radiation therapy and chemotherapy
- Psychological and social needs

The person's psychological and social needs are great. Anger, fear, and depression are common. Disfigurement from surgery may cause the person to feel unwhole, unattractive, or unclean. The person and family need much emotional support. Talk to the person. Do not avoid the person because you are uncomfortable. Use touch to communicate that you care. Listen to the person. Often the person needs to talk and have someone listen. Being there when needed is important. You may not have to say anything. Just be there to listen. (See Focus on Children.)

MUSCULOSKELETAL DISORDERS

Musculoskeletal disorders affect the ability to move about. Some are caused by injury. Others result from aging.

Arthritis

Arthritis means joint *(arth)* inflammation *(itis)*. It is the most common joint disease. Pain and decreased mobility occur in the affected joints. There are two basic types of arthritis.

Osteoarthritis (degenerative joint disease)

This type of arthritis occurs with aging. Joint injury and obesity are other causes. The hips, knees, and spine commonly are affected. These joints bear the body's weight. Joints in the fingers and thumbs also can be affected. Symptoms are joint stiffness and pain. Joint stiffness occurs with rest and lack of motion. Pain occurs with weight-bearing and joint motion. Severe pain can interfere with rest and sleep. Cold weather and dampness seem to increase the symptoms. Bony growths called *Heberden's nodes* (Fig. 30-4) are common in the fingers.

Osteoarthritis has no cure. Treatment involves relieving pain and stiffness. Doctors often order aspirin for pain. Local heat or local cold applications may be ordered. For obese persons, weight loss is stressed. A low-fat, low-calorie diet often is ordered. When the condition is advanced, the person may need a cane or walker. Assistance with daily activities is given as needed. Sometimes joint replacement surgery is necessary (see p. 705).

Rheumatoid arthritis

Rheumatoid arthritis (RA) is a chronic disease. It occurs at any age and is more common in women. Connective tissue throughout the body is affected. The disease affects the heart, lungs, eyes, kidneys, and skin. However, mainly the joints are affected. Smaller joints in the fingers, hands, and feet are affected first (Fig. 30-5). Eventually, larger joints are involved (wrists, elbows, and shoulders;

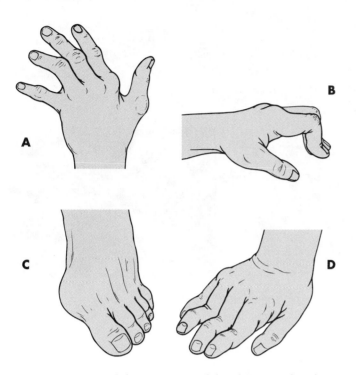

Fig. 30-5 *Finger deformities caused by rheumatoid arthritis.* *(From Lewis SM, Collier IC, Heitkemper MM:* Medical-surgical nursing: assessment and management of clinical problems, *ed 4, St Louis, 1996, Mosby.)*

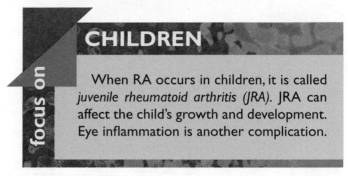

ankles, knees, and hips). Joint inflammation usually occurs on both sides of the body. For example, if the right wrist is involved, so is the left wrist.

Severe inflammation causes very painful and swollen joints. The person restricts movement with severe pain. As the disease progresses, more and more joints become involved. Changes in other organs eventually occur.

Signs and symptoms of RA include:
- Pain, redness, warmth, and swelling in the joint area
- Joint stiffness upon awakening and after inactivity
- Limitation of joint motion
- Fever
- Fatigue
- Loss of appetite
- Weight loss
- Muscle aches

Treatment goals are to maintain joint motion, control pain, and prevent deformities. Rest is balanced with exercise. Bedrest is needed if several joints are involved and when fever is present. Turning and repositioning are done every 2 hours. Good body alignment is essential. Positioning to prevent contractures and deformities promotes comfort. Bed boards, a bed cradle, trochanter rolls, and pillows are used for alignment and positioning. Adequate sleep—8 to 10 hours—is needed each night. Morning and afternoon rest periods also are necessary.

Range-of-motion exercises are done. Walking aids may be needed. Splints may be applied to the affected body parts. Safety measures to prevent falls are practiced.

The doctor orders drugs for pain. Local heat or local cold applications may be ordered. Back massages are relaxing. Joint replacement surgery may be indicated.

Emotional support and reassurance are needed. The disease is chronic. Death from other organ involvement is always possible. A good attitude is important. Being active is important. The more that persons can do for themselves, the better off they are. A person may need someone to talk to. You must be a good listener when the person needs to talk. (See Focus on Children.)

Total joint replacement

Arthroplasty is the surgical replacement *(plasty)* of a joint *(arthro)*. Ankle, knee, hip, shoulder, wrist, finger, and toe joints can be replaced. The diseased joint is removed and replaced with a prosthesis (Fig. 30-6, p. 706). The surgery relieves pain and restores joint motion.

Osteoporosis

Osteoporosis is a bone *(osteo)* disorder in which the bone becomes porous and brittle *(porosis)*. Bones are fragile and break easily. Bones of the spine, hips, and wrists are affected most often. Osteoporosis is common in older persons and in women after menopause. The ovaries do not produce the hormone *estrogen* after menopause. The lack of estrogen results in bone changes. Lack of dietary calcium is also a major cause of osteoporosis. Smoking, high alcohol intake, and lack of exercise also are risk factors. Bedrest and immobility are other causes because they do not allow for proper bone use. For bone to form properly, it must bear weight. If not, calcium is absorbed and the bone becomes porous and brittle.

Signs and symptoms of osteoporosis include low back pain, gradual loss of height, and stooped posture. Fractures are a major threat. Sometimes bones are so brittle that the slightest stress can cause a fracture. Turning in bed or getting up from a chair can cause a fracture. Fractures are a great risk if the person falls or has an accident.

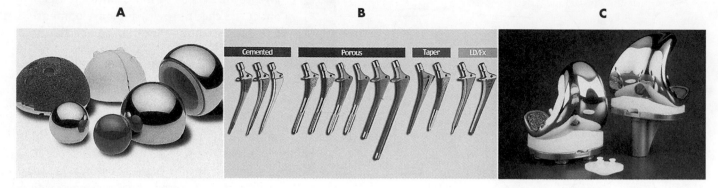

Fig. 30-6 A, *Hip replacement prosthesis cups.* **B,** *Hip replacement prosthesis stems.* **C,** *Knee replacement prosthesis.* (*Courtesy Zimmer, A Bristol-Myers Squibb Company, Warsaw, Indiana.*)

Prevention is important. Calcium, estrogen replacement therapy, and exercise are key. The diet must contain enough calcium. Often doctors order calcium and vitamin supplements. Estrogen is often ordered for women after menopause. Exercise that involves weight bearing is best. Walking, jogging, dancing, and stair climbing are examples. Good posture is also important. Some people wear a back brace or corset or need walking aids. Protect the person from falls and accidents (see Chapter 10). Always turn and reposition the person gently.

Fractures

A **fracture** is a broken bone. Tissues around the fracture (muscles, blood vessels, nerves, and tendons) are usually injured. Fractures are open or closed (Fig. 30-7). A **closed fracture (simple fracture)** means the bone is broken but the skin is intact. An **open fracture (compound fracture)** means the broken bone has come through the skin.

Fractures are caused by falls and accidents. Bone tumors, metastatic cancer, and osteoporosis are other causes. Signs and symptoms of a fracture are:

- Pain
- Swelling
- Limited movement and loss of function
- Bruising and color changes in the skin at the fracture site
- Bleeding (internal or external)

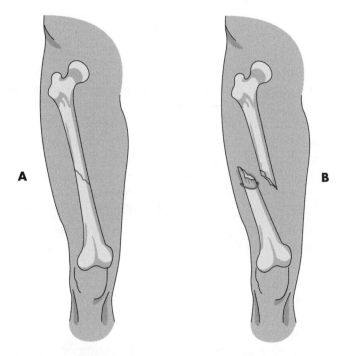

Fig. 30-7 A, *Closed fracture.* **B,** *Open fracture.* (*From Beare PG, Myers, JL:* Principles and practice of adult health nursing, *ed 3, St Louis, 1998, Mosby.*)

The bone has to heal. The bone ends are brought into normal position. This is called *reduction. Closed reduction* involves moving the bone back into place. The skin is not opened. *Open reduction* involves surgery. The bone is exposed and brought back into alignment. Nails, rods, pins,

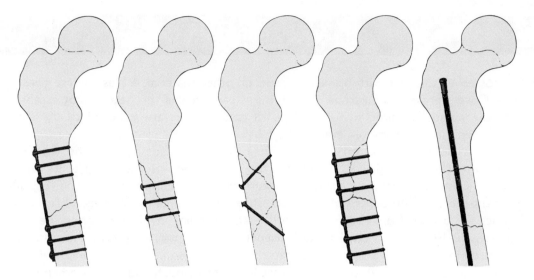

Fig. 30-8 *Devices used to reduce a fracture.* *(From Beare PG, Myers, JL:* Principles and practice of adult health nursing, *ed 3, St Louis, 1998, Mosby.)*

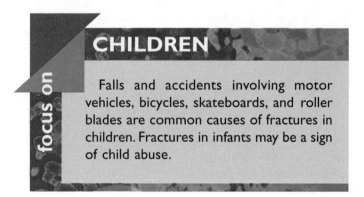

CHILDREN

focus on

Falls and accidents involving motor vehicles, bicycles, skateboards, and roller blades are common causes of fractures in children. Fractures in infants may be a sign of child abuse.

screws, plates, or wires are used to keep the bone in place (Fig. 30-8). After reduction, the fracture is immobilized. That is, movement of the bone ends is prevented. This is done with a cast or traction. (See Focus on Children.)

Cast care

Casts are made of plaster of paris, plastic, or fiberglass. The cast covers all or part of an extremity (Fig. 30-9). Before the doctor applies a cast, the extremity is covered with stockinette. This protects the skin. Casting material comes in rolls. The rolls are moistened and wrapped around the part. Plastic and fiberglass casts dry quickly. A plaster of paris cast needs 24 to 48 hours to dry. It is odorless, white, and shiny when dry. When wet, it is gray and cool and has a musty smell. The rules listed in Box 30-2 on p. 708 are for cast care.

Text continued on p. 710

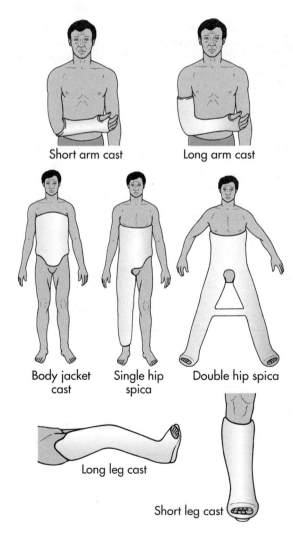

Short arm cast

Long arm cast

Body jacket cast

Single hip spica

Double hip spica

Long leg cast

Short leg cast

Fig. 30-9 *Common casts.* *(From Lewis SM, Collier IC, Heitkemper MM:* Medical-surgical nursing: assessment and management of clinical problems, *ed 4, St Louis, 1996, Mosby.)*

BOX 30-2

RULES FOR CAST CARE

- Do not cover the cast with blankets, plastic, or other material. A plaster cast gives off heat as it dries. Covers prevent the escape of heat. Burns can occur if the heat cannot escape.
- Turn the person as directed by the RN. All cast surfaces are exposed to the air at one time or another. Turning promotes even drying.
- Do not place a wet cast on a hard surface. A hard surface flattens the cast. The cast must maintain its shape. Use pillows to support the entire length of the cast (Fig. 30-10).
- Support a wet cast with your palms when turning and positioning the person (Fig. 30-11). Fingers can dent the cast. The dents can cause pressure areas that can lead to skin breakdown.
- Protect the person from rough edges of the cast. Petaling involves covering the cast edges with tape (Fig. 30-12, p. 710). If stockinette is used, the doctor pulls it up over the cast. The stockinette is secured in place with a roll of cast material.
- Keep a plaster cast dry. A wet plaster cast loses its shape. It must be protected from moisture from the perineal area. The RN may apply a waterproof material around the perineal area once the cast is dry.
- Do not let the person insert anything into the cast. Itching often occurs under the cast and causes an intense desire to scratch. Items used for scratching (pencils, coat hangers, knitting needles, back scratchers) can open the skin. An infection can develop. Items used for scratching can also wrinkle the stockinette. The object can be lost in the cast. Both can cause pressure and lead to skin breakdown.
- Elevate a casted arm or leg on pillows. This reduces swelling.
- Have enough help when turning and repositioning the person. Plaster casts are heavy and awkward. Balance is lost easily.
- Position the person as directed by the RN.
- Report these signs and symptoms immediately:
  - Pain—warns of a pressure ulcer, poor circulation, or nerve damage
  - Swelling and a tight cast—a sign of reduced blood flow to the part
  - Pale skin—a sign of reduced blood flow to the part
  - Cyanosis—a sign of reduced blood flow to the part
  - Odor—a sign of infection
  - Inability to move the fingers or toes—a sign of pressure on a nerve
  - Numbness—a sign of pressure on a nerve or reduced blood flow to the part
  - Temperature changes—cool skin means poor circulation; hot skin means inflammation
  - Drainage on or under the cast—a sign of infection under the cast
  - Chills, fever, nausea, and vomiting—may signal an infection under the cast

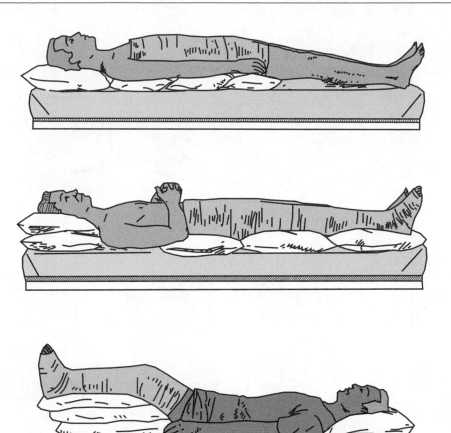

Fig. 30-10 *Pillows support the entire length of the wet cast.* *(From Harkness GH, Dincher JR: Medical-surgical nursing: total patient care, ed 9, St Louis, 1996, Mosby.)*

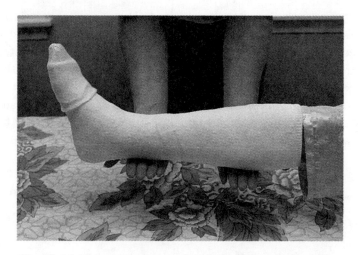

Fig. 30-11 *The cast is supported with the palms during lifting.*

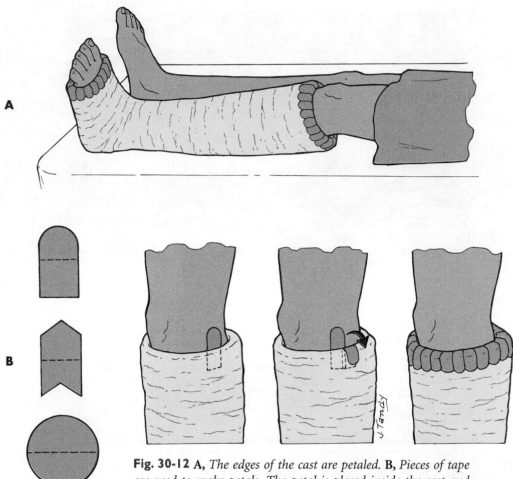

Fig. 30-12 A, *The edges of the cast are petaled.* **B,** *Pieces of tape are used to make petals. The petal is placed inside the cast and then brought over the edge.*

Traction

Traction is used to reduce and immobilize fractures. A steady pull from two directions keeps the fractured bone in place. Traction is used also for muscle spasms, to correct or prevent deformities, and for other musculoskeletal injuries. Weights, ropes, and pulleys are used (Fig. 30-13). Traction can be applied to the neck, arms, legs, or pelvis.

A doctor applies traction to the skin or to the bone. With *skin traction,* bandages and strips of material are applied to the skin. Weights are attached to the material or bandage (see Fig. 30-13). Traction applied directly to the bone is called *skeletal traction.* It is used for some arm and leg fractures. A pin, nail, or wire is inserted through the bone (Fig. 30-14). For traction to the cervical spine, tongs are applied to the skull (Fig. 30-15). Weights are attached to the device.

The rules listed in Box 30-3 on p. 712 apply when caring for a person in traction.

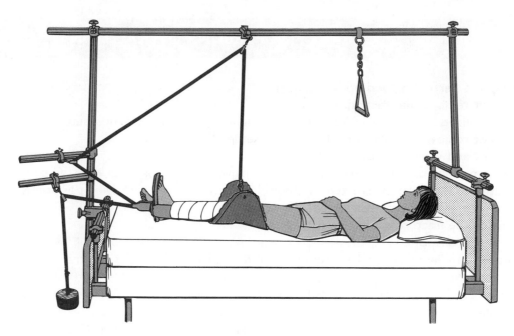

Fig. 30-13 *Traction setup. Note the weights, pulleys, and ropes.* *(From Phipps WJ, Cassmeyer VL, Sands JK, Lehman MK: Medical-surgical nursing: concepts and clinical practice, ed 5, St Louis, 1995, Mosby.)*

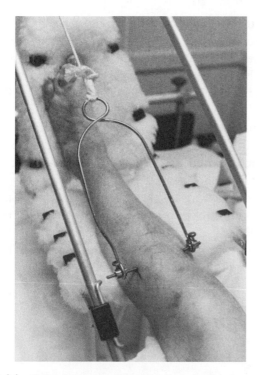

Fig. 30-14 *Skeletal traction is attached to the bone.* *(From Phipps WJ, Cassmeyer VL, Sands JK, Lehman MK: Medical-surgical nursing: concepts and clinical practice, ed 5, St Louis, 1995, Mosby.)*

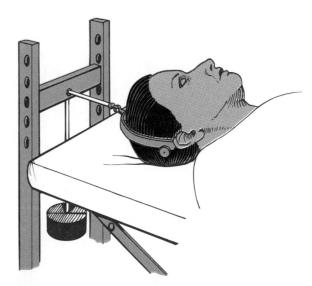

Fig. 30-15 Tongs are inserted into the skull for traction to the cervical spine. *(From Phipps WJ, Cassmeyer VL, Sands JK, Lehman MK: Medical-surgical nursing: concepts and clinical practice, ed 5, St Louis, 1995, Mosby.)*

BOX 30-3

CARING FOR PERSONS IN TRACTION

- Keep the person in good body alignment.
- Do not remove the traction.
- Keep weights off the floor. Weights must hang freely from the traction setup (see Fig. 30-13).
- Do not remove weights from the traction setup.
- Do not add weights to the traction setup.
- Perform range-of-motion exercises for the uninvolved body parts as directed by the RN.
- Position the person as directed by the RN. Usually only the back-lying position is allowed. Slight turning is allowed with some types of traction.
- Provide the fracture pan for elimination.
- Give skin care often.
- Put bottom linens on the bed from the top down. The person uses the trapeze to raise the body off the bed.
- Check pin, nail, wire, or tong sites for redness, drainage, or odors. Report any observations to the RN immediately.
- Observe for the signs and symptoms listed under cast care (see Box 30-2). Report these observations to the RN immediately.

Hip fractures

Fractured hips are common in older persons, especially older women (Fig. 30-16). They are especially serious because healing is slower in older people. The person may have other disorders. These disorders and slow healing may complicate the person's condition and care. The person is also at great risk for postoperative complications. These include pneumonia, atelectasis, urinary tract infections, and thrombi in the leg veins. The person can die from these complications. The person is also at risk for pressure ulcers, constipation, and confusion.

Open reduction is usually required. The fracture is fixed in position with a pin, nail, plate, screw, or prosthesis (Fig. 30-17). The person needs preoperative and postoperative care as described in Chapter 27. The person also requires the care described in Box 30-4 on p. 714. (See Focus on Home Care on p. 715.)

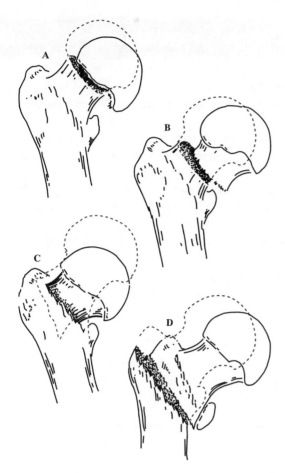

Fig. 30-16 *Hip fractures.* *(From Phipps WJ, Cassmeyer VL, Sands JK, Lehman MK:* Medical-surgical nursing: concepts and clinical practice, *ed 5, St Louis, 1995, Mosby.)*

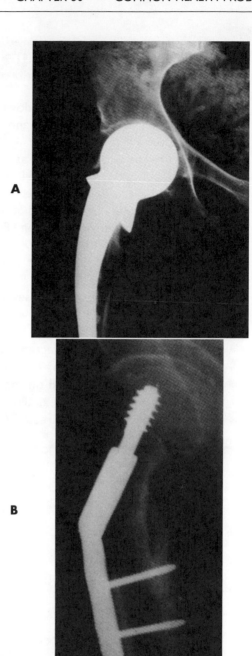

Fig. 30-17 A, *Hip fracture repaired with a prosthesis.* **B,** *Hip fracture repaired with a hip nail.* *(From Thompson JM; et al:* Mosby's Clinical Nursing, *ed 4, 1997.)*

BOX 30-4

CARE OF THE PERSON WITH A HIP FRACTURE

- Give good skin care. Skin breakdown can occur rapidly.
- Encourage incentive spirometry and coughing and deep breathing exercises as directed by the RN. See Chapter 21.
- Turn and reposition the person as directed by the RN. The doctor's orders for turning and positioning depend on the type of fracture and the surgery performed. Usually the person is not positioned on the operative side.
- Keep the operated leg abducted at all times. The leg is abducted when the person is supine, being turned, or in a side-lying position (Fig. 30-18, A). Pillows or abductor splints are used as directed (Fig. 30-18, B).
- Prevent external rotation of the hip (turning outward). Use trochanter rolls or abduction splints as directed.
- Perform range-of-motion exercises as directed (see Chapter 22). Do not exercise the affected leg.
- Provide a straight-backed chair with armrests when the person is to be up. The person needs a high, firm seat. A low, soft chair is not used.
- Place the chair on the unaffected side.
- Assist the RN in transferring the person from the bed to the chair as directed.
- Do not let the person stand on the operated leg unless allowed by the doctor.
- Support and elevate the leg as directed when the person is in the chair.
- Apply elastic stockings as directed (see Chapter 27).

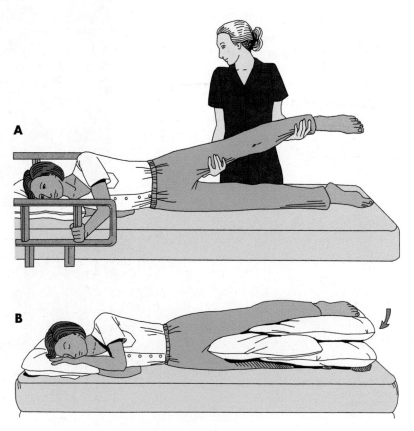

Fig. 30-18 A, *The hip is abducted when the person is turned.* **B,** *Pillows are used to maintain the hip in abduction.* (*From Lewis SM, Collier IC, Heitkemper MM:* Medical-surgical nursing: assessment and management of clinical problems, *ed 4, St Louis, 1996, Mosby.*)

HOME CARE

The prosthesis can dislocate (move out of place) with adduction, internal rotation (turning inward), and severe hip flexion. Lying on the affected side, sitting in a low seat, sitting with the legs crossed, bending from the waist, and putting on shoes and socks or stockings involve these movements. Therefore such movements are avoided for 6 weeks after surgery. An occupational therapist helps the person learn to do activities of daily living. Assistive devices are used for dressing (see Chapter 33). The person needs a raised toilet seat for elimination and a shower chair for bathing. The person uses a pillow or abductor splint between the legs when in bed. Muscle-strengthening exercises also are needed. A physical therapist helps the person with the exercises. A walker usually is needed for ambulation.

LONG-TERM CARE

Older persons often require rehabilitation after a hip fracture. If home care is not possible, the person requires long-term care. Unless complications develop, the person usually returns home after successful rehabilitation. As in home care, adduction, internal rotation, and severe hip flexion are avoided.

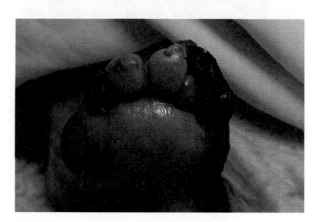

Fig. 30-19 *Gangrene.*

Loss of a Limb

An **amputation** is the removal of all or part of an extremity. Usually the part is removed surgically. Traumatic amputations can occur from vehicle and workplace accidents. Severe injuries, bone tumors, severe infections, and circulatory disorders may require amputations.

Gangrene is a condition in which there is death of tissue. It can result from infection, injuries, and circulatory disorders. These conditions interfere with blood supply to the tissues. The tissues do not get enough oxygen and nutrients. Poisonous substances and waste products build up in the affected tissues. Tissue death results. The tissue becomes black, cold, and shriveled (Fig. 30-19) and eventually falls off. If untreated, gangrene spreads through the body and causes death.

All or part of an extremity may be amputated. Fingers, the hand, forearm, or entire arm may be removed. Toes, the foot, lower leg, upper and lower leg, or entire leg may be amputated.

Much support is needed. A major psychological adjustment is necessary. The person's life is affected by the amputation. Appearance, activities of daily living, moving about, and work are some areas affected.

At some point most persons with amputations are fitted with a prosthesis. A prosthesis is an artificial replacement for a missing body part (Fig. 30-20, p. 716). The stump is conditioned so the prosthesis fits. Stump conditioning involves shrinking and shaping the stump into a cone shape. An elastic stocking or bandage is used to shrink and shape the stump (Fig. 30-21, p. 716). Exercises are ordered to strengthen the other limbs. Physical therapists help the person use the prosthesis. Occupational therapy is necessary if the stump or prosthesis is used for activities of daily living.

The person may feel that the limb is still there or may complain of pain in the amputated part. This is called *phantom limb pain.* The exact cause is unknown. However, it is a normal reaction. The sensation may occur only for a short time after surgery. However, some persons have phantom limb pain for many years.

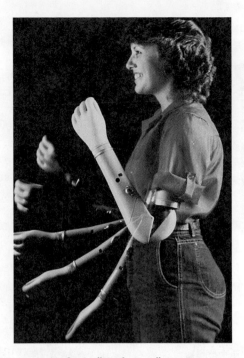

Fig. 30-20 *Arm prosthesis, "Utah Arm." (Courtesy Motion Control, Inc, Subsidiary of Fillauer, Salt Lake City, Utah.)*

NERVOUS SYSTEM DISORDERS

Nervous system disorders can affect mental and physical functions. They can affect the ability to speak, understand, feel, see, hear, touch, think, control bowels and bladder, and move.

Stroke

The American Heart Association (AHA) defines stroke as a cardiovascular disease affecting the blood vessels that supply blood to the brain. Blood supply to a part of the brain is suddenly interrupted. Brain cells in the area affected do not get oxygen and nutrients. Brain damage occurs. Functions controlled by that part of the brain are lost or impaired. A ruptured blood vessel is one cause of stroke. This causes hemorrhage (excessive bleeding) into the brain. Blood clots are another cause. A blood clot obstructs blood flow to the brain. A stroke is also called a *cerebrovascular accident (CVA)* or *brain attack.*

Stroke is the third leading cause of death in the United States. It is the leading cause of disability in adults. Stroke is a medical emergency. The person needs immediate medical attention. (See Chapter 35 for emergency care.)

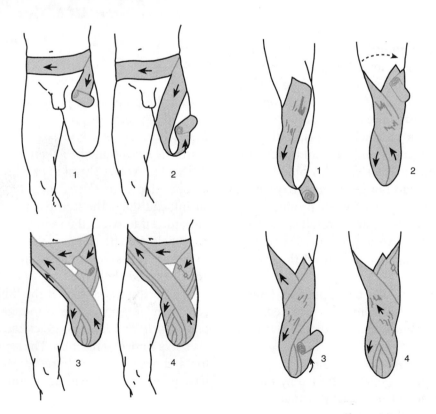

Fig. 30-21 *A midthigh amputation is bandaged to shrink and shape the stump. (From Phipps WJ, Cassmeyer VL, Sands JK, Lehman MK:* Medical-surgical nursing: concepts and clinical practice, *ed 5, St Louis, 1995, Mosby.)*

WARNING SIGNS OF STROKE (CVA, BRAIN ATTACK)

- Sudden weakness or numbness of the face, arm, or leg on one side of the body
- Sudden dimness or loss of vision, particularly in one eye
- Loss of speech, or trouble talking or understanding speech
- Sudden, severe headaches with no known cause
- Unexplained dizziness, unsteadiness, or sudden falls (especially with any of the other signs)

From American Heart Association, 1997.

Box 30-5 lists the warning signs of stroke. Sometimes the warning signs last a few minutes. This is called a *transient ischemic attack (TIA)*. (*Transient* means temporary or short term. *Ischemic* means to hold back *[ischein]* blood *[hemic]*.) Blood supply to the brain is interrupted for a short time. Sometimes a TIA occurs before a stroke. The person having a TIA needs medical attention. The TIA warns of a stroke.

Stroke is more common among persons over 65 years of age. However, it does occur in young and middle-age adults. A common cause of stroke is hypertension (high blood pressure). Other risk factors include diabetes, family history of stroke, hardening of the arteries, smoking, heart disease, and stress. Lack of exercise and high alcohol intake also are risk factors. So is race. Black men and women are at greater risk than white persons.

Signs and symptoms vary. Warning signs may occur (see Box 30-5). Dizziness, ringing in the ears, headache, nausea and vomiting, and memory loss also can occur. The stroke may occur suddenly. Unconsciousness, noisy breathing, high blood pressure, slow pulse, redness of the face, seizures, and paralysis on one side of the body (**hemiplegia**) may occur. The person may lose bowel and bladder control and the ability to speak. **Aphasia** is the inability *(a)* to speak *(phasia)*.

If the person survives, some brain damage is likely. The functions lost depend on the area of brain damage (Fig. 30-22). The effects of a stroke include:
- Loss of hand, arm, leg, or body control
- Loss of face control
- Hemiplegia

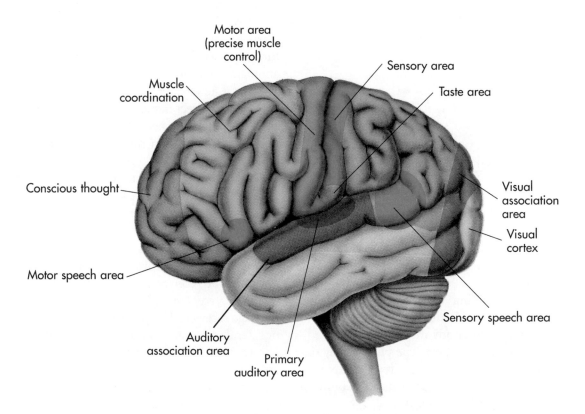

Fig. 30-22 *Functions lost from a stroke depend on the area of brain damage.* (*Modified from Thibodeau GA, Patton KT:* The human body in health & disease, *ed 2, St Louis, 1997, Mosby.*)

BOX 30-6

CARE OF THE PERSON WITH A STROKE (CVA, BRAIN ATTACK)

- Use the lateral position to prevent aspiration.
- Encourage coughing and deep breathing.
- Keep the bed in semi-Fowler's position.
- Turn and reposition the person at least every 2 hours.
- Meet food and fluid needs.
- Elastic stockings are ordered to prevent thrombi (blood clots) in the legs.
- Perform range-of-motion exercises to prevent contractures.
- A catheter may be inserted or a bladder training program started.
- A bowel training program may be necessary.
- Practice safety precautions. Check with the RN about the use of bed rails.
- Assist with self-care activities. Encourage the person to do as much as possible.
- Establish communication methods. Use Magic Slates, pencil and paper, a picture board, or other methods. Limit questions to those that have "yes" or "no" answers. Speak slowly. Allow the person time to respond. (See Chapter 6.)
- Give good skin care to prevent pressure ulcers.
- Speech therapy, physical therapy, and occupational therapy are ordered. Assistive devices are used as necessary (see Chapter 33).
- Give emotional support and encouragement. Give praise for even the slightest accomplishment.

- Changing emotions (the person can cry easily, sometimes for no reason)
- Difficulty swallowing (**dysphagia** means difficulty [dys] swallowing [phagia])
- Dimmed vision
- Aphasia
- Slow or slurred speech
- Changes in perception (sight, touch, movement, thought)
- Impaired memory
- Urinary frequency, urgency, or incontinence
- Depression
- Frustration

These effects change the person's behavior. The person may forget about or ignore the weaker side. This is from loss of movement and feeling on that side. If vision is affected, the person may not see that side of the body. The person may not recognize or know how to use familiar items. Activities of daily living and other tasks are difficult. The person may forget what to do and how to do it. If the person does know, the body may not respond.

Rehabilitation starts immediately. The person may depend partially or totally on others for care. The RN uses the nursing process to meet the person's needs. Common care measures are listed in Box 30-6.

Aphasia

There are two basic types of aphasia. **Expressive aphasia** involves difficulty expressing or sending out thoughts. There are problems with speaking, spelling, counting, gesturing, or writing. The person thinks one thing but says another. For example, the person thinks about food but asks for a newspaper. People are called the wrong names even when correct names are known. Or the person thinks clearly but cannot speak. Some produce only sounds and no words. The person may cry or swear for no apparent reason.

Receptive aphasia relates to receiving information. The person has trouble understanding what is said or read. Everyday objects are not recognized. The person may not know how to use a fork, toilet, water glass, TV, telephone, or other items. The person may not recognize people.

Remember, for communication to occur, the message sent must be received and correctly interpreted. The person with *receptive* aphasia simply cannot interpret the message received. The person with *expressive* aphasia cannot send messages. Some people have both expressive and receptive aphasia. This is called **expressive-receptive aphasia.**

HOME CARE

Many stroke survivors return home. A partner or family members assist with the person's care. Home nursing services are often needed. The care measures in Box 30-6 continue in the home. The RN and therapists also recommend changes in the home setting that will help the person function.

LONG-TERM CARE

Some stroke survivors need long-term care. Some persons need rehabilitation and are able to return home. Long-term care often is permanent for survivors who totally depend on others for care. Many measures listed in Box 30-6 are part of the person's care.

Persons with aphasia have many emotional needs. Frustration, depression, and anger are common. Communication is important for functioning and relationships with others. Remember, the person wants to communicate but cannot. You need to be patient and kind. (See Focus on Home Care and Focus on Long-Term Care.)

Parkinson's Disease

Parkinson's disease is a slow, progressive disorder with no cure. Degeneration of a part of the brain occurs. The disease is usually seen in persons over 50 years of age. Signs and symptoms are a masklike expression, tremors, pill-rolling movements of the fingers, a shuffling gait, stooped posture, impaired balance, stiff muscles (rigidity), slow movements, and drooling. Difficulty swallowing and chewing, bowel and bladder problems, sleep problems, and depression can occur. Some patients have memory loss, slow thinking, and emotional changes (fear and insecurity). Speech changes include slurred, monotone, and soft speech. Some patients talk too fast or repeat what they said.

The doctor orders drugs that are specific for Parkinson's disease. Exercise and physical therapy are ordered. These help the person improve strength, posture, balance, and mobility. The person may need help with eating and other self-care activities. Measures to promote normal elimination are practiced. Safety practices are followed to prevent injury. Remember, mental function may not be affected. Talk to and treat the person as an adult.

Multiple Sclerosis

Multiple sclerosis (MS) is a progressive disease. The myelin sheath (which covers the nerves), the spinal cord, and the white matter in the brain are destroyed. Nerve impulses are not sent to and from the brain in a normal manner. Functions are impaired or lost.

Symptoms start between the ages of 20 and 40. Women are affected more than men. The onset is gradual. Blurred or double vision occurs first. Muscle weakness and difficulty with balance and walking occur. Tremors, numbness and tingling, loss of feeling, speech impairment, dizziness, and poor coordination eventually occur. So do urinary incontinence, anal incontinence or constipation, and behavior changes. The person's condition worsens over many years. Blindness, contractures, paralysis of all extremities (quadriplegia), loss of bowel and bladder control, and respiratory muscle weakness are among the person's many problems. The person becomes totally dependent on others for care. Anger and depression are common.

There is no known cure. Persons are kept active as long as possible. They need to do as much for themselves as possible. Nursing care depends on the person's needs and condition. Skin care, hygiene, and range-of-motion exercises are important. Measures are taken to prevent injury and to promote bowel and bladder elimination. Turning, positioning, coughing, and deep breathing also are important. Complications from bed rest are prevented. (See Focus on Home Care on p. 720.)

Head Injuries

Injuries can occur to the scalp, skull, and brain tissue. Some injuries are minor. They cause only temporary loss of consciousness. Others are more serious. Brain tissue is bruised or torn. Bleeding can occur in the brain or surrounding structures. Permanent brain damage or death may result.

focus on

HOME CARE

At first the person may need help with housekeeping tasks to avoid fatigue. As mobility decreases, the person depends more on others. Eventually the person becomes bedridden and depends on others for basic needs. The nursing care plan reflects the person's changing needs. Occupational and physical therapists often are involved in the person's care. The National Multiple Sclerosis Society can provide resources for the person and family.

CHILDREN

Birth injuries are a major cause of head trauma in newborns. As a child grows older, motor vehicle accidents, biking accidents, and falls are the major causes of brain damage. According to the National SAFE KIDS Campaign, falling is the greatest home danger for infants and toddlers. Falling down stairs and falling from windows are common accidents. See Chapter 10 for safety practices for infants and children and for how to prevent falls.

Head injuries are caused by falls, vehicle accidents, workplace accidents, and sports injuries. Other body parts often are injured. Spinal cord injuries are likely. If the person survives a severe head injury, some permanent damage is likely. Paralysis, mental retardation, personality changes, speech problems, breathing difficulties, and loss of bowel and bladder control may be permanent. Rehabilitation is required. Nursing care depends on the person's needs and remaining abilities. (See Focus on Children.)

Spinal Cord Injuries

Spinal cord injuries can permanently damage the nervous system. Common causes are stab or bullet wounds, motor vehicle accidents, workplace accidents, falls, or sports injuries. Cervical traction often is necessary (see Fig. 30-15). The person in cervical traction is placed on a Stryker frame or rotation bed. These devices keep the spine straight while the person is turned.

The type of damage depends on the level of injury. The higher the level of injury, the greater the loss of function (Fig. 30-23). With lumbar injuries, muscle function in the legs is lost. Injuries at the thoracic level cause loss of muscle function below the chest. Persons with injuries at the lumbar or thoracic levels are paraplegics. **Paraplegia** is paralysis of the legs. Cervical injuries cause loss of function to the arms, chest, and all muscles below the chest. Persons with these injuries are quadriplegics. **Quadriplegia** is paralysis of the arms, legs, and trunk.

If the person survives, rehabilitation is necessary. The person's needs and the rehabilitation program depend on the functions lost and remaining abilities. Attention is given to emotional needs. These persons have severe emotional reactions to paralysis and the loss of function. Paralyzed persons generally need the care listed in Box 30-7 on p. 721. (See Focus on Long-Term Care and Focus on Home Care on p. 721.)

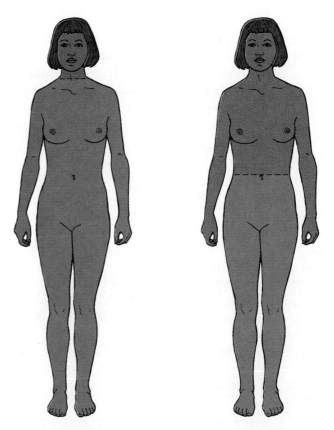

Fig. 30-23 *The shaded areas indicate the areas of paralysis.*

focus on LONG-TERM CARE

Persons with spinal cord injuries often enter special rehabilitation centers. There they learn to function at their highest possible level. The person learns to use self-help and assistive devices and other special equipment. The person needs the care listed in Box 30-7.

focus on HOME CARE

Rehabilitation often continues when the person goes home. The RN, physical therapist, and occupational therapist suggest changes in the home to meet the person's needs. Ramps for wheelchair use usually are needed. So are changes in the kitchen, bathroom, and bedroom. For example, the refrigerator door may need to open from the other side. Kitchen shelves may need rearranging. A raised toilet seat, safety rails by the toilet and tub, bathtub seats, and tub transfer benches may help the person. The person may need a hospital bed, overbed trapeze, and a bedside commode. Furniture in all rooms may need rearranging to allow wheelchair access.

The person may need assistance with activities of daily living and with housekeeping tasks. The RN instructs you in the person's care and reviews the nursing care plan with you.

BOX 30-7 — CARE OF PERSONS WITH PARALYSIS

- Prevent falls. Keep bed rails up, the bed in low position, and the call bell within reach. Check the person often if he or she cannot use the call bell.
- Prevent burns. Check bath water, heat applications, and food for the proper temperature.
- Turn and reposition the person at least every 2 hours.
- Give skin care and other measures to prevent pressure ulcers.
- Maintain good body alignment at all times. Use pillows, trochanter rolls, foot boards, and other devices as needed.
- Carry out bowel and bladder training programs.
- Perform range-of-motion exercises to maintain muscle function and prevent contractures. Assist with other exercises as ordered.
- Assist with food and fluids as needed. Provide self-help devices as ordered. Feed the person if necessary.
- Give emotional and psychological support. The person's care may involve psychiatrists or psychologists.
- Physical therapy, occupational therapy, and vocational rehabilitation are ordered. They help the person regain independent functioning to the extent possible.

EAR DISORDERS

The ear is important for hearing and balance. Middle ear infections, Ménière's disease, and hearing loss are presented in this section.

Otitis Media

Otitis media is infection *(itis)* of the middle *(media)* ear *(ot)*. The infection is acute or chronic. Chronic otitis media can damage the tympanic membrane (eardrum) or the ossicles (see Fig. 7-12). The eardrum and ossicles are needed for hearing. Permanent hearing loss can occur from chronic otitis media.

Fluid buildup occurs in the ear. It causes pain and hearing loss. Other signs and symptoms include fever and ringing in the ears (**tinnitus**). Antibiotics usually are ordered by the doctor. (See Focus on Children.)

Ménière's Disease

Ménière's disease involves increased fluid in the inner ear. The increased fluid causes pressure in the middle ear. There are three symptoms. Vertigo is the major symptom. **Vertigo** means dizziness. The person feels whirling and spinning sensations. The person must lie down. Severe dizziness can cause nausea and vomiting. The other main symptoms are ringing in the ears (tinnitus) and hearing loss.

The doctor can order drugs for the person. Sometimes a low-salt diet can decrease the amount of fluid in the ear. Safety is important during vertigo. The person must lie down. Falls are prevented. Bed rails usually are ordered. The head is kept still, and the person avoids turning the head. To talk to the person, stand directly in front of him or her. When movement is necessary, the person moves slowly. Bright or glaring lights are avoided. Assist with ambulation. The person should not walk alone in case vertigo occurs.

Hearing Problems

Hearing losses range from slight hearing impairments to complete deafness. Clear speech, responding to others, safety, and awareness of surroundings all require hearing. Many people deny having difficulty hearing. This is because hearing loss often is associated with aging.

Effects on the person

Infants with hearing impairments often fail to start talking. Lack of attention and failing grades are early signs of poor hearing in children. The obvious signs of hearing impairment in children and adults include:

- Speaking too loudly
- Leaning forward to hear

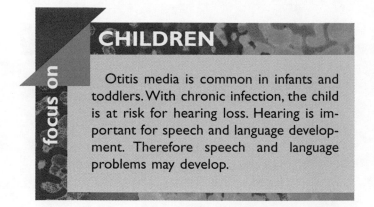

focus on CHILDREN

Otitis media is common in infants and toddlers. With chronic infection, the child is at risk for hearing loss. Hearing is important for speech and language development. Therefore speech and language problems may develop.

- Turning and cupping the better ear toward the speaker
- Answering questions or responding inappropriately
- Asking for words to be repeated

Psychological and social effects are less obvious. People may give wrong answers or responses. Therefore they tend to avoid social situations. This is to avoid embarrassment. However, loneliness, boredom, and feeling left out often result. Only parts of conversations are heard. People with hearing loss may become suspicious. They think they are being talked about or that others are talking softly on purpose. Some control conversations to avoid answering questions. Straining and working to hear can cause fatigue, frustration, and irritability.

Hearing loss may cause speech problems. How you pronounce words and the volume of your voice depend on how you hear yourself. Hearing loss may result in slurred speech and improper pronunciation. Monotone speech and dropping word endings also may occur.

Communicating with the person

Hearing-impaired persons may wear hearing aids or read lips. They also watch facial expressions, gestures, and body language. Some people learn sign language (Figs. 30-24, p. 723 and 30-25, p. 724). Some hearing-impaired people have *hearing* dogs. The dog alerts the person to such things as ringing phones, doorbells, sirens, or oncoming cars. Certain measures are needed when communicating with the person. The measures listed in Box 30-8, p. 724 can help the person hear or speech-read (lip-read).

The person may have speech problems. Understanding what the person is saying can be hard. Do not assume that you understand what the person says. Do not pretend to understand to avoid embarrassing the person. Serious problems can result if you assume or pretend to understand. Follow the guidelines in Box 30-9, p. 725 to communicate with the speech impaired person.

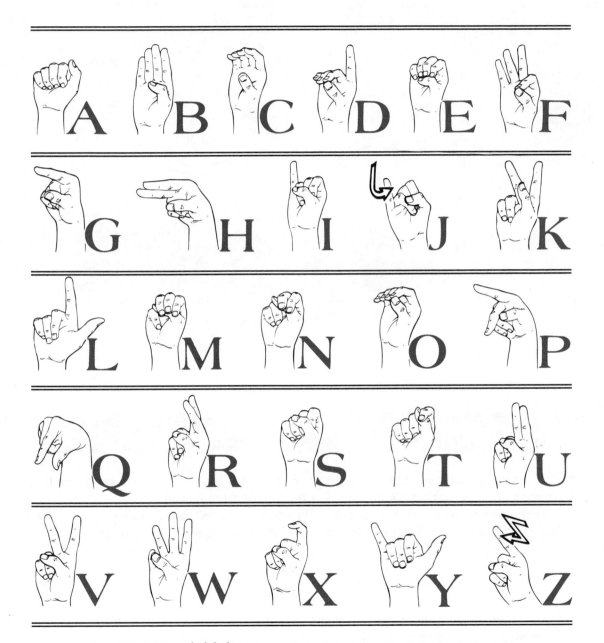

Fig. 30-24 *Manual alphabet. (Courtesy National Association of the Deaf, Silver Springs, Md.)*

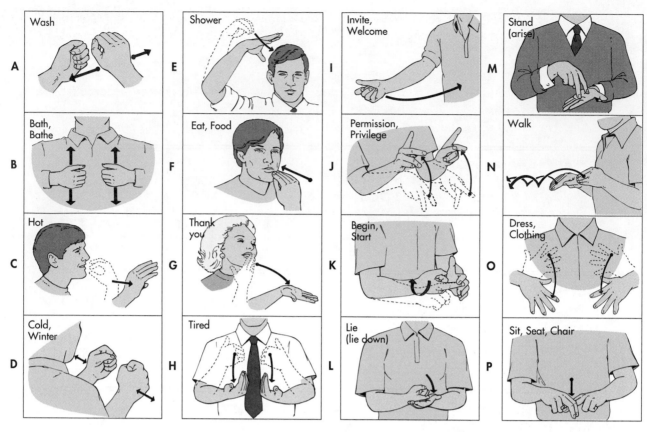

Fig. 30-25 *Sign language.*

BOX 30-8

COMMUNICATING WITH THE HEARING-IMPAIRED PERSON

- Gain attention, and alert the person to your presence. Raise an arm or hand or lightly touch the person's arm. Do not startle or approach the person from behind.
- Face the person directly when speaking. Do not turn or walk away while you are talking.
- Stand or sit in good light. Shadows and glares affect the person's ability to see your face clearly.
- Speak clearly, distinctly, and slowly.
- Speak in a normal tone of voice. Do not shout.
- Do not cover your mouth, smoke, eat, or chew gum while talking. These things affect mouth movements.
- Stand or sit on the side of the better ear.
- State the topic of conversation first.
- Use short sentences and simple words.
- Write out important names and words.
- Say things in a different way if the person does not seem to understand.
- Keep conversations and discussions short to avoid tiring the person.
- Repeat and rephrase statements as needed.
- Be alert to the messages sent by your facial expressions, gestures, and body language.
- Reduce or eliminate background noises.

COMMUNICATING WITH THE SPEECH-IMPAIRED PERSON

- Listen, and give the person your full attention.
- Ask the person questions to which you know the answer. This helps you to become familiar with the person's speech.
- Determine the subject being discussed. This helps you to understand main points.
- Ask the person to repeat or rephrase statements if necessary.
- Repeat what the person has said. Ask if you have understood correctly.
- Ask the person to write down key words or the message.
- Watch the person's lip movements.
- Watch facial expressions, gestures, and body language for clues about what is being said.

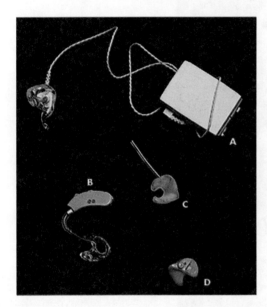

Fig. 30-26 *Types of hearing aids.* **A,** *Older aid with a battery pack worn on the body and a wire connected to the ear mold.* **B,** *Behind-the-ear battery with ear mold.* **C,** *Small ear canal mold with battery.* **D,** *Newer, smaller mold worn in the ear. (Courtesy OSF, St Joseph Medical Center, Bloomington, Ill.)*

Hearing aids

A *hearing aid* makes sounds louder (Fig. 30-26). It does not correct or cure the hearing problem. Hearing ability does not improve. However, the person hears better because the hearing aid makes sounds louder. Both background noise and speech are louder. The measures for communicating with hearing-impaired persons apply to those with hearing aids.

Hearing aids operate on batteries. There is an *on* and *off* switch. Sometimes hearing aids do not seem to work properly. Often only simple measures are needed to get them to work:

- Check if the hearing aid is *on*.
- Check the battery position.
- Insert a new battery if needed.
- Clean the earmold if necessary.

There are many different types of hearing aids. They are expensive. They are handled carefully and cared for properly. *Check with the RN before washing or cleaning a hearing aid. Also follow the manufacturer's instructions for proper care and use.* Only the earmold is washed. It is usually washed daily with soap and water. The battery is removed at night. When not in use, the hearing aid is turned off.

EYE DISORDERS

Vision problems occur at all ages. Problems range from very mild vision loss to complete blindness. Vision loss is sudden or gradual in onset. One or both eyes are affected. Surgery, eyeglasses, or contact lenses are often necessary.

Glaucoma

With glaucoma, fluid pressure within the eye is increased. This damages the optic nerve. The result is vision loss with eventual blindness. The disease is gradual or sudden in onset. Signs and symptoms include tunnel vision (Fig. 30-27, p. 726), blurred vision, and halos around lights. Eye discomfort and aching also occur. With sudden onset, the person also has severe eye pain, nausea, and vomiting. Glaucoma is a major cause of blindness. Blacks and persons over 40 years of age are at risk.

Treatment involves drug therapy and possibly surgery. The goal is to prevent further damage to the optic nerve. Damage that has already occurred cannot be reversed.

Cataract

Cataract is an eye disorder in which the lens becomes cloudy (opaque). The cloudiness prevents light from entering the eye (Fig. 30-28, p. 727). Cataract comes from the

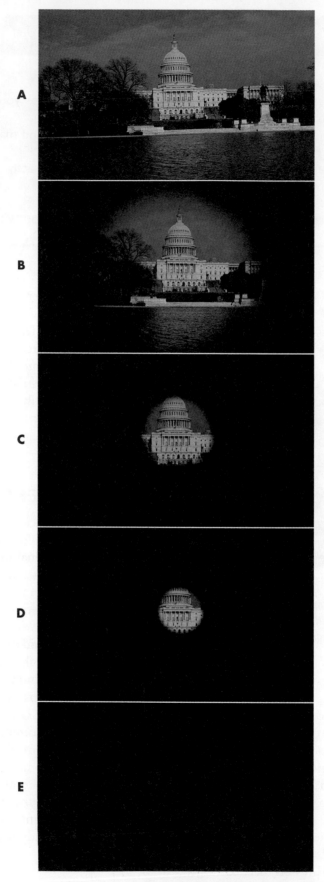

Fig. 30-27 **A,** *Normal vision.* **B,** *Tunnel vision.* **C, D, E,** *Vision loss continues with eventual blindness.*

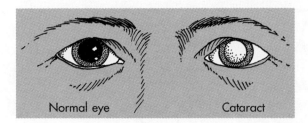

Fig. 30-28 *The left eye has a cataract.* *(From Phipps WJ, Cassmeyer VL, Sands JK, Lehman MK:* Medical-surgical nursing: concepts and clinical practice, *ed 5, St Louis, 1995, Mosby.)*

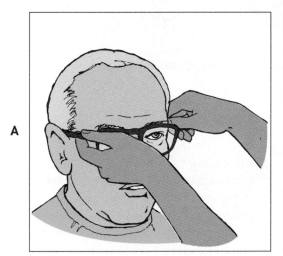
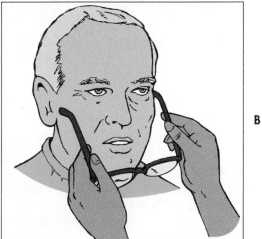

Fig. 30-29 A, *Remove eyeglasses by holding the frames in front of both ears.* **B,** *Lift the frames from the ears, and bring the glasses down away from the face.*

Greek word that means *waterfall*. Trying to see is like looking through a waterfall. Gradual blurring and dimming of vision occur. The person is sensitive to light and glares. A cataract can occur in one or both eyes. Aging is the most common cause. Persons age 60 and older are at risk.

Surgery is the only treatment. A tiny incision is made into the eye. The cloudy lens is removed. A plastic lens is implanted into the eye. Vision returns to near normal.

The person may have to wear an eye shield or patch a day or two after surgery. The shield protects the eye from injury. Measures for the blind person are practiced when an eye shield is worn. The person may have vision loss in the other eye from a cataract or other causes.

Corrective Lenses

Eyeglasses and contact lenses are prescribed to correct vision problems. Often eyeglasses are worn only for certain activities, such as reading or seeing at a distance. Some people wear them all the time while awake. Contact lenses usually are worn continuously while awake.

Eyeglasses

Lenses are made of hardened glass or plastic. They are made to prevent shattering. Wash glass lenses with warm water, and dry them with soft tissue. Plastic lenses are easily scratched. Use special cleaning solutions, tissues, and cloths to clean and dry them.

Glasses are costly. Protect them from breakage or other damage (Fig. 30-29). Put them in their case when they are not worn. Put the case in the drawer of the bedside stand to prevent loss or damage to the glasses.

Contact lenses

Contact lenses fit directly on the eye. Many people like contacts because they cannot be seen. However, contacts are easily lost. Depending on the type of lens, contacts can be worn for 12 to 24 hours or for 1 week.

Artificial Eyes

Removal of an eye is sometimes necessary because of injury or disease. The person is then fitted with an ocular

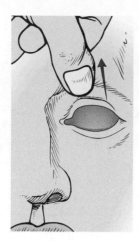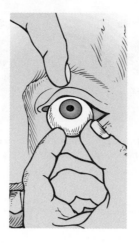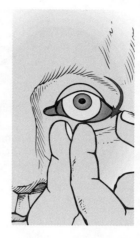

Fig. 30-30 *Inserting an artificial eye.* *(From Lewis SM, Collier IC, Heitkemper MM:* Medical-surgical nursing: assessment and management of clinical problems, *ed 4, St Louis, 1996, Mosby.)*

prosthesis, or artificial eye (Fig. 30-30). The artificial eye is made of plastic or glass. It matches the other eye in color and shape. Some prostheses are permanent implants, and others are removable. If the prosthesis is removable, the person is taught to remove, clean, and insert it. The person performs routine care of the prosthesis.

The artificial eye is the person's property. As with dentures, eyeglasses, and other valuables, you must protect it from loss or damage. Practice the following measures if the eye is removed and will not be reinserted:

- Wash the eye with a mild soap and warm water. Then rinse it well.
- Line a container with a soft cloth or 4 × 4 gauze. This prevents scratches and damage to the eye.
- Fill the container with water or a saline (salt) solution.
- Place the eye in the container. Close the container.
- Label the container with the person's name and room number.
- Place the labeled container in the drawer in the bedside stand.
- Wash the eye socket with warm water or saline. Use a washcloth or gauze square to clean the eye socket. Use a gauze square to remove excess moisture.
- Wash the eyelid with mild soap and warm water. Clean from the inner to the outer aspect of the eyelid (see Fig. 14-9 on p. 308). Dry the eyelid.

The person is blind on the side of the artificial eye. Vision in the other eye may be normal or impaired.

Blindness

Birth defects, accidents, and eye diseases are among the many causes of blindness. It is also a complication of some diseases. The level of blindness varies. Some blind persons cannot sense light and have no usable vision. These persons are totally blind. Others sense some light but have no usable vision. Still others have some usable vision but cannot read newsprint. The legally blind person sees at 20 feet what a person with normal vision sees at 200 feet.

A person's life is seriously affected by the loss of sight. Physical and psychological adjustments are hard and long. Special education and training are needed. Moving about, activities of daily living, reading braille, and using a guide dog all require training.

Braille is a method of writing that uses raised dots. Dots are arranged to represent each letter of the alphabet. The first 10 letters also represent the numbers 0 through 9 (Fig. 30-31). The person feels the arrangement of dots with the fingers (Fig. 30-32). Many books, magazines, and newspapers are available in braille. So are typewriters and computer keyboards.

Braille is hard to learn, especially for many older persons. Entire books and articles are available on compact disks and tapes. They are bought in bookstores or borrowed from libraries.

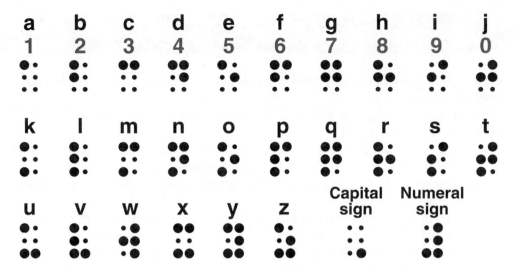

Fig. 30-31 *Braille.*

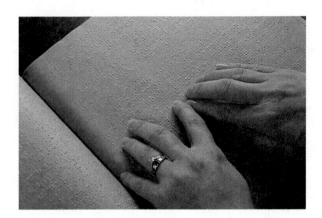

Fig. 30-32 *Braille is "read" with the fingers.*

HOME CARE

focus on

The practices listed in Box 30-10 apply in the home setting. A safe environment also is important. Outdoor walks and stairs must be free of toys, ice, and snow. Remember, furniture, closets, drawers, shelves, and other items are arranged to meet the person's needs. Always replace items where you found them. Avoid rearranging the person's belongings.

The blind person is taught to move about using a white cane with a red tip or a guide dog. Both are recognized worldwide as signs that the person is blind. The dog serves as the eyes of the blind person. The dog recognizes danger and guides the person through traffic.

Treat the blind person with respect and dignity—not with pity. Most blind people adjust well. They lead independent lives. Some have been blind for a long time and others for a short time. The practices in Box 30-10 on p. 730 are necessary for all blind persons. (See Focus on Home Care.)

BOX 30-10

CARING FOR THE BLIND PERSON

- Ask the person how much he or she can see. Do not assume the person is totally blind or that the person has some vision.
- Ask the person what type of lighting he or she prefers. Provide enough lighting. Tell the person when the lights are on or off.
- Adjust blinds and shades to adjust lighting for glares. Sunny days and bright, snowy days cause glares.
- Face the person when speaking. Speak slowly and clearly.
- Use a normal tone of voice. Do not shout or speak loudly. Blindness does not mean the person is hearing impaired.
- Identify yourself when you enter the room. Give your name, title, and reason for being there. Do not touch the person until you have indicated your presence in the room.
- Identify others in the room. Explain where each person is located and what the person is doing.
- Address the person by name. This lets the person know that you are directing a comment or question to him or her.
- Do not avoid using the words "see," "look," or "read."
- Orient the person to the room. Describe the layout. Also, identify the location and purpose of furniture and equipment.
- Let the person move about and touch and locate furniture and equipment if able.
- Do not leave the person alone in the middle of a room. Make sure the person can reach a wall, chair, table, or sofa.
- Do not rearrange furniture and equipment.
- Keep doors open or shut, never partially open.
- Give step-by-step explanations of procedures as you perform them. Indicate when the procedure is over.
- Offer assistance. Simply say "May I help you?" Respect the person's answer.
- Tell the person when you are leaving the room.
- Assist the person in ambulating by walking slightly ahead of him or her (Fig. 30-33). Offer your right or left arm. Tell the person which arm you are offering so he or she can take your arm. Never push, pull, or guide the person in front of you.
- Walk at a normal pace when guiding the person.
- Let the person know when you are coming to a curb or steps. Let the person know if you will step up or down.
- Inform the person of doors, turns, furniture, and other obstructions when assisting with ambulation.
- Give specific directions. For example, say "right behind you," "on your left," or "in front of you." Avoid phrases like "over here" or "over there."
- Keep hallways and walkways free of carts, equipment, toys, and other items.
- Assist in food selection by reading the menu to the person.
- Avoid plates, napkins, place mats, and tablecloths with patterns and designs. These items should be solid colors and provide contrast. For example, a white plate is placed on dark place mat or tablecloth.
- Explain the location of food and beverages on the tray. Use the face of a clock (see Fig. 19-7, p. 460), or guide the person's hand to each item on the tray.
- Cut meat, open containers, butter bread, and perform other similar activities if needed.
- Keep the call bell within the person's reach.
- Provide a radio, compact disks or audiotapes, television, and braille books for entertainment.
- Let the person perform self-care if able.

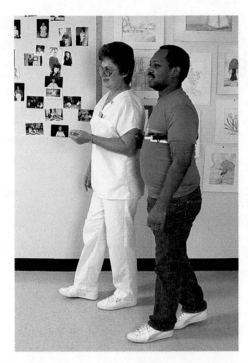

Fig. 30-33 *The blind person walks slightly behind the assistive person. He takes the assistant's arm.*

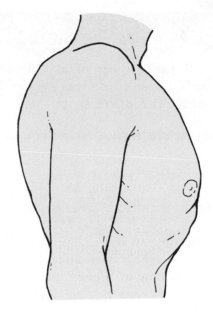

Fig. 30-34 *Barrel chest from emphysema.*

RESPIRATORY DISORDERS

The respiratory system brings oxygen (O_2) into the lungs and removes carbon dioxide (CO_2) from the body. Respiratory disorders interfere with this function and threaten life.

Chronic Obstructive Pulmonary Disease

Three disorders are grouped under chronic obstructive pulmonary disease (COPD). They are chronic bronchitis, emphysema, and asthma. These disorders interfere with the exchange of O_2 and CO_2 in the lungs. They obstruct airflow.

Chronic bronchitis

Chronic bronchitis occurs after repeated episodes of bronchitis (inflammation of the bronchi). Cigarette smoking is the major cause. Air pollution and industrial dusts are other causes. *Smoker's cough* in the morning is usually the first symptom. At first the cough is dry. Eventually the person coughs up mucus, which may contain pus. The cough becomes more frequent as the disease progresses. The person has difficulty breathing and tires easily. The mucus and inflamed breathing passages *obstruct* airflow into the lungs. Therefore the body cannot get normal amounts of oxygen.

The person must stop smoking. Oxygen therapy and breathing exercises often are ordered. Respiratory tract infections are prevented. If one occurs, prompt treatment is essential.

Emphysema

In emphysema the alveoli enlarge. Walls of the alveoli are less elastic. They do not expand and shrink normally with inspiration and expiration. As a result, some air is trapped in the alveoli during expiration. Trapped air is not exhaled. As the disease progresses, more alveoli are involved. Therefore more air is trapped. The normal exchange of O_2 and CO_2 cannot occur in affected alveoli. Chronic bronchitis and emphysema often occur together.

Cigarette smoking is the most common cause. Signs and symptoms include shortness of breath and smoker's cough. At first, shortness of breath occurs with exertion. As the disease progresses, it occurs at rest. Sputum may contain pus. As more air is trapped in the lungs, the person develops a *barrel chest* (Fig. 30-34). Persons usually prefer to sit upright and slightly forward. Breathing is easier in this position.

The person must stop smoking. Respiratory therapy, breathing exercises, oxygen, and drug therapy are ordered.

Asthma

Air passages narrow with asthma. Dyspnea results. Allergies and emotional stress are common causes. Episodes occur suddenly and are called *asthma attacks*. The person also has shortness of breath, wheezing, coughing, rapid pulse, perspiration, and cyanosis. The person is very frightened during the attack. Fear causes the attack to become worse.

Drugs are used to treat asthma. Emergency room treatment may be necessary for severe attacks. The person and family are taught how to prevent asthma attacks. Repeated attacks can damage the respiratory system.

Pneumonia

Pneumonia is an inflammation of lung tissue. Alveoli in the affected area fill with fluid. Because of fluid in the alveoli, O_2 and CO_2 are not exchanged normally.

Pneumonia is caused by bacteria, viruses, aspiration, or immobility. The person is very ill. Fever, chills, painful cough, chest pain on breathing, and a rapid pulse occur. Cyanosis may be present. Sputum is clear, green, yellow, or rust colored. The color depends on the cause.

Drugs are ordered for infection and pain. Fluids are encouraged because of fever. Fluids also help to thin mucous secretions. Thin secretions are easier to cough up. Oxygen may be necessary. Most persons prefer semi-Fowler's position for breathing. Standard Precautions are followed. Transmission-Based Precautions may be necessary, depending on the cause. Mouth care is important. Frequent linen changes are needed because of fever. (See Focus on Children and Focus on Older Persons.)

Tuberculosis

Tuberculosis (TB) is a bacterial infection. The lungs are affected. However, TB can occur also in the kidney and bones. TB was a major cause of death in the early 1900s. TB drug therapy was introduced in the 1940s and 1950s. A dramatic decline in the number of TB cases resulted. However, TB still occurs and is a major health problem. In the late 1980s the number of cases began to increase.

The bacteria causing TB are spread by airborne droplets (see Chapter 11). Bacteria are spread when the person coughs, sneezes, speaks, or sings. Others in the environment can inhale the bacteria. Persons who have close, frequent contact with an infected person are at risk. TB is more likely to occur in close, crowded areas such as inner-city neighborhoods. Persons with human immunodeficiency virus (HIV) infection (p. 742-743) also are at risk.

Sometimes the bacteria do not produce an infection until many years later. The person may not have symptoms at first. The disease is found when a routine chest x-ray examination is done or when a TB skin test is required for a job. Early signs and symptoms are tiredness, loss of appetite, weight loss, fever, and night sweats. Coughing occurs. The cough is more frequent as the disease progresses. Sputum production also increases. Chest pain occurs.

Treatment involves drugs for TB. Hospital care usually is not necessary. Persons with TB need to cover their nose and mouth with tissues when coughing or sneezing. Tissues are flushed down the toilet or placed in a paper bag and burned. In health care agencies, tissues are placed in a biohazard bag and disposed of following agency policy. Handwashing after contact with sputum is essential. Standard Precautions and Airborne Precautions are practiced.

CARDIOVASCULAR DISORDERS

Cardiovascular disorders are the leading causes of death in the United States. Problems occur in the heart or in the blood vessels.

Hypertension

Hypertension *(high blood pressure)* is a condition in which the blood pressure is abnormally high. The systolic pressure is 140 mm Hg or higher. Or the diastolic pressure is 90 mm Hg or higher. Elevated measurements must

BOX 30-11

RISK FACTORS FOR HYPERTENSION

- Age—the risk increases with aging beginning at about age 35
- Sex—younger men are at greater risk than younger women; the risk increases for women after menopause
- Race—blacks are at greater risk than whites
- Family history—tends to run in families
- Obesity—related to lack of exercise and atherosclerosis
- Stress—increased sympathetic nervous system activity
- Cigarette smoking—nicotine narrows blood vessels
- High-salt diet—sodium causes fluid retention; increased fluid raises the blood volume
- Alcohol—increases chemical substances in the body that increase blood pressure
- Lack of exercise—leads to obesity
- Atherosclerosis—arteries narrow because of fatty buildup in the vessels

occur on two different occasions. Risk factors are listed in Box 30-11. Narrowed blood vessels are a common cause. When vessels narrow, the heart pumps with more force to move blood through the vessels. Kidney disorders, head injuries, some complications of pregnancy, and tumors of the adrenal gland can also cause hypertension.

Hypertension can damage other body organs. The heart may enlarge so it can pump with more force. Blood vessels in the brain may burst and cause a stroke. Blood vessels in the eyes and kidneys may be damaged.

At first, hypertension may not cause signs or symptoms. Usually it is discovered when blood pressure is measured. Signs and symptoms develop as the disorder progresses. Headache, blurred vision, and dizziness may be reported. Complications of hypertension include stroke, heart attack, kidney (renal) failure, and blindness.

Certain drugs can lower blood pressure. The person needs to exercise, get enough rest, and quit smoking. A sodium-restricted diet also may be ordered. If the person is overweight, a low-calorie diet is ordered.

Coronary Artery Disease

The coronary arteries are in the heart. They supply the heart with blood. In coronary artery disease (CAD), the coronary arteries narrow. One or all of the arteries may be affected. Because of narrowed vessels, the heart muscle gets less blood. The most common cause is atherosclerosis. In atherosclerosis, fatty material collects on the arterial walls (Fig. 30-35). The arteries narrow and obstruct blood flow. Blood flow through an artery may be totally blocked. Permanent damage occurs in the part of the heart receiving its blood supply from that artery.

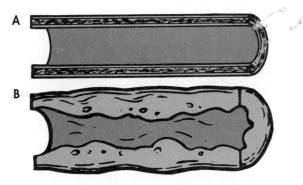

Fig. 30-35 A, *Normal artery.* **B,** *Fatty deposits collect on the walls of arteries in atherosclerosis.*

CAD is the leading cause of death in the United States. Risk factors include:
- Sex (male gender)
- Age (more common in older persons)
- Obesity
- Cigarette smoking
- Lack of exercise
- A diet high in fat and cholesterol
- Hypertension
- Family history of CAD
- Uncontrolled diabetes (see p. 738)

The major complications of CAD are angina pectoris and myocardial infarction (heart attack). Treatment involves reducing risk factors. Nothing can be done about the person's sex, age, and family history. However, efforts are directed at losing weight, regular exercise, no smoking, and eating a healthy diet. Controlling blood pressure and diabetes also is important.

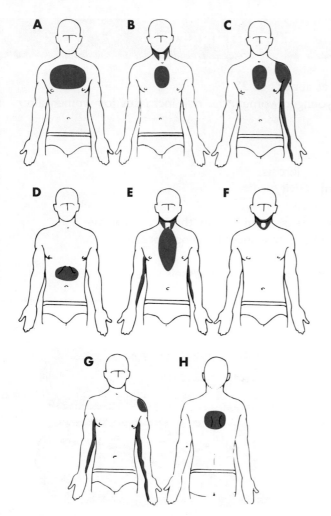

Fig. 30-36 *Shaded areas show where the pain of angina pectoris is located. (From Phipps WJ, Cassmeyer VL, Sands JK, Lehman MK:* Medical-surgical nursing: concepts and clinical practice, *ed 5, St Louis, 1995, Mosby.)*

Angina pectoris

Angina *(pain)* pectoris *(chest)* means chest pain. The chest pain is from reduced blood flow to a part of the heart muscle (myocardium). Commonly called *angina*, it occurs when the heart needs more oxygen. Normally, blood flow to the heart increases when the heart's need for oxygen increases. Physical exertion, a heavy meal, emotional stress, and excitement increase the heart's need for oxygen. In CAD, narrowed vessels prevent increased blood flow.

Signs and symptoms include chest pain. The pain may be described as a tightness or discomfort in the left side of the chest. Pain may radiate to other sites (Fig. 30-36). Pain in the left jaw and down the inner aspect of the left arm is common. The person may be pale, feel faint, and perspire. Dyspnea may be present. These signs and symptoms cause the person to stop activity and rest. Rest often relieves the symptoms in 3 to 15 minutes. Rest re-

duces the heart's need for oxygen. Therefore normal blood flow is achieved and heart damage is prevented.

Besides rest, a drug called *nitroglycerin* is taken to relieve angina. A nitroglycerin tablet is taken when an angina attack occurs. The tablet is put under the tongue. It dissolves under the tongue and is rapidly absorbed into the bloodstream. Most doctors want the tablets kept at the bedside. The person takes a tablet when one is needed and then tells the nurse. The person does not have to wait for someone to answer the call bell and then for a nurse to get the tablet. The person needs the tablets nearby at all times. This includes when the person goes to physical therapy, occupational therapy, the x-ray department, the dining room, lounge, or other parts of the agency.

Persons are taught to avoid things likely to cause angina pectoris. These include overexertion, heavy meals and overeating, and emotional times. They need to stay indoors during cold weather or during hot, humid weather. Exercise programs supervised by doctors are helpful.

Some people need coronary artery bypass surgery. The surgery bypasses the diseased part of the artery (Fig. 30-37) and increases blood flow to the heart. Many persons with angina pectoris eventually have heart attacks. Chest pain that is not relieved by rest and nitroglycerin may have a more serious cause.

Myocardial infarction

A myocardial infarction (MI) is caused by lack of blood supply to the heart muscle (myocardium). Tissue death occurs (infarction). Common terms for MI are *heart attack, coronary, coronary thrombosis,* and *coronary occlusion.* Blood flow to the myocardium is suddenly interrupted. Atherosclerosis or a thrombus (blood clot) obstructs blood flow through an artery. The area of damage may be small or large (Fig. 30-38). Sudden cardiac death *(cardiac arrest)* can occur (see Chapter 35).

The person has one or more signs and symptoms listed in Box 30-12. Myocardial infarction is an emergency. Efforts are directed at relieving pain, stabilizing vital signs, giving oxygen, and calming the person. Many drugs are given. The person is treated in a coronary care unit (CCU). The unit has emergency equipment and drugs needed during cardiac arrest. Measures are taken to prevent life-threatening complications.

The person is in the CCU for 2 to 3 days. When stable, the person is transferred. Activity is increased gradually. Drug therapy and measures to prevent complications are continued. A cardiac rehabilitation program is planned. It includes an exercise program, teaching about drugs, dietary changes, and sexual activity. Life-style changes may be necessary. The goal of cardiac rehabilitation is to prevent another heart attack. (See Focus on Home Care on p. 735.)

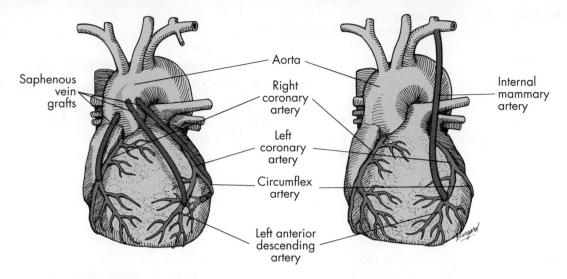

Fig. 30-37 *Coronary artery bypass surgery.* (*From Phipps WJ, Cassmeyer VL, Sands JK, Lehman, MK: Medical-surgical nursing: concepts and clinical practice, ed 5, St Louis, 1995, Mosby.*)

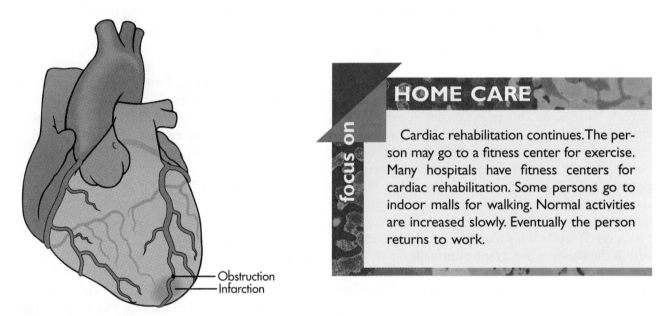

Fig. 30-38 *Myocardial infarction.* (*From Lewis SM, Collier IC: Medical-surgical nursing: assessment & management of clinical problems, ed 4, St Louis, 1996, Mosby. By permission of Mayo Foundation, Rochester, Minn.*)

HOME CARE

focus on

   Cardiac rehabilitation continues. The person may go to a fitness center for exercise. Many hospitals have fitness centers for cardiac rehabilitation. Some persons go to indoor malls for walking. Normal activities are increased slowly. Eventually the person returns to work.

BOX 30-12

SIGNS AND SYMPTOMS OF MYOCARDIAL INFARCTION

- Sudden, severe chest pain
- Pain is usually on the left side
- Pain described as crushing, stabbing, or squeezing; some describe pain in terms of someone sitting on the chest
- Pain may radiate to the neck and jaw, and down the arm or to other sites
- Pain is more severe and lasts longer than angina pectoris
- Pain is not relieved by rest and nitroglycerin
- Indigestion

- Dyspnea
- Nausea
- Dizziness
- Perspiration
- Pallor
- Cyanosis
- Cold and clammy skin
- Low blood pressure
- Weak and irregular pulse
- Fear and apprehension
- A feeling of doom

Heart Failure

Heart failure or congestive heart failure (CHF) occurs when the heart cannot pump blood normally. Blood backs up and causes congestion of tissues. Left-sided heart failure, right-sided heart failure, or both can occur.

When the heart's left side fails to pump efficiently, blood backs up into the lungs. Signs and symptoms of respiratory congestion occur. These include dyspnea, increased sputum, cough, and gurgling sounds in the lungs. Also, blood is not pumped out of the heart to the rest of the body in adequate amounts. Organs do not get enough blood. Signs and symptoms occur from effects on the organs. Poor blood flow to the brain causes confusion, dizziness, and fainting. Poor blood flow to the kidneys causes reduced kidney function and decreased urinary output. The skin becomes pale or cyanotic. Blood pressure falls. A very severe form of left-sided failure is *pulmonary edema* (fluid in the lungs). Pulmonary edema is an emergency. Death can occur.

With right-sided failure, blood backs up into the venae cavae and into the venous system. Feet and ankles swell. Neck veins bulge. Liver congestion causes decreased liver function. The abdomen becomes congested with fluid. The right side of the heart cannot pump blood to the lungs efficiently. Normal blood flow does not occur from the lungs to the left side of the heart. Less blood than normal is pumped from the left side of the heart to the rest of the body. As with left-sided heart failure, the body's organs have a reduced blood supply. The signs and symptoms described in the previous paragraph eventually occur.

Heart failure usually is caused by a weakened heart. Myocardial infarction and hypertension are common causes. Damaged heart valves are another cause.

Heart failure can be treated and controlled. Drugs strengthen the heart and reduce the amount of fluid in the body. A sodium-restricted diet is ordered. Oxygen is given. Most persons prefer semi-Fowler's or Fowler's position for breathing. You may be involved in these aspects of the person's care:

- Maintaining bedrest or a limited activity program
- Measuring intake and output
- Measuring weight daily
- Restricting fluids as ordered by the doctor
- Giving good skin care to prevent skin breakdown
- Performing range-of-motion exercises
- Assisting with transfers or ambulation
- Assisting with self-care activities
- Maintaining good body alignment
- Applying elastic stockings

(See Focus on Children and Focus on Home Care.)

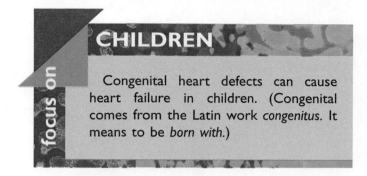

focus on CHILDREN

Congenital heart defects can cause heart failure in children. (Congenital comes from the Latin work *congenitus*. It means to be *born with*.)

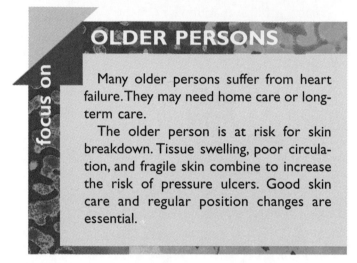

focus on OLDER PERSONS

Many older persons suffer from heart failure. They may need home care or long-term care.

The older person is at risk for skin breakdown. Tissue swelling, poor circulation, and fragile skin combine to increase the risk of pressure ulcers. Good skin care and regular position changes are essential.

DISORDERS OF THE URINARY SYSTEM

The kidneys, ureters, bladder, and urethra are the major structures of the urinary system. Disorders can occur in one or more of these structures.

Urinary Tract Infections

Urinary tract infections (UTIs) are common. They can occur in the bladder or in a kidney. Infection in one area can lead to infection of the entire system. Normally the urinary system is sterile. It has no pathogens or nonpathogens. Microbes can enter the urinary system through the urethra. Catheterization, urological examinations, sexual intercourse, and poor perineal hygiene are common causes. UTI is a common nosocomial infection (see Chapter 11).

Women are at greater risk for UTIs than are men. Women have a shorter urethra, which microbes can easily enter. In men, prostate gland secretions offer protection from UTIs. (See Focus on Older Persons on p. 737.)

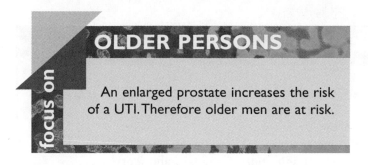

OLDER PERSONS

focus on

An enlarged prostate increases the risk of a UTI. Therefore older men are at risk.

Cystitis

Cystitis is inflammation *(itis)* of the bladder *(cyst)*. It is caused by bacteria. The person may have one or more of the following:

- Urinary frequency
- Urgency
- Dysuria—difficult or painful *(dys)* urination *(uria)*
- Pain
- Foul-smelling urine
- Hematuria—blood *(hemat)* in the urine *(uria)*
- Pyuria—pus *(py)* in the urine *(uria)*

Antibiotics are the treatment of choice.

Pyelonephritis

Pyelonephritis is inflammation *(itis)* of the kidney *(nephr)* pelvis *(pyelo)*. Infection is the most common cause. Chills, fever, back pain, and nausea and vomiting occur. So do the signs and symptoms of cystitis. Treatment consists of antibiotics and fluids.

Renal Calculi

Renal calculi are kidney *(renal)* stones *(calculi)*. White men between the ages of 20 and 40 have the greatest risk. Bedrest and immobility also are risk factors. Stones vary in size. Signs and symptoms include:

- Severe, cramping pain in the back and side; pain can occur also in the abdomen, thigh, and urethra
- Nausea and vomiting
- Fever and chills
- Dysuria—difficult or painful *(dys)* urination *(uria)*
- Urinary frequency and urgency
- Oliguria—scant *(olig)* urine *(uria)*
- Hematuria—blood *(hemat)* in the urine *(uria)*

Treatment involves pain relief and forcing fluids. The person needs to drink about 4000 ml of fluid a day. Forcing fluids helps promote passage of the stone through the urine. All urine is strained (see Chapter 17). Surgical removal of the stone may be necessary.

Renal Failure

In renal failure (kidney failure) the kidneys do not function or are severely impaired. Waste products are not removed from the blood. Fluids are retained in the body. Heart failure and hypertension easily result. Renal failure may be acute or chronic. The person is very ill.

Acute renal failure

Acute renal failure occurs suddenly. Severe decreased blood flow to the kidneys is a common cause. The many causes of decreased blood flow to the kidneys include postoperative bleeding, bleeding from trauma, myocardial infarction (heart attack), severe congestive heart failure, burns, and severe allergic reactions.

At first the person has *oliguria* (scant amount of urine). Urine output is less than 400 ml in 24 hours. This is followed by *anuria* (absence of urine). It can last a few days to 2 weeks. Then diuresis occurs. *Diuresis* means the process *(esis)* of passing *(di)* the urine *(ur)*. Large amounts of urine are produced. Urine output ranges from 1000 to 5000 ml a day. Kidney function improves and returns to normal during the recovery phase. This phase can take anywhere from 1 month to 1 year. Some persons develop chronic renal failure.

Every system is affected by the buildup of waste products in the blood. Death can occur.

The doctor orders drug therapy, restricted fluids, and diet therapy. The person's diet is low in protein, high in carbohydrates, and low in potassium. The nurse plans for the person's physical and psychological needs. The person's care plan is likely to include:

- Measuring and recording urine output every hour; an output of less than 30 ml per hour is reported to the RN immediately
- Measuring and recording intake and output
- Restricting fluid intake
- Daily weight measurements with the same scale
- Turning and repositioning at least every 2 hours
- Measures to prevent pressure ulcers
- Frequent oral hygiene
- Measures to prevent infection
- Coughing and deep breathing exercises
- Measures to meet the person's emotional needs

Chronic renal failure

In chronic renal failure the kidneys cannot meet the body's needs. Nephrons of the kidney are slowly destroyed over many years. Hypertension and diabetes are the most common causes. Infections, urinary tract obstructions, and tumors are other causes.

BOX 30-13

SIGNS AND SYMPTOMS OF CHRONIC RENAL FAILURE

- Yellow, tan, or dusky skin
- Dry, itchy skin
- Thin, brittle skin
- Bruises
- Bad breath (halitosis)
- Stomatitis (inflammation of the mouth)
- Nausea and vomiting
- Loss of appetite
- Diarrhea or constipation
- Bleeding tendencies
- Susceptibility to infection
- Hypertension
- Congestive heart failure
- Gastric ulcers
- Irregular pulse
- Abnormal breathing patterns
- Burning sensation in the legs and feet
- Muscle twitching
- Leg cramps at night
- Fatigue
- Headache
- Convulsions
- Confusion
- Coma

BOX 30-14

CARE OF THE PERSON IN CHRONIC RENAL FAILURE

- A diet low in protein, potassium, and sodium
- Fluid restriction
- Measuring blood pressure in the supine, sitting, and standing positions
- Measuring weight daily (with the same scale)
- Measuring and recording intake and output
- Turning and repositioning
- Measures to prevent pressure ulcers
- Range-of-motion exercises
- Measures to prevent itching (bath oils, lotions, and creams)
- Measures to prevent injury and bleeding
- Frequent oral hygiene
- Measures to prevent infection
- Measures to prevent diarrhea or constipation
- Measures to meet the person's emotional needs
- Measures to promote rest

Signs and symptoms appear when 80% to 90% of kidney function is lost. Every body system is affected by the buildup of waste products in the blood. Box 30-13 lists some of the signs and symptoms that occur.

Treatment includes fluid restriction, diet therapy, drugs, and dialysis. **Dialysis** is the process of removing waste products from the blood. It is a complex process. Specially trained nurses perform the procedure. Some persons have kidney transplants.

Nursing measures for the person in chronic renal failure are listed in Box 30-14.

THE ENDOCRINE SYSTEM

The endocrine system is made of glands. The endocrine glands secrete hormones that affect other organs and glands. The most common endocrine disorder is diabetes mellitus.

Diabetes Mellitus

In this disorder the body cannot use sugar properly. Insulin is needed for the proper use of sugar. Insulin is secreted by the pancreas. In diabetes mellitus, the pancreas does not secrete enough insulin. Sugar builds up in the blood. Cells do not have enough sugar for energy. Therefore cells cannot perform their functions.

Diabetes mellitus occurs in children and adults. Risk factors include obesity and a family history of diabetes. The risk increases after age 40.

There are three types of diabetes mellitus:

- *Insulin-dependent diabetes mellitus (IDDM or type 1)*—occurs most often in children and young adults. The pancreas does not secrete insulin. The person needs daily insulin injections. Onset is rapid.
- *Non-insulin-dependent diabetes mellitus (NIDDM or type 2)*—occurs in adults over 40 years of age. The pancreas secretes insulin. However, the body cannot use it effectively. Onset is slow.
- *Gestational diabetes mellitus (GDM)*—develops during pregnancy. (Gestation comes from the Latin word *gestare,* which means to *bear.*) It usually disappears after the baby is born. However, the woman is at risk for NIDDM.

Signs and symptoms include increased urine production, increased thirst, hunger, weight loss, and extreme tiredness. Blurred vision is common. Frequent infections and slow healing of sores is common in persons with NIDDM. In both types, blood tests show increased sugar levels.

If diabetes is not controlled, complications occur. These include blindness, renal failure, nerve damage, hypertension, and circulatory disorders. Circulatory disorders can lead to stroke, heart attack, and slow wound healing. Foot and leg wounds are very serious. Infection and gangrene can occur and require amputation of the part.

Risk factors include a family history of the disease. Obesity is also a risk factor. Blacks, Hispanics, and Native Americans are at risk. So are older persons.

Insulin-dependent diabetes is treated with daily insulin therapy, diet, and exercise. The amount of sugar in the diet is limited (see Chapter 19). Meals are served on time to balance insulin needs. Remember, food raises the blood sugar and insulin lowers blood sugar. The person needs to eat all foods served.

Non-insulin-dependent diabetes is treated with diet and exercise. The number of calories and sugar in the diet are restricted. Overweight persons need to lose weight. Oral medications may be ordered. Some persons need insulin.

Both types require blood glucose monitoring (see Chapter 25). Good foot care is very important. Corns, blisters, and calluses on the feet can lead to an infection and amputation.

Hypoglycemia (insulin shock) occurs with too much insulin. **Hypoglycemia** means low *(hypo)* sugar *(glyc)* in the blood *(emia)*. Hyperglycemia (diabetic coma) develops if a person does not get enough insulin. **Hyperglycemia** means high *(hyper)* sugar *(glyc)* in the blood *(emia)*. Table 30-1 on p. 740 lists the causes, signs, and symptoms of hypoglycemia and hyperglycemia. Both can lead to death if not corrected. (See Focus on Children.)

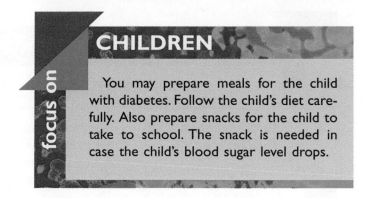

focus on CHILDREN

You may prepare meals for the child with diabetes. Follow the child's diet carefully. Also prepare snacks for the child to take to school. The snack is needed in case the child's blood sugar level drops.

DIGESTIVE DISORDERS

The digestive system breaks down food for absorption by the body. It also eliminates solid wastes. Some digestive disorders were discussed in Chapter 18: diarrhea, constipation, flatulence, anal incontinence, and care of persons with colostomies and ileostomies.

Vomiting

Vomiting is the act of expelling stomach contents through the mouth. It is a sign of illness or injury. It can be life-threatening. The vomitus (material vomited) can be aspirated and obstruct the airway. Shock can also occur if large amounts of blood are vomited. The following measures are practiced:

- Use Standard Precautions and follow the Bloodborne Pathogen Standard.
- Turn the person's head well to one side. This prevents aspiration.
- Place a kidney basin under the person's chin.
- Remove the vomitus from the person's immediate environment.
- Let the person perform oral hygiene. This helps eliminate the taste of vomitus.
- Eliminate odors.
- Change linens as necessary.
- Observe vomitus for color, odor, and undigested food. Vomitus that looks like coffee grounds contains digested blood. This indicates bleeding.
- Measure the amount of vomitus. Report the amount to the RN. Note the amount on the I&O record.
- Save a specimen for laboratory study.
- Do not discard vomitus until it is observed by the RN.

TABLE 30-1	HYPOGLYCEMIA AND HYPERGLYCEMIA		
		Causes	Signs and Symptoms
	Hypoglycemia (insulin shock)	Too much insulin Omitting a meal Eating too little food Increased exercise Vomiting	Hunger Weakness Trembling Perspiration Headache Dizziness Rapid pulse Low blood pressure Confusion Cold, clammy skin Convulsions Unconsciousness
	Hyperglycemia (diabetic coma)	Undiagnosed diabetes Not enough insulin Eating too much food Too little exercise Stress (e.g., from surgery, illness, emotional upset)	Weakness Drowsiness Thirst Hunger Frequent urination Flushed face Sweet breath odor Slow, deep, and labored respirations Rapid, weak pulse Low blood pressure Dry skin Headache Nausea and vomiting Coma

COMMUNICABLE DISEASES

Communicable diseases (contagious or infectious diseases) can be transmitted from one person to another. They can be transmitted in the following ways:

- Direct—from the infected person
- Indirect—from dressings, linens, or surfaces
- Airborne—from the person through sneezing or coughing
- Vehicle—through ingestion of contaminated food, water, drugs, blood, or fluids
- Vector—from animals, fleas, and ticks

This section discusses hepatitis, acquired immunodeficiency sydrome (AIDS), and sexually transmitted diseases. Table 30-2 outlines common childhood communicable diseases. Standard Precautions and Transmission-Based Precautions are followed.

Hepatitis

Hepatitis is an inflammation of the liver. The major types of hepatitis are:

- *Hepatitis A*—is spread by the fecal-oral route. Food, water, or drinking or eating vessels can be contaminated with feces. The virus is ingested when eating or drinking contaminated food or water. It is ingested also when eating or drinking from a contaminated vessel. Causes include poor sanitation, crowded living conditions, poor nutrition, and poor hygiene. Handle bedpans, feces, and rectal thermometers carefully. Good handwashing is essential for everyone.
- *Heptatitis B*—is caused by the hepatitis B virus (HBV). The virus is present in blood and body fluids (saliva, semen, vaginal secretions) of infected persons. It is transmitted by needle sharing among

	COMMON COMMUNICABLE CHILDHOOD DISEASES	
Disease	Transmission	Signs and Symptoms
Chickenpox (varicella)	Direct contact and airborne contact with respiratory secretions; direct contact with skin lesions	Fever, rash, skin lesions
Diphtheria	Direct or indirect contact with respiratory secretions and skin lesions from the person or a carrier	Sore throat, fever, nasal discharge, enlarged lymph glands in the neck, cough, hoarseness, patches (lesions) on the tonsils, pharynx, larynx, nasal membranes, skin
Measles (rubeola)	Direct or indirect contact with nasal secretions	Fever, cough, rash, inflammation of the mucous membranes of the nose, nasal discharge; bronchitis
Mumps	Direct contact with saliva droplets	Fever, headache, swollen salivary glands, earache
Pertussis (whooping cough)	Airborne or direct contact with droplets from the respiratory tract	Fever, sneezing, severe cough at night, coughs are short and rapid followed by a "whoop" or crowing sound with inhalation
Poliomyelitis	Airborne or direct contact with respiratory secretions; direct contact with feces	Fever, sore throat, headache, nausea and vomiting, loss of appetite, abdominal pain, neck and spinal stiffness, paralysis
Rubella (German measles)	Airborne or direct contact with secretions from the nose and pharynx	Fever, headache, loss of appetite, nasal inflammation, sore throat, cough, rash
Scarlet fever	Airborne or direct contact with nasal and pharyngeal secretions	Fever, chills, headache, vomiting, abdominal pain, red and swollen tonsils and pharynx, rash

TABLE 30-2

IV drug users. The virus is spread also by sexual contact, especially anal sex. (The HBV vaccine is discussed in Chapter 11.)
- *Hepatitis C*—is caused by a virus spread through needle sharing and sexual contact.
- *Hepatitis D*—occurs in persons infected with HBV. Persons who receive frequent blood transfusions are at risk.
- *Hepatitis E*—occurs in countries with poor sanitation. It is spread by the fecal-oral route.

Hepatitis can be mild or can cause death. The signs and symptoms of hepatitis are listed in Box 30-15 on p. 742. Treatment involves bedrest and a healthful diet. The person is not allowed to drink alcohol. Full recovery takes about 8 weeks.

You must protect yourself and others from the hepatitis virus. Standard Precautions and the Bloodborne Pathogen Standard are followed. Transmission-Based Precautions are ordered as necessary (see Chapter 11). (See Focus on Children on p. 742.)

BOX 30-15

SIGNS AND SYMPTOMS OF HEPATITIS

- Loss of appetite
- Weakness, fatigue, exhaustion
- Nausea and vomiting
- Fever
- Skin rash
- Dark urine
- Jaundice (yellowish color to the skin and whites of the eyes)
- Light-colored stools
- Headache
- Chills
- Abdominal pain
- Muscle aches

focus on CHILDREN

Hepatitis A is more common in preschool and school-age children. Poor hygiene practices after defecation lead to contamination of eating and drinking vessels. Also, young children often put their hands into their mouths.

Acquired Immunodeficiency Syndrome

AIDS is caused by a virus. The virus is called the human immunodeficiency virus (HIV). The virus attacks the immune system. The person's ability to fight other diseases is affected. AIDS has no cure at present. It eventually leads to death.

The virus is spread through certain body fluids—blood, semen, vaginal secretions, and breast milk. HIV is not spread by saliva, tears, sweat, sneezing, coughing, insects, or casual contact. AIDS is transmitted mainly by:

- Unprotected anal, vaginal, or oral sex with an infected person ("unprotected" is without a latex condom)
- Needle-sharing among IV drug users
- HIV-infected mothers before or during childbirth
- HIV-infected mothers through breast-feeding

The virus enters the bloodstream through the rectum, vagina, penis, or mouth. Small breaks in the mucous membrane of the vagina or rectum may occur when the penis, finger, or other objects are inserted. Gum disease can cause breaks in the mucous membrane of the gums. The breaks in the mucous membrane of the mouth, vagina, or rectum provide a route for the virus to enter the bloodstream.

Intravenous drug users transmit AIDS through the use of contaminated needles and syringes. The virus is carried in the contaminated blood left in needles or syringes. When needles and syringes are used by others, contaminated blood enters their bloodstream.

Infection can occur also when infected body fluids come in contact with open areas on the skin. Babies can become infected during pregnancy, shortly after birth, or from breast-feeding.

The virus is very fragile. It cannot live outside the body. Therefore HIV is not spread by casual, everyday contact. Such contact includes using public telephones, restrooms, or water fountains. Other forms of casual contact include talking to, hugging, or dancing with an infected person. HIV is not transmitted by food prepared by the infected person.

Signs and symptoms of AIDS are listed in Box 30-16. Some persons infected with HIV do not develop AIDS for as long as 10 to 15 years. They may not show signs or symptoms of the disease. However, they are carriers of the virus. They can spread the disease to others.

Persons with AIDS develop other diseases. Their bodies do not have the ability to fight disease. Their immune system, which fights diseases, is damaged. The person is at risk for pneumonia, Kaposi's sarcoma (a type of cancer), and central nervous system damage. The person with central nervous system damage may show memory loss, loss of coordination, paralysis, mental health disorders, and dementia.

You may care for persons with AIDS or who are HIV carriers (Box 30-17). You may have contact with the person's blood and body fluids. Mouth-to-mouth contact is possible during cardiopulmonary resuscitation (CPR). Certain precautions are necessary to protect yourself and others from the AIDS virus. Standard Precautions and the Bloodborne Pathogen Standard are followed. *These precautions apply when caring for all persons.* Remember, you may care for a person who has the HIV virus but shows no symptoms. You may also care for a person who has not yet been diagnosed as having AIDS. (See Focus on Older Persons on p. 744.)

BOX 30-16

SIGNS AND SYMPTOMS OF ACQUIRED IMMUNODEFICIENCY SYNDROME (AIDS)

- Loss of appetite
- Weight loss
- Fever
- Night sweats
- Diarrhea
- Painful or difficulty swallowing
- Tiredness, extreme or constant
- Skin rashes
- Swollen glands in the neck, underarms, and groin
- Cough
- Sores or white patches in the mouth or on the tongue
- Purple blotches or bumps on the skin that look like bruises but do not disappear
- Confusion
- Forgetfulness
- Dementia (see Chapter 32)

BOX 30-17

CARING FOR THE PERSON WITH AIDS

- Practice Standard Precautions.
- Follow the Bloodborne Pathogen Standard.
- Provide daily hygiene. Avoid harsh soaps that irritate the skin.
- Provide oral hygiene before meals and at bedtime. Make sure the person uses a toothbrush with soft bristles.
- Provide oral fluids as ordered.
- Measure and record intake and output.
- Measure weight daily.
- Have the person perform deep breathing and coughing exercises as ordered.
- Practice measures to prevent pressure ulcers.
- Assist with range-of-motion exercises and ambulation as ordered.
- Encourage the person to perform self-care as able. The person may need assistive devices (walkers, commode, eating devices).
- Encourage the person to be as active as possible.
- Change linens, gowns, or pajamas as often as needed when fever is present.
- Be a good listener and provide emotional support.

OLDER PERSONS

AIDS is often viewed as a young person's disease. Plus people often think that older persons are not sexually active and do not consider them to be at risk for AIDS. Except for childbirth and breast-feeding, older persons do get and spread AIDS in the same ways as younger persons do.

The disease is often missed during diagnosis. Aging and other diseases can mask the signs and symptoms of AIDS. Often the person dies without the disease being diagnosed.

Sexually Transmitted Diseases

Sexually transmitted diseases (STDs) are spread by sexual contact (Table 30-3). Some people are not aware of being infected. Others know but do not seek treatment. Embarrassment is a common reason for not seeking treatment.

The genital area is usually associated with STDs. However, other areas may be involved. These areas include the rectum, ears, mouth, nipples, throat, tongue, eyes, and nose. Most STDs are spread by sexual contact. The use of condoms helps prevent the spread of STDs. The use of condoms is very important for preventing the spread of HIV and AIDS. Some STDs are spread also through a break in the skin, by contact with infected body fluids (blood, sperm, saliva), or by contaminated blood or needles.

Standard Precautions are necessary. The Bloodborne Pathogen Standard also is followed.

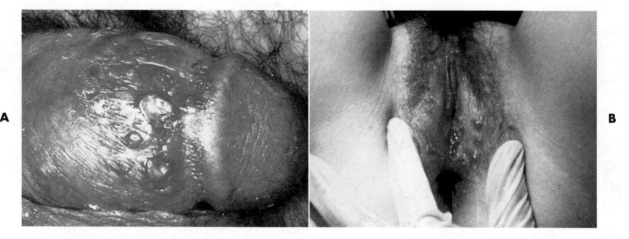

Fig. 30-39 *Genital herpes.* **A,** *Sores on the penis.* **B,** *Sores on the perineum.* *(Courtesy USPHS, Washington, DC.)*

TABLE 30-3

SEXUALLY TRANSMITTED DISEASES

Disease	Signs and Symptoms	Treatment
Genital herpes	Painful, fluid-filled sores on or near the genitalia (Fig. 30-39) The sores may have a watery discharge Itching, burning, and tingling in the genital area Fever Swollen glands	No known cure Medications can be given to control discomfort
Venereal warts	Male—Warts appear on the penis, anus, or genitalia Female—Warts appear near the vagina, cervix, labia	Application of special ointment that causes the warts to dry up and fall off Surgical removal may be necessary if the ointment is not effective
AIDS (acquired immunodeficiency syndrome)	See p. 742-743	See p. 742-743
Gonorrhea	Burning on urination Urinary frequency and urgency Vaginal discharge in the female Urethral discharge in the male	Antibiotic medications
Syphilis	*Stage 1*—10 to 90 days after exposure Painless chancre on the penis, in the vagina, or on genitalia; the chancre also may be on the lips or inside the mouth or anywhere else on the body *Stage 2*—About 2 months after the chancre General fatigue, loss of appetite, nausea, fever, headache, rash, sore throat, bone and joint pain, hair loss, lesions on the lips and genitalia *Stage 3*—3 to 15 years after infection Damage to the cardiovascular system and central nervous system, blindness	Antibiotic medications

REVIEW QUESTIONS

Circle the best *answer.*

1 Which is *not* a warning sign of cancer?

   a Painful, swollen joints

   b A sore that does not heal

   c Unusual bleeding or discharge from a body opening

   d Nagging cough or hoarseness

2 Martha Powers has arthritis. Care does *not* include

   a Measures to prevent contractures

   b Range-of-motion exercises

   c A cast or traction

   d Assistance with activities of daily living

3 A cast needs to dry. Which is *false?*

   a The cast is covered with blankets or plastic.

   b The person is turned as directed so the cast dries evenly.

   c The entire length of the cast is supported with pillows.

   d The cast is supported by the palms when lifted.

4 A person has a cast. Which are reported immediately?

   a Pain, numbness, or inability to move the fingers or toes

   b Chills, fever, or nausea and vomiting

   c Odor, cyanosis, or temperature changes of the skin

   d All of the above

5 A person is in traction. You should do the following *except*

   a Perform range-of-motion exercises as directed

   b Keep the weights off the floor

   c Remove the weights if the person is uncomfortable

   d Give skin care at frequent intervals

6 After a hip pinning, the operated leg is

   a Abducted at all times

   b Adducted at all times

   c Externally rotated at all times

   d Flexed at all times

7 Martha Powers has osteoporosis. She is at risk for

   a Fractures

   b An amputation

   c Phantom limb pain

   d All of the above

8 A person has had a stroke. The RN tells you to do the following. Which should you question?

   a Elevate the head of the bed to a semi-Fowler's position.

   b Do range-of-motion exercises every 2 hours.

   c Turn, reposition, and give skin care every 2 hours.

   d Keep the bed in the highest horizontal position.

9 Receptive aphasia means that the person

   a Cannot talk

   b Cannot write

   c Has trouble understanding messages

   d All of the above

10 A person has Parkinson's disease. Which is *false?*

   a Parkinson's disease affects part of the brain.

   b The person's mental function is affected first.

   c Signs and symptoms include stiff muscles, slow movements, and a shuffling gait.

   d The person is protected from injury.

11 A person has multiple sclerosis. Which is *false?*

   a Nerve impulses are sent to and from the brain in a normal manner.

   b Symptoms begin in young adulthood.

   c There is no cure.

   d The person is eventually paralyzed and totally dependent on others for care.

12 Persons with head or spinal cord injuries require

   a Rehabilitation

   b Speech therapy

   c Long-term care

   d Psychiatric care

REVIEW QUESTIONS—cont'd

13 Mr. Young has Ménière's disease. It is important to prevent

a Infection
b Falls
c Constipation
d All of the above

14 Mr. Young has hearing loss. You can do the following *except*

a State the topic of discussion
b Chew gum while talking
c Use short sentences and simple words
d Write out important names and words

15 A person has a speech problem. You should

a Pretend to understand so the person is not embarrassed
b Have the person write out all messages
c Ask the person to repeat or rephrase statements when necessary
d All of the above

16 Mr. Young's hearing aid does not seem to be working. First, you should

a See if it is turned on
b Wash the entire instrument with soap and water
c Have it repaired
d Remove the batteries

17 Mr. Young has a cataract. Which is *true?*

a Surgery is the only treatment.
b There is no cure.
c He will become blind.
d There is pressure in the eye.

18 Mr. Young is not wearing his eyeglasses. They should be

a Soaked in a cleansing solution
b Kept within his reach
c Put in the case and in the top drawer of the bedside stand
d Placed on the overbed table

19 Mr. Goldman is blind. You should do the following *except*

a Identify yourself when you enter the room
b Move equipment and furniture to provide variety
c Explain procedures step by step
d Have him walk behind you

20 You can provide for Mr. Goldman's safety by

a Keeping doors partially open
b Informing him of steps and curbs
c Rearranging furniture
d All of the above

21 A person has emphysema. Which is *false?*

a The person has dyspnea only with activity.
b Cigarette smoking is the most common cause.
c The person will probably breathe easier sitting upright and slightly forward.
d Sputum may contain pus.

22 A person has hypertension. Which complication can occur?

a Stroke
b Heart attack
c Renal failure
d All of the above

23 A person has hypertension. Treatment will probably include the following *except*

a No smoking and regular exercise
b A high-sodium diet
c A low-calorie diet if the person is obese
d Medications to lower the blood pressure

24 A person has angina pectoris. Which is *true?*

a Damage to the heart muscle occurs.
b The pain is described as crushing, stabbing, or squeezing.
c The pain is relieved with rest and nitroglycerin.
d All of the above

REVIEW QUESTIONS—cont'd

25 A person is having a myocardial infarction. You know that
- a The person is having a heart attack
- b This is an emergency situation
- c The person may have a cardiac arrest
- d All of the above

26 A person has heart failure. The following measures have been ordered. Which should you question?
- a Encourage fluids
- b Measure intake and output
- c Measure weight daily
- d Perform range-of-motion exercises

27 A person has cystitis. This is
- a A kidney infection
- b Kidney stones
- c A urinary tract infection
- d An inflammation of the bladder

28 A person has chronic renal failure. Care will include all of the following *except*
- a A diet low in protein, potassium, and sodium
- b Measuring urinary output every hour
- c Measures to prevent pressure ulcers
- d Measuring weight daily

29 Which is not a sign of diabetes mellitus?
- a Increased urine production
- b Weight gain
- c Hunger
- d Increased thirst

30 Martha Powers has diabetes. She needs all of the following *except*
- a Her meals served on time
- b Good foot care
- c Oral insulin
- d Diet therapy

31 Vomiting is dangerous because of
- a Aspiration
- b Cardiac arrest
- c Fluid loss
- d Stroke

32 AIDS and hepatitis require
- a Airborne Precautions
- b Droplet Precautions
- c Standard Precautions
- d Contact Precautions

REVIEW QUESTIONS—cont'd

33 AIDS is usually spread by contact with infected
   a Blood
   b Urine
   c Tears
   d Saliva

34 These statements are about HIV and AIDS. Which is *false?*
   a Standard Precautions are practiced and the Blood Pathogen Standard is followed.
   b There may be signs and symptoms of central nervous system damage.
   c The person is at risk for infection.
   d The person always shows some signs and symptoms.

35 Which statement is *false?*
   a STDs are usually spread by sexual contact.
   b STDs can affect the genital area and other parts of the body.
   c Signs and symptoms of STDs are always obvious.
   d Some STDs result in death.

Answers to these questions are on p. 854.

31
Mental Health Problems

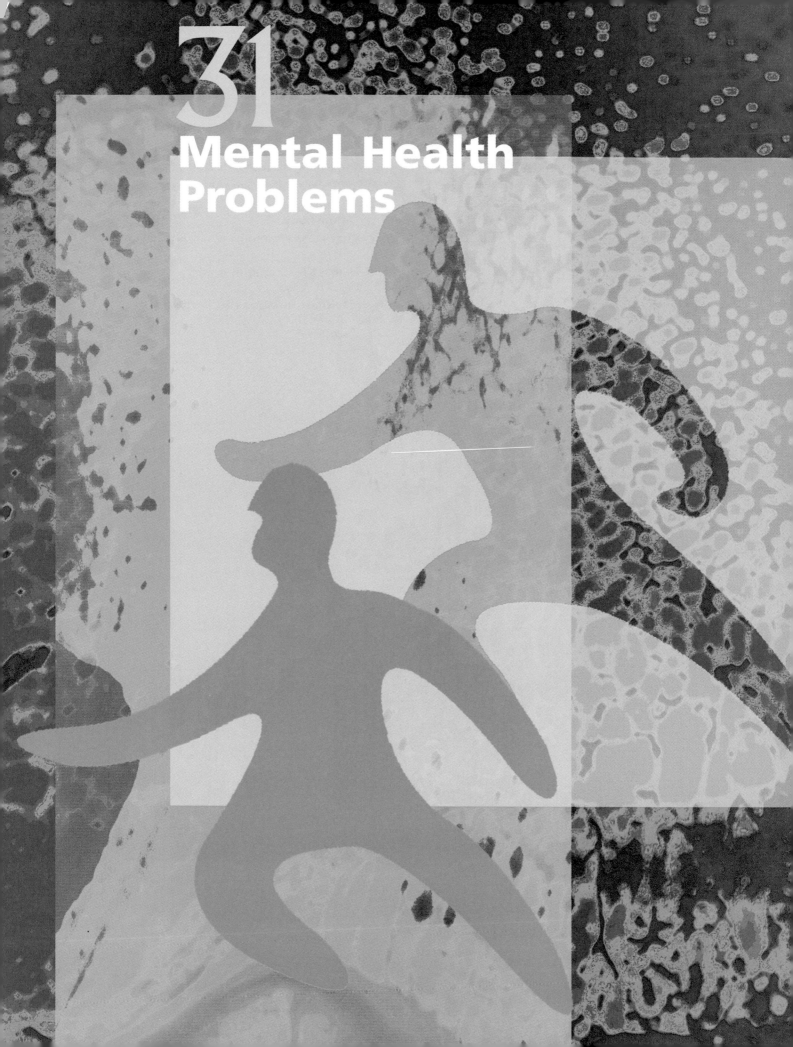

OBJECTIVES

- Define the key terms in this chapter
- Explain the difference between mental health and mental illness
- List the causes of mental illness
- Explain how personality develops
- Describe three levels of awareness
- Describe anxiety and three anxiety disorders
- Understand the defense mechanisms used to relieve anxiety
- Describe common phobias
- Explain schizophrenia
- Describe bipolar disorder and depression
- Describe three personality disorders
- Describe substance abuse, anorexia nervosa, and bulimia
- Describe the care required by a person with a mental health disorder

KEY TERMS

affect Feelings and emotions

anxiety A vague, uneasy feeling that occurs in response to stress

compulsion The uncontrolled performance of an act

conscious Awareness of the environment and experiences; the person knows what is happening and can control thoughts and behaviors

defense mechanism An unconscious reaction that blocks unpleasant or threatening feelings

delusion A false belief

delusion of grandeur An exaggerated belief about one's own importance, wealth, power, or talents

delusion of persecution A false belief that one is being mistreated, abused, or harassed

ego The part of the personality dealing with reality; deals with thoughts, feelings, good sense, and problem solving

emotional illness Mental illness, mental disorder, psychiatric disorder

hallucination Seeing, hearing, or feeling something that is not real

id The part of the personality at the unconscious level; concerned with pleasure

mental Relating to the mind; something that exists in the mind or is performed by the mind

mental disorder Mental illness; emotional illness, psychiatric disorder

mental health A state of mind in which the person copes with and adjusts to the stresses of everyday living in ways acceptable to society

mental illness A disturbance in the person's ability to cope or adjust to stress; behavior and functioning are impaired; mental disorder, emotional illness, psychiatric disorder

obsession A persistent thought or idea

panic An intense and sudden feeling of fear, anxiety, terror, or dread

paranoia A disorder (*para*) of the mind (*noia*); false beliefs (delusions) and suspicion about a person or situation

personality The set of attitudes, values, behaviors, and traits of a particular person

phobia Fear, panic, or dread

psychiatric disorder Mental illness, mental disorder, emotional illness

Key Terms continued on p. 752

psychosis A serious mental disorder; the person does not view or interpret reality correctly

schizophrenia Split *(schizo)* mind *(phrenia)*

stress The response or change in the body caused by any emotional, physical, social, or economic factor

stressor Any emotional, physical, social, or economic factor that causes stress

subconscious Memory, past experiences, and thoughts of which the person is not aware; they can be easily recalled

superego The part of the personality concerned with what is right and wrong

unconscious Experiences and feelings that cannot be remembered

The whole person has physical, social, psychological, and spiritual parts. Each part affects the other. A physical problem has social, mental, and spiritual effects. Likewise, mental health problems affect the person physically, socially, and spiritually. A social problem can have physical, mental health, and spiritual effects.

You will assist the RN in caring for persons who have physical problems. In turn, emotional or mental health problems may develop. Mentally ill persons often have physical problems resulting from mental illness.

BASIC CONCEPTS

Mental health and mental illness are opposites. However, like physical health and illness, there are levels of seriousness. The common cold is at one extreme. The person has chills, fever, and respiratory congestion. At the other extreme is a life-threatening illness. Mental health has the same extremes.

Mental Health

Mental relates to the mind. It is something that exists in the mind or is done by the mind. Therefore mental health involves the mind. Definitions of mental health and mental illness vary among textbooks and cultures. Most definitions include the concept of stress. In this textbook, these definitions are used:

- **Stress**—the response or change in the body caused by any emotional, physical, social, or economic factor.
- **Mental health**—a state of mind in which the person copes with and adjusts to the stresses of everyday living in ways acceptable to society.
- **Mental illness**—a disturbance in the person's ability to cope or adjust to stress. The person's behavior and functioning are impaired. **Mental disorder, emotional illness,** and **psychiatric disorder** also mean mental illness.

Mental health disorders have many causes. Some result when the person cannot cope or adjust to stress. Others are caused by chemical imbalances in the body. Some are genetic in origin. (Genes are found in chromosomes. Characteristics from parents are passed on to children through genes contained in the chromosomes.) Other causes include drug or substance abuse. Social and cultural factors can also lead to mental illness.

Personality

Personality is the set of attitudes, values, behaviors, and traits of a person. Personality development starts at birth. It is affected by many factors. They include genes, culture, environment, parenting, and social experiences.

Maslow's theory of basic needs (see Chapter 5) affects personality development. Lower level needs must be met before higher level needs. Safety and security, love and belonging, esteem, and self-actualization needs cannot be met unless the physical needs are met. A child who grows up hungry, neglected, cold, or abused will not feel safe and secure. Higher level needs cannot be met. Unmet needs at any age affect personality development.

The growth and development tasks presented in Chapter 8 also affect personality development. Remember, there is a sequence, order, and pattern to growth and development. Certain developmental tasks must be accomplished at each stage. Each stage lays the foundation for the next stage.

Sigmund Freud's theory of personality development involves the id, ego, and superego. To understand his theory, you need to understand three levels of awareness:

- **Conscious**—awareness of the environment and experiences. The person knows what is happening and can control thoughts and behavior.
- **Subconscious**—the memory, past experiences, and thoughts of which the person is not aware. Such thoughts, experiences, and memory are easily recalled.
- **Unconscious**—experiences and feelings that cannot be remembered.

The **id** part of the personality is at the unconscious level. The id is concerned with pleasure. The need for pleasure must be satisfied almost right away. The id deals

BOX 31-1

SIGNS AND SYMPTOMS OF ANXIETY

- A "lump" in the throat
- "Butterflies" in the stomach
- Rapid pulse
- Rapid respirations
- Increased blood pressure
- Rapid speech
- Voice changes
- Dry mouth
- Perspiration
- Nausea
- Diarrhea
- Urinary frequency
- Urinary urgency
- Poor attention span
- Difficulty following directions
- Difficulty sleeping
- Loss of appetite

with hunger, comfort, sex, and warmth. People are not aware that they behave and act in ways to satisfy the id.

The **ego** deals with reality—with what is happening in the person's world. Thoughts, feelings, reasoning, good sense, and problem-solving occur in the ego. The ego decides what to do and when.

The **superego** is concerned with right and wrong. Morals and values are in the superego. The superego judges what the ego thinks and does. It is like a parent helping a child look at behaviors.

Anxiety

Anxiety is a vague, uneasy feeling. It is a response to stress. The person may not know the source or cause of the uneasy feeling. The person has a sense of danger or harm. Danger or harm may be real or imagined. Anxiety is usually a normal emotion. The person acts to relieve the unpleasant feeling. Anxiety generally occurs when the person's needs are not met. Anxiety is seen in all mental health disorders.

The many signs and symptoms of anxiety are listed in Box 31-1. They depend on the degree of anxiety. Persons with mental health disorders have higher levels of anxiety.

Anxiety level depends on the stressor. A **stressor** is any emotional, physical, social, or economic factor that causes stress. Past experiences with the same or a similar stressor affect how a person reacts. The number of stressors also affects the person's reaction. A stressor at one time in a person's life may produce only mild anxiety.

The same stressor may produce a higher level of anxiety at another time.

Coping and defense mechanisms are used to relieve anxiety. Common coping mechanisms include eating, drinking, smoking, exercising, talking about the problem, and fighting. Some people play music, go for a walk, take a hot bath, or want to be alone. Some coping mechanisms are healthier than others.

Defense mechanisms are unconscious reactions that block unpleasant or threatening feelings. Defense mechanisms protect the ego. They are used by everyone. Some use of defense mechanisms is normal. They relieve anxiety. Persons with mental health disorders use defense mechanisms poorly. Box 31-2 on p. 754 describes the common defense mechanisms.

MENTAL HEALTH DISORDERS

There are many types of mental health disorders. Some affect thinking; others affect mood. There are anxiety disorders and personality disorders. Substance abuse and eating disorders also are mental health problems. Changes in the brain are another cause. Dementia can occur (see Chapter 32).

Anxiety Disorders

Persons with anxiety disorders have a high degree of anxiety. Signs and symptoms depend on the anxiety level.

Panic disorder

Panic is the highest level of anxiety. **Panic** is an intense and sudden feeling of fear, anxiety, terror, or dread. It occurs suddenly with no obvious reason. The person cannot function and has severe signs and symptoms of anxiety. *Panic attacks* can last for a few minutes or for hours. They can occur several times a week.

Phobic disorders

Phobia means fear, panic, or dread. The person with a phobia has an intense fear of an object or situation. Common phobias are described in Box 31-3 on p. 755.

Obsessive-compulsive disorder

An **obsession** is a persistent thought or idea. The thought or idea may be violent. **Compulsion** is the uncontrolled performance of an act. The person knows the act is wrong but has much anxiety if the act is not done. Some eating disorders are obsessive-compulsive. The person is obsessed with thoughts of food and eats constantly. Constant handwashing because of mysophobia (fear of dirt or contamination) is another act. Some obsessive-compulsive disorders involve violent acts.

BOX 31-2

DEFENSE MECHANISMS

Compensation—to compensate means to make up for, replace, or substitute. Compensation means to make up for or substitute a strength for a weakness.

Example: A boy is not good in sports. But he learns to play the guitar well.

Conversion—to convert means to change. Conversion is when an emotion is expressed or changed into a physical symptom.

Example: A girl knows she will have to read out loud in school today. She does not want to go to school. She complains of a stomach ache.

Denial—to deny means to refuse to accept or believe something that is true or correct. Denial is when the person refuses to face or accept something that is unpleasant or threatening.

Example: A man had a heart attack. He is told to quit smoking and to eat a low-fat diet. He continues to smoke and eat fatty foods.

Displacement—to displace means to move or take the place of. Displacement is when an individual moves behaviors or emotions from one person, place, or thing to another person, place, or thing. The behavior or emotion is directed at a safe person, place, or thing.

Example: You are angry with your supervisor. Instead of yelling at your supervisor, you yell at a friend.

Identification—to identify means to relate or recognize. Identification is when a person assumes the ideas, behaviors, and traits of another person.

Example: A little girl admires her neighbor who is a high school cheerleader. The little girl practices cheerleading in her back yard.

Projection—to project means to blame or assign responsibility to another. Projection is blaming another person or object for one's own unacceptable behavior, emotions, ideas, or wishes.

Example: Two girls are in the same class. One fails a test. She blames the other girl for not helping her study.

Rationalization—to rationalize means to give some acceptable reason or excuse for one's behavior or actions. The real reason is not given. Rational means sensible, reasonable, or logical.

Example: A student does not study for a test and gets a poor grade. She says that the teacher is too hard and doesn't like her.

Reaction formation—a person acts in a way that is opposite to what he or she truly feels.
Example: A man does not like his boss. He buys the boss an expensive gift for Christmas.

Regression—to regress means to move back or to retreat. Regression means to retreat or move back to an earlier time or condition.

Example: A 3-year-old wants to drink from a baby bottle when a new baby comes into the family.

Repression—to repress means to hold down or keep back. Repression is keeping unpleasant or painful thoughts or experiences from the conscious mind. Such thoughts and experiences are in the unconscious mind and cannot be recalled or remembered.

Example: A little girl was sexually abused by her father. She is now 33 years old and has no memory of the event.

BOX 31-3

COMMON PHOBIAS

Agoraphobia—*agora* means marketplace. *Fear of being in an open, crowded, or public place.*

Algophobia—*algo* means pain. *Fear of being in pain or seeing others in pain.*

Aquaphobia—*aqua* means water. *Fear of water.*

Claustrophobia—*claustro* means closing. *Fear of being in or being trapped in an enclosed or narrow space.*

Gynephobia—*gyne* means woman. *Fear of women.*

Laliophobia—*lalio* means to talk or babble. *Fear of talking because of the fear of stuttering.*

Mysophobia—*myso* means anything that is disgusting. *Fear of the slightest uncleanliness; fear of dirt or contamination.*

Nyctophobia—*nycto* means night or darkness. *Fear of night or darkness.*

Photophobia—*photo* pertains to light. *Fear of light with the need to avoid light places.*

Pyrophobia—*pyro* means fire. *Fear of fire.*

Xenophobia—*xeno* means strange. *Fear of strangers.*

Schizophrenia

Schizophrenia means split *(schizo)* mind *(phrenia)*. You need to know the following terms to understand schizophrenia:

- **Psychosis** means a serious mental disorder. The person does not view or interpret reality correctly.
- **Delusion** is a false belief. A person believes he or she is God, a movie star, or some other person.
- **Hallucination** is seeing, hearing, or feeling something that is not real. A person may see animals, insects, or people that are not present.
- **Paranoia** means a disorder *(para)* of the mind *(noia)*. The person has false beliefs (delusions) and is suspicious about a person or situation. For example, the person believes his or her food and drinks are poisoned.
- **Delusion of grandeur** is an exaggerated belief about one's own importance, wealth, power, or talents. For example, a man believes he is Superman or a woman believes she is the Queen of England.
- **Delusion of persecution** is the false belief that one is being mistreated, abused, or harassed. For example, a person believes that someone is "out to get" him or her.

The person with schizophrenia has a disorder of the mind (psychosis). Thinking and behavior are disturbed. The person has delusions (false beliefs) and hallucinations (seeing, hearing, or feeling things that are not real). The person has difficulty relating to others and may be paranoid (suspicion about a person or situation). The person's responses are inappropriate. Communication is disturbed. The person may ramble or repeat what another says. Sometimes speech cannot be understood. The person may withdraw from others and the world. That is, the person lacks interest in others and is not involved with people or society. The person may sit for hours alone without moving, speaking, or responding. Some persons *regress*. To regress means to retreat or move back to an earlier time or condition. For example, it is normal for a 5-year-old to regress back to bedwetting when a new baby comes into the family. It is not normal for an adult to have the behaviors of an infant or child. However, that is often seen in schizophrenia.

Affective Disorders

Affect relates to feelings and emotions. Affective disorders involve feelings, emotions, and moods. There are two major affective disorders.

Bipolar disorder

Bipolar means two *(bi)* poles or ends *(polar)*. The person with bipolar disorder has extreme mood swings. Depression is at one extreme. Mania (elation) is at the other extreme. The person may:

- Be more depressed than manic
- Be more manic than depressed
- Alternate between depression and mania

When depressed, the person is very sad and feels lonely, worthless, empty, and hopeless. Self-esteem is low. The person may think about suicide.

In the manic phase, the person is excited, has much energy, and is very busy. The person cannot sleep and does not take time to eat or tend to self-care needs. Delusions of grandeur are common.

Major depression

The person is very unhappy, lacks motivation, and feels unwanted. These feelings are extreme. Problems with concentration occur. Body functions are depressed. Sleeping problems and inactivity are common. Constipation can occur.

Personality Disorders

The individual with a personality disorder has rigid, inflexible, and maladaptive behaviors. To *adapt* means to change or adjust. *Mal* means bad, wrong, or ill. *Maladaptive* means to change or adjust in the wrong way. Because of their behaviors, individuals with personality disorders cannot function well in society. Personality disorders include:

- *Abusive personality*—the person copes with anxiety by abusing others. Behavior may be violent.
- *Paranoid personality*—the person is very suspicious. There is distrust of others.
- *Antisocial personality*—the person has poor judgment, lacks responsibility, and is hostile. The person has no loyalty to any person or group. Morals and ethics are lacking. The person blames others for actions and behaviors. The rights of others are not considered. The person has no guilt and does not learn from past experiences or punishment. The person is often in trouble with law enforcement authorities.

Substance Abuse

Substance abuse occurs when a person physically or psychologically depends on drugs or alcohol. Alcohol is abused more than any other drug or substance. Both legal and illegal drugs are abused. Legal drugs are approved for use in the United States. Doctors prescribe them. Illegal drugs are not approved for use. They are obtained through illegal means. Commonly abused drugs are listed in Box 31-4. Abused substances affect the central nervous system. Some have a depressing effect. Others stimulate the nervous system. All affect the mind and thinking.

Eating Disorders

Eating disorders involve disturbances in eating behaviors. The two common eating disorders are anorexia nervosa and bulimia.

Anorexia nervosa

Anorexia means no *(a)* appetite *(orexis)*. *Nervosa* relates to *nerves* or *emotions*. Anorexia nervosa occurs when a person has an abnormal fear of weight gain and obesity. The person refuses to eat. The disorder is most common in adolescent girls. The person believes she is fat despite body weight and appearance. She has a poor self-image. Sleep problems, depression, and amenorrhea occur. *Amenorrhea* means lack of *(a)* monthly *(meno)* flow *(rrhea)*. In other words, she stops having monthly menstrual periods. There also may be suicidal thoughts. The person with anorexia nervosa is severely emaciated (Fig. 31-1). *Emaciation* means extreme leanness from disease or poor nutrition.

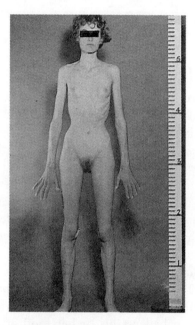

Fig. 31-1 *Emaciation from anorexia nervosa.* (*From Forbes CD, Jackson WF:* A color atlas and text of clinical medicine, *London, 1993, Mosby.*)

BOX 31-4

COMMONLY ABUSED SUBSTANCES

Narcotics
- Heroin (Horse; Smack)
- Morphine (Duramorph; MS-Contin; Roxanol; Oramorph SR)
- Codeine (Tylenol with Codeine; Empirin with Codeine; Robitussin A-C; Fiorinal with Codeine; APAP with Codeine)
- Hydrocodone (Tussionex; Vicodin; Hycodan; Lorcet)
- Hydromorphone (Dilaudid)
- Oxycodone (Percodan; Percocet; Tylox; Roxicet; Roxicodone)
- Methadone (Dolophine; Methadose)
- Fentanyl (Innovar, Sublimaze, Alfenta, Sufenta; Duragesic)
- Other narcotics (Opium, Darvon, Demerol)

Depressants
- Chloral Hydrate (Noctec; Somnox; Felsules)
- Barbiturates (Amytal; Fiorinal; Nembutal; Seconal; Tuinal; Phenobarbital; Pentobarbital)
- Benzodiazepines (Ativan; Dalmane; Diazepam; Librium; Xanax; Serax; Valium; Tranxene; Verstran; Versed; Halcion; Paxipam; Restoril)
- Glutethimide (Doriden)
- Other depressants (Equanil; Miltown; Noludar; Placidyl; Valmid)

Stimulants
- Cocaine (Coke, Flake, Snow, Crack)
- Amphetamine/Methamphetamine (Biphetamine; Desoxyn; Dexedrine; Obetrol; Ice)
- Methylphenidate (Ritalin)
- Other stimulants (Adipex; Didrex; Ionamin; Melfiat; Plegine; Captagon; Sanorex; Tenuate; Tepanil; Prelu-2; Preludin)

Cannabis
- Marijuana (Pot; Acapulco Gold; Grass; Reefer; Sinsemilla; Thai Sticks)
- Tetrahydrocannabinol (THC; Marinol)
- Hashish and hashish oil (Hash; Hash Oil)

Hallucinogens
- LSD (Acid; Microdot)
- Mescaline and Peyote (Mescal; Buttons, Cactus)
- Amphetamine variants (2,5-DMA; STP; MDA; MDMA; Ecstacy; DOM; DOB)
- Phencyclidine (PCE; PCPy; TCP; PCP; Hog; Loveboat; Angel Dust)
- Other Hallucinogens (Bufotenin; Ibogaine; DMT; DET; Psilocybin; Psilocyn)

Anabolic Steroids
- Testosterone (Depo-Testosterone; Delatestryl)
- Nandrolene (Nortestosterone; Durabolin; Deca-Durobolin; Deca)
- Oxymetholone (Anadrol-50)

Modified from U.S. Department of Justice, Drug Enforcement Agency.

Bulimia

Bulimia comes from the Greek words that mean ox *(bous)* and hunger *(limos)*. The person with bulimia craves food. Constant eating or binge eating can occur. After eating, the person induces vomiting. That is, the body is purged (rid) of the food eaten. Some persons with bulimia take diuretics. Diuretics cause the kidneys to produce large amounts of urine. Extra fluid in the body is lost. This results in weight loss. Laxative abuse may occur. Laxatives are drugs that rid the intestines of feces through defecation.

CARE OF PERSONS WITH MENTAL HEALTH DISORDERS

Treatment of mental health disorders involves having the person explore his or her thoughts and feelings. This is done through psychotherapy, group therapy, occupational therapy, art therapy, and family therapy. Often drugs are ordered for anxiety or depression.

The RN uses the nursing process to meet the person's needs. The needs of the total person must be met. This includes the person's physical, safety and security, and emotional needs.

Communication is important. You need to review p. 56 in Chapter 4 and pp. 96-102 in Chapter 6. Be alert to nonverbal communication. This includes the person's nonverbal communication and your own.

REVIEW QUESTIONS

Circle the best answer.

1 Patty has a mental health problem. The doctor says that she is under stress. Stress is

  a The way she copes with and adjusts to everyday living

  b A response or change in the body caused by some factor

  c A mental or emotional disorder

  d A thought or idea

2 The doctor asks Patty's parents about her personality development. Personality is

  a The id and the ego

  b A person's attitudes, values, behaviors, and traits

  c The coping and defense mechanisms used by a person

  d All of the above

3 The doctor says that Patty has many unpleasant experiences in her subconscious. You know that Patty

  a Can remember those experiences

  b Cannot remember those experiences

  c Is aware of those experiences

  d Is projecting those experiences to others

4 Which part of Patty's personality is concerned with right and wrong?

  a The id

  b The ego

  c The superego

  d The conscious

5 Patty uses defense mechanisms. Defense mechanisms are used to

  a Blame others

  b Make excuses for behavior

  c Return to an earlier time

  d Block unpleasant feelings

6 These statements are about defense mechanisms. Which is *false?*

  a Mentally healthy persons do not use defense mechanisms.

  b Defense mechanisms protect the ego.

  c Defense mechanisms relieve anxiety.

  d All of the above

7 Patty also has phobias. A phobia is

  a A serious mental disorder

  b A false belief

  c An intense fear of an object or situation

  d Feelings and emotions

8 Patty believes she is married to a rock singer. She is constantly trying to telephone him. This behavior is a

  a Delusion

  b Hallucination

  c Compulsion

  d Obsession

9 Patty's belief that she is married to a rock singer is called a

  a Fantasy

  b Delusion of grandeur

  c Delusion of persecution

  d Hallucination

10 Patty believes that her parents are against her marriage. This belief is called a

  a Fantasy

  b Delusion of grandeur

  c Delusion of persecution

  d Hallucination

11 Patty's roommate has bipolar disorder. This means that the person

  a Is very suspicious

  b Has poor judgment, lacks responsibility, and is hostile

  c Is very unhappy and feels unwanted

  d Has severe mood swings

12 A person has an abusive personality. You know that the person

  a Abuses drugs or alcohol

  b Has an eating disorder

  c Has bulimia

  d May have violent behavior

Answers to these questions are on p. 854.

32
Confusion and Dementia

- Define the key terms in this chapter
- Describe confusion and its causes
- List the measures that help confused persons
- Explain the difference between delirium, depression, and dementia
- Describe Alzheimer's disease
- Describe the signs, symptoms, and behaviors associated with Alzheimer's disease
- Explain the care required by persons with Alzheimer's disease
- Describe the effects of Alzheimer's disease on the family

KEY TERMS

delirium A state of temporary but acute mental confusion that comes on suddenly

delusion A false belief

dementia An illness that affects memory, thinking, and behavior and is caused by changes in the brain

hallucination Seeing, hearing, or feeling something that is not real

pseudodementia False *(pseudo)* disorder of the mind *(dementia)*

sundowning Increased signs, symptoms, and behaviors of Alzheimer's disease during hours of darkness

Some changes in the brain and nervous system occur normally with aging (Box 32-1, p. 762). Certain diseases also can cause changes in the brain. No matter the cause, changes in the brain can affect the person's cognitive function. (*Cognitive* relates to knowledge.) Cognitive functioning relates to memory, thinking, reasoning, ability to understand, judgment, and behavior.

CONFUSION

Confusion has many causes. Diseases, infections, losses of hearing and sight, and drug reactions are major causes. Brain injury and changes from aging are other causes. With aging, there is reduced blood supply to the brain and progressive loss of brain cells. Sometimes personality and mental changes result. Memory and judgment are lost. The person may not know people, the time, or the place. Gradual loss in the ability to perform activities of daily living is common. So are behavior changes. Anger, restlessness, depression, and irritability may occur.

Acute confusion (delirium) occurs suddenly. It is usually caused by infection, illness, injury, or medications. It can occur postoperatively. Treatment is aimed at the cause of the confusion. Usually acute confusion is temporary.

Confusion caused by physical changes cannot be cured. Some measures help to improve the person's functioning (Box 32-2, p. 762). The person's physical and safety needs must be met.

DEMENTIA

Dementia is a condition affecting memory, thinking, and behavior. It is caused by changes in the brain. The prefix *de* means *off of, out of,* or *from. Mentia* comes from the Latin word for *mind.* Common signs and symptoms are anxiety, personality changes, and difficulty learning. Alzheimer's disease is the most common type of dementia. Other types and causes of dementia are listed in Box 32-3 on p. 763.

Persons with signs and symptoms of dementia need to see a doctor. To determine the cause and type of problem, the doctor orders many tests. Treatment depends on the cause and problem. Some dementias can be reversed. When the cause is removed, so are the signs and symptoms of dementia. Treatable causes include:

- Drugs
- Alcohol
- Delirium
- Depression

BOX 32-1

CHANGES IN THE NERVOUS SYSTEM FROM AGING

- Loss of brain cells
- Slower nerve conduction
- Slower response and reaction times
- Slower reflexes
- Decreased vision and hearing
- Decreased senses of taste and smell
- Reduced sense of touch and sensitivity to pain
- Reduced blood flow to the brain
- Changes in sleep patterns
- Shorter memory
- Forgetfulness
- Confusion
- Dizziness

- Tumors
- Heart, lung, and blood vessel problems
- Head injuries
- Infection
- Vision and hearing problems

Permanent dementias result from changes in the brain. Parkinson's disease and cerebrovascular disease cause permanent changes in the brain. Multi-infarct dementia (MID) is caused by many *(multi)* strokes. The stroke leaves an area of brain damage called an *infarct*. Alzheimer's disease is the most common type of permanent dementia.

Pseudodementia means false *(pseudo)* dementia. The person has the signs and symptoms of dementia. However, changes in the brain do not occur. This can occur with delirium and depression.

BOX 32-2

CARING FOR THE CONFUSED PERSON

- Follow the person's care plan to meet basic needs.
- Provide for the person's safety.
- Face the person, and speak clearly and slowly.
- Call the person by name every time you are in contact with him or her.
- State your name, and show your name tag.
- Tell the person the date and time each morning. Repeat the information as often as necessary during the day or evening.
- Explain what you are going to do and why.
- Give clear and simple answers to questions.
- Ask clear and simple questions. Allow enough time for the person to respond.
- Give short, simple instructions.
- Keep calendars and clocks with large numbers in the person's room and in nursing areas (Fig. 32-1).
- Encourage the person to wear glasses and a hearing aid if needed.
- Use touch to communicate (see Chapter 6).
- Allow the person to place familiar objects and pictures within view.
- Provide newspapers and magazines. Read to the person if appropriate.
- Discuss current events with the person.
- Provide access to television and radios.
- Maintain the day-night cycle. Open curtains, shades, and drapes during the day, and close them at night. Use a night-light at night. Encourage the person to wear regular clothes during the day rather than gowns or pajamas.
- Maintain a calm, relaxed, and peaceful atmosphere. Prevent loud noises, rushing, and congested hallways and dining rooms.
- Maintain the person's routine. Meals, bathing, exercise, television programs, and other activities are on a schedule. This promotes a sense of order and anticipation of what to expect.
- Do not rearrange furniture or the person's belongings.
- Encourage the person to participate in self-care activities.
- Be consistent.
- Remind the person of holidays, birthdays, and other special events.

BOX 32-3

TYPES AND CAUSES OF DEMENTIA

- Alcoholism—alcohol depresses the brain
- AIDS-related dementia—see Chapter 30
- Brain tumors—see Chapter 30
- Cerebrovascular disease—diseased blood vessels *(vascular)* in the brain *(cerebro)*
- Delirium—a temporary state of acute confusion
- Depression—see text on this page
- Drugs—some drugs affect how the brain functions
- Huntington's disease—a nervous system disease
- Infection—see Chapter 11
- Multi-infarct dementia—many *(multi)* strokes leave areas of brain damage *(infarct)*
- Multiple sclerosis—see Chapter 30
- Parkinson's disease—see Chapter 30
- Stroke—see Chapter 30
- Syphilis—see Chapter 30
- Trauma and head injury—see Chapter 30

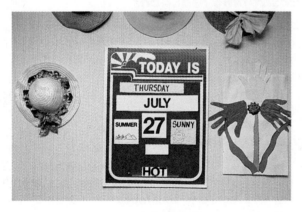

Fig. 32-1 *A large calendar is within the person's view.*

Delirium and Depression

Delirium and depression can be mistaken for dementia. They can occur alone or with dementia. Or the person with dementia can also suffer from delirium and depression.

Delirium

Delirium is a state of temporary but acute mental confusion. It comes on suddenly. Delirium is common in older persons with acute or chronic illnesses. Infections, heart and lung diseases, poor nutrition, and hormone disorders are common causes. Hypoglycemia is also a cause (see Chapter 30). Alcohol can cause delirium. So can many types of drugs. Delirium is an emergency. The cause must be identified and treated. Signs and symptoms of delirium include:

- Anxiety
- Disorientation
- Tremors
- Hallucinations (see p. 755)
- Delusions (see p. 755)
- Disturbances in attention
- Decline in level of consciousness

Depression

Depression is the most common mental health problem in older persons. It is often overlooked when the person has physical problems. A correct diagnosis is important. Otherwise the person does not receive proper treatment. The person and family both experience unnecessary emotional, physical, social, and financial discomfort.

Some signs and symptoms of depression are also signs of aging. They also are the side effects of some drugs. Signs and symptoms of depression include:

- Sadness
- Inactivity
- Difficulty thinking
- Problems concentrating
- Feelings of despair
- Problems sleeping
- Changes in appetite
- Fatigue
- Agitation

ALZHEIMER'S DISEASE

Alzheimer's disease (AD) is a brain disease. Brain cells that control intellectual function are damaged. Memory, thinking, judgment, and behavior are affected. Mood and personality changes are seen. The person has difficulty with work and everyday functions. The person also has problems with family and social relationships.

Gradual in onset, the disease progresses over 3 to 20 years. It gets worse and worse. AD occurs in both men and women. Though more common in older persons, it also occurs in younger people. Some people in their 40s and 50s have AD. The risk increases after the age of 65. The cause is unknown. However, a family history of AD and Down syndrome are risk factors. (Down syndrome is a congenital disease [congenital means to be born with]. The child has mental retardation and many physical defects.)

Signs of AD

According to the Agency for Health Care Policy and Research, the classic sign of AD is gradual loss of short-term memory. Other early signs include:

- Problems finding or speaking the right word
- Not recognizing objects
- Forgetting how to use simple, everyday things (like using a pencil)
- Forgetting to turn off the stove, close windows, or lock doors
- Mood and personality changes
- Agitation
- Poor judgment

AD affects the person's ability to perform complex and simple tasks. Problems with complex tasks appear first. The person has problems using the telephone, driving a car, managing money, planning meals, and working. As the disease progresses, problems occur with simple tasks. The person has problems with bathing, dressing, eating, using the toilet, and walking.

Stages of AD

The stages of AD are described in Box 32-4. Signs and symptoms are more severe with each stage. The following problems are common. The disease ends in death.

Wandering

Persons with AD are disoriented to person, time, and place. They may wander from home or the agency and not find their way back. They may be with caregivers one moment and gone the next. Judgment is poor. They cannot tell what is safe or dangerous. They are in danger of accidents. A person may walk into traffic or into a nearby river, lake, or forest. If they are not properly dressed, exposure is a risk in cold climates.

Sundowning

Sundowning occurs in the late afternoon and evening hours. As daylight ends and darkness occurs, confusion, restlessness, and other symptoms increase. Behavior is worse after the sun goes down. Sundowning may relate to fatigue or hunger. Inadequate light may cause the person to see things that are not there. Persons with AD may be afraid of the dark.

Hallucinations

An hallucination is seeing, hearing, or feeling something that is not really there. Senses are dulled. Affected persons see animals, insects, or people that are not present. Some hear voices. They may feel bugs crawling on their bodies or feel that they are being touched.

Delusions

Delusions are false beliefs. People with AD may think they are God, a movie star, or some other person. Some believe they are in jail, are going to be murdered, or are being attacked. A person may believe that the caregiver is actually someone else. Many other false beliefs can occur.

Catastrophic reactions

Catastrophic reactions are extreme responses. The person reacts as if a disaster or tragedy has occurred. The person may scream, cry, or be agitated or combative. These reactions often occur when there is too much stimuli at one time. Eating, music or television playing, and being asked questions all at one time can overwhelm the person.

Agitation and restlessness

The agitated and restless person may pace, hit, or yell. Such behaviors may be the result of pain or discomfort, anxiety, lack of sleep, too much or too little stimuli, hunger, or the need to eliminate. A calm, quiet setting and meeting basic needs help calm the person.

Caregivers can cause agitation and restlessness. A caregiver may rush the person or be impatient. Or a caregiver's communication may give mixed verbal and nonverbal messages. Caregivers always need to look at how their behaviors affect other persons.

Aggression and combativeness

Aggressive and combative behaviors occur in some persons. They may result from agitation and restlessness. Examples include hitting, pinching, grabbing, biting, or

BOX 32-4

STAGES OF ALZHEIMER'S DISEASE

Stage 1

- Memory loss—forgetfulness; forgets recent events
- Difficulty finding words, finishing thoughts, following directions, and remembering names
- Poor judgment; bad decisions (including when driving motor vehicle)
- Disoriented to time and place
- Lack of spontaneity—less outgoing or interested in things
- Blames others for mistakes, forgetfulness, and other problems
- Moodiness
- Difficulty performing everyday tasks

Stage 2

- Restlessness; increases during the evening hours
- Sleep disturbances
- Memory loss increases—may not know family and friends
- Dulled senses—cannot tell the difference between hot and cold; cannot recognize dangers
- Bowel and bladder incontinence
- Needs assistance with activities of daily living—problems with bathing, feeding, and dressing self; afraid of bathing; will not change clothes
- Loses impulse control—may use foul language, have poor table manners, be sexually aggressive, or be rude
- Movement and gait disturbances—walks slowly; has a shuffling gait
- Communication problems—cannot follow directions; has problems with reading, writing, and math; speaks in short sentences or single words; statements may not make sense
- Repeats motions and statements—may move things back and forth constantly; may say the same thing over and over again
- Agitation—behavior may be violent

Stage 3

- Seizures (see Chapter 35)
- Cannot communicate—may groan, grunt, or scream
- Does not recognize self or family members
- Depends totally on others for all activities of daily living
- Disoriented to person, time, and place
- Totally incontinent of urine and feces
- Cannot swallow—choking and aspiration are risks
- Sleep disturbances increase
- Becomes bed bound—cannot sit or walk
- Coma
- Death

swearing. Such behaviors are frightening to caregivers, to others in the home, or to patients and residents. Sometimes aggressive and combative behaviors are part of the person's personality.

Screaming

Persons with AD have communication problems. At first the person has difficulty finding the right words. As the AD progresses, the person may speak only short sentences or one word. Often the person's speech is not understandable.

The person may scream to communicate. Screaming is seen in persons who are very confused and have poor communication skills. The person may scream a word or a name. Or the person may just make screaming sounds.

Screaming has many causes. Possible causes include hearing and vision problems, pain or discomfort, fear, and fatigue. Too much or not enough stimulation can cause the person to scream. Sometimes the person reacts to a caregiver or family member by screaming.

A calm, quiet setting is helpful. Soft music can calm the person. If it is safe for the person to have them, make sure hearing aids and eyeglasses are worn. Sometimes the person is comforted by a family member. Many patients have favorite caregivers. That person may be able to calm the person. If the person responds to touch, use touch to calm him or her.

Abnormal Sexual Behaviors

Sexual behaviors are labeled abnormal because of how and when they occur. Remember, persons with AD are disoriented to person, time, and place. Therefore sexual behaviors may involve the wrong person, the wrong place, and the wrong time. They also have lost the ability to control behavior. Normally they would know not to undress or expose themselves in front of others. They would know not to masturbate or engage in sexual pleasures in public. Normally they would know their sexual partners. Persons with AD often mistake a sexual partner for someone else. The person kisses and hugs the other person.

Sexual behaviors may mean that the person's sexual needs are not being met. Touching, scratching, and rubbing the genitals can signal infection, pain, or discomfort involving the urinary or reproductive systems. Poor hygiene is another cause. So is being wet or soiled from urine or feces.

The RN encourages the person's sexual partner to show affection. The couple's normal practices are encouraged. Examples include hand holding, hugging, kissing, and touching. When a person masturbates in public, lead the person to his or her room. Provide privacy, and make sure the person is safe. Good hygiene is important to prevent itching. If the person urinates or has a bowel movement, make sure the person is cleaned quickly and thoroughly. Do not let the person stay wet or soiled.

The RN needs to assess the person for urinary or reproductive system problems. The doctor is contacted as necessary.

Repetitive Behaviors

Repetitive means to repeat over and over again. Persons with AD repeat the same motions over and over again. For example, the person folds the same napkin over and over. Or the person says the same words or asks the same question over and over. Such behaviors are usually harmless. They do not hurt the person. However, they can annoy the caregivers and the family.

The person is allowed to continue harmless acts. Music and TV can distract the person. Taking the person for a walk can help. Such measures also are useful when the person repeats words or questions.

Care of the Person With AD

Alzheimer's disease is frustrating to the person, family, and caregivers. Usually the person is cared for at home until symptoms are severe. Adult day care may help. Care in a nursing center often is required. The person may develop other illnesses and need hospital care. Thus you may care for a person with AD in an adult day care setting or in a hospital, nursing center, or private home. The person needs your support and understanding. So does the family.

Remember, people with AD do not choose to be forgetful, incontinent, agitated, or rude. Nor do they choose to have all of the other behaviors, signs, and symptoms of the disease. They have no control over what is happening to them. The disease causes the behaviors. Thus when the person does something that a healthy individual would not do, remember that the disease is responsible, not the person.

The RN uses the nursing process to plan measures to meet the person's specific needs. The person's safety, personal hygiene, nutrition and fluids, elimination, and activity needs must be met. So must the need for comfort and sleep. Many of the measures listed in Box 32-5 will be part of the person's care plan.

Your observations are important. The person can develop other health problems. Injuries can occur. However, the person may not know there is pain, fever, constipation, incontinence, or other signs and symptoms. You need to carefully observe the person. Report any change in the person's usual behavior to the RN.

Infection is a major risk in persons with AD. Remember, the person's ability to give full attention to activities

Text continued on p. 770

BOX 32-5

CARE OF THE PERSON WITH ALZHEIMER'S DISEASE

Environment

- Follow established routines.
- Avoid changing rooms or roommates.
- Place picture signs on rooms, bathrooms, dining rooms, and other areas (Fig. 32-2, p. 769).
- Keep personal items where the person can see them.
- Stay within the person's sight to the extent possible.
- Place memory aids (large clocks and calendars) where the person can see them.
- Keep noise levels low.
- Play music and show movies from the person's past.
- Keep tasks and activities simple.

Communication

- Approach the person in a calm, quiet manner.
- Follow the rules of communication described in Chapter 4.
- Practice measures to promote communication (see Chapter 6).
- Provide simple explanations of all procedures and activities.
- Give consistent responses.

Safety

- Remove harmful, sharp, and breakable objects from the environment. This includes knives, scissors, glass, dishes, razors, and tools.
- Provide plastic eating and drinking utensils. This helps prevent breakage and cuts.
- Place safety plugs in electrical outlets.
- Keep cords and electrical equipment out of reach.
- Childproof caps should be on medicine containers and household cleaners.
- Store household cleaners and medicines in locked storage areas.
- Remove knobs from stoves, or place childproof covers on the knobs.
- Remove dangerous appliances and power tools from the home.
- Remove firearms from the home.
- Store keys to the car or other motor vehicle in a safe place.
- Supervise the person who smokes.
- Store cigarettes, cigars, pipes, matches and other smoking materials in a safe place.
- Practice safety measures to prevent falls (see Chapter 10).
- Practice safety measures to prevent fires (see Chapter 10).
- Practice safety measures to prevent burns (see Chapter 10).
- Practice safety measures to prevent poisoning (see Chapter 10).

Wandering

- Make sure doors and windows are securely locked. Locks are often placed at the top and bottom of doors (Fig. 32-3, p. 769). The person is not likely to look for a lock at the top or bottom of the door.
- Make sure door alarms are turned on. The alarm goes off when the door is opened. These are common in nursing centers.
- Make sure the person wears an ID bracelet at all times.
- Exercise the person as ordered. Adequate exercise often reduces wandering.
- Do not restrain the person. Restraints require a doctor's order. They also tend to increase confusion and disorientation.

Continued

BOX 32-5

CARE OF THE PERSON WITH ALZHEIMER'S DISEASE—cont'd

- Do not argue with the person who wants to leave. Remember, the person does not understand what you are saying.
- Go with the person who insists on going outside. Make sure he or she is properly dressed. Guide the person inside after a few minutes (Fig. 32-4, p. 769).
- Let the person wander in enclosed areas if provided. Many nursing centers have enclosed areas where residents can walk about (Fig. 32-5, p. 769). These areas provide a safe place for the person to wander.

Sundowning
- Provide a calm, quiet setting late in the day. Treatments and activities should be done early in the day.
- Do not restrain the person.
- Encourage exercise and activity early in the day.
- Make sure the person has eaten. Hunger can increase restlessness.
- Promote urinary and bowel elimination. A full bladder or constipation can increase restlessness.
- Do not try to reason with the person. Remember, he or she cannot understand what you are saying.
- Do not ask the person to tell you what is bothering him or her. The person's ability to communicate is impaired. He or she does not understand what you are asking. The person cannot think or speak clearly.

Hallucinations and Delusions
- Do not argue with the person. He or she does not understand what you are saying.
- Reassure the person. Tell him or her that you will provide protection from harm.
- Distract the person with some item or activity.
- Use touch to calm and reassure the person (Fig. 32-6, p. 769).

Basic Needs
- Provide for the person's food and fluid needs (see Chapter 19). Provide finger foods. Cut food and pour liquids as needed.
- Provide good skin care (see Chapter 14). Keep the person's skin free of urine and feces.
- Promote urinary and bowel elimination (see Chapters 17 and 18).
- Promote exercise and activity during the day (see Chapter 22). This helps reduce wandering and sundowning behaviors. The person may also sleep better.
- Reduce the person's intake of coffee, tea, and cola drinks. These contain caffeine. Caffeine is a stimulant. It can increase the person's restlessness, confusion, and agitation.
- Provide a quiet, restful setting (see Chapter 16). Soft music is better in the evening than loud television programs. Play music during care activities such as bathing and during meals.
- Promote personal hygiene (see Chapter 14). Do not force the person into a shower or tub. People with AD are often afraid of bathing. Try bathing the person when he or she is calm. Use the bathing method preferred by the person (tub bath, shower, bed bath). Provide for privacy and keep the person warm. Do not rush the person.
- Provide oral hygiene (see Chapter 14).
- Have equipment ready for any procedure ahead of time. This reduces the amount of time the person is involved in care measures.
- Observe for signs and symptoms of other disorders or diseases (see Chapter 4).
- Protect the person from infection (see Chapter 11).

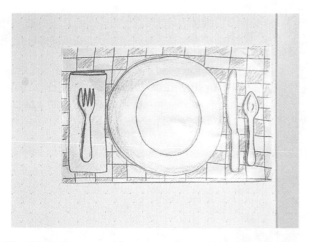

Fig. 32-2 *Signs provide cues to the person with dementia.*

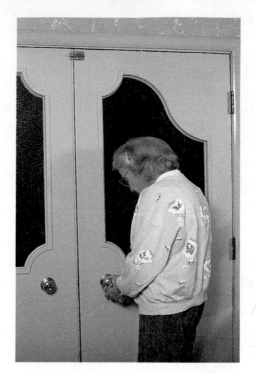

Fig. 32-3 *A slide lock is at the top of the door. The person tries to open the lock on the knob.*

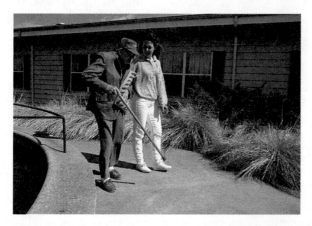

Fig. 32-4 *Walk outside with the person who wanders. Then guide him back inside.*

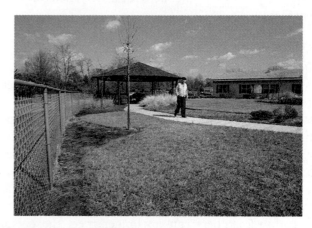

Fig. 32-5 *An enclosed garden allows persons with AD to wander in a safe setting.*

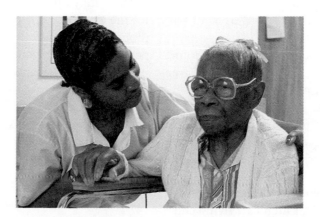

Fig. 32-6 *Use touch to calm a person with Alzheimer's disease.*

of daily living is greatly reduced. Infection can occur from poor hygiene. This includes poor skin care, oral hygiene, and perineal care after bowel and bladder elimination. Inactivity and immobility can lead to pneumonia and pressure ulcers.

Besides the measures listed in Box 32-5, other activities and therapies are ordered. These are intended to make the person feel useful, worthwhile, and active. They help the person's self-esteem. The therapist may work with one person, a small group, or a large group. Therapies and activities focus on the person's strengths and past successes. For example:

- A person used to cook. The person is given the task of cleaning vegetables.
- A person was a good dancer. Activities are planned so the person can dance.
- A person likes to clean. The person helps dust furniture.

Crafts, exercise, meal preparation, and household chores are among the activities planned for the person. All activities are supervised. Sing-alongs, reminiscing, and board games are other activities. (See Focus on Long-Term Care.)

The Family

Persons with AD may live at home or with children or other family members. Care is given by family members in the household. Or arrangements are made for a family member or someone else to stay with the person. Health professionals can help family members cope with the situation or help meet the person's needs. Home health care may help for awhile. Adult day care is another option. The decision for long-term care is usually made when:

- Family members can no longer meet the person's needs
- The person with AD no longer knows the caregiver
- Family members have health problems
- Money problems occur
- The person has behaviors that are dangerous to self or others

Diagnostic tests, doctor's visits, medicines, and home care are costly. Long-term care is even more expensive. The person's medical care can drain family finances.

The family has special needs. Care of the person at home or in a nursing center is stressful. There are physical, emotional, social, and financial stresses. Children find themselves in the *sandwich generation*. They are in the middle—between their own children who need to be taken care of and an ill parent who needs care. The stress of caring for two families is great. Often caregiving children have jobs too.

focus on LONG-TERM CARE

Many long-term care centers have special nursing units for AD residents. The setting is designed to meet the special needs of persons with AD.

focus on HOME CARE

Home care is an option for many families. Sometimes the family needs someone to prepare the patient's meals. Help is often needed with bathing and elimination. The family may need someone to supervise the patient while family members work, do errands, or need time to themselves. The amount and kind of care depends on the patient's needs and the family's ability to provide care.

Caring for loved ones can be exhausting. Caregivers need much support and encouragement. Many join AD support groups. These groups are sponsored by hospitals, nursing centers, and the Alzheimer's Association. The Alzheimer's Association has chapters in cities and towns across the country. Support groups offer encouragement, advice, and ideas about care. Group members share their feelings, anger, frustration, guilt, and other emotions.

The family often feels helpless. No matter what is done for the loved one, the person only gets worse. Much time, money, energy, and emotion are needed to care for the person. Anger and resentment may result. Then the family feels guilty because of their anger and resentment. They know that the person did not choose to develop the disease. The family also knows that the person does not choose to have the signs, symptoms, and behaviors of the disease. They may be frustrated and angry that the loved one can no longer show love or affection. How would you feel if your mother, father, or partner did not recognize you? Sometimes the person's behavior is embarrassing.

LONG-TERM CARE

Quality of life is important for all persons with confusion and dementia. Those in nursing centers have the same rights under the Omnibus Budget Reconciliation Act of 1987 (OBRA) as other residents. Confused and demented residents may not know or be able to exercise their rights. However, the family is aware of the resident's rights. They need to know that their loved one's rights are protected. The family also needs to know that the loved one is treated with respect and dignity.

Confused and demented residents have the right to privacy and confidentiality. You must protect the person from exposure. Only those involved in the person's care are present for care and procedures. The resident is allowed to visit with others in private. When family and friends visit, they are given space for a private visit. Confidentiality is also important. The resident's care and condition are not shared with others.

Even confused and demented residents have the right to personal choice. Some can still make simple choices. For example, a person may be able to choose between wearing a dress or slacks. Choosing to watch or not watch television may be a simple choice. Others cannot make choices themselves. The family may do so. Bath times, menus, clothing, activities, and other aspects of care may be chosen by the family.

The resident has the right to keep and use personal possessions. Some items comfort the resident. A pillow, blanket, afghan, or sweater may be important to the person. The resident may not be able to tell you why or even recognize the item. Still, it is important. Personal items kept by the resident need to be safe. You must also protect the person's property from loss or damage.

Confused and demented residents must be kept free from abuse, mistreatment, and neglect. Caring for these people can be very frustrating. The person's behaviors may be difficult to deal with. Family and staff can become short-tempered and angry. The resident must be protected from abuse (see Chapter 2). Report any signs of abuse to the RN right away. You need to be patient and calm when caring for these residents. Talk with the RN if you find yourself becoming frustrated. Sometimes an assignment change is needed for a while.

All residents have the right to be free from restraints. Remember, restraints require a doctor's order. They are used only when it is the best way to protect the resident. They are not used for staff convenience. Restraints can make confusion and demented behaviors worse. The RN tells you when to use restraints.

Activity and a safe setting promote quality of life. Box 32-5 identifies safety measures for confused and demented residents. These residents also need activities that are safe, calm, and quiet. The recreation therapist and other health team members will find activities that are best for each confused or demented resident. These are part of the person's care plan.

The family has to learn some of the same care measures and procedures that you learn. They need to learn how to bathe, feed, dress, and give oral hygiene to the person. They also need to learn how to provide a safe setting. The RN and support group will help them learn to give necessary care. (See Focus on Home Care on p. 770 and Focus on Long-Term Care above.)

REVIEW QUESTIONS

Circle the best *answer.*

1 You must protect the confused person from
   a Danger
   b Infection
   c Incontinence
   d Constipation

2 Joe Dunn has dementia. Dementia describes
   a A false belief
   b An illness caused by changes in the brain
   c Seeing, hearing, or feeling something that is not real
   d Alzheimer's disease

3 Joe Dunn was diagnosed with AD. Which is *true?*
   a AD occurs only in older persons.
   b Diet and medications can control the disease.
   c AD and delirium are the same.
   d AD ends in death.

4 Which are not signs or symptoms of AD?
   a Memory loss, poor judgment, and sleep disturbances
   b Loss of impulse control and the ability to communicate
   c Wandering or having delusions and hallucinations
   d Delirium and depression

5 Sundowning means that
   a The person becomes sleepy when the sun sets
   b Behaviors become worse in the late afternoon and evening hours
   c Behavior improves at night
   d The person is in the third stage of the disease

6 Joe Dunn is screaming. You know that this is
   a An agitated reaction
   b His way of communicating
   c Caused by a delusion
   d A repetitive behavior

7 AD support groups do the following *except*
   a Provide care
   b Offer encouragement and care ideas
   c Provide support for the family
   d Promote the sharing of feelings and frustrations

8 Joe Dunn tends to wander. You should do the following *except*
   a Make sure doors and windows are locked
   b Make sure he wears an ID bracelet
   c Help him with exercise as ordered
   d Restrain him

REVIEW QUESTIONS—cont'd

9 Safety is important for Joe Dunn. Which is *false?*

   a Safety plugs are placed in electrical outlets.

   b Cleaners and medications should be out of his reach.

   c He can keep smoking materials.

   d Sharp and breakable objects are removed from his environment.

10 You have been assigned to care for Joe Dunn. Which is *false?*

   a It is possible to reason with him.

   b Touch can calm and reassure him.

   c A calm, quiet environment is important.

   d Assistance is needed with activities of daily living.

Answers to these questions are on p. 854.

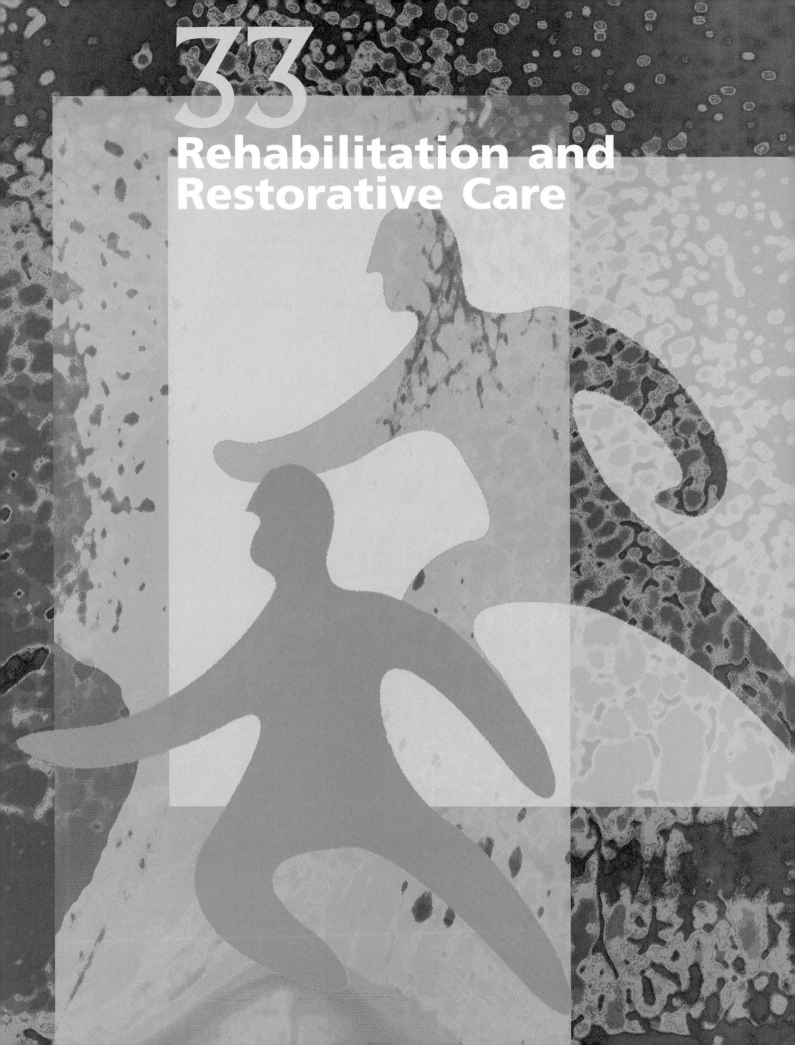

33
Rehabilitation and Restorative Care

- Define the key terms in this chapter
- Describe how rehabilitation involves the whole person
- Identify the complications that are prevented for successful rehabilitation
- Identify how to help disabled persons perform activities of daily living
- Identify the common reactions to rehabilitation
- Describe how rehabilitation can help a person work
- Identify the members of the rehabilitation team
- List the common rehabilitation services
- Explain your responsibilities and how to promote quality of life during the rehabilitation process

activities of daily living (ADL) Self-care activities a person performs daily to remain independent and to function in society

disability Any lost, absent, or impaired physical or mental function

prosthesis An artificial replacement for a missing body part

rehabilitation The process of restoring the person to the highest level of physical, psychological, social, and economic functioning possible; restorative care

restorative care Rehabilitation

Disease, injury, and surgery can result in loss of function or loss of a body part. So can birth injuries and birth defects. Often more than one function is lost. Daily activities such as eating, bathing, dressing, and walking are hard or seem impossible. Some persons cannot work. Others cannot care for children or family.

Disability is any lost, absent, or impaired physical or mental function. It is caused by an acute or chronic illness or problem. An acute problem has a short course. Recovery is complete. A fracture is an acute problem. A chronic problem has a long course. The problem is controlled—not cured—with treatment. Diabetes and coronary artery disease are chronic health problems. Disabilities are short-term or long-term.

Rehabilitation is the process of restoring the person to the highest level of physical, psychological, social, and economic functioning possible. The focus is on improving the person's abilities. For some persons the goal is to return to work. For others, self-care is the goal. Sometimes improvement is not possible. Then the focus is on maintaining the highest level of function possible and preventing further disability. **Restorative care** is another term for rehabilitation. Box 33-1, on p. 776 lists some common health problems that require rehabilitation.

REHABILITATION AND THE WHOLE PERSON

The rehabilitation process involves the whole person. An illness or injury has physical, psychological, and social effects. So does a disability. How would you feel if an illness left you paralyzed from the waist down? Would you be angry, afraid, or depressed? Would you deny it happened? Could you dance, shop, or go to school? Could you attend church services or visit family and friends in their homes? Could you drive a car? Could you return to work? Could you find another job with your remaining skills?

Rehabilitation helps a person adjust to the disability physically, psychologically, socially, and economically. Abilities—what the person can do—are stressed. (See Focus on Children and Focus on Older Persons on p. 776.)

COMMON HEALTH PROBLEMS REQUIRING REHABILITATION

- Alcoholism
- Amputation
- Brain tumor
- Burns
- Cerebral palsy
- Chronic obstructive pulmonary disease
- Head injury
- Myocardial infarction (heart attack)
- Parkinson's disease
- Spinal cord injury
- Spinal cord tumor
- Stroke (brain attack)
- Substance abuse

focus on
CHILDREN

Disabilities in children occur from birth defects or from illness, injury, or surgery. They can affect normal growth and development (see Chapter 8). Factors important for normal growth and development include hand skills, mobility, communication, play, and relationships with parents, family, and peers. A disability can affect one or more of these factors.

focus on
OLDER PERSONS

Rehabilitation often takes longer in older persons than in other age-groups. Changes from aging affect healing, mobility, vision and hearing, and other functions (see Chapter 8). Older persons often have chronic health problems that interfere with or slow recovery. They also are at higher risk for injuries. Many do not have money or insurance coverage for rehabilitation.

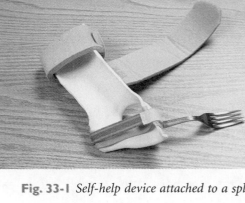

Fig. 33-1 *Self-help device attached to a splint.*

Physical Aspects

Rehabilitation begins when the person seeks health care. It starts with preventing complications. Complications can occur from bedrest or from prolonged illness or recovery. Bowel and bladder problems are prevented. Contractures and pressure ulcers are prevented with good body alignment, turning and repositioning, range-of-motion exercises, and supportive devices (see Chapters 12 and 22). Good skin care also prevents pressure ulcers (see Chapter 14).

Bladder training is described in Chapter 17. The method used depends on the person's problems, abilities, and needs. The RN explains the method planned for the person.

Bowel training is described in Chapter 18. It involves gaining control of bowel movements and developing a regular pattern of elimination. Fecal impaction, constipation, and fecal incontinence are prevented.

Self-care is a major goal. **Activities of daily living (ADL)** refer to self-care activities. ADLs are performed daily by the person to remain independent and to function in society. ADLs include bathing, oral hygiene, eating, bowel and bladder elimination, and moving about. A person's ability to do self-care and the need for self-help devices are evaluated.

Disease, injury, and birth defects can affect the hands, wrists, and arms. Self-help devices often are needed. Special eating devices include glass holders, plate guards, and silverware with curved handles or cuffs (see Fig. 19-5 on p. 454). Some devices attach to a special splint (Fig. 33-1). Electric toothbrushes are helpful for persons who cannot perform the back-and-forth motions needed for brushing teeth. Longer handles are attached to combs, brushes, and sponges. There also are self-help devices for preparing meals, dressing, writing, dialing telephones, and many other tasks (Fig. 33-2).

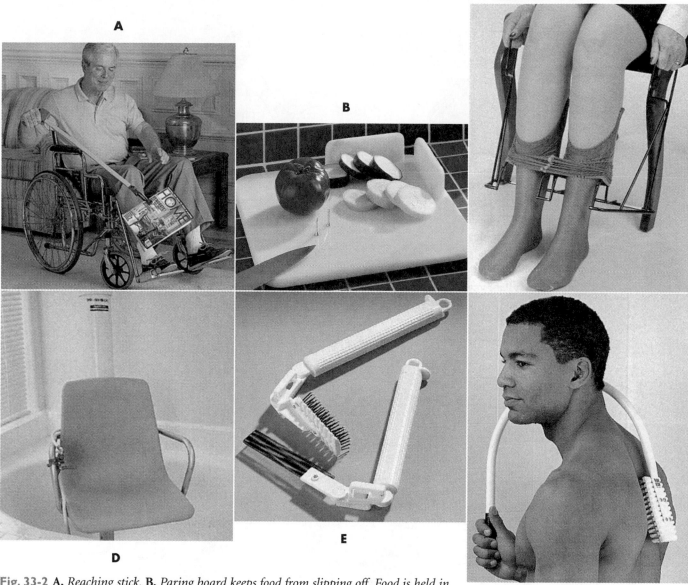

Fig. 33-2 A, *Reaching stick.* **B,** *Paring board keeps food from slipping off. Food is held in place by two prongs in the center of the board.* **C,** *Stocking helper.* **D,** *Bath lift chair swivels for getting into and out of the tub.* **E,** *Comb and brush with extended handles.* **F,** *Shower brush with curved handle. (Courtesy BISSEL Healthcare Corp/Fred Sammons, Inc, Bolingbrook, Ill.)*

Some persons have to learn how to walk with supportive devices. The person is taught to use crutches or a walker, cane, or brace. If both legs are paralyzed or amputated, a wheelchair is used. Persons with hemiplegia also need a wheelchair. If possible, the person learns how to transfer to and from the wheelchair using a transfer board (Fig. 33-3). The person learns to transfer to and from the bed, toilet, bathtub, and sofas and chairs and in and out of cars (Fig. 33-4, pp. 778-779).

Prostheses are helpful for persons with missing body parts. A **prosthesis** is an artificial replacement for a missing body part (see Chapter 30). A person can usually be fitted with an artificial arm or leg. The person learns to use the prosthesis. *Text continued on p. 780*

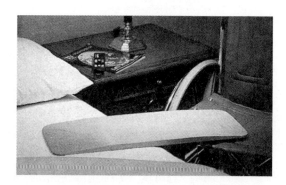

Fig. 33-3 *A transfer board is used to transfer from a bed to a chair. (Courtesy Northcoast Medical, San Jose, Calif.)*

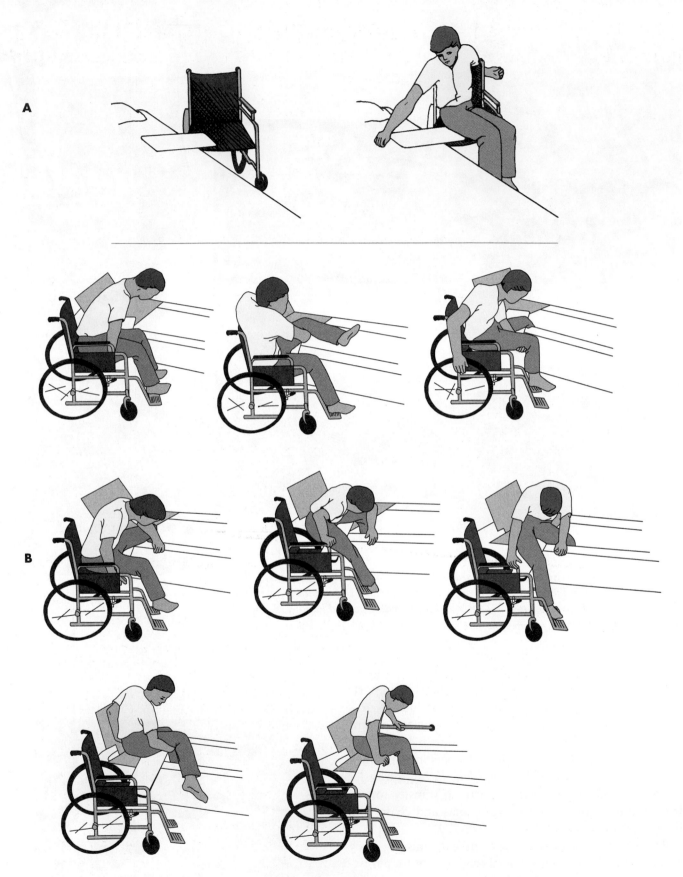

Fig. 33-4 A, *The person transfers from the wheelchair to the bed.* **B,** *A transfer from the wheelchair to the bathtub.* (*From Hoeman SP:* Rehabilitation/restorative care in the community, *St Louis, 1990, Mosby*).

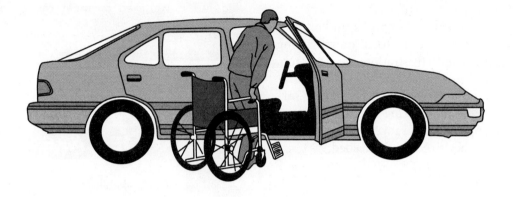

C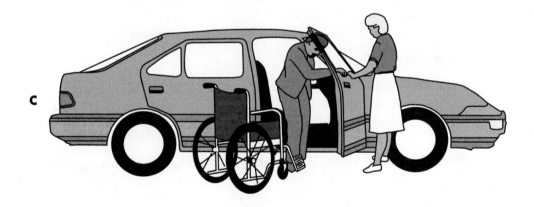

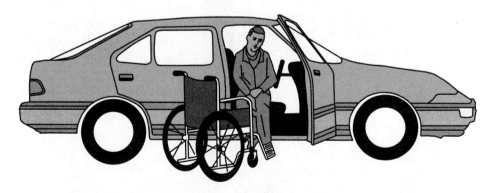

Fig. 33-4, cont'd C, *A transfer to the car. The person has left-side paralysis.*

Psychological and Social Aspects

A disability often affects self-esteem and relationships. Appearance and function changes may cause the person to feel unwhole, unattractive, or unclean. At first the person may refuse to accept the disability. The person may be depressed, angry, and hostile.

The person's attitude, acceptance of limits, and motivation are important. The person must focus on remaining abilities. Discouragement and frustration are common. Progress may be slow. Learning each new task is a reminder of the disability. Old fears and emotions may surface. The person needs help accepting the disability and the resulting limits. Support, reassurance, encouragement, and sensitivity from the health team are needed.

Economic Aspects

Some persons cannot return to their jobs. The person is assessed for work skills, past work history, interests, and talents. A job skill may be restored or a new one learned. The goal is for the person to become gainfully employed. Assistance often is given in finding a job.

THE REHABILITATION TEAM

Rehabilitation is a team effort. The team includes the person, doctor, nursing team, other health team members (see Chapter 1), and the family. All help the person to become independent.

The team meets often to discuss the person's progress. Goals are set for the person. The person helps in goal setting. Changes are made as needed. The person and family are encouraged to attend the meetings.

REHABILITATION SERVICES

The person may need extended hospital care. Some need subacute or long-term care. Others are treated as outpatients. Home care agencies and day care centers often provide rehabilitation services. Some people are transferred to rehabilitation centers. There are centers for persons who are blind, deaf, mentally retarded, physically disabled, or mentally ill or who have speech problems. (See Focus on Children, Focus on Home Care, and Focus on Long-Term Care.)

focus on **CHILDREN**

Federal laws require that schools provide needed therapies. In-school therapy is required to meet the child's learning needs.

focus on **HOME CARE**

The rehabilitation team assesses the person's home setting (Box 33-2). Changes in the home are made to meet the person's needs. Some individuals require personal attendants 24 hours a day.

focus on **LONG-TERM CARE**

The Omnibus Budget Reconciliation Act of 1987 (OBRA) requires that nursing centers provide rehabilitation services. Services required by a resident's comprehensive care plan must be provided. If a resident requires physical therapy, it must be provided. If occupational therapy is required, it must be provided. The same holds for speech and other therapies. All services require a doctor's order.

BOX 33-2

HOME ASSESSMENT

Outdoors
- Where is parking located? What is the distance from the parking area to the door?
- Where is the mailbox?
- Where is the motor vehicle stored?
- What is the width of doors?
- Can the person turn a key?
- Can the person open and close doors?
- Are ramps needed?
- Are handrails needed?
- Are entrances lighted?
- Does the person have access to private or public transportation?
- Can the person operate a motor vehicle?
- What is the width and height of ramps and sidewalks?

Indoors
- Are there floor obstructions?
- Are there steps in the home? Where are they located?
- How is furniture arranged?
- Can the person use the furniture?
- Where are telephones located?
- Can the person raise and lower windows?
- How are floors covered (wall-to-wall carpeting, tile, hardwood floors, throw rugs)?
- Can the person use a wheelchair throughout the home?
- Where is the fuse or circuit-breaker box located?
- Can the person control the heat?
- Are walkways, doors, and halls wide enough for the person to use a wheelchair?
- Is there an elevator in an apartment or condominium building?

Kitchen
- Does the person have access to the stove, sink, cupboards, storage areas, work space, refrigerator, and other appliances?
- What is the height of the sink and countertops?
- Is there an opening under the sink for wheelchair access?
- Can the person turn faucets on and off?
- Can the person use the microwave?
- Can the person reach stove knobs?
- Are appliances arranged conveniently for the person?

Bathroom
- What is the height of the sink, toilet, shower, and tub?
- Can the person reach the faucets?
- Can the person turn the faucets on and off?
- Is there space for using a wheelchair and other assistive devices?
- Can the person get into and out of the tub or shower?
- Are there grab bars by the toilet, shower, and tub?

(Modified from Hoeman SP: *Rehabilitation nursing: process and application*, ed 2, St Louis, 1996, Mosby.)

Continued

BOX 33-2

HOME ASSESSMENT—cont'd

Bedroom

- What is the height of the person's bed?
- Can the person access the closet? Can the person reach rods and shelves?
- Can the person transfer in and out of bed safely? Is there enough space around the bed for the person to move?
- How is furniture arranged?
- Does the furniture arrangement allow for the use of a wheelchair or assistive devices?

Safety

- Is the house number clearly visible and readable during an emergency?
- Are deadbolts and locks secure? Can the person use the locks?
- Can the person see and talk to a visitor at the door without being seen?
- Are steps, porch, and front door lighted?
- Are the steps, porch, and front door protected from rain, sleet, and snow?
- Is there a nonslip doormat?
- Can the person use the telephone?
- Are emergency telephone numbers available?
- Can the person control water temperature?
- Do electrical outlets have childproof covers?
- Where are the smoke detectors? Are they working?
- Are rooms and hallways well-lighted?
- Can the person control indoor and outdoor lighting?
- Can the person exit the home in an emergency?
- Is oxygen used in the home? Are safety measures for the use of oxygen in place?
- Does the person have access to the telephone, television, radio, and lights while in bed?
- Are space heaters used in the home? Are safety measures in place?
- Does the person have good judgment for cooking and stove use?
- Is there a safe play area for children?
- Can the person safely dispose of blood, body fluids, secretions, and excretions?
- Is there a pest-free method of trash storage?

QUALITY OF LIFE

Successful rehabilitation improves the person's quality of life. A hopeful and winning attitude helps motivate the person. However, the process can be slow and frustrating. Promoting quality of life helps the person's attitude.

The person's rights are protected. The right to privacy is important. The person relearns old or practices new skills in private. Other persons do not need to watch. They do not need to see mistakes, falls, spills, or clumsiness. Nor do they need to see the person's anger or tears. Privacy protects the person's dignity and promotes self-respect.

Personal choice gives the person control. Not being able to control body movements or functions is very frustrating. Persons are allowed and encouraged to control the other aspects of their lives to the extent possible. You need to allow personal choice whenever possible. Sad and depressed persons may not want to make choices. Encourage them to do so. Making choices helps them have control of those things that affect them.

The person is part of the rehabilitation team. The team plans and evaluates the person's program. Being part of the team allows the individual personal choice in planning care.

The person has the right to be free from abuse and mistreatment. Rehabilitation is often a slow process. Sometimes improvement is not seen for weeks. Learning how to use an assistive device takes time. Learning to speak again after a stroke can take a long time. So can learning how to dress when there is paralysis. What seems so simple to you can be very hard for the person. Repeated explanations and demonstrations may have no or little results. You may become impatient and short with the person. Or you may see such behavior from other team members or the family. You must protect the person from physical and mental abuse and mistreatment. No one can shout, scream, or yell at the person. Nor can they hit or strike the person. The person cannot be called names. Unkind remarks must not be made. You must report signs of abuse or mistreatment to the RN.

You must deal with your own anger and frustration. Remember that the person wants to function and control movements. The person does not choose loss of function. If the process frustrates you, just think how the person must feel. Discuss your feelings with the RN. The RN can suggest ways to help you control your feelings. Perhaps you can be reassigned for a while.

Taking part in activities promotes quality of life. The person is encouraged to join in group activities. Often persons are concerned about how others view the disability. Provide support and reassurance. Remind the person that others have disabilities. Other persons are likely to provide support and understanding because of their own disabilities. Allow personal choice in activities. The person usually chooses those that are of interest and that are the least threatening.

The environment promotes quality of life. It must be safe and meet the person's needs. The setting may need changes because of disabilities. Location of the overbed table or the bedside stand may need to be changed. The person may need a special chair. If the call bell cannot be used, another way is needed to communicate with the staff. These and other changes are suggested by all health team members. The RN or therapist explains the need and purpose of the change to the person and family.

YOUR RESPONSIBILITIES

Your role as a member of the rehabilitation team has value. An RN directs you in performing care activities. Box 33-3 on p. 784 lists your responsibilities. Many procedures and care measures already learned are part of the person's care. Safety, communication, legal, and ethical aspects apply in rehabilitation. The many rules described throughout this book also apply, regardless of the disability.

BOX 33-3

RESPONSIBILITIES OF ASSISTIVE PERSONNEL IN REHABILITATION

- Follow the RN's instructions and directions very carefully.
- Report early signs and symptoms of complications such as pressure ulcers, contractures, and bowel and bladder problems.
- Keep the person in good body alignment at all times (see Chapter 12).
- Practice measures to prevent pressure ulcers (see Chapter 14).
- Turn and reposition the person as directed (see Chapter 12).
- Perform range-of-motion exercises as instructed (see Chapter 22).
- Encourage the person to perform as many ADLs as possible and to the extent possible.
- Give genuine praise when even a little progress is made.
- Provide emotional support and reassurance.
- Practice the techniques developed by members of the rehabilitation team when assisting the person. This helps you understand what the person needs to do.
- Know how to apply self-care devices used by the person.
- Try to understand and appreciate the person's situation, feelings, and concerns.
- Do not pity the person or give sympathy.
- Focus on the person's abilities, not the disabilities.
- Remember that muscles atrophy if they are not used.
- Practice the task that the person must do. This helps you guide and direct the person.
- Know how to use and operate special equipment used in the person's rehabilitation program.
- Convey an attitude of hopefulness to the person and family.

REVIEW QUESTIONS

Circle the best answer.

1 Rehabilitation is concerned with
a What the person cannot do
b What the person can do
c The whole person
d The person's rights

2 Mrs. Lund's rehabilitation begins with preventing
a Angry feelings
b Contractures and pressure ulcers
c Illness and injury
d Loss of self-esteem

3 Mrs. Lund has weakness on her right side. ADLs are
a Done by Mrs. Lund to the extent possible
b Done by the nursing staff
c Postponed until she can use her right side
d Supervised by a therapist

4 Which reaction is Mrs. Lund likely to experience?
a Feelings of being undesirable
b Anger and hostility
c Depression
d All of the above

5 Which statement is *false?*
a Disabled people can never work again.
b Disabled people may need to learn a new job skill.
c The disabled person is evaluated to determine the ability to work.
d Disabled people are often given help in finding a job.

6 Which statement is *false?*
a Sympathy and pity help the person adjust to the disability.
b You should know how to apply self-care devices.
c You should know how to use equipment used in the person's care.
d An attitude of hopefulness must be conveyed to the person.

7 Mrs. Lund requires speech therapy after a stroke. Therapy should be provided in private.
a True
b False

8 Mrs. Lund is learning to use a walker. She asks to have music played. You should
a Tell her music is not allowed
b Choose some music
c Ask Mrs. Lund to choose some music
d Ask a therapist to choose some music

9 Mrs. Lund is told that she cannot have dessert until she does her exercises. This is abuse and mistreatment.
a True
b False

10 Mrs. Lund's right side is weak. The call bell is on her right side. You move it to the left side of the bed. You have promoted her quality of life by
a Protecting her from abuse and mistreatment
b Allowing personal choice
c Providing for her safety
d All of the above

Answers to these questions are on p. 854.

34

Caring for Mothers and Newborns

- Define the key terms in this chapter
- Describe how to meet an infant's safety and security needs
- Identify the signs and symptoms of illness in infants
- Explain how to help mothers with breast-feeding
- Describe three forms of baby formulas
- Explain how to bottle-feed babies
- Explain how to burp a baby
- Describe how to give cord care
- Describe the purposes of circumcision, the necessary observations, and the required care
- Explain how to bathe infants
- Explain why infants are weighed
- Describe the care needed by mothers during the postpartum period
- Perform the procedures described in this chapter

KEY TERMS

circumcision The surgical removal of foreskin

episiotomy Incision *(otomy)* into the perineum

lochia The vaginal discharge that occurs during the postpartum period

postpartum After *(post)* childbirth *(partum)*

rooting reflex The baby turns his or her head when the cheek or mouth is stroked; the head is turned toward the direction of the stimulus, and the baby starts to suck

umbilical cord The structure that carries blood, oxygen, and nutrients from the mother to the fetus

You may care for new mothers and newborns. They usually stay in the hospital only a short while. Some need home care after discharge. Common reasons for home care include:

- Complications in the mother before or after childbirth
- Help with childcare when other young children are in the home
- Multiple births (e.g., twins, triplets)
- Help with meals and housekeeping

Babies are helpless. They depend on others for their basic needs. Besides physical needs, babies have safety and security and love and belonging needs. A review of growth and development will help you care for newborns and infants (see Chapter 8).

INFANT SAFETY AND SECURITY

Babies cannot protect themselves. Like everyone else, babies need to feel safe and secure. They feel secure when warm and when wrapped and held snugly. Babies cry to communicate. They cry when wet, hungry, hot or cold, tired, uncomfortable, or in pain. Responding to their cries and feeding them when hungry promote safety and security. Infant safety is discussed in Chapter 10. The measures listed in Box 34-1 on p. 788 are also important for hospital or home care.

Signs and Symptoms of Illness

Your observations are important for the infant's safety and well-being. Babies can become ill quickly. Signs and symptoms may be sudden. Therefore you must be very alert. Box 34-2 on p. 789 lists the signs and symptoms that are reported to the RN immediately.

Tell the RN when a sign or symptom began. You may need to take an infant's or child's temperature, pulse, and respirations (see Chapter 23). Axillary temperatures are taken on infants. Tympanic, rectal, or axillary temperatures are taken on children younger than 5 years. The RN tells you which method to use for the child. Apical pulses are taken on infants and young children.

Text continued on p. 790

BOX 34-1

INFANT SAFETY

- Follow the safety measures listed in Chapter 10.
- Keep the baby warm. Check windows for drafts. Close windows securely.
- Keep your fingernails short. Do not wear rings or bracelets. Long nails and jewelry can scratch the baby.
- Use both hands to lift a newborn.
- Hold the baby securely. Use the cradle hold, football hold, or shoulder hold (Fig. 34-1).
- Support the baby's head and neck when lifting or holding the baby (see Fig. 34-1). Neck support is necessary for the first 3 months after birth.
- Handle the baby with gentle, smooth movements. Avoid sudden or jerking movements. Do not startle the baby.
- Hold and cuddle infants. This is comforting and helps them learn to feel love and security.
- Talk, sing, or play with the baby often. Be sure to talk to the baby during the bath, dressing, and diapering.
- Respond to the baby's crying. Babies cry when they are hungry, uncomfortable, wet, frightened, or tired or when they want attention. Crying is how they communicate. Responding to their cries helps them feel safe and secure.
- Do not leave a baby unattended on a table, bed, sofa, highchair, or other high surface. Keep one hand on the baby if you must look away (see Fig. 10-1, p. 160).
- Use safety straps for babies in an infant seat or highchair. Do not use safety straps on changing tables. The baby can roll off the table and strangle on the straps.
- Make sure the crib is within hearing distance of the caregivers.
- Keep crib rails up at all times.
- Do not put a pillow, quilts, or soft toys in the crib. They can cause suffocation.
- Lay babies on their backs or in a side-lying position for sleep. The back-lying position is preferred. *Do not lay babies on their stomachs for sleep. This can interfere with chest expansion and breathing. The baby can suffocate.* If the side-lying position is used, bring the baby's lower arm forward (Fig. 34-2). This prevents the baby from rolling onto the stomach. Infants can lie on their stomach when awake.
- Keep pins and small objects out of the baby's reach.
- Do not shake powders directly over the baby. The powder can get into the baby's eyes and lungs. Shake some on your hand away from the baby.

A   B   C

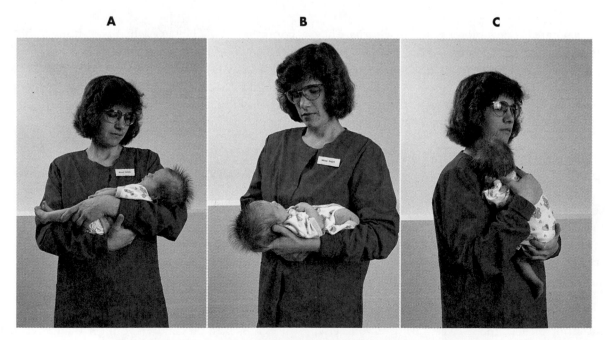

Fig. 34-1 A, *The cradle hold.* **B,** *The football hold.* **C,** *The shoulder hold.*

BOX 34-2

SIGNS AND SYMPTOMS OF ILLNESS IN BABIES

- The baby has jaundice—a yellowish color to the skin and whites of the eyes.
- The baby looks sick.
- The baby has redness or drainage around the cord stump or circumcision.
- The baby has a high temperature (see Chapter 23).
- The baby is limp and slow to respond.
- The baby cries all the time or does not stop crying.
- The baby is flushed, pale, or perspiring.
- The baby has noisy, rapid, difficult, or slow respirations.
- The baby is coughing or sneezing.
- The baby has reddened or irritated eyes.
- The baby turns his or her head to one side or puts a hand to one ear (signs of an earache).
- The baby screams for a long time.
- The baby has skipped feedings.
- The baby has vomited most of the feeding or vomits between feedings.
- The baby has hard, formed stools or watery stools.
- The baby has a rash.

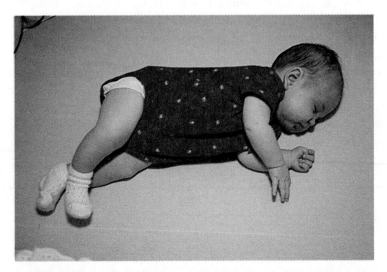

Fig. 34-2 *The baby's lower arm is brought forward in the side-lying position. This prevents the baby from rolling onto the stomach.*

BOX 34-3

HELPING WITH BREAST-FEEDING

- Practice Standard Precautions. Remember, human immunodeficiency virus (HIV) can be transmitted through breast milk (see Chapters 11 and 30).
- Help the mother wash her hands. Handwashing is necessary before she handles her breasts.
- Help the mother to a comfortable position. She may want to nurse sitting up in bed, in a chair, or in the side-lying position (Fig. 34-3).
- Change the baby's diaper if necessary. Bring the baby to the mother.
- Make sure the mother holds the baby close to her breast.
- Have the mother stroke the baby's cheek closest to the breast (Fig. 34-4). This stimulates the **rooting reflex.** The baby turns his or her head when the cheek or mouth is stroked. The head is turned toward the direction of the stimulus, and the baby starts to suck. If the right cheek is stroked, the baby turns the head to the right.
- Have the mother keep breast tissue away from the baby's nose with her thumb (Fig. 34-5).
- Give her a baby blanket to cover the baby and her breast. This promotes privacy during the feeding.
- Encourage nursing from both breasts at each feeding. If the baby finished the last feeding at the right breast, the baby starts the next feeding at the left breast.
- Remind her how to remove the baby from the breast. She needs to break the seal or suction between the baby and the breast. She can press a finger down on her breast close to the baby's mouth. Or she can insert a finger into a corner of the baby's mouth (Fig. 34-6).
- Help the mother burp the baby if necessary (see p. 795). The baby is burped after nursing at each breast.
- Have the mother put a diaper pin on the bra strap of the breast last used. This reminds her which breast to use at the next feeding.
- Change the baby's diaper after the feeding.
- Lay the baby in the crib if he or she has fallen asleep. *Remember to lay the baby on his or her back or in the side-lying position. Do not lay the baby on his or her stomach.*
- Encourage the mother to wear a nursing bra day and night. The bra supports the breasts and promotes comfort.
- Encourage the mother to place cotton pads in the bra. The pads absorb leaking milk.
- Have the mother apply cream (if prescribed) to her nipples after each feeding. The cream prevents nipples from drying and cracking.
- Help the mother straighten clothing after the feeding if necessary.
- Remind the mother to wash her breasts with a clean washcloth and warm water. Soap is not used. It can cause the nipples to dry and crack.

HELPING MOTHERS BREAST-FEED

Many mothers breast-feed their babies. Breast-fed babies usually nurse every 2 to 3 hours. They are fed on demand. In other words, they are fed when hungry, not on a schedule. At first, babies nurse for a short time (5 minutes at each breast). Eventually, nursing time takes up to 30 minutes.

RNs help new mothers learn to breast-feed. They also teach breast care. Mothers and babies learn how to nurse in a very short time. If the mother or baby is having problems breast-feeding, you must call the RN.

Mothers may need help getting ready to breast-feed. They may need help with positioning. You may be responsible for bringing babies to mothers. You must help as needed. When you leave the room, make sure the call bell is within reach. The mother and baby need privacy during breast-feeding. Box 34-3 describes how you can help with breast-feeding. (See Focus on Home Care on p. 791.)

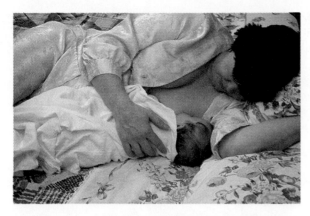

Fig. 34-3 *A mother nursing in the side-lying position.*

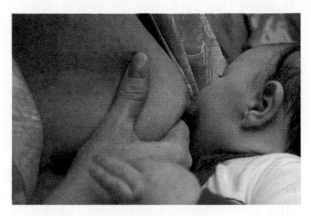

Fig. 34-4 *The mother strokes the baby's cheek with her breast. This stimulates the rooting reflex.*

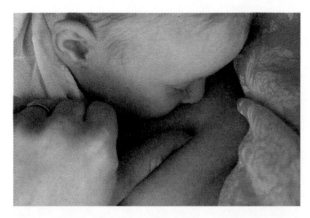

Fig. 34-5 *The thumb is used to keep breast tissue away from the baby's nose.*

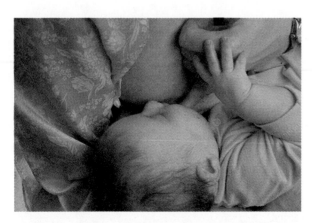

Fig. 34-6 *The mother inserts a finger in the baby's mouth to remove the baby from the breast.*

focus on HOME CARE

When the mother is nursing, stay within hearing distance in case she needs help.

The nursing mother needs good nutrition. If you are providing home care, you may need to plan meals and grocery shop. Remember the following when planning meals or grocery shopping:

- Calorie intake may be increased. The RN tells you how much to increase the mother's calorie intake.
- The mother should drink 6 or more cups of milk a day. She can drink whole, 2%, or skim milk.
- Include foods high in calcium in the diet.
- The mother should avoid spicy and gas-forming foods. They can cause cramping and diarrhea in the infant. She should avoid onions, garlic, spices, cabbage, brussels sprouts, asparagus, and beans. Chocolate, cola beverages, and coffee also can cause cramping and diarrhea.

✦ BOTTLE-FEEDING BABIES

Formula is given to babies who are not breast-fed. The doctor prescribes the formula. It provides the essential nutrients needed by the infant.

Formula comes in three forms. The *ready-to-feed* form is ready to use. It is poured directly from the can into the baby bottle (Fig. 34-7). Water is added to *powdered* and *concentrated* formula. Container directions tell how much formula to use and how much water to add. Bottles are prepared one at a time or in batches for the whole day. Extra bottles are capped (Fig. 34-8) and stored in the refrigerator. These bottles are used within 24 hours.

Babies must be protected from infection. Therefore baby bottles, caps, and nipples must be as clean as possible. Disposable equipment is used in hospitals. Reusable equipment may be used in homes. Reusable bottle-feeding equipment is carefully washed in hot, soapy water or in a dishwasher. Complete rinsing is needed to remove all soap. Some mothers use plastic nursers. They require plastic liners that are used once and then discarded.

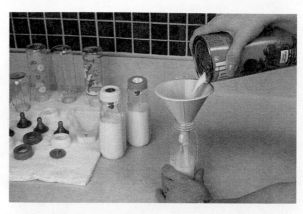

Fig. 34-7 *Ready-to-feed formula is poured from the can into the bottle. A funnel is used to prevent spilling.*

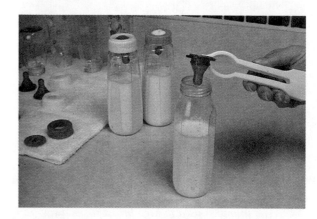

Fig. 34-8 *Bottles are capped for storage in the refrigerator.*

CLEANING BABY BOTTLES

PRE-PROCEDURE

1 Wash your hands.

2 Collect the following:

- Bottles, nipples, and caps

- Funnel

- Can opener

- Bottle brush

- Dishwashing soap

- Other items used to prepare formula

- Towel

PROCEDURE

3 Wash the bottles, nipples, caps, funnel, and can opener in hot, soapy water. Wash other items used to prepare formula.

4 Clean inside baby bottles with the bottle brush (Fig. 34-9).

5 Squeeze hot, soapy water through the nipples (Fig. 34-10). This removes formula from them.

6 Rinse all items thoroughly in hot water. Squeeze hot water through the nipples to remove soap.

7 Lay a clean towel on the countertop.

8 Stand the bottles upside down to drain. Place the nipples, caps, and other items on the towel. Let the items dry.

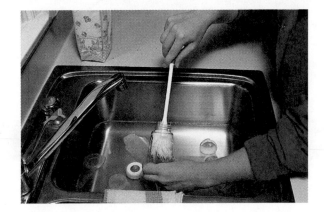

Fig. 34-9 *A bottle brush is used to clean the inside of the bottle.*

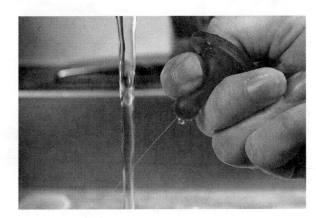

Fig. 34-10 *Water is squeezed through the nipples during cleaning.*

Feeding the Baby

Babies want to be fed every 3 to 4 hours. The amount of formula taken increases as they grow older. The RN or the mother tells you how much formula a baby needs at each feeding. Babies usually take as much formula as they need. The baby stops sucking and turns away from the bottle when satisfied.

Babies are not given cold formula out of the refrigerator. A bottle is warmed before the feeding. You can warm the bottle in a pan of water. The formula should feel warm. Test the temperature by sprinkling a few drops on the inside of your wrist (Fig. 34-11). Do not set the bottle out to warm at room temperature. This takes too long and allows the growth of microbes. Do not heat formula in microwave ovens. The formula can heat unevenly and burn the baby's mouth.

The guidelines in Box 34-4 will help you bottle-feed babies.

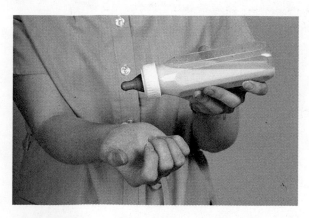

Fig. 34-11 *Formula should feel warm on the wrist.*

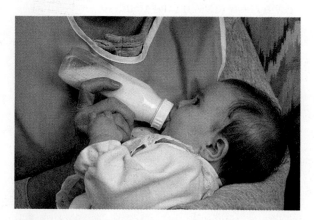

Fig. 34-12 *The bottle is tilted so that formula fills the bottle neck and nipple.*

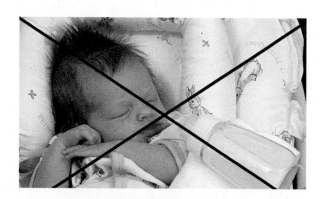

Fig. 34-13 *Do not prop the bottle to feed the baby.*

BOX 34-4

BOTTLE-FEEDING BABIES

- Warm the bottle so the formula feels warm to your wrist.
- Assume a comfortable position for the feeding.
- Hold the baby close to you. Relax and snuggle the baby.
- Tilt the bottle so that the neck of the bottle and the nipple are always filled (Fig. 34-12). Otherwise some air is in the neck or nipple. The baby sucks air into the stomach. The air causes cramping and discomfort.
- Do not prop the bottle and lay the baby down for the feeding (Fig. 34-13).
- Burp the baby when he or she has taken half the formula (see p. 795). Also burp the baby at the end of the feeding.
- Do not leave the baby alone with a bottle.
- Discard remaining formula.
- Wash the bottle, cap, and nipple after the feeding (see *Cleaning Baby Bottles*, p. 793).

Burping the Baby

Babies take in air when they nurse. Bottle-fed babies take in more air than breast-fed babies. Air in the stomach and intestines causes cramping and discomfort. This can lead to vomiting. Burping helps to get rid of the air. Most babies burp in the middle and after the feeding.

Burping a baby is sometimes called *bubbling.* There are two ways to position the baby for burping (Fig. 34-14). One way is to hold the infant over your shoulder. First place a clean diaper or towel over your shoulder. This protects your clothing if the baby "spits up." You can also support the baby in a sitting position on your lap. The towel or diaper is held in front of the baby. To burp the baby, gently pat or rub the baby's back with circular motions. Do this for 2 to 3 minutes.

✦ DIAPERING

Babies urinate several times a day. Breast-fed babies usually have bowel movements after feedings. Bottle-fed babies may have 3 bowel movements a day. Stools are usually soft and unformed. Hard, formed stools mean the baby is constipated. This is reported to the RN immediately. Watery stools mean diarrhea. Diarrhea is very serious in infants. Their water balance can be upset quickly (see Chapter 20). Tell the RN immediately if you suspect a baby has diarrhea.

Diapers are changed when wet or soiled. Changing the diaper after a feeding is usually a good idea. Cloth and disposable diapers are available. Cloth diapers are washed, dried, and folded for reuse. They are washed daily or every 2 days with a laundry detergent made especially for baby clothes. Putting them through the wash cycle a second time without detergent helps remove all soap. If possible, hang diapers outside to dry. This gives them a fresh, clean smell. Cloth diapers are available with Velcro fasteners. Diaper pins are not needed. The danger of sticking the baby or yourself with a diaper pin is avoided.

Disposable diapers are placed in the trash. They are not flushed down the toilet. The use of disposable diapers is more costly.

Changing diapers often helps prevent diaper rash. Moisture, feces, and chemicals from urine irritate the baby's skin. When changing diapers, make sure the baby is clean and dry before applying a clean diaper. If a diaper rash develops, tell the RN immediately. The RN will tell you what to do.

Text continued on p. 798

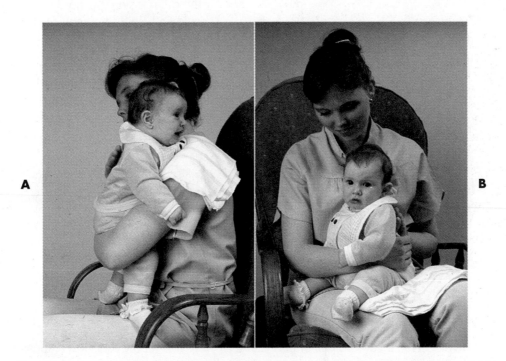

Fig. 34-14 A, *Hold the baby over a shoulder for burping.* **B,** *Support the baby in the sitting position for burping.*

DIAPERING A BABY

PRE-PROCEDURE

1   Wash your hands.

2   Collect the following:

   • Gloves

   • Clean diaper

   • Waterproof changing pad

   • Washcloth

   • Disposable wipes or cotton balls

   • Basin of warm water

   • Baby soap

   • Baby lotion or cream

3   Place the changing pad under the baby.

PROCEDURE

4   Put on the gloves.

5   Unfasten the dirty diaper. Place diaper pins out of the baby's reach.

6   Wipe the genital area with the front of the diaper (Fig. 34-15). Wipe from the front to the back.

7   Fold the diaper so urine and feces are well inside. Set the diaper aside.

8   Clean the genital area from front to back. Use a wet washcloth, disposable wipes, or cotton balls. Wash with mild soap and water if there is a lot of feces or if the baby has a rash. Rinse thoroughly, and pat the area dry.

9   Give cord care, and clean the circumcision at this time (see p. 798).

10   Apply cream or lotion to the genital area and buttocks. Do not use too much. Caking can occur.

11   Raise the baby's legs. Slide a clean diaper under the buttocks.

12   Fold a cloth diaper so extra thickness is in the front for a boy (Fig. 34-16, *A*). For girls, fold the diaper so the extra thickness is at the back (Fig. 34-16, *B*).

13   Bring the diaper between the baby's legs.

14   Make sure the diaper is snug around the hips and abdomen. It should be loose near the penis if the circumcision has not healed. The diaper should be below the umbilicus if the cord stump has not healed.

15   Secure the diaper in place. Use the plastic tabs on disposable diapers (Fig. 34-17, *A*). Make sure the tabs stick in place. Use baby pins or Velcro strips for cloth diapers. Pins should point away from the abdomen (Fig. 34-17, *B*).

16   Apply plastic pants if cloth diapers are worn. Do not use plastic pants with disposable diapers. They already have waterproof protection.

17   Put the baby in the crib, infant seat, or other safe location.

POST-PROCEDURE

18   Rinse feces from the cloth diaper in the toilet.

19   Store used cloth diapers in a covered pail or plastic bag. Take the disposable diaper to the trash.

20   Remove the gloves, and wash your hands.

21   Note and report your observations.

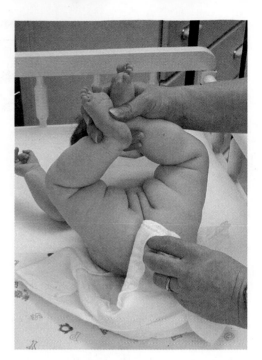

Fig. 34-15 *The front of the diaper is used to clean the genital area.*

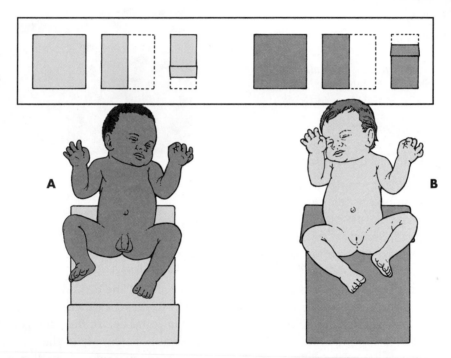

Fig. 34-16 **A,** *A cloth diaper is folded in front for boys.* **B,** *The diaper has a fold in the back for girls.*

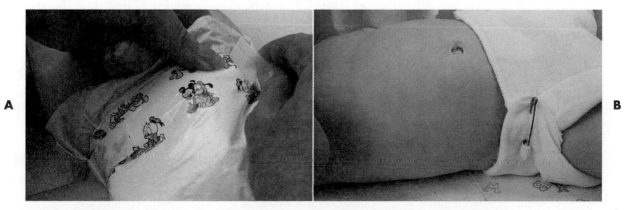

Fig. 34-17 **A,** *A disposable diaper is secured in place with plastic tabs.* **B,** *Pins are used to secure cloth diapers. Pins point away from the abdomen.*

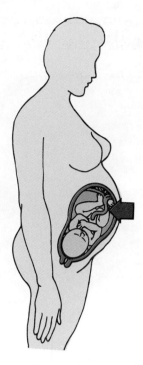

Fig. 34-18 *The umbilical cord connects the mother and fetus.* *(From Wernig J, Sorrentino SA:* The homemaker-home health aide, *St Louis, 1989, Mosby.)*

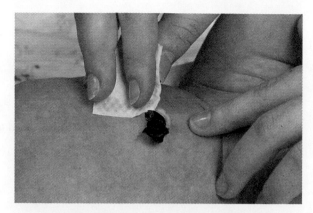

Fig. 34-19 *The cord stump is wiped at the base with alcohol.*

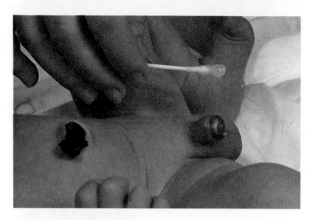

Fig. 34-20 *Petroleum jelly is applied to the circumcised penis.*

CARE OF THE UMBILICAL CORD

The **umbilical cord** connects the mother and the fetus (unborn baby). It carries blood, oxygen, and nutrients from the mother to the fetus (Fig. 34-18). The umbilical cord is not needed after birth. Shortly after delivery, the doctor clamps and cuts the cord. A stump of cord is left on the baby. The stump dries up and falls off in 7 to 10 days. Slight bleeding can occur when the cord comes off.

The cord provides an area for the growth of microbes. You need to keep it clean and dry. Cord care is done at each diaper change. Cord care is continued for 1 to 2 days after the cord comes off. It consists of the following:

* Keep the stump dry. Do not get the stump wet.
* Wipe the base of the stump with alcohol (Fig. 34-19). Use an alcohol wipe or a cotton ball moistened with alcohol. The alcohol promotes drying.
* Keep the diaper below the cord as in Figure 34-17. This prevents the diaper from irritating the stump. It also keeps the cord from becoming wet from urine.
* Report any signs of infection. These include redness or odor or drainage from the stump.
* Give sponge baths until the cord falls off. Then the baby can have a tub bath.
* Do not pull the cord off—even if looks ready to fall off.

CIRCUMCISION

Boys are born with foreskin on the penis. The surgical removal of foreskin is called a **circumcision** (see Fig. 17-11, p. 385). The procedure allows good hygiene and is thought to prevent cancer of the penis. It is usually done in the hospital before the baby goes home. Circumcision is a religious ceremony in the Jewish faith.

The penis will look red, swollen, and sore. However, the circumcision should not interfere with urination. You must carefully check for signs of bleeding and infection. There should be no odor or drainage. You should check the diaper for bleeding. The area should completely heal in 10 to 14 days.

The penis is thoroughly cleaned at each diaper change. Cleaning is especially important if the baby has had a bowel movement. Mild soap and water or commercial wipes are used. The diaper is loosely applied. This prevents the diaper from irritating the penis. Some doctors advise applying petroleum jelly to the penis. This protects the penis from urine and feces. It also prevents the penis from sticking to the diaper. A cotton swab is used to apply the petroleum jelly (Fig. 34-20). The RN tells you if other measures are needed.

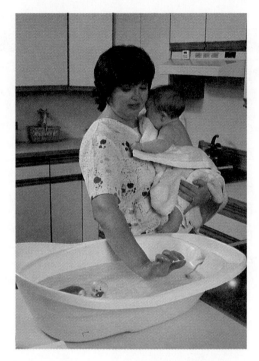

Fig. 34-21 *The wrist is used to test the temperature of the bath water.*

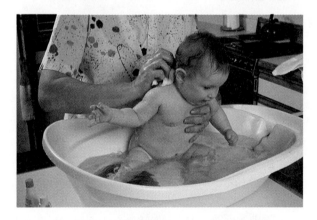

Fig. 34-22 *The baby is given a tub bath.*

✦ BATHING AN INFANT

A bath is important for cleanliness. Though babies do not get very dirty, they need good skin care. Baths comfort and relax babies. They also provide a wonderful time to hold, touch, and talk to babies. Stimulation is important for development. Being touched and held help babies learn safety, security, and love and belonging.

Planning is an important part of the bath. You cannot leave the baby alone if you forget something. Therefore you need to gather equipment, supplies, and the baby's clothes before you start the bath. Everything you need must be within your reach.

Safety measures are also very important:
- Never leave the baby alone on a table or in the bathtub.
- Always keep one hand on the baby if you must look away for a moment.
- Hold the baby securely throughout the bath. Babies are very slippery when they are wet. A wet, squirming baby is hard to hold.
- Room temperature should be 75° to 80° F for the bath. Turn up the thermostat and close windows and doors about 20 minutes before the bath. The room temperature may be uncomfortable for you. You may want to remove a sweater or lab coat or roll up your sleeves before starting the bath.
- Water temperature needs special attention. Babies have delicate skin and are easily burned. Bath water temperature should be 100° to 105° F (38° to 40.5° C). Bath water temperature is measured with a bath thermometer. If one is not available, test the water temperature with the inside of your wrist (Fig. 34-21). The water should feel warm and comfortable to your wrist.

(See Focus on Home Care.)

There are two bath procedures for babies. Sponge baths are given until the baby is about 2 weeks old. They are given until the cord stump falls off and the umbilicus and circumcision heal. *The cord must not get wet.* The tub bath is given after the cord site and circumcision heal (Fig. 34-22).

Text continued on p. 802

GIVING A BABY A SPONGE BATH

PRE-PROCEDURE

1 Wash your hands.

2 Place the following items in your work area:

   • Bath basin

   • Bath thermometer

   • Bath towel

   • Two hand towels

   • Receiving blanket

   • Washcloth

   • Clean diaper

   • Clean clothing for the baby

   • Cotton balls

   • Baby soap

   • Baby shampoo

   • Baby lotion

   • Gloves

PROCEDURE

3 Fill the bath basin with warm water. Water temperature should be 100° to 105° F (38° to 40.5° C). Measure water temperature with the bath thermometer or use the inside of your wrist. The water should feel warm and comfortable on your wrist.

4 Provide for privacy.

5 Identify the baby. Check the ID bracelet against the assignment sheet.

6 Undress the baby. Leave the diaper on.

7 Wash the baby's eyes (Fig. 34-23):

   a Dip a cotton ball into the water.

   b Squeeze out excess water.

   c Wash one eye from the inner part to the outer part.

   d Repeat this step for the other eye with a new cotton ball.

8 Moisten the washcloth. Clean the outside of the ear and then behind the ear. Repeat this step for the other ear. Be gentle.

9 Rinse and squeeze the washcloth. Make a mitt with the washcloth (see Fig. 14-8, p. 308).

10 Wash the baby's face (Fig. 34-24). Clean inside the nostrils with the washcloth. *Do not use cotton swabs to clean inside the ears.* Pat the face dry.

11 Pick up the baby. Hold the baby over the bath basin using the football hold. Support the baby's head and neck with your wrist and hand.

12 Wash the baby's head (Fig. 34-25):

   a Squeeze a small amount of water from the washcloth onto the baby's head.

   b Apply a small amount of baby shampoo to the head.

   c Wash the head with circular motions.

   d Rinse the head by squeezing water from a washcloth over the baby's head. Be sure to rinse thoroughly. Avoid getting soap in the baby's eyes.

   e Use a small hand towel to dry the head.

13 Lay the baby on the table.

14 Put on the gloves.

15 Remove the diaper.

16 Wash the front of the body. Use a soapy washcloth. You may also apply soap to your hands and wash the baby with your hands (Fig. 34-26). Do not get the cord wet. Rinse thoroughly. Pat dry. Be sure to wash and dry all creases and folds.

17 Turn the baby to the prone position. Repeat step 16 for the back and buttocks.

GIVING A BABY A SPONGE BATH—cont'd

PROCEDURE—cont'd

18 Give cord care, and clean the circumcision.

19 Apply baby lotion to the baby's body as directed by the RN.

20 Put a clean diaper and clean clothes on the baby.

21 Remove the gloves.

22 Wrap the baby in the receiving blanket. Put the baby in the crib or other safe location.

POST-PROCEDURE

23 Clean and return equipment and supplies to the proper place. Do this step when the baby is settled.

24 Wash your hands.

25 Note and report your observations.

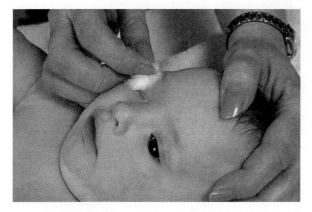

Fig. 34-23 *The baby's eyes are washed with cotton balls. The eye is cleaned from the inner to the outer part.*

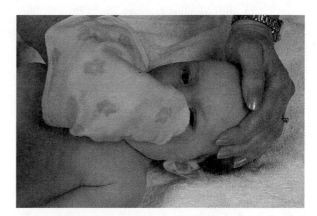

Fig. 34-24 *The baby's face is washed with a mitted washcloth.*

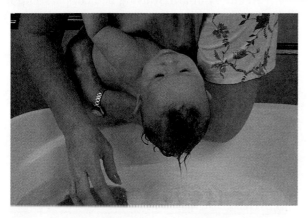

Fig. 34-25 *The baby's head is washed over the basin.*

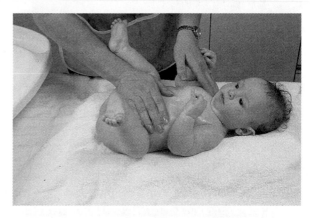

Fig. 34-26 *The hands are used to wash the baby.*

GIVING A BABY A TUB BATH

PROCEDURE

1 Follow steps 1 through 15 in the sponge bath procedure (see p. 800).

2 Hold the baby as in Figure 34-27:

a Place your right hand under the baby's shoulders. Your thumb should be over the baby's right shoulder. Your fingers should be under the right arm.

b Use your left hand to support the baby's buttocks. Slide your left hand under the thighs. Hold the right thigh with your left hand.

3 Lower the baby into the water feet first.

4 Wash the front of the baby's body. Be sure to wash all folds and creases. Rinse thoroughly.

5 Reverse your hold. Use your left hand to hold the baby.

6 Wash the baby's back as in Figure 34-22. Rinse thoroughly.

7 Reverse your hold again. Use your right hand to hold the baby.

8 Wash the genital area.

9 Lift the baby out of the water and onto a towel.

10 Wrap the baby in the towel. Also cover the baby's head.

11 Pat the baby dry. Be sure to dry all folds and creases.

12 Follow steps 19-25 of the sponge bath (p. 801).

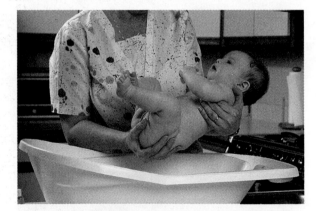

Fig. 34-27 *The baby is held for the tub bath.*

NAIL CARE

The baby's fingernails and toenails are kept short. Otherwise, the baby can scratch himself or herself and others. Nails are best cut when the baby is sleeping. The baby is quiet and will not squirm or fuss. Use nail clippers or file nails with an emery board. If using nail clippers, clip nails straight across as for an adult (see Fig. 15-7 on p. 341).

✦ WEIGHING AN INFANT

PRE-PROCEDURE

1 Wash your hands.

2 Collect the following:

   • Baby scale

   • Paper for the scale

   • Items for diaper changing (see *Diapering a Baby*, p. 796)

PROCEDURE

3 Identify the baby. Check the ID bracelet against the assignment sheet.

4 Place the paper on the scale. Adjust the scale to zero (0).

5 Put on the gloves.

6 Undress the baby, and remove the diaper. Clean the genital area.

7 Lay the baby on the scale. Keep one hand over the baby to prevent falling.

8 Read the digital display (Fig. 34-28), or move the pointer until the scale is balanced.

9 Diaper and dress the baby. Lay the baby in the crib.

10 Remove and discard the gloves.

POST-PROCEDURE

11 Return the scale to its proper place.

12 Wash your hands.

13 Report your observations to the RN.

14 Record the weight according to agency policy.

✦ WEIGHING INFANTS

Infants are weighed at birth. The birth weight is the baseline for measuring the infant's growth. The RN uses weight measurements in the assessment step of the nursing process. It is used also to evaluate how much breast milk was taken during breast-feeding. The baby is weighed before and after breast-feeding. The difference in the weights is the amount of milk taken in during breast-feeding. The RN uses this information to determine if the baby is getting enough milk.

The RN tells you when to weigh the baby. You must meet the baby's safety needs. Protect the baby from chills. Keep the room warm and free of drafts. Also protect the baby from falling. Always keep a hand over the baby when taking the weight measurement. Remember to keep one hand on the baby if you need to look away. Breast-fed babies wear the same diaper, clothes, and blanket for each weight measurement.

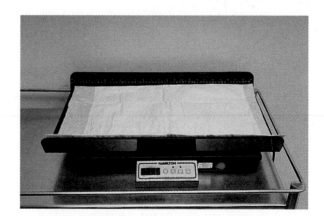

Fig. 34-28 *Digital infant scale.*

CARE OF THE MOTHER

Postpartum means after *(post)* childbirth *(partum)*. The postpartum period starts with birth of the baby. It ends 6 weeks later. The mother's body returns to its normal state during this time. The mother adjusts physically and emotionally to childbirth.

The uterus returns almost to its pre-pregnant size. This is called *involution of the uterus.* If the mother does not breast-feed, she can expect a menstrual period within 3 to 8 weeks. The mother can get pregnant again unless she practices birth control measures.

A vaginal discharge occurs during the postpartum period. It is called **lochia.** (Lochia comes from the Greek word *lochos,* which means *childbirth.*) Lochia consists of blood and other substances left in the uterus from childbirth. The lochia changes color and decreases in amount during the postpartum period:

- *Lochia rubra*—is dark or bright red *(rubra)* discharge. It is mainly blood and is seen during the first 3 to 4 days.
- *Lochia serosa*—is pinkish brown *(serosa)* drainage. It lasts until about 10 days after birth.
- *Lochia alba*—is whitish *(alba)* drainage. It continues for 2 to 6 weeks after birth.

Lochia increases with breast-feeding and activity. When she stands after lying or sitting, the mother may feel a gush of lochia. The mother wears a sanitary napkin to absorb the lochia. Normally, lochia smells like menstrual flow. Foul-smelling lochia is a sign of infection.

Good perineal care is important. Sanitary pads are changed often. When wiping after elimination, the mother wipes from front to back. Sanitary napkins are applied and removed from front to back. Good handwashing is essential after perineal care, changing sanitary napkins, and elimination. Standard Precautions are followed.

Some mothers have episiotomies. An **episiotomy** is an incision *(otomy)* into the perineum. (*Episeion* is from the Greek word meaning *pubic region.*) The doctor performs this procedure during childbirth. The incision increases the size of the vaginal opening for delivery of the baby. The incision is sutured after the delivery. The doctor may order sitz baths for comfort and hygiene (see Chapter 29). Practice Standard Precautions when helping the mother with sitz baths. As with other incisions, complications can develop. These include infection and wound separation (dehiscence). Tell the RN immediately if the mother complains of pain, discomfort, or a discharge.

If the mother delivered the baby by *cesarean section (C-section),* she has an abdominal incision. With a cesarean section, the doctor makes an incision into the abdominal wall. The baby is delivered through the incision. This is done:

- When the baby must be delivered to save the baby's or mother's life
- When the baby is too large to pass through the birth canal
- When the mother has a vaginal infection that could be transmitted to the baby
- When a normal vaginal delivery will be difficult for the baby or mother

The C-section incision needs to heal. See Chapter 28 for wound healing and wound care.

The mother has emotional reactions after childbirth. Hormone changes, life-style changes, and lack of sleep can cause her to have mood swings. So can frequent visits and telephone calls from friends and family. This is especially true if they interfere or offer advice and opinions about parenting. The mother can help herself by resting when the baby is sleeping. She needs to take time for herself and her partner. She is likely to feel better after pampering herself with a shower, washing and styling her hair, and getting dressed. These can be done while the baby is sleeping.

Complications can occur at any time during pregnancy, labor, and delivery. They also can occur during the postpartum period. Box 34-5 lists the signs and symptoms of postpartum complications. Report any sign or symptom to the RN immediately.

BOX 34-5 SIGNS AND SYMPTOMS OF POSTPARTUM COMPLICATIONS

- Fever of 100.4° F or greater
- Abdominal or perineal pain
- Foul-smelling vaginal discharge
- Bleeding from an episiotomy or cesarean-section incision
- Redness, swelling, or drainage from an episiotomy or cesarean-section incision
- Saturating a sanitary napkin within 1 hour of application
- Red lochia after lochia has changed color to pinkish-brown or white
- Burning on urination
- Leg pain, tenderness, or swelling
- Sadness or feelings of depression
- Breast pain, tenderness, or swelling

REVIEW QUESTIONS

Circle the best *answer.*

1 A newborn's head is supported for the first
   a 7 to 10 days   c 3 months
   b Month   d 6 months

2 Andrew is a newborn. When holding him you should do the following *except*
   a Hold him securely   c Sing and talk to him
   b Cuddle him   d Hold him on his stomach

3 Which is *false?*
   a Andrew's crib should be within hearing distance of caregivers.
   b Andrew should have a pillow for sleep.
   c Andrew should be positioned on his back for sleep.
   d Crib rails should be up at all times.

4 Report the following to the RN *except*
   a Andrew looks flushed and is perspiring
   b Andrew has watery stools
   c Andrew's eyes are red and irritated
   d Andrew spits up a small amount when burped

5 Andrew is breast-fed. The mother should do the following *except*
   a Wash her hands
   b Hold Andrew close to her breast
   c Stimulate the rooting reflex
   d Clean her breasts with soap and water

6 A breast-fed baby is burped
   a Every 5 minutes
   b After nursing from one breast
   c After nursing from both breasts
   d After the feeding

7 Andrew is being switched to bottle-feedings. You do the grocery shopping. Which formula should you buy?
   a The one that is on sale
   b The ready-to-feed type
   c The one ordered by the doctor
   d The powdered form

8 You are to warm Andrew's bottle. Which is *true?*
   a The bottle is warmed for 5 minutes in the microwave.
   b The formula should warm at room temperature.
   c The formula should feel warm on your wrist.
   d The formula is warmed in a pan for 5 minutes.

9 When bottle-feeding Andrew, you should
   a Burp him every 5 minutes
   b Save remaining formula for the next feeding
   c Tilt the bottle so that formula fills the neck of the bottle and the nipple
   d Leave him alone with the bottle

10 Andrew's diapers are changed whenever he is wet.
   a True
   b False

11 Andrew's cord has not yet healed. His diaper should be
   a Loose over the cord
   b Snug over the cord
   c Below the cord
   d Disposable

12 Andrew's cord stump is cleaned with
   a Soap and water
   b Baby shampoo
   c Plain water
   d Alcohol

REVIEW QUESTIONS—cont'd

13 Andrew's cord and the circumcision are cleaned
a Once a day
b When he has a bowel movement
c Three times a day
d At every diaper change

14 Andrew's cord and circumcision have not healed. He should have a sponge bath.
a True
b False

15 Bath water for Andrew should be
a 85° to 90° F
b 90° to 95° F
c 95° to 100° F
d 100° to 105° F

16 Which should you use to wash Andrew's eyes?
a A mitted washcloth
b Alcohol wipes
c A cotton swab
d Cotton balls

17 Cotton swabs are used to clean inside Andrew's ears.
a True
b False

18 Andrew is being breast-fed. He is weighed with his diaper on.
a True
b False

19 A mother has a red vaginal discharge the first few days after childbirth. This
a Is her menstrual flow
b Signals a postpartum complication
c Is lochia rubra
d Is from her episiotomy

20 A cesarean delivery involves
a A vaginal incision
b A perineal incision
c An abdominal incision
d A normal delivery through the birth canal

Answers to these questions are on p. 854.

35

Basic Emergency Care

- Define the key terms in this chapter
- Describe the general rules of emergency care
- Identify the signs of cardiac arrest and obstructed airway
- Describe basic life support and basic life support procedures
- Explain the difference between internal and external hemorrhage
- Explain how to control hemorrhage
- Identify the signs of and emergency care for shock
- Describe two types of seizures and how to care for a person during a seizure
- Describe burns, their causes, and emergency care
- Identify the common causes of and emergency care for fainting
- Describe the signs of and emergency care for stroke
- Perform the procedures described in this chapter

KEY TERMS

anaphylaxis A life-threatening sensitivity to an antigen

cardiac arrest The heart and breathing stop suddenly and without warning

convulsion A seizure

fainting The sudden loss of consciousness from an inadequate blood supply to the brain

first aid Emergency care given to an ill or injured person before medical help arrives

hemorrhage The excessive loss of blood in a short period of time

respiratory arrest Breathing stops but the heart still pumps blood for several minutes

seizure Violent and sudden contractions or tremors of muscles; convulsion

shock A condition that results when there is not enough blood supply to organs and tissues

Emergencies can occur anywhere. They happen in health care agencies, homes, and public places and on highways. Knowing what to do can mean the difference between life and death. This chapter describes some common emergencies and the basic care that is given. You are encouraged to take a first aid course from the National Safety Council or the American Red Cross. A basic life support course given by the American Heart Association, National Safety Council, or the American Red Cross is also recommended. These courses prepare you to give care in emergency situations.

GENERAL RULES OF EMERGENCY CARE

First aid is the emergency care given to an ill or injured person before medical help arrives. The goals of first aid are to:

- Prevent death
- Prevent injuries from becoming worse

When an emergency occurs, the local emergency medical services (EMS) system must be activated. The system involves emergency personnel (paramedics, emergency medical technicians) who are trained and educated to give emergency care. They know how to treat, stabilize, and transport persons with life-threatening conditions. Their emergency vehicles have the equipment, supplies, and drugs used in emergencies. Emergency personnel communicate by telephone or two-way radio with doctors based in hospital emergency rooms. The doctors tell them what to do. In many areas the EMS system is activated by dialing 911. Calling the local fire or police department or the telephone operator also activates the system.

Each emergency is different. However, the rules in Box 35-1 on p. 810 apply to any emergency.

BOX 35-1

GENERAL RULES OF EMERGENCY CARE

- Know your limits. Do not do more than you are able. Do not perform an unfamiliar procedure. Do what you can under the circumstances.
- Stay calm. This helps the person feel more secure.
- Practice Standard Precautions and follow the Bloodborne Pathogen Standard to the extent possible.
- Check for signs of life-threatening problems. Check for breathing, a pulse, and bleeding.
- Keep the person lying down or in the position in which he or she was found. Moving the person could make an injury worse.
- Perform necessary emergency measures.
- Call for help or tell someone to activate the emergency medical services (EMS) system. An operator will send emergency vehicles and personnel to the scene. *Do not hang up until the operator has hung up.* Give the operator the following information:
  - Your location—street address and city or town you are in. Give names of cross streets or roads and landmarks if possible
  - Telephone number you are calling from
  - What happened (e.g., heart attack, accident)—police, fire equipment, and ambulances may be needed
  - How many people need help
  - Condition of victims, any obvious injuries, and any life-threatening situations
  - What aid is being given
- Do not remove the person's clothing unless you have to. If you must remove clothing, tear or cut garments along the seams.
- Keep the person warm. Cover the person with a blanket. Or use coats and sweaters.
- Reassure those who are conscious. Explain what is happening and that you called for help.
- Do not give the person any food or fluids.
- Do not move the person. Emergency personnel are trained to do so.
- Keep bystanders away from the person. Bystanders tend to stare, give advice, and comment about the person's condition. The person may think the situation is worse than it really is. Also, the person's privacy is invaded by onlookers.

BASIC LIFE SUPPORT

When the heart and breathing stop, the person is clinically dead. Blood is not circulated through the body. Permanent brain damage and other organ damage occur within minutes. Sometimes death is expected. Death is expected in persons suffering from terminal illnesses. However, the heart and breathing can stop suddenly and without warning. This is a state of **cardiac arrest**.

Cardiac arrest is a sudden, unexpected, and dramatic event. It can occur while driving, shoveling snow, playing golf or tennis, watching television, eating, and sleeping. Cardiac arrest can occur anywhere and at any time. Common causes include heart disease, drowning, electrical shock, severe injury, airway obstruction, and drug overdose. The person suffers permanent brain damage unless breathing and circulation are restored.

Respiratory arrest is when breathing stops but the heart still pumps blood for several minutes. Causes of respiratory arrest include drowning, stroke, obstructed airway, drug overdose, electrocution, lightning strike, smoke inhalation, suffocation, heart attack (myocardial infarction), coma, and other injuries. If breathing is not restored, cardiac arrest occurs. If the person still has a pulse, rescue breathing (p. 811) can prevent cardiac arrest.

Basic life support (BLS) involves preventing or promptly recognizing cardiac arrest or respiratory arrest. BLS procedures support breathing and circulation. These life-saving measures require speed, skill, and efficiency. Prompt activation of the EMS system is also part of BLS.

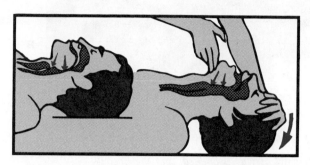

Fig. 35-1 *The head-tilt/chin-lift maneuver is used to open the airway. One hand is on the victim's forehead, and pressure is applied to tilt the head back. The fingers of the other hand are placed under the chin. The chin is lifted forward with the fingers.*

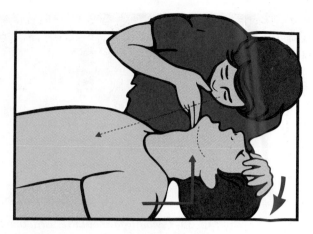

Fig. 35-2 *Determine breathlessness by* looking *to see if the chest rises and falls,* listening *for the escape of air, and* feeling *for the flow of air.*

NOTE: *The American Heart Association, National Safety Council, and American Red Cross certify individuals to perform basic life support procedures. The basic life support procedures that follow are presented as information. They do not replace certification training. You are encouraged to take a basic life support course offered by one of these organizations.*

Cardiopulmonary Resuscitation

There are three major signs of cardiac arrest—no pulse, no breathing, and unconsciousness. The person's skin is cool, pale, and gray. The person has no blood pressure.

Cardiopulmonary resuscitation (CPR) must be started as soon as cardiac arrest occurs. CPR provides oxygen to the brain, heart, kidneys, and other organs until more advanced emergency care can be given. CPR has three basic parts (the ABCs of CPR):

- Airway
- Breathing
- Circulation

The person must be supine on a hard, flat surface. The arms are positioned at the sides. If turning is necessary, use the logrolling procedure (see Chapter 12). The person may have other injuries. Therefore the person is turned as a unit to prevent twisting of the spinal cord.

Airway

The respiratory passages (airway) must be open to restore breathing. The airway is often blocked or obstructed during cardiac arrest. The person's tongue falls toward the back of the throat and blocks the airway. The *head-tilt/chin-lift maneuver* is used to open the airway (Fig. 35-1):

- Place one hand on the person's forehead.
- Apply pressure on the forehead with the palm to tilt the head back.

- Place the fingers of the other hand under the bony part of the chin.
- Lift the chin forward as the head is tilted backward with the other hand.

When the airway is open, check for vomitus, loose dentures, or other foreign bodies. These can obstruct the airway during rescue breathing. Remove dentures, and wipe vomitus away with your index and middle fingers. Wear disposable gloves, or cover your fingers with a cloth. Although you must not waste time, try to protect the dentures from loss or damage.

Breathing

Air is not inhaled when breathing stops. The person must get oxygen. Otherwise, permanent brain and organ damage occur. Breathing is done for the person. This is called *rescue breathing.* Before you start rescue breathing, determine breathlessness (Fig. 35-2). It should take 3 to 5 seconds to do the following:

- Maintain an open airway.
- Place your ear over the person's mouth and nose.
- Observe the person's chest.
  - *Look* to see if the chest rises and falls.
  - *Listen* for the escape of air.
  - *Feel* for the flow of air on your cheek

Mouth-to-mouth resuscitation (Fig. 35-3, p. 812) is the most common method of rescue breathing. The airway is kept open to give mouth-to-mouth resuscitation. Pinch the person's nostrils shut with the thumb and index finger of the hand on the forehead. Shutting the nostrils prevents the escape of air from the nose. After taking a deep breath, place your mouth tightly over the person's mouth. Slowly blow air into the person's mouth. You should see the person's chest rise as the lungs fill with air.

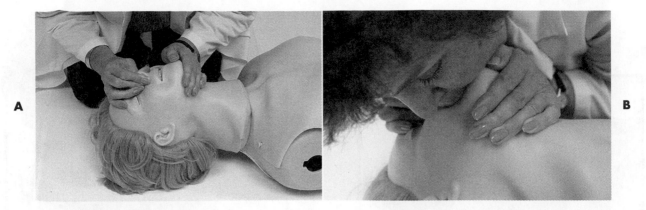

Fig. 35-3 *Mouth-to-mouth resuscitation.* **A,** *The person's airway is opened, and the nostrils are pinched shut.* **B,** *The person's mouth is sealed by the rescuer's mouth.*

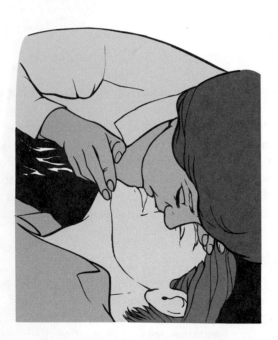

Fig. 35-4 *Mouth-to-nose resuscitation.*

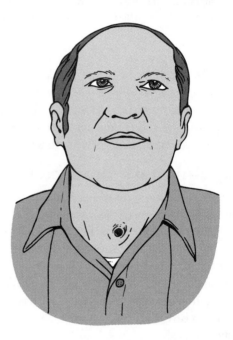

Fig. 35-5 *A stoma in the neck. The person breathes air in and out of the stoma.*

You should also hear air escape when the person exhales. After giving a ventilation, remove your mouth from the person's mouth. Then take in a quick, deep breath.

Mouth-to-mouth resuscitation is not always indicated or possible. The *mouth-to-nose* technique is used when:

- You cannot ventilate the victim's mouth
- You cannot open the mouth
- You cannot make a tight seal for mouth-to-mouth resuscitation
- The mouth is severely injured

The mouth is closed for mouth-to-nose resuscitation. The head-tilt/chin-lift method is used to open the airway. Pressure is placed on the chin to close the mouth. To give the ventilation, place your mouth over the person's nose and blow air into the nose (Fig. 35-4). After the ventilation, remove your mouth from the person's nose.

Some people breathe through an opening *(stoma)* in the neck (Fig. 35-5). They need *mouth-to-stoma* ventilation during cardiac or respiratory arrest. You will seal your mouth around the stoma and blow air into the stoma (Fig. 35-6). Before giving mouth-to-mouth or mouth-to-nose resuscitation, always check to see if a person has a stoma. Other methods of rescue breathing are not effective if the person has a stoma.

Barrier devices prevent contact with the person's mouth and blood, body fluids, secretions, or excretions.

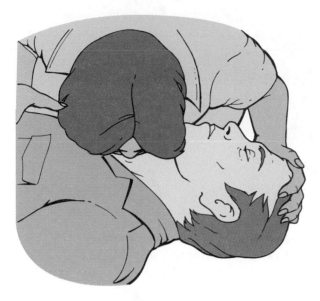

Fig. 35-6 *Mouth-to-stoma resuscitation.*

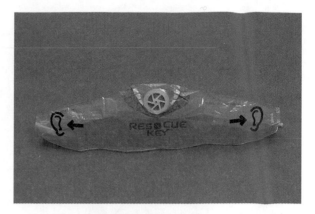

Fig. 35-7 *Mask device.*

Mask devices are available (Fig. 35-7). *Mouth-to-barrier device* is another method of rescue breathing. The barrier device is placed over the person's mouth and nose. Make sure you have a tight seal. Then breathe into the barrier device.

When CPR is started, give two breaths at first. Exhale after each breath. Then give breaths at a rate of 10 to 12 breaths per minute. During one-rescuer CPR, give two breaths after every 15 chest compressions. During two-rescuer CPR, give a breath after every 5 chest compressions.

Circulation

Blood flow to the brain and other organs must be maintained. Otherwise, permanent damage results. The heart has stopped beating in cardiac arrest. Therefore blood must be pumped through the body in some other way. Artificial circulation is accomplished by chest compression. Each chest compression forces blood through the circulatory system.

Before starting chest compressions, determine pulselessness. Use the carotid artery on the side near you to check for pulselessness. To find the carotid pulse, place the tips of your index and middle fingers on the person's trachea (windpipe). Then slide your fingertips down off the trachea to the groove of the neck (Fig. 35-8).

The heart lies between the sternum (breastbone) and the spinal column. When pressure is applied to the sternum, the sternum is depressed. This compresses the heart between the sternum and spinal column (Fig. 35-9). For effective chest compressions, the person must be supine and on a hard, flat surface.

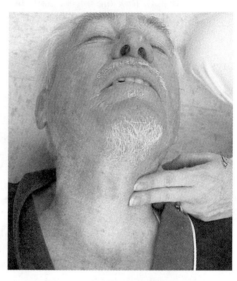

Fig. 35-8 *Locating the carotid pulse. Index and middle fingers are placed on the trachea. The fingers are moved down into the groove of the neck where the carotid pulse is located.*

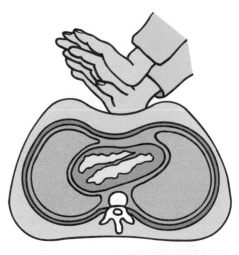

Fig. 35-9 *The heart lies between the sternum and spinal cord. The heart is compressed when pressure is applied to the sternum.* (From Rosen P et al: Emergency medicine: concepts and clinical practice, ed 2, St Louis, 1992, Mosby.)

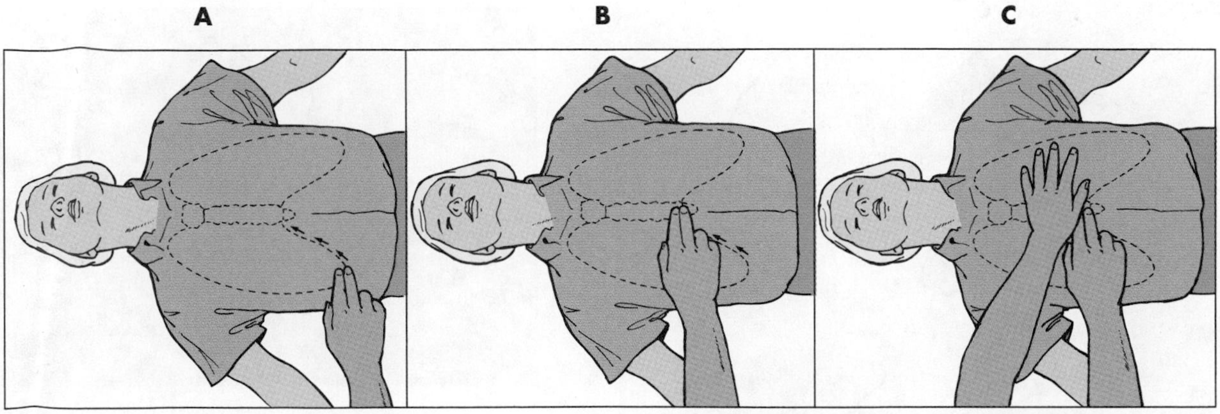

A	B	C

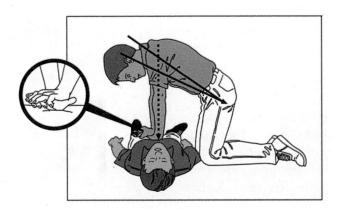

Fig. 35-10 *Proper hand position for cardiopulmonary resuscitation (CPR).* **A,** *Locate the rib cage.* **B,** *Run the fingers along the rib cage to the notch.* **C,** *Place the heel of your other hand next to your index finger.*

Fig. 35-11 *Position of the shoulders for CPR.*

Proper hand position is important for chest compressions. The process for locating hand position for adults is shown in Figure 35-10:

- Use your index and middle fingers to locate the lower part of the person's rib cage on the side near you.
- Then run your fingers up along the rib cage to the notch at the center of the chest. The notch is where the ribs and sternum meet.
- Place the heel of your other hand on the lower half of the sternum next to your index finger.
- Remove your index and middle fingers from the notch.
- Place that hand on the hand already on the sternum.
- Extend or interlace your fingers. Keep your fingers off the chest.

You must be positioned properly for chest compressions. Your elbows are straight. Your shoulders are directly over the person's chest (Fig. 35-11). Exert firm downward pressure to depress the sternum about $1\frac{1}{2}$ to 2 inches in the adult. Then release pressure without removing your hands from the chest. Give compressions in a regular rhythm.

✦ *Performing CPR*

You must determine if cardiac arrest or fainting has occurred. CPR is done only for cardiac arrest. CPR is done when there is unresponsiveness, breathlessness, and pulselessness. That is, the person does not respond, is not breathing, and has no pulse. Basic life support for the adult involves the following sequence:

1. Determine unresponsiveness. Tap or gently shake the person, and shout, "Are you OK?" If there is no response, the person is unconscious.
2. *Activate the EMS system immediately if the person is unresponsive.*
3. Determine breathlessness. *Look* at the person's chest to see if it rises and falls. *Listen* for the escape of air during expiration. *Feel* for the flow of air.
4. Open the airway, and give two breaths if the person is not breathing.
5. Determine pulselessness.
6. Start chest compressions if the person has no pulse.

You can do CPR alone or with another person. *Never practice CPR on another person.* You can cause serious damage. Mannequins are used to learn CPR.

✦ ADULT CPR—ONE RESCUER

PROCEDURE

1 Check for unresponsiveness.

2 Activate the EMS system.

3 Position the person supine. Logroll the person so there is no twisting of the spine. The person must be on a hard, flat surface. Place the person's arms alongside the body.

4 Open the airway. Use the head-tilt/chin-lift maneuver.

5 Check for breathlessness.

6 Give 2 breaths. Each should be 1½ to 2 seconds long. Let the person's chest deflate between breaths.

7 Check for pulselessness. Check the carotid pulse for 5 to 10 seconds. Use your other hand to keep the airway open with the head-tilt maneuver.

8 Give chest compressions if the person has no pulse. Give compressions at a rate of 80 to 100 per minute. Give 15 compressions and then 2 breaths:

   a Establish a rhythm, and count out loud (try: "1 and, 2 and, 3 and, 4 and, 5 and, 6 and, 7 and, 8 and, 9 and, 10 and, 11 and, 12 and, 13 and, 14 and, 15").

   b Open the airway, and give 2 breaths.

   c Repeat this step until you have given 4 cycles of 15 compressions and 2 breaths.

9 Check for a carotid pulse (3 to 5 seconds).

10 Continue CPR if the person has no pulse. Begin with chest compressions.

11 Continue the cycle of 15 compressions and 2 breaths. Check for a pulse every few minutes.

12 Repeat steps 10 and 11 as long as necessary.

ADULT CPR— TWO RESCUERS

PROCEDURE

1   Perform one-person CPR until a helper arrives.

2   Continue chest compressions. The helper says, "I know CPR. Can I help?"

3   Indicate that you want help. Ask that the EMS system be activated, if not already done.

4   Do not stop chest compressions. The helper kneels on the other side of the person. The two-rescuer procedure starts after you complete a cycle of 15 compressions and 2 breaths.

5   Stop compressions for 3 to 5 seconds. The helper checks for a carotid pulse. The helper states, "No pulse."

6   Perform two-person CPR (Fig. 35-12) as follows:

  a   The helper gives 2 breaths.

  b   Give chest compressions at a rate of 80 to 100 per minute. Count out loud in a rhythm (try: "1 and, 2 and, 3 and, 4 and, 5").

  c   The helper gives a breath immediately after the fifth compression. Pause for the breath. Continue chest compressions after the breath.

  d   A breath is given after every fifth compression.

7   Stop compressions after 1 minute. Your helper checks for a carotid pulse. After the first minute, compressions are stopped every few minutes to check for breathing and circulation. Compressions are stopped for only 5 seconds.

8   Call for a switch in positions when you are tired.

9   Change positions quickly:

  a   Helper gives a breath after you give the fifth compression.

  b   Helper moves down to kneel at the person's shoulder and finds the proper hand position.

  c   You move to the person's head after giving the fifth compression.

  d   Check for a carotid pulse (3 to 5 seconds).

  e   Say, "No pulse."

  f   Give one breath before your helper starts chest compressions.

10 Give 1 breath after every fifth compression.

11 Switch positions when the person giving the compressions is tired. Check for a pulse and breathing at every position change.

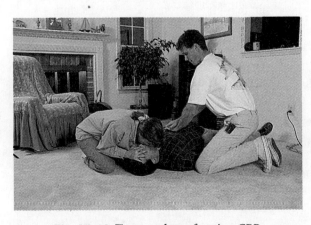

Fig. 35-12 *Two people performing CPR.*

✦ Basic Life Support for Infants and Children

Cardiac arrest caused by heart disease is rare in children. More common causes involve diseases and injuries that lead to respiratory arrest or circulatory failure. Sudden infant death syndrome (SIDS), respiratory diseases, airway obstruction, drowning, infection, and nervous system diseases are the most common causes of cardiac arrest in children under 1 year of age. Injuries are the most common cause in children older than 1 year. They include motor vehicle injuries, street injuries, bicycle injuries, drowning, burns, and firearm injuries.

Sequence of BLS for infants and children

Basic life support for infants and young children (1 to 8 years) also involves determining unresponsiveness, activating the EMS system, and determining breathlessness and pulselessness. However, there are some important differences from the adult procedures:

- Injuries are a likely cause of respiratory or cardiac arrest. Head, neck, and spinal cord injury are possible. Therefore do not move or shake the child to determine responsiveness. Check unresponsiveness by tapping or shouting to get a response.
- Shout for help, or send a second rescuer to activate the EMS system.
- If you are alone, provide basic life support for 1 minute before activating the EMS system. This can prevent respiratory arrest from advancing to cardiac arrest.
- If there are no injuries and if the person is small, carry the person to the telephone. This makes calling the EMS system easier.
- Move any person from a dangerous location. Also move the person if you cannot perform CPR where the person is lying.
- If you must move the person, make sure the head does not roll, twist, or tilt. Hold the head and body straight without twisting. Use the logrolling procedure to turn the person.
- Use the head-tilt/chin-lift maneuver for infants and children. Do not hyperextend the head as in the adult. Rather, tilt the head to a normal (neutral) or *sniffing* position (Fig. 35-13).
- If neck injury is suspected, use the jaw-thrust maneuver (Fig. 35-14):
  1. Place two or three fingers under each side of the lower jaw at the angle of the jaw.
  2. Use your other finger to lift the jaw upward and outward.
  3. Rest your elbows on the surface on which the infant or child is lying.

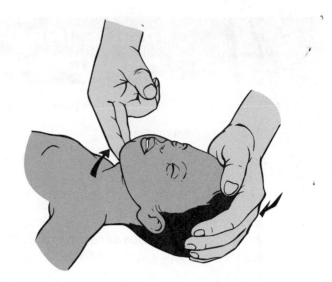

Fig. 35-13 *The head-tilt/chin-lift maneuver is used for infants. The infant's head is not tilted as far back as that of the adult. The infant's head is in a neutral or "sniffing" position.*

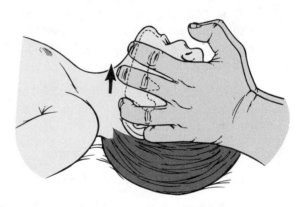

Fig. 35-14 *The jaw-thrust maneuver. Place two or three fingers on the lower jaw. Use your other fingers to lift the jaw upward and outward.*

- Keep the airway open throughout CPR. Only use one hand for chest compressions. Keep the other hand on the forehead to maintain the head tilt. For children, use both hands for the head-tilt/chin-lift maneuver when giving breaths.
- In children under 1 year of age, use the brachial pulse to determine pulselessness.
- Give 20 breaths and 100 chest compressions per minute.

CPR FOR INFANTS AND CHILDREN (UNDER 8 YEARS OF AGE)

PROCEDURE

1 Check for unresponsiveness.

2 Activate the EMS system if help is available. Otherwise, activate the EMS system after 1 minute of CPR.

3 Logroll the child onto his or her back. Support the head and neck when turning the child. Position the child supine on a hard, flat surface.

4 Open the airway. Use the head-tilt/chin-lift maneuver. Do not hyperextend the head. Extension of the head usually opens an infant's or child's airway (see Fig. 35-13).

5 Check for breathlessness.

6 Give 2 slow breaths. Use enough force to make the chest rise. Take 1 to $1\frac{1}{2}$ seconds for each breath. Cover an infant's nose and mouth with your mouth when giving a breath (Fig. 35-15). Let the chest deflate between breaths.

7 Check for pulselessness. Use the brachial artery for infants and the carotid artery for children. Keep the airway open.

8 Give chest compressions to an *infant:*

   a Locate hand position (Fig. 35-16).

   • Draw an imaginary line between the nipples.

   • Place your index finger just under the imaginary line.

   • Place your middle and ring fingers next to your index finger. The area for chest compression is below your middle and ring fingers.

   b Give compressions using your middle and ring fingers. Compress the sternum $\frac{1}{2}$ to 1 inch at least 100 times per minute. Release pressure after each compression. Do not remove your fingers from the chest.

   c Count out loud in a rhythm (try: "1, 2, 3, 4, 5").

   d Give 1 breath after every fifth compression.

   e Check for a brachial pulse after 20 cycles of 5 compressions and 1 breath (about 1 minute).

   f Activate the EMS system if there is no pulse.

   g Continue chest compressions and ventilation if there is no pulse.

   h Check for a pulse every few minutes.

9 Give chest compressions to a *child* (use the adult method if the child is large or older than age 8):

   a Locate proper hand position (Fig. 35-17):

   • Run your middle finger up along the rib cage to the notch at the center of the chest.

   • Mark the notch with your middle finger.

   • Place your index finger next to your middle finger.

   • Place the heel of the same hand next to where the index finger was located.

   b Depress the sternum 1 to $1\frac{1}{2}$ inches with the heel of your hand. Keep your fingers off the chest. Keep the airway open with your other hand.

   c Give 80 to 100 compressions per minute. Count out loud in a rhythm (try: "1 and, 2 and, 3 and, 4 and, 5").

   d Give a breath after every fifth compression.

   e Check for a carotid pulse after 20 cycles of 5 compressions and 1 breath.

   f Activate the EMS system if there is no pulse.

   g Continue chest compressions and breaths if there is no pulse.

   h Check for a pulse every few minutes.

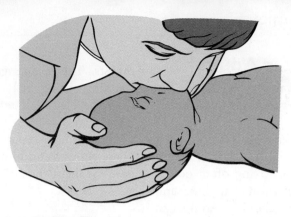

Fig. 35-15 *Cover the infant's mouth and nose during mouth-to-mouth resuscitation.*

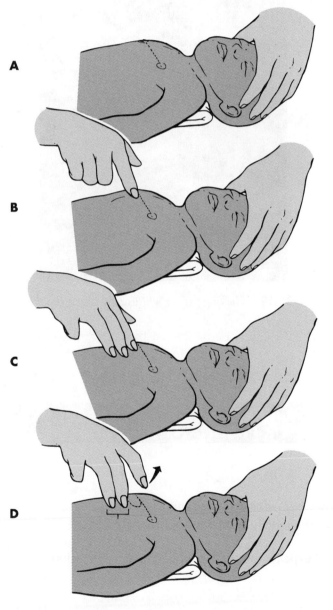

A

B

C

D

Fig. 35-16 *Locating hand position for infant chest compressions.* **A,** *Draw an imaginary line between the nipples.* **B,** *The index finger is placed just under the line.* **C,** *The middle and ring fingers are placed next to the index finger.* **D,** *The area for chest compressions is under the middle and ring fingers.*

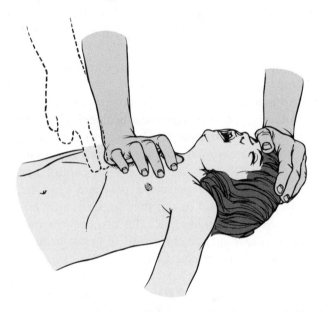

Fig. 35-17 *The heel of one hand is used for CPR on a child. The heel is placed over the lower end of the sternum as for an adult.*

⚜ Obstructed Airway in Adults

Airway obstruction (choking) can lead to cardiac arrest. Air cannot pass through the air passages to the lungs. The body does not get oxygen.

Foreign bodies can cause airway obstruction. This often occurs during eating. Meat is the most common food causing airway obstruction. Choking often occurs on large, poorly chewed pieces of meat. Laughing and talking while eating can also cause choking. Adults can choke on dentures. Excessive alcohol intake is another cause.

Airway obstruction can occur in unconscious persons. Common causes are aspiration of vomitus and the tongue falling back into the airway. These can occur during cardiac arrest.

Foreign bodies can cause partial or complete airway obstruction. With *partial obstruction*, the person moves some air in and out of the lungs. The person is conscious. Forceful coughing often removes the object. The EMS system is activated if the partial obstruction is not relieved.

With *complete airway obstruction*, the person clutches at the throat (Fig. 35-18). The person cannot breathe, speak, or cough. The person is pale and cyanotic. Air does not move in and out of the lungs. If conscious, the person is very apprehensive. The obstruction must be removed immediately, before cardiac arrest occurs. Obstructed airway is an emergency. The EMS system must be activated.

The *Heimlich maneuver* is used to relieve an obstructed airway caused by a foreign body. It involves abdominal thrusts. The maneuver is performed with the person standing, sitting, or lying down. The *finger sweep* is used with the Heimlich maneuver when an adult becomes unconscious.

The Heimlich maneuver is not effective in extremely obese persons and in pregnant women. Chest thrusts are used for them (Box 35-2).

Text continued on p. 824

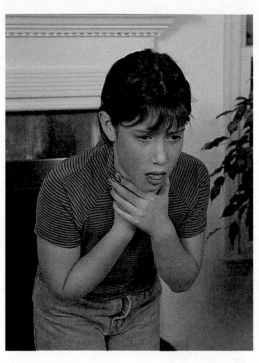

Fig. 35-18 *A choking person will usually clutch the throat.*

BOX 35-2

OBSTRUCTED AIRWAY:
CHEST THRUSTS FOR OBESE OR PREGNANT PERSONS

The Victim Is Sitting or Standing
1. Stand behind the victim.
2. Place your arms under the victim's underarms. Wrap your arms around the victim's chest.
3. Make a fist. Place the thumb side of the fist on the middle of the sternum (breastbone).
4. Grasp the fist with your other hand.
5. Give backward chest thrusts until the object is expelled or the victim becomes unconscious.

The Victim Is Lying Down or Unconscious
1. Position the victim supine.
2. Kneel next to the victim's body.
3. Position your hands as for external chest compression.
4. Give chest thrusts until the object is expelled or the victim becomes unconscious.

CLEARING THE OBSTRUCTED AIRWAY— THE PERSON IS STANDING OR SITTING

PROCEDURE

1 Ask the person if he or she is choking.

2 Determine if the person can cough or speak.

3 Perform the Heimlich maneuver if the person is choking (Fig. 35-19, p. 822):

 a Stand behind the person.

 b Wrap your arms around the person's waist.

 c Make a fist with one hand.

 d Place the thumb side of the fist against the abdomen. The fist is in the middle above the navel and below the end of the sternum (breastbone).

 e Grasp your fist with your other hand.

 f Press your fist and hand into the person's abdomen with a quick, upward thrust.

 g Repeat the abdominal thrust until the object has been expelled or the person loses consciousness.

4 Lower the unconscious person to the floor or ground.

5 Activate the EMS system.

6 Do the finger sweep maneuver to check for a foreign object (Fig. 35-20, p. 820).

 a Open the person's mouth. Use the tongue-jaw lift maneuver (see Fig. 35-20, *A*):

 • Grasp the tongue and lower jaw with your thumb and fingers.

 • Lift the lower jaw upward.

 b Insert your other index finger into the mouth along the side of the cheek and deep into the throat (Fig. 35-20, *B*). Your finger should be at the base of the tongue.

 c Form a hook with your index finger.

 d Try to dislodge and remove the object. Do not push it deeper into the throat.

 e Grasp and remove the object if it is within reach.

7 Open the airway with the head-tilt/chin-lift maneuver.

8 Give 2 breaths.

9 Reposition the person's head if you could not ventilate the person. Give 2 breaths.

10 Give up to 5 abdominal thrusts. (See *Clearing the Obstructed Airway—The Person is Lying Down*, p. 23.)

11 Repeat steps 6 through 10 (finger sweeps, rescue breathing, and abdominal thrusts) until the object is expelled or emergency medical personnel arrive.

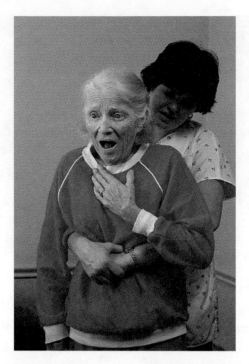

Fig. 35-19 *Abdominal thrusts with the person standing.*

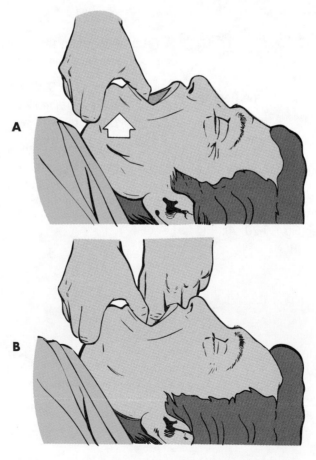

Fig. 35-20 A, *The person's tongue is grasped, and the jaw is lifted forward with one hand.*
B, *The index finger of the other hand is used to check for a foreign object.*

CLEARING THE OBSTRUCTED AIRWAY— THE PERSON IS LYING DOWN

PROCEDURE

1 Ask the person if he or she is choking.

2 Determine if the person can cough or speak.

3 Perform the Heimlich maneuver if the person is choking (Fig. 35-21):

  a Position the person supine.

  b Kneel next to the person's thighs.

  c Place the heel of one hand against the abdomen. It should be in the middle above the navel and below the end of the sternum (breastbone).

  d Place your second hand on top of your first.

  e Press your fist and hand into the abdomen with a quick, upward thrust.

  f Repeat abdominal thrusts until the object has been expelled or the person loses consciousness.

4 Activate the EMS system if the person becomes unconscious.

5 Do the finger sweep maneuver to check for a foreign object. See step 6 in *Clearing the Obstructed Airway—The Person Is Standing or Sitting.*

6 Open the airway with the head-tilt/chin-lift maneuver.

7 Give 2 breaths.

8 Reposition the person's head if you could not ventilate the person. Give 2 breaths

9 Give up to 5 abdominal thrusts.

10 Repeat steps 5 through 10 (finger sweeps, rescue breathing, abdominal thrusts) until the object is expelled or emergency medical personnel arrive.

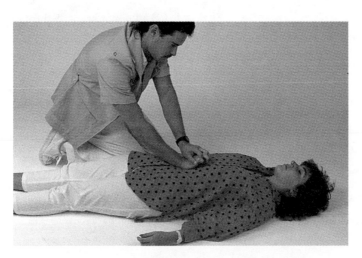

Fig. 35-21 *Abdominal thrusts with the victim lying down.*

Finding an unconscious adult

You may find an adult unconscious. You did not see the person lose consciousness, and you do not know the cause. You cannot assume the cause is choking. Therefore you need to establish unresponsiveness and attempt rescue breathing. Abdominal thrusts are done if you cannot ventilate the person. Then the finger sweep maneuver is used.

CLEARING THE OBSTRUCTED AIRWAY— THE UNCONSCIOUS ADULT

PROCEDURE

1 Check for unresponsiveness.

2 Activate the EMS system.

3 Logroll the person to the supine position with his or her face up. The person's arms should be at the sides.

4 Open the airway. Use the head-tilt/chin-lift maneuver.

5 Give 2 breaths. Reposition the person's head and open the airway if you could not ventilate. Give 2 breaths.

6 Do the Heimlich maneuver if you could not ventilate the person. See *Clearing The Obstructed Airway—The Person Is Lying Down*.

7 Do the finger sweep maneuver to check for a foreign object. See step 6 in *Clearing the Obstructed Airway—The Person Is Standing or Sitting*.

8 Repeat steps 4 through 7 until the object is expelled or emergency personnel arrive.

✦ Obstructed Airway in Children

Children have choked on small objects such as pieces of hot dogs, marbles, hard candy, peanuts, and grapes. Peanut butter and popcorn also can cause choking. So can coins and small toys and toy parts.

As with the adult, airway obstruction may be partial or complete. If the child has a strong cough, encourage the child to continue coughing. Try to relieve the obstruction if the cough weakens or when respiratory difficulty increases. Loss of consciousness is another reason to relieve the obstruction. Activate the EMS system if the child is in distress or loses consciousness.

As with adults, you may find a child or infant unconscious. You cannot assume the cause is choking on a foreign object.

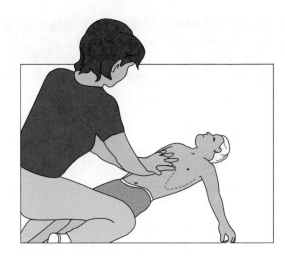

Fig. 35-22 *The Heimlich maneuver performed on an unconscious child.*

✦ CLEARING AN OBSTRUCTED AIRWAY—THE CONSCIOUS CHILD (UNDER 8 YEARS OF AGE)

PROCEDURE

1 Stand behind the child.

2 Wrap your arms under the child's underarms and around the chest.

3 Make a fist with one hand. Place the thumb side of the fist against the child's abdomen. The fist should be in the middle, above the navel and below the end of the sternum (breastbone).

4 Grab the fist with the other hand.

5 Give a quick inward and upward thrust.

6 Repeat the abdominal thrusts until the object is expelled or the child loses consciousness.

7 Lay the child down if he or she loses consciousness.

8 Call for help, and ask someone to activate the EMS system.

9 Use the tongue-jaw lift maneuver to lift the chin.

10 Look for a foreign object.

11 Remove the foreign object with the finger sweep maneuver *only if you can see the object.*

12 Open the airway. Use the head-tilt/chin-lift maneuver.

13 Give 2 breaths. Reposition the child's head if you could not ventilate the child. Give 2 more breaths.

14 Do the Heimlich maneuver if you could not ventilate the child (Fig. 35-22).

   a Kneel beside the child or straddle the hips if he or she is on the floor.

   b Place the heel of one hand against the child's abdomen. The hand is in the middle and slightly above the navel and below the end of the sternum (breastbone).

   c Place your other hand directly on top of your fist.

   d Give up to 5 quick, upward abdominal thrusts.

15 Repeat steps 9 through 14 for 1 minute. *Activate the EMS system after 1 minute if you are alone.*

16 Continue steps 9 through 14 until the object is expelled or emergency personnel arrive.

CLEARING AN OBSTRUCTED AIRWAY—THE UNCONSCIOUS CHILD (UNDER 8 YEARS OF AGE)

PROCEDURE

1 Establish unresponsiveness.

2 Ask someone to activate the EMS system.

3 Open the airway. Use the head-tilt/chin-lift maneuver.

4 Give 2 breaths. Reposition the child's head if you could not ventilate the child. Give 2 more breaths.

5 Give up to 5 abdominal thrusts (see Fig. 35-22).

6 Use the tongue-jaw lift maneuver to lift the chin.

7 Look for a foreign object.

8 Remove the foreign object with the finger sweep maneuver *only if you can see the object.*

9 Repeat steps 3 through 8 for 1 minute. *Activate the EMS system after 1 minute if you are alone.*

10 Continue steps 3 through 8 until the object is expelled or emergency personnel arrive.

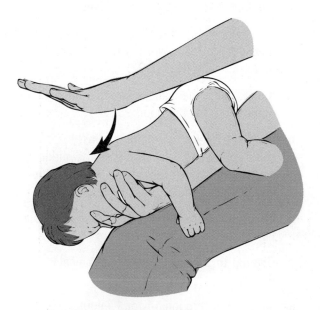

Fig. 35-23 *The infant is held face down and supported with one hand and forearm. The rescuer supports her arm on her thigh. Back blows are given with the heel of one hand. The blows are given between the infant's shoulder blades.*

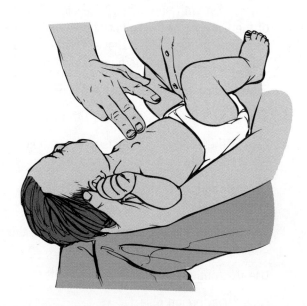

Fig. 35-24 *The infant is positioned on the rescuer's thigh for chest thrusts. Hand position for chest thrusts in the infant is the same as for chest compressions.*

CLEARING AN OBSTRUCTED AIRWAY— THE CONSCIOUS INFANT

PROCEDURE

1 Determine if the infant has an airway obstruction.

2 Hold the infant face down over your forearm. Support your arm on your thigh. The infant's head should be lower than the trunk. Hold the infant's jaw to support the head.

3 Give up to 5 back blows with the heel of one hand. Give the blows between the infant's shoulder blades (Fig. 35-23).

4 Turn the infant. Support the infant's head, neck, jaw, and chest with one hand. Support the back with your other hand.

5 Place the infant over your thigh. The baby's head is lower than the trunk.

6 Give chest thrusts (Fig. 35-24):

   a Locate hand position as for chest compressions.

   b Give up to 5 downward chest thrusts (chest compressions).

7 Repeat steps 2 through 6 until the object is expelled or the child loses consciousness.

8 Call out for help if the child loses consciousness. Ask someone to activate the EMS system.

9 Use the tongue-jaw lift maneuver to lift the chin.

10 Look for a foreign object. Remove the foreign object with the finger sweep maneuver *only if you see the object.*

11 Open the airway. Use the head-tilt/chin-lift maneuver.

12 Give 2 breaths.

13 Reposition the head if you could not ventilate. Give 2 breaths.

14 Repeat up to 5 back blows and up to 5 chest thrusts.

15 Use the tongue-jaw lift maneuver to lift the chin. Look for a foreign object. Remove the object with the finger sweep maneuver *only if you see the object.*

16 Repeat steps 11 through 15 for 1 minute. Activate the EMS system.

17 Continue steps 11 through 15 until the object is expelled or emergency personnel arrive.

18 Check for breathing and a pulse when the object is expelled.

19 Do the following if the infant has a pulse after the object is expelled:

   a Keep the airway open.

   b Give 20 breaths per minute if the infant is not breathing.

20 Start CPR if the infant has no pulse.

CLEARING AN OBSTRUCTED AIRWAY—THE UNCONSCIOUS INFANT

PROCEDURE

1 Establish unresponsiveness.

2 Call for help. Ask someone to activate the EMS system.

3 Open the airway. Use the head-tilt/chin-lift maneuver.

4 Determine breathlessness.

5 Give 2 breaths.

6 Reposition the head if you could not ventilate. Give two breaths.

7 Call out for help. Ask someone to activate the EMS system.

8 Give up to 5 back blows.

9 Give up to 5 chest thrusts.

10 Use the tongue-jaw lift maneuver to lift the chin.

11 Look for a foreign object. *Use the finger sweep maneuver only if you see the object.*

12 Open the airway. Use the head-tilt/chin-lift maneuver.

13 Give 2 breaths.

14 Repeat steps 8 through 13 for 1 minute. Activate the EMS system.

15 Continue steps 8 through 13 until the object is expelled or emergency personnel arrive.

16 Check for breathing and a pulse when the object is expelled.

17 Do the following if the infant has a pulse after the object is expelled:

    a Keep the airway open.

    b Give 20 breaths per minute if the infant is not breathing.

18 Start CPR if the infant has no pulse.

Recovery Position

The recovery position is a side-lying position (Fig. 35-25). It is used when the person is breathing and has a pulse. Logroll the person into the recovery position, keeping the head, neck, and spine straight. Then keep the person in good alignment. An arm supports the head. This position keeps the airway open and prevents aspiration. *Do not use this position if the person might have neck injuries or other trauma.*

Self-Administered Heimlich Maneuver

You yourself may choke. You can perform the Heimlich maneuver to relieve the obstructed airway. To do so:

- Make a fist with one hand.
- Place the thumb side of the fist above your navel and below the lower end of the sternum.
- Grasp your fist with your other hand.
- Press inward and upward quickly.
- Press the upper abdomen against a hard surface if the thrust did not relieve the obstruction. Use the back of a chair, a table, or a railing.
- Use as many thrusts as needed.

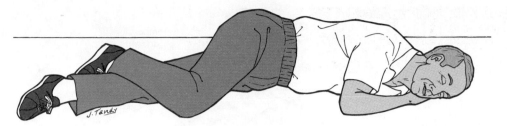

Fig. 35-25 *Recovery position.*

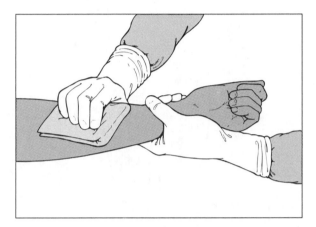

Fig. 35-26 *Apply direct pressure to the wound to stop bleeding. Place your hand over the wound.* (*From Parcel GS, Rinear CE:* Basic emergency care of the sick and injured, *ed 4, 1990, McGraw Hill.*)

HEMORRHAGE

Life and body functions require an adequate blood supply. Blood must circulate through the body. If a blood vessel is torn or cut, bleeding occurs. The larger the blood vessel, the greater the bleeding and blood loss. **Hemorrhage** is the excessive loss of blood in a short period of time. If the bleeding is not stopped, death results.

Hemorrhage may be internal or external. You cannot see internal hemorrhage. Bleeding occurs inside the body into tissues and body cavities. Pain, shock (see p. 830), vomiting blood, coughing up blood, and loss of consciousness are signs of internal hemorrhage. There is little you can do for internal bleeding. Activate the EMS system. Then keep the person warm, flat, and quiet until medical help arrives. Do not give fluids. Follow Standard Precautions and the Bloodborne Pathogen Standard in case the person vomits or coughs up blood.

External bleeding is usually seen. However, it may be hidden by clothing. Hemorrhage may be from an injured artery or vein. Bleeding from an artery is bright red and occurs in spurts. There is a steady flow of blood from a vein. External bleeding must be stopped. You can do the following to control external hemorrhage:

- Activate the EMS system.
- Practice Standard Precautions, and follow the Bloodborne Pathogen Standard. Wear gloves if possible.
- Place a sterile dressing directly over the wound. Use any clean material (handkerchief, towel, cloth, or sanitary napkin) if you do not have a sterile dressing.
- Apply pressure with your hand directly over the bleeding site (Fig. 35-26). Do not release the pressure until the bleeding is controlled.
- If direct pressure does not control bleeding, apply pressure over the artery above the bleeding site (Fig. 35-27, p. 830). For example, if bleeding is from the lower arm, apply pressure over the brachial artery. The brachial artery supplies blood to the lower arm. Use your first three fingers to apply pressure on the artery.

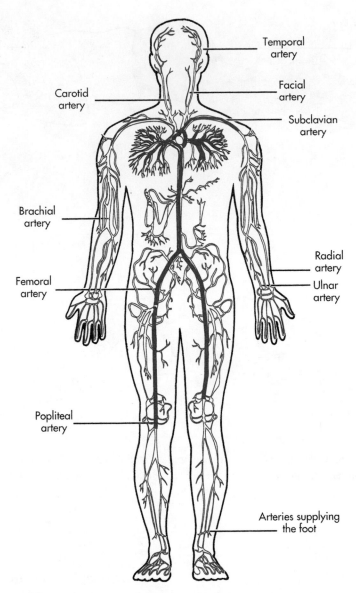

Fig. 35-27 *Pressure points to control bleeding. (From Kidd PS, Sturt P: Mosby's emergency nursing reference, St Louis, 1996, Mosby.)*

SHOCK

Shock results when there is not enough blood supply to organs and tissues. Blood loss, heart attack (myocardial infarction), burns, and severe infection can cause shock. Signs and symptoms include:

- Low or falling blood pressure
- Rapid and weak pulse
- Rapid respirations
- Cold, moist, and pale skin
- Thirst
- Restlessness
- Confusion and loss of consciousness as shock worsens

Shock is possible in any person who is acutely ill or injured. Do the following to prevent and treat shock:

- Keep the person lying down.
- Maintain an open airway.
- Control hemorrhage.
- Keep the person warm. Place a blanket over and under the person if possible.
- Reassure the person.
- Activate the EMS system.

Anaphylactic Shock

Some people are allergic or sensitive to various substances such as foods, insects, chemicals, and drugs. Many people are allergic to penicillin. Remember, an antigen is a substance that the body reacts to (see Chapter 20). The body fights or attacks the antigen by releasing chemicals. The reaction may be a local area of redness, swelling, or itching. Or the reaction can involve the entire body.

Anaphylaxis is life-threatening sensitivity to an antigen. It comes from the Greek words that mean without *(ana)* protection *(phylaxis)*. In severe cases, anaphylactic shock can occur within seconds. Signs and symptoms include:

- Sweating
- Shortness of breath
- Low blood pressure
- Irregular pulse
- Respiratory congestion
- Swelling of the larynx (laryngeal edema)
- Hoarseness
- Dyspnea

Anaphylactic shock is an emergency. The EMS system must be activated. The person needs special drugs to reverse the allergic reaction. Until emergency help arrives, keep the person lying down. Also keep the airway open. CPR is necessary if cardiac arrest occurs.

SEIZURES

Seizures (convulsions) are violent and sudden contractions of muscles. The muscle contractions are involuntary. Seizures are caused by an abnormality in the brain. Causes include head injuries during birth or from trauma, high fever, brain tumors, poisoning, seizure disorders, and central nervous system infections. Lack of blood flow to the brain can also cause seizures.

The major types of seizures are *partial seizures* and *generalized seizures*. Only a part of the brain is involved with a partial seizure. A body part may jerk. Or the person has hearing or vision problems or stomach discomfort. The person does not lose consciousness.

With generalized seizures, the whole brain is involved. The *generalized tonic-clonic seizure (grand mal seizure)* has two phases. The tonic phase is first. The person loses consciousness. If standing or sitting, the person falls to the floor. The body is rigid because all muscles contract at once. The clonic phase is next. Muscle groups contract and relax. This causes jerking and twitching movements of the body. Urinary and fecal incontinence may occur. After the seizure, the person usually falls into a deep sleep. The person may have confusion and headache on awakening.

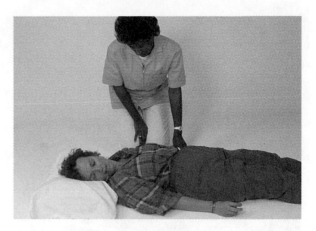

Fig. 35-28 *Protect the person's head during a seizure.*

The *generalized absence (petit mal) seizure* usually lasts a few seconds. There is loss of consciousness, twitching of the eyelids, and staring. No first aid is necessary.

You cannot stop a seizure. However, you can protect the person from injury during a seizure. The following measures are performed for a generalized tonic-clonic seizure:

- Call for help.
- Lower the person to the floor. This protects the person from falling.
- Place a folded blanket, towel, cushion, pillow, or other soft item under the person's head (Fig. 35-28). Cradle the person's head in your lap if a soft item is not available. This prevents the person's head from striking the hard surface of the floor.
- Turn the person onto his or her side. Make sure the head is turned to the side.
- Loosen tight clothing around the person's neck. This includes ties, scarves, or collars. Also loosen tight neck jewelry.
- Move furniture, equipment, and sharp objects away from the person. The person may strike these objects during the uncontrolled body movements.
- Do not try to restrain body movements during the seizure.
- Summon medical help. Do not leave the person during the seizure.
- Do not put your fingers between the person's teeth. The person can bite down on your fingers during the seizure.

(See Focus on Children on p. 832.)

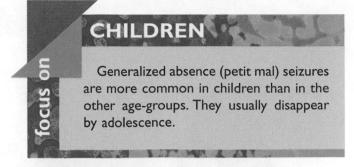

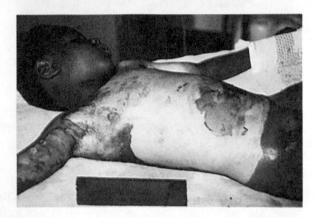

Fig. 35-29 *Full-thickness burn from flames. (Courtesy St. John's Mercy Hospital, St Louis, Mo.)*

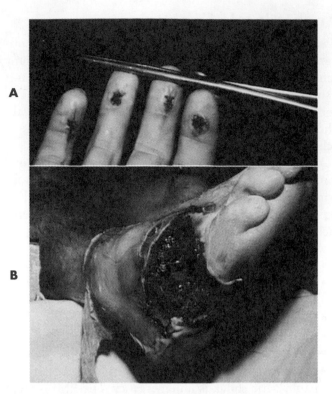

Fig. 35-30 *An electrical burn.* **A,** *The electrical current enters through the hand.* **B,** *The electrical current exits through the foot. (From JEMS, March 1992, p 514, JEMS Communications, Inc, Carlsbad, Calif.)*

BURNS

Burns can severely disable a person (Fig. 35-29). They can also cause death. Most burn injuries occur in the home. Common causes of burns and fires are:

- Scalds from hot liquids
- Playing with matches and lighters
- Electrical injuries (Fig. 35-30)
- Cooking accidents (barbecues, microwaves, stoves, ovens)
- Falling asleep while smoking
- Fireplaces
- Space heaters
- No smoke detectors or nonfunctioning smoke detectors
- Sunburn
- Chemicals

The skin has two layers: the dermis and epidermis. Burns are described as partial thickness or full thickness. *Partial-thickness burns* involve the dermis and part of the epidermis. These burns are very painful. Nerve endings are exposed. *Full-thickness burns* involve the dermis and the entire epidermis. The fat layer, muscle, and bone may be injured or destroyed. Full-thickness burns are not painful. Nerve endings are destroyed.

Burns vary in seriousness. Burn size and depth, the body part involved, and the person's age affect the severity of the burn. Burns to the face, eyes, ears, hands, and feet are more serious than burns to an arm or leg.

Activate the EMS system as soon as possible. Emergency care of burns includes the following:

- Do not touch the person if he or she is in contact with an electrical source. Have the power source turned off, or remove the electrical source first. Use an object that does not conduct electricity (rope or wood) to remove the electrical source.
- Remove the person from the fire or burn source.
- Stop the burning process. Extinguish flames with water, or roll the person in a blanket. Or use a coat, sheet, or towel.
- Remove hot clothing that is not sticking to the skin. Also remove jewelry and any tight clothing. If you cannot remove hot clothing, cool the clothing with water.
- Provide basic life support as needed. This includes activating the EMS system.
- Cover the burn wounds with a clean, moist covering. You can use towels, sheets, or any other clean cloth. Keep the covering wet.

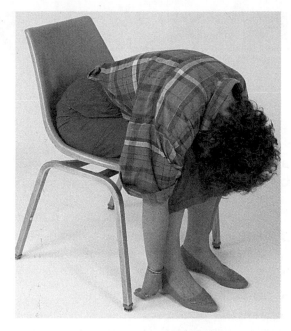

Fig. 35-31 *The person bends forward and places the head between the knees to prevent fainting.*

- Do not put oil, butter, salve, or ointments on the burns.
- Cover the person with a blanket or coat to prevent heat loss.

(See Focus on Children and Focus on Older Persons.)

FAINTING

Fainting is the sudden loss of consciousness from an inadequate blood supply to the brain. Hunger, fatigue, fear, and pain are common causes. Some people faint at the sight of blood or injury. Standing in one position for a long time or being in a warm, crowded room can lead to fainting. Dizziness, perspiration, and blackness before the eyes are warning signals. The person looks pale. The pulse is weak. Respirations are shallow if consciousness is lost. Emergency care for fainting includes the following:

- Have the person sit or lie down before fainting occurs.
- If sitting, the person bends forward and places his or her head between the knees (Fig. 35-31).
- If the person is lying down, elevate the legs.
- Loosen tight clothing.

- Keep the person lying down if fainting has occurred.
- Do not let the person get up until symptoms have subsided for about 5 minutes.
- Help the person to a sitting position after recovery from fainting. Observe for symptoms of fainting.

STROKE

Stroke (cerebrovascular accident, brain attack) was described in Chapter 30. A stroke occurs when the brain is suddenly deprived of its blood supply. Usually only part of the brain is affected. A stroke may be caused by a thrombus, an embolus, or cerebral hemorrhage. Cerebral hemorrhage is caused by the rupture of a blood vessel in the brain.

The signs of stroke vary. They depend on the size and location of brain injury. Loss of consciousness or semi-consciousness, rapid pulse, labored respirations, elevated blood pressure, vomiting, and hemiplegia are signs of stroke. The person may have aphasia (the inability to speak). Seizures may occur.

Emergency care includes the following:

- Turn the person onto the affected side. The affected side is limp, and the cheek appears puffy.
- Elevate the head without flexing the neck.
- Loosen tight clothing.
- Keep the person quiet and warm.
- Reassure the person.
- Activate the EMS system.

REVIEW QUESTIONS

Circle the best *answer.*

1 The goals of first aid are to
   a   Call for help and keep the person warm
   b   Prevent death and prevent injuries from becoming worse
   c   Stay calm and perform emergency measures
   d   Reassure the person and keep bystanders away

2 When giving first aid, you should
   a   Be aware of your own limitations
   b   Move the person
   c   Give the person fluids
   d   Perform any necessary emergency measures

3 The person is in cardiac arrest. Cardiac arrest is
   a   The same as stroke
   b   The sudden stopping of heart action and breathing
   c   The sudden loss of consciousness
   d   The condition that results when there is inadequate blood supply to the organs and tissues of the body

4 Which is *not* a sign of cardiac arrest?
   a   No pulse
   b   No breathing
   c   A sudden drop in blood pressure
   d   Unconsciousness

5 You are to give mouth-to-mouth rescue breathing. You should do the following *except*
   a   Pinch the person's nostrils shut
   b   Place your mouth tightly over the person's mouth
   c   Blow air into the person's mouth as you exhale
   d   Cover the person's nose with your mouth

6 External chest compressions are performed on an adult. The chest is compressed
   a $\frac{1}{2}$ to 1 inch with the index and middle fingers
   b   1 to $1\frac{1}{2}$ inches with the heel of one hand
   c $1\frac{1}{2}$ to 2 inches with two hands
   d   With one hand in the middle of the sternum

7 Which does *not* determine breathlessness?
   a   Looking to see if the chest rises and falls
   b   Counting respirations for 30 seconds
   c   Listening for the escape of air
   d   Feeling for the flow of air

8 Which is used to feel for a pulse during adult CPR?
   a   The apical pulse
   b   The brachial pulse
   c   The carotid pulse
   d   The dorsalis pedis pulse

9 How many breaths are given at the beginning of CPR?
   a   One
   b   Two
   c   Three
   d   Four

10 You are performing adult CPR alone. Which is *false?*
   a   Give two breaths after every 15 compressions
   b   Check for a pulse after 1 minute
   c   Give one breath after every fifth compression
   d   Count out loud

11 Adult CPR is being given by two people. Breaths are given
   a   After every fifth compression
   b   After every fifteenth compression
   c   After every compression
   d   Only when the positions are changed

12 External cardiac compressions are given to an infant at a rate of
   a   60 per minute
   b   75 per minute
   c   80 per minute
   d   100 per minute

13 The most common cause of obstructed airway in adults is
   a   A loose denture
   b   Meat
   c   Marbles
   d   Candy

REVIEW QUESTIONS—cont'd

14 If airway obstruction occurs, the person usually

 a Clutches at the throat

 b Can speak, cough, and breathe

 c Is calm

 d Has a seizure

15 The Heimlich maneuver is used to relieve an obstructed airway. Which is *false?*

 a The person can be standing, sitting, or lying down.

 b A fist is made with one hand.

 c The thrusts are given inward and upward at the lower end of the sternum.

 d The hands are positioned in the middle between the waist and lower end of the sternum.

16 An adult has an obstructed airway. Poking motions are used with the finger-sweep maneuver.

 a True

 b False

17 Arterial bleeding is suspected. Arterial bleeding

 a Cannot be seen

 b Occurs in spurts

 c Is dark red

 d Oozes from the wound

18 A person is hemorrhaging from the left forearm. The first action is to

 a Lower the body part

 b Apply pressure to the brachial artery

 c Apply direct pressure to the wound

 d Cover the person

19 A person is in shock. The signs of shock are

 a Rising blood pressure, rapid pulse, and slow respirations

 b Rapid pulse, rapid respirations, and warm skin

 c Falling blood pressure; rapid pulse and respirations; and skin that is cold, moist, and pale

 d Falling blood pressure; slow pulse and respirations; thirst; restlessness; and warm, flushed skin

20 A person in shock needs

 a Mouth-to-mouth resuscitation

 b To be kept lying down

 c Clothes removed

 d To be placed in Trendelenburg position

21 These statements relate to generalized tonic-clonic seizures. Which is *false?*

 a There is contraction of all muscles at once.

 b Lowering the person to the floor stops the seizure.

 c The person's head must be protected during the seizure.

 d There is loss of consciousness during the seizure.

22 A person was burned. There are no complaints or signs of pain. You know that

 a The burn is minor

 b The burn is partial thickness

 c The burn is full thickness

 d The dermis was destroyed

23 Burns are covered with

 a A clean, moist cloth or dressing

 b Butter, oil, or salve

 c Water

 d Nothing

24 A person is about to faint. You should *not*

 a Take the person outside for some fresh air

 b Have the person sit or lie down

 c Loosen tight clothing

 d Elevate the legs if the person is lying down

25 Emergency care of the person having a stroke includes the following *except*

 a Positioning the person on the affected side

 b Giving the person sips of water

 c Loosening tight clothing

 d Keeping the person quiet and warm

Answers to these questions are on p. 854.

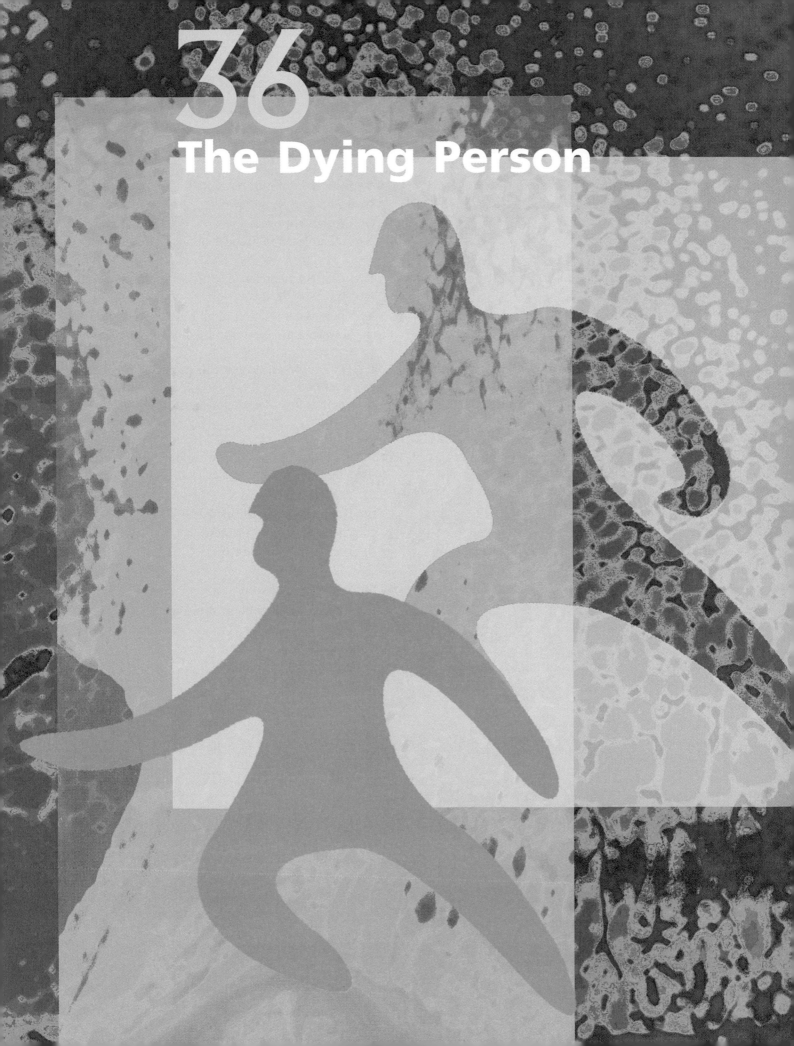

36

The Dying Person

- Define the key terms in this chapter
- Describe terminal illness
- Identify the psychological forces that influence living and dying
- Explain how culture and religion influence attitudes about death
- Describe how different age-groups view death
- Describe the five stages of dying
- Explain how to meet the dying person's psychological, social, and spiritual needs
- Explain how you can help meet the physical needs of the dying person
- Describe the needs of the family during the dying process
- Describe hospice care
- Explain the importance of the Patient Self-Determination Act
- Explain what is meant by a *do not resuscitate* order
- Explain how to promote quality of life for the dying person
- Identify the signs of approaching death and the signs of death
- Perform the procedure described in this chapter

KEY TERMS

advance directive A written document stating a person's wishes about health care when that person can no longer make his or her own decisions

postmortem After *(post)* death *(mortem)*

reincarnation The belief that the spirit or soul is reborn in another human body or in another form of life

rigor mortis The stiffness or rigidity *(rigor)* of skeletal muscles that occurs after death *(mortis)*

terminal illness An illness or injury for which there is no reasonable expectation of recovery

Dying people are cared for in hospitals, long-term care centers, or at home. Many are in hospice programs (see p. 841). Death can occur suddenly and without warning. Often it is expected.

The health team members see death often. Many are unsure of their feelings about death. They are uncomfortable with dying persons and the subject of death. Dying persons represent helplessness and failure to cure. They also remind us of our own eventual death.

You must examine your feelings about death. Your attitudes about death and dying affect the care you give. You will help meet the dying person's physical, psychological, social, and spiritual needs. Therefore you need to understand the dying process. Then you can approach the dying person with care, kindness, and respect.

TERMINAL ILLNESS

Many illnesses and diseases can be cured or controlled. Others have no cure. Many injuries can be repaired. Others are so serious that the body cannot function. Recovery is not expected. The disease or injury ends in death. An illness or injury for which there is no reasonable expectation of recovery is a **terminal illness.**

Doctors cannot predict the exact time of death. A person may have days, weeks, months, or years to live. Predictions have been wrong. People expected to live for only a short time have lived for years. Others were expected to live for a longer time. They died sooner than expected.

Modern medicine has found cures or has prolonged life in many cases. Future research will bring new cures.

However, two very powerful psychological forces influence living and dying. They are hope and the will to live. People have died sooner than expected or for no apparent reason when they lost hope or the will to live.

ATTITUDES ABOUT DEATH

Experiences, culture, religion, and age influence a person's attitude about death. Many people fear death. Others do not believe they will die. Some look forward to and accept death. Attitudes and beliefs about death often change as a person grows older. They are also affected by changing circumstances.

Dying people are usually cared for in health agencies or at home. The family is often involved in the person's care. Family members usually gather at the bedside to comfort the person and to say their last farewells. The family also comforts each other. When death occurs, the funeral director is called to take the body to the funeral home. There the body is prepared for funeral practices.

Many adults and children never have had contact with a dying person. Nor were they present when death occurred. Some have not attended a visitation or funeral. They have not seen the process of dying and death. Therefore it is frightening, morbid, and a mystery.

Culture and Religion

American practices and attitudes are different from those of other cultures (Box 36-1). In some cultures, dying people are cared for at home by the family. Some families care for the body after death and prepare it for burial.

Attitudes about death are closely related to culture and religion. Some believe that life after death is free of suffering and hardship. They also believe in future reunion with family and loved ones. Many believe there is punishment and suffering in the afterlife for sins and misdeeds. Others do not believe in the afterlife. They believe death is the end of life. There are also religious beliefs about the form of the human body after death. Some believe the body keeps its physical form. Others believe that only the spirit or soul is present in the afterlife. **Reincarnation** is the belief that the spirit or soul is reborn into another human body or into another form of life. Many people strengthen their religious beliefs when dying. Religion also provides comfort for the dying person and the family.

Beliefs About Death

Adults fear pain and suffering, dying alone, and the invasion of privacy. They also fear loneliness and separation from family and loved ones. They worry about who

focus on CHILDREN

Ideas about death change as people grow older. Infants and toddlers have no concept of death. Children between the ages of 3 and 5 years start to be curious and have ideas about death. They recognize the death of family members or pets and notice dead birds or bugs. They think death is temporary. Children often blame themselves when someone or something dies. They see the death as punishment for being bad. When children ask questions about death, adults often give answers that cause fear and confusion. Children who are told, "He is sleeping," may be afraid to go to sleep.

Children between the ages of 5 and 7 years know death is final. They do not think that they will die. Death happens to other people. They also think death can be avoided. Children associate death with punishment and body mutilation. It is associated also with witches, ghosts, goblins, and monsters. These ideas come from fairy tales, cartoons, movies, video games, and television.

focus on OLDER PERSONS

Older persons usually have fewer fears than younger adults. They accept that death will occur. They have had more experiences with dying and death. Many have lost family members and friends. Some welcome death as freedom from pain, suffering, and disability. Death also means reunion with those who have died first. Like younger adults, older persons often fear dying alone.

will care for and support those left behind. Adults often resent death. This is particularly true when it interferes with plans, hopes, dreams, and ambitions. (See Focus on Children and Focus on Older Persons.)

BOX 36-1

TOP TEN COUNTRIES OF ORIGIN OF IMMIGRANTS TO THE UNITED STATES*: DEATH RITES

Country	Death Rites
Mexico	Small children may not be part of dying and death rituals. Family members take turns staying around the clock with the dying person in the hospital. Grief can be expressive; for example, *el ataque* consists of hyperkinetic (increased muscle movement) or seizure-type behavior patterns. These behavior patterns serve to release emotions.
Vietnam	Quality of life is more important than length of life because of beliefs in reincarnation. There is also the expectation of less suffering in the next life. Therefore dying persons are helped to recall their past good deeds and to achieve a fitting mental state. Autopsies are allowed. Cremation is preferred. Death at home is preferred over death in the hospital. Upon death the body is washed and wrapped in clean white sheets. In some areas a coin or jewels (a wealthier family) and rice (a poorer family) are put in the dead person's mouth. This is from the belief that they will help the soul go through the encounters with gods and devils and the soul will be born rich in the next life. Relatives sew small pillows to place under the neck, feet, and wrists of the body. The body is placed in a coffin, and burial is in the ground.
Philippines	The person is protected from knowing about a poor prognosis because it will only add to his or her suffering. After death, emotional grief responses may occur.
Former Soviet Union	The family is told first of a serious prognosis. They decide if the person should be informed.
Dominican Republic	No information
Mainland China	The Chinese have an aversion to death and to anything concerning death. Autopsy and disposal of the body are individual preferences and are not prescribed by religion. Euthanasia is allowed. Donation of body parts is encouraged. The eldest son is responsible for all arrangements for the deceased. The deceased is initially buried in a coffin. After 7 years the body is exhumed and cremated. The urn is reburied in the tomb. White clothing is worn for mourning.
India	Hindu persons may make indirect references to their own deaths, often accepting God's will. The person's desire to be clearheaded as death approaches must be assessed in planning medical treatment. Providing a time and place for prayer is essential for the family and the person. Prayer helps them deal with anxiety and conflict. The Hindu priest or anyone present may read from the Holy Sanskrit books. Some priests tie strings (signifying a blessing) around the neck or wrist. After death the priest pours water into the mouth of the deceased. Families may prefer that only Hindus touch the body and may wash the body themselves. Blood transfusions, organ transplants, and autopsies are allowed. Cremation is preferred. Reincarnation is a Hindu belief.
El Salvador	No information
Poland	The body is not embalmed. It is placed in the home for the wake. Church services and ground burial follow. Feelings of grief may be verbally expressive.
United Kingdom	No information

From Geissler EM: *Pocket guide to cultural assessment*, St Louis, 1994, Mosby.
*Information obtained from U.S. Dept. of Immigration and Naturalization Services.

THE STAGES OF DYING

Dr. Elisabeth Kübler-Ross described five stages of dying. They are denial, anger, bargaining, depression, and acceptance:

- *Denial* is the first stage. Persons refuse to believe they are dying. "No, not me" is a common response. The person believes a mistake was made. Information about the illness or injury is not heard. The person cannot deal with any problem or decision about the illness or injury. This stage can last for a few hours, days, or much longer. Some people are still in denial when they die.
- *Anger* is the second stage of dying. The person thinks "Why me?" People in this stage feel anger and rage. They envy and resent those who have life and health. Family, friends, and the health team are usually targets of anger. They blame others. Fault is found with those who are loved and needed the most. The health team and family may have a hard time dealing with persons during this stage. Remember that anger is a normal, healthy reaction. Do not take the person's anger personally. You must control any urge to attack back or avoid the person.
- *Bargaining* is the third stage. Anger has passed. The person now says "Yes, me, but. . . ." Often there is bargaining with God for more time. Promises are made in exchange for more time. The person may want to see a child marry, see a grandchild, have one more Christmas, or live for an important event. Usually more promises are made as the person makes "just one more" request. This stage may not be obvious to you. Bargaining is usually done privately and on a spiritual level.
- *Depression* is the fourth stage. The person thinks "Yes, me" and is very sad. There is mourning over things that were lost and the future loss of life. The person may cry or say little. Sometimes the person talks about people and things that will be left behind.
- *Acceptance* of death is the fifth and final stage of dying. The person is calm and at peace. The person has said what needs to be said. Unfinished business is completed. The person is ready to accept death. A person may be in this stage for many months or years. Reaching the acceptance stage does not mean death is near.

Dying persons do not always pass through all five stages. A person may never get beyond a certain stage. Some people move back and forth between stages. For example, a person who has reached acceptance may move back to bargaining. Then the person may move forward to acceptance. Some people are in one stage until death.

PSYCHOLOGICAL, SOCIAL, AND SPIRITUAL NEEDS

Dying people continue to have psychological, social, and spiritual needs. They may want family and friends present. They may want to talk about the fears, worries, and anxieties of dying. Some want to be alone. Often they want to talk to a nursing team member. Persons often need to talk during the night. Things are quiet, distractions are few, and there is more time to think.

Listening and touch are two very important aspects of communication when dealing with the dying person:

- *Listening.* The dying person is the one who needs to talk, express feelings, and share worries and concerns. Just being there and listening help to meet the person's psychological and social needs. Do not worry about saying the wrong thing. Nor should you worry about finding the right words to comfort and cheer the person. Nothing really must be said. Being there for the person is what counts.
- *Touch.* Touch can convey caring and concern when words cannot. Sometimes a person does not want to talk but needs you nearby. Do not feel that you need to talk. Silence, along with touch, is a powerful and meaningful way to communicate.

Spiritual needs are important. The person may wish to see a priest, rabbi, minister, or other cleric. The person may also want to participate in religious practices. Privacy is provided during prayer and spiritual moments. Courtesy is given to the clergy. The person is allowed to have religious objects nearby (medals, pictures, statues, or religious books and writings). You must handle these items like other valuables.

PHYSICAL NEEDS

Dying may take a few minutes, hours, days, or weeks. There is general slowing of body processes, weakness, and changes in levels of consciousness. The person is allowed to be as independent as possible. As the person's condition weakens, the nursing team helps meet basic needs. The person may totally depend on others for basic needs and activities of daily living. Every effort is made to promote the person's physical and psychological comfort. The person is allowed to die in peace and with dignity.

Vision, Hearing, and Speech

Vision blurs and gradually fails. The person naturally turns toward light. A darkened room may frighten the person. The eyes may be half open. Secretions often collect in the corners of the eyes. Because of failing vision, explain what is being done to the person or in the room.

The room should be well lit. However, avoid bright lights and glares. Good eye care is essential (see Chapter 14). If the eyes stay open, a nurse may apply a protective ointment. Then the eyes are covered with moistened pads to prevent injury.

Hearing is one of the last functions lost. Many people hear until the moment of death. Even if unconscious, the person may hear. Always assume that the dying person or any unconscious person can hear. Speak in a normal voice, provide reassurance and explanations about care, and offer words of comfort. Avoid topics that could upset the person.

Speech becomes difficult. It may be hard to understand the person. Sometimes the person cannot speak. The nursing team needs to anticipate the person's needs. The person is not asked questions that have long answers. "Yes" or "no" questions are asked. These are kept to a minimum. Though speech may be hard or impossible, you must still talk to the person.

Mouth, Nose, and Skin

Oral hygiene is essential for comfort. Routine mouth care is given if the person can eat and drink. Frequent oral hygiene is given as death approaches and when there is difficulty taking oral fluids. Oral hygiene is also important if mucus collects in the mouth and the person cannot swallow.

Crusting and irritation of the nostrils can occur. Common causes are increased nasal secretions, an oxygen cannula, or a nasogastric (NG) tube. The nose is carefully cleaned. The nurse may have you apply a lubricant to the nostrils.

Circulation fails and body temperature rises as death approaches. Though body temperature rises, the skin is cool, pale, and mottled (blotchy). Perspiration increases. Good skin care, bathing, and the prevention of pressure ulcers are necessary. Linens and gowns are changed whenever needed because of perspiration. Although the skin feels cool, only light bed coverings are needed. Blankets may make the person feel warm and cause restlessness.

Elimination

Dying persons may have urinary and fecal incontinence. Waterproof bed protectors are used. Perineal care is given as necessary. Some persons are constipated and have urinary retention. Doctors may order enemas and Foley catheters.

Comfort and Positioning

Measures are taken to promote comfort. Good skin care, personal hygiene, back massages, and oral hygiene help to increase comfort. Some persons have severe pain.

The nurse gives pain medications ordered by the doctor. Frequent position changes promote comfort. So does good body alignment using supportive devices. Care is taken when turning the person. You may need help to turn the person slowly and gently. Persons with breathing difficulties usually prefer semi-Fowler's position.

The Person's Room

The person's room should be as pleasant as possible. It should be well lit and well ventilated. Unnecessary equipment is removed. Some equipment is upsetting to look at (suction machines, drainage containers). If possible, these items are kept out of the person's sight. The room should be near the nurse's station. The person can be watched more carefully.

Mementos, pictures, cards, flowers, religious objects, and other significant items comfort and reassure the person. Arranging them within the person's view is appreciated. The person and family are allowed to arrange the room as they wish. This helps meet the needs of love, belonging, and self-esteem. The room should be comfortable, pleasant, and reflect the person's choices. This promotes physical and mental comfort.

THE FAMILY

The family is going through a hard time. It may be very hard to find the right words to comfort them. You can show your feelings to the family by being available, courteous, and considerate. Also use touch to show your concern.

The family usually spends a lot of time with their loved one. Normal visiting hours do not apply if the person is dying. You must respect the person's and family's right to privacy. They need as much time together as possible. However, you cannot neglect the person's care just because the family is present. Most agencies let family members help give care. If they do not want to help, you can suggest that they take a break for a beverage or meal.

The family may be very tired, sad, and tearful. They need support and understanding. Watching a loved one die is very painful. So is dealing with the eventual loss of that person. The family is given every possible courtesy and respect. They may find comfort in a visit from a member of the clergy. You need to communicate this request to the nurse immediately.

HOSPICE CARE

Hospice care is an option for the terminally ill (see Chapter 1). Hospices are concerned with the physical, emotional, social, and spiritual needs of dying persons and their families. Care does not focus on cures or life-saving procedures. Rather, pain relief and comfort measures are stressed. The goal of hospice care is to improve the dying person's quality of life.

A hospice may be part of a hospital or nursing center or a separate agency. Many hospices offer home care. Follow-up care and support groups for survivors are other hospice services.

LEGAL ISSUES AND QUALITY OF LIFE

Much attention is given to the right to die. Many people do not want to be kept alive by machines or other measures. Consent must be given for any treatment. People make their own decisions when they are able. Some make their wishes about prolonging death known before the time comes.

The Patient Self-Determination Act

The Patient Self-Determination Act gives persons the right to accept or refuse medical treatment. They also have the right to make advance directives. An **advance directive** is a written document stating a person's wishes about health care when that person can no longer make his or her own decisions. Advance directives usually forbid certain types of care if there is no hope of recovery. Living wills and durable power of attorney are common advance directives.

All health care agencies must inform all persons on admission of the right to advance directives. This information must be in writing. The person's medical record must document whether the person has made advance directives. The law also protects the person's quality of care. Quality of care cannot be less because the person has made advance directives.

Living wills

A living will is a person's written statement about the use of life-sustaining measures. Life-sustaining measures are those that support or maintain life. Tube feedings, ventilators, and cardiopulmonary resuscitation (CPR) are some examples. These measures and other machines keep the person alive when death is likely. A living will instructs doctors:
- Not to start measures that prolong dying
- To remove measures that prolong dying

Durable power of attorney

Durable power of attorney for health care is another type of advance directive. The power to make decisions about health care is given to another person. Usually this is a family member or friend. Sometimes it is a lawyer. A person may no longer be able to make decisions about his or her own health care. Then the person with durable power of attorney has the legal authority to do so.

"Do Not Resuscitate" Orders

When death is sudden and unexpected, every effort is made to save the person's life. CPR is started (see Chapter 35) and an emergency *code* is called. Nurses, doctors, and emergency staff rush to the person's bedside. They bring emergency and life-saving equipment with them. CPR and other life-support measures are continued until the person is resuscitated or until the doctor declares the person dead.

Doctors often write *do not resuscitate (DNR)* or *no code* orders for terminally ill persons. This means that no attempts will be made to resuscitate the person. The person will be allowed to die in peace and with dignity. The orders are often written after consulting with the person or family. Some advance directives address resuscitation.

Quality of Life

A person has the right to die in peace and with dignity. Box 36-2 contains the dying person's bill of rights. (See Focus on Long-Term Care on p. 845.)

BOX 36-2

THE DYING PERSON'S BILL OF RIGHTS

- I have the right to be treated as a living human being until I die.
- I have the right to maintain a sense of hopefulness, however changing its focus may be.
- I have the right to be cared for by those who can maintain a sense of hopefulness, however changing this might be.
- I have the right to express my feelings and emotions about my approaching death, in my own way.
- I have the right to participate in decisions concerning my care.
- I have the right to expect continuing medical and nursing attention even though "cure" goals must be changed to "comfort" goals.
- I have the right not to die alone.
- I have the right to be free from pain.
- I have the right to have my questions answered honestly.
- I have the right not to be deceived.
- I have the right to have help from and for my family accepting my death.
- I have the right to die in peace and dignity.
- I have the right to retain my individuality and not be judged for my decisions, which may be contrary to the beliefs of others.
- I have the right to discuss and enlarge my religious and/or spiritual experiences, regardless of what they may mean to others.
- I have the right to expect that the sanctity of the human body will be respected after death.
- I have the right to be cared for by caring, sensitive, knowledgeable people who will attempt to understand my needs and will be able to gain some satisfaction in helping me face my death.

Modified from Barbus AJ: *Am J Nurs* 75(1):99, 1975.

SIGNS OF DEATH

There are signs of approaching death. They may occur rapidly or slowly.

- Movement, muscle tone, and sensation are lost. This usually starts in the feet and legs. It eventually spreads to the rest of the body. When the mouth muscles relax, the jaw drops. The mouth may stay open. There is often a peaceful facial expression.
- Peristalsis and other gastrointestinal functions slow down. There may be abdominal distention, fecal incontinence, impaction, nausea, and vomiting.
- Circulation fails, and body temperature rises. The person feels cool or cold, looks pale, and perspires heavily. The pulse is fast, weak, and irregular. Blood pressure starts to fall.

- The respiratory system fails. Cheyne-Stokes, slow, or rapid and shallow respirations are observed. Mucus collects in the respiratory tract. This causes the *death rattle* that is heard.
- Pain decreases as the person loses consciousness. However, some people are conscious until the moment of death.

The signs of death include no pulse, respirations, or blood pressure. The pupils are fixed and dilated. A doctor determines that death has occurred and pronounces the person dead.

LONG-TERM CARE

focus on

The dying person also has rights under the Omnibus Budget Reconciliation Act of 1987 (OBRA). You must protect the person's right to privacy and confidentiality. Remember, do not expose the person unnecessarily. The person has the right not to have his or her body seen by others. Proper draping and screening procedures are important.

The person and family or other visitors have the right to visit in private. The dying person may be too weak to leave the bed or room. Therefore the roommate may have to leave the room. The nurse tries to work out a plan that satisfies both roommates. The dying person may need a private room. This gives the person and family privacy. The family can also stay as long as they like.

The right to confidentiality is important. This right is protected before and after death. The person's condition and diagnoses are shared only with those involved with the person's care. The person's final moments and cause of death also are kept confidential. So are statements, conversations, and family reactions.

The dying person has the right to be free from abuse, mistreatment, and neglect. Some health team members avoid the dying person. They are uncomfortable with death and dying. Others have superstitions or religious beliefs about being near dying people. Abuse and mistreatment may occur. Family members or health team members may be the sources of such actions. The person may be too weak to report the abuse or mistreatment. Or the person may feel that punishment is deserved for needing so much care. The person has the right to receive kind and respectful care before and after death. Be sure to report signs of abuse, mistreatment, or neglect to the RN.

Freedom of restraint applies to the dying person. Restraints are used only if ordered by the doctor. Dying persons are often too weak to be dangerous to themselves or others.

You must protect the individual's personal possessions. The person may want certain photos and religious items nearby. Religious items may include medals, a rosary, religious books or writings, a crucifix, and candles. Such items should be provided if possible. The person's property must be protected from loss or damage before and after death. They may be passed on as family treasures or mementos.

Nursing center residents have the right to a safe and homelike environment. They usually depend on others for safety. The health team must keep the environment safe and homelike. Remember, the center is the person's home. Try to keep equipment and supplies out of view. Also try to keep the room free of unpleasant odors and noises. Do your best to keep the room neat and clean.

The right to personal choice is especially important. Remember, the person has the right to be involved in treatment and care. The dying person may refuse treatment. The person may also have a living will. The person may not be mentally able to be involved in treatment decisions. The family or legal representative will act on the person's behalf. The decision may be to allow the person to die with peace and dignity. The health team needs to respect choices to refuse treatment or not prolong life.

✦ CARE OF THE BODY AFTER DEATH

Care of the body after (post) death (mortem) is called **postmortem** care. A nurse gives postmortem care. You may be asked to assist. The care begins as soon as the doctor pronounces the person dead. Standard Precautions and the Bloodborne Pathogen Standard are followed.

You may have contact with infected blood, body fluids, secretions, or excretions.

Postmortem care is done to maintain the body's appearance. Discoloration and skin damage are prevented. Postmortem care also includes gathering valuables and personal items for the family. The right to privacy and the right to be treated with dignity and respect apply after death.

Within 2 to 4 hours after death, rigor mortis develops. **Rigor mortis** is the stiffness or rigidity *(rigor)* of skeletal muscles. It occurs after death *(mortis)*. Postmortem care involves positioning the body in normal alignment before rigor mortis sets in. The family may want to see the body before it is taken to the morgue or funeral home. The body should appear in a comfortable and natural position for this viewing.

In some agencies the body is prepared only for viewing. Postmortem care is completed later by the funeral director.

Repositioning of the body is often required during postmortem care. The repositioning is done to bathe soiled areas and to put the body in good alignment. Movement of the body can cause remaining air in the lungs, stomach, and intestines to be expelled. When air is expelled, the body produces sounds. Do not be alarmed or frightened by these sounds. They are normal and expected.

✦ ASSISTING WITH POSTMORTEM CARE

PRE-PROCEDURE

1. Wash your hands.

2. Collect the following:

   - Postmortem kit if used in your agency (shroud or body bag, gown, two tags, gauze squares, and safety pins)

   - Valuables list

   - Waterproof bed protectors

   - Wash basin

   - Bath towels

   - Washcloth

   - Tape

   - Dressings

   - Gloves

   - Cotton balls

3. Provide for privacy.

4. Raise the bed to its highest level.

5. Make sure the bed is flat.

PROCEDURE

6. Put on the gloves.

7. Position the body supine. Arms and legs are straight. Put a pillow under the head and shoulders (Fig. 36-1, p. 846).

8. Close the eyes. Gently pull the eyelids over the eyes. Apply a moistened cotton ball gently over the eyelids if the eyes will not stay closed.

9. Insert dentures if it is agency policy. If not, put them in a labeled denture container.

10. Close the mouth. Place a rolled towel under the chin to support the mouth in the closed position if necessary.

11. Follow agency policy about jewelry. Remove all jewelry except for wedding rings if this is agency policy. List the jewelry that was removed. Place the jewelry and the list in an envelope for the family.

12. Place a cotton ball over the wedding ring. Secure it in place with tape.

13. Remove drainage bottles, bags, and containers. Leave tubes and catheters in place if an autopsy is to be performed. Ask the RN about removal of tubes.

14. Bathe soiled areas with plain water. Dry thoroughly.

15. Place a bed protector under the buttocks.

16. Remove soiled dressings, and replace them with clean ones.

17. Put a clean gown on the body. Make sure the body is positioned as in step 7.

Continued

✦ ASSISTING WITH POSTMORTEM CARE—cont'd

PROCEDURE—cont'd

18 Brush and comb the hair if necessary.

19 Fill out the ID tags. Tie one to an ankle or to the right big toe.

20 Cover the body to the shoulders with a sheet if the family will view the body.

21 Gather all of the person's belongings. Put them in a bag labeled with the person's name.

22 Remove all used supplies, equipment, and linens except the shroud and the other ID tag. Make sure the room is neat. Adjust lighting so it is soft.

23 Remove the gloves, and wash your hands.

24 Let the family view the body. Provide for privacy. Ask the RN to give the person's belongings to the family.

25 Get a stretcher if the body will be taken to the morgue.

26 Put on another pair of gloves.

27 Place the body on the shroud or in the body bag or cover the body with a sheet after the family has left the room. Apply the shroud as in Figure 36-2:

a Bring the top down over the head.

b Fold the bottom up over the feet.

c Fold the sides over the body.

28 Secure the shroud in place with safety pins or tape.

29 Attach the second ID tag to the shroud or body bag.

30 Take the body to the morgue:

a Move the body onto the stretcher with the help of co-workers.

b Have the doors to other rooms along the hallway closed.

c Transport the body to the morgue. Leave the denture cup with the body.

d Return the stretcher to its proper place.

31 Leave the body on the bed if it will be taken directly to the funeral home. Leave the denture cup with the body. Close the door, or pull the privacy curtain around the bed.

POST-PROCEDURE

32 Remove the gloves, and wash your hands.

33 Strip the person's unit after the body is removed. Wear gloves for this step.

34 Wash your hands.

35 Report the following to the RN:

• The time the body was taken by the funeral director

• What was done with dentures

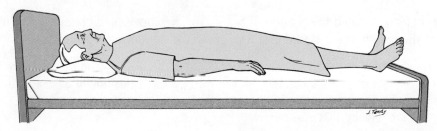

Fig. 36-1 *The body is in the dorsal recumbent position. Arms are straight at the sides. There is a pillow under the head and shoulders.*

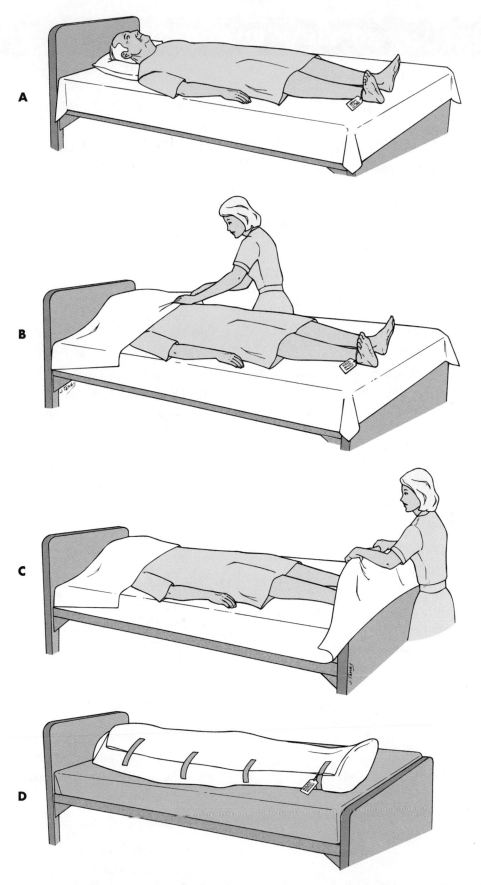

Fig. 36-2 *Applying a shroud.* **A,** *Place the body on the shroud.* **B,** *Bring the top of the shroud down over the head.* **C,** *Fold the bottom over the feet.* **D,** *Fold the sides over the body, tape or pin the sides together, and attach the ID tag.*

REVIEW QUESTIONS

Circle the best *answer.*

1 Which is *true?*

    a Death from terminal illness is sudden and unexpected.

    b Doctors know when death will occur.

    c An illness is terminal when there is no reasonable hope of recovery.

    d All severe injuries result in death.

2 Which psychological forces influence living and dying?

    a Hope and the will to live

    b Reincarnation and belief in the afterlife

    c Denial and anger

    d Bargaining and depression

3 These statements relate to attitudes about death. Which is *false?*

    a Dying people are often cared for in health agencies.

    b Attitudes about death are influenced by religion.

    c Infants and toddlers understand death.

    d Young children often blame themselves when someone dies.

4 Reincarnation is the belief that

    a There is no afterlife

    b The spirit or soul is reborn into another human body or another form of life

    c The body keeps its physical form in the afterlife

    d Only the spirit or soul is present in the afterlife

5 Children between the ages of 5 and 7 years view death as

    a Temporary

    b Final

    c Adults do

    d Going to sleep

6 Adults and the older persons usually fear

    a Dying alone

    b Reincarnation

    c The five stages of dying

    d All of the above

7 Persons in the stage of denial

    a Are angry

    b Make "deals" with God

    c Are sad and quiet

    d Refuse to believe they are dying

8 Jenny Parker is dying. At one point she tried to gain more time. She was in the stage of

    a Anger

    b Bargaining

    c Depression

    d Acceptance

9 When caring for Jenny Parker, you should

    a Use touch and listen

    b Do most of the talking

    c Keep the room darkened

    d Speak in a loud voice

10 As death nears, the last sense lost is

    a Sight

    b Taste

    c Smell

    d Hearing

11 Jenny Parker's care includes the following *except*

    a Eye care

    b Mouth care

    c Active range-of-motion exercises

    d Position changes

12 Jenny Parker is positioned in

    a The supine position

    b The Fowler's position

    c Good body alignment

    d The dorsal recumbent position

13 A "do not resuscitate" order was written for Jenny Parker. This means that

    a CPR will not be done

    b She has a living will

    c Life-prolonging measures will be carried out

    d She will be kept alive as long as possible

REVIEW QUESTIONS—cont'd

14 Which are *not* signs of approaching death?
a Rapid pulse and slowing of gastrointestinal functions
b Loss of movement and muscle tone
c Increased pain and blood pressure
d Cheyne-Stokes respirations and the death rattle

15 The signs of death are
a Convulsions and incontinence
b No pulse, respirations, or blood pressure
c Loss of consciousness and convulsions
d Open eyes, no muscle movements, and rigid body

16 Postmortem care is done
a After rigor mortis sets in
b After the doctor pronounces the person dead
c When the funeral director arrives for the body
d After the family has viewed the body

Answers to these questions are on p. 854.

ANSWERS TO REVIEW QUESTIONS

Chapter 1: Health Care Today

1 c
2 c
3 b
4 a
5 c
6 True
7 True
8 True
9 False
10 True

Chapter 2: Roles and Functions of Assistive Personnel

1 False
2 True
3 False
4 False
5 False
6 False
7 False
8 d
9 c
10 a
11 b
12 a
13 a
14 a
15 b
16 a
17 c
18 b
19 a
20 a
21 d
22 a
23 d
24 c
25 a
26 b
27 a
28 c

Chapter 3: Work Ethics

1 True
2 True
3 False
4 True

5 True
6 True
7 False
8 False
9 True
10 False
11 c
12 d
13 c
14 d
15 b
16 d
17 c
18 b
19 c
20 d
21 c
22 b
23 a
24 a
25 b
26 c
27 d
28 d

Chapter 4: Communicating With the Health Team

1 True
2 False
3 False
4 False
5 True
6 False
7 False
8 a
9 d
10 b
11 b
12 c
13 c
14 b
15 c
16 d
17 d
18 b
19 c
20 d
21 b

Chapter 5: The Whole Person and Basic Needs

1 c
2 d
3 c
4 b
5 c
6 b
7 d
8 a
9 c
10 a
11 b
12 d

Chapter 6: Communicating With the Person

1 b
2 d
3 c
4 a
5 c
6 a
7 a
8 d
9 a
10 c

Chapter 7: Body Structure and Function

1 a
2 b
3 d
4 c
5 c
6 a
7 b
8 c
9 d
10 d
11 b
12 a
13 b
14 b
15 b
16 c
17 d
18 a
19 d
20 a
21 b

Chapter 8: Growth and Development

1 b
2 c
3 d
4 b
5 d
6 a
7 b
8 a
9 c
10 c
11 c
12 c
13 a
14 b
15 c
16 a
17 d
18 c
19 d
20 a
21 d
22 d

Chapter 9: Sexuality

1 a
2 d
3 c
4 a
5 b
6 b
7 d
8 b
9 d
10 b

Chapter 10: Safety

1 False
2 True
3 True
4 True
5 True
6 False
7 True
8 True
9 False
10 True
11 True
12 True
13 True
14 True
15 True

16 False
17 True
18 True
19 True
20 False
21 True
22 True
23 True
24 True
25 d
26 d
27 c
28 a
29 a
30 d
31 d
32 b
33 c
34 a
35 a
36 c
37 d
38 d
39 b
40 b
41 c
42 c

Chapter 11: Infection Control

1 False
2 True
3 False
4 False
5 False
6 False
7 True
8 True
9 False
10 True
11 b
12 d
13 d
14 b
15 d
16 c
17 a
18 d
19 c
20 a
21 d
22 b
23 d
24 c

Chapter 12: Body Mechanics

1 False
2 True
3 True
4 False
5 True
6 True
7 True
8 True
9 False
10 True
11 False
12 True
13 False
14 False
15 True
16 False
17 True
18 False
19 False
20 True

Chapter 13: Bedmaking

1 True
2 False
3 True
4 False
5 False
6 True
7 True
8 True
9 True
10 True
11 True
12 True
13 True
14 False
15 False

Chapter 14: Cleanliness and Skin Care

1 True
2 False
3 False
4 False
5 False
6 False
7 False
8 True
9 False

10	False
11	False
12	False
13	True
14	True
15	True
16	True
17	True
18	d
19	b
20	b
21	c
22	c
23	d
24	c

Chapter 15: Personal Care and Grooming

1	d
2	c
3	a
4	d
5	c
6	b
7	b
8	d
9	b
10	b
11	a
12	a

Chapter 16: Comfort, Rest, and Sleep

1	a
2	c
3	d
4	c
5	a
6	b
7	c
8	d
9	b
10	a
11	c
12	a
13	b
14	b

Chapter 17: Urinary Elimination

1	b
2	d
3	a
4	b
5	b
6	a
7	a
8	c
9	a
10	c
11	b
12	a
13	d
14	c
15	d
16	b
17	a
18	c
19	d
20	b

Chapter 18: Bowel Elimination

1	a
2	b
3	d
4	a
5	c
6	d
7	b
8	c
9	b
10	d
11	d
12	a

Chapter 19: Nutrition

1	False
2	True
3	False
4	False
5	True
6	False
7	True
8	b
9	a
10	a
11	d
12	d
13	c

14	a
15	c
16	a
17	c
18	b
19	b
20	a
21	b
22	d
23	b
24	d
25	d
26	a
27	b
28	c

Chapter 20: Fluids and Blood

1	a
2	c
3	c
4	b
5	d
6	b
7	b
8	d
9	d
10	b
11	a
12	b
13	c
14	a
15	c
16	a
17	d
18	b
19	c
20	d
21	c
22	a
23	b
24	a

Chapter 21: Oxygen Needs

1	a
2	c
3	c
4	b
5	d
6	c
7	d
8	a

9	b
10	a
11	b
12	d
13	b
14	d
15	d
16	c
17	a
18	a
19	c
20	b
21	b
22	d
23	b
24	c
25	d

Chapter 22: Exercise and Activity

1	a
2	b
3	c
4	d
5	b
6	c
7	a
8	b
9	c
10	b
11	False
12	False
13	True
14	False
15	True

Chapter 23: Measuring Vital Signs

1	c
2	b
3	d
4	c
5	a
6	a
7	c
8	d
9	b
10	c
11	a
12	b

Chapter 24: Obtaining an Electrocardiogram

1	b
2	b
3	a
4	a
5	d
6	c
7	a
8	b
9	c
10	d
11	a
12	d

Chapter 25: Collecting and Testing Blood Specimens

1	c
2	d
3	d
4	a
5	b
6	a
7	b
8	c
9	a
10	c
11	a
12	c

Chapter 26: Assisting With the Physical Examination

1	b
2	d
3	c
4	a
5	b
6	c

Chapter 27: The Surgical Patient

1	c
2	d
3	b
4	a
5	a
6	c
7	c

8	a
9	b
10	c
11	d
12	a
13	a
14	a
15	False
16	True
17	False
18	False
19	True
20	True
21	True
22	False
23	True
24	True

Chapter 28: Wound Care

1	b
2	c
3	a
4	a
5	a
6	b
7	a
8	d
9	c
10	c
11	d
12	a
13	a
14	c

Chapter 29: Heat and Cold Applications

1	d
2	b
3	d
4	b
5	c
6	b
7	d
8	a
9	d
10	c
11	a
12	b

Chapter 30: Common Health Problems

1 a
2 c
3 a
4 d
5 c
6 a
7 a
8 d
9 c
10 b
11 a
12 a
13 b
14 b
15 c
16 a
17 a
18 c
19 b
20 b
21 a
22 d
23 b
24 c
25 d
26 a
27 d
28 b
29 b
30 c
31 a
32 c
33 a
34 d
35 c

Chapter 31: Mental Health Problems

1 b
2 b
3 a
4 c
5 d
6 a
7 c
8 a
9 b
10 c
11 d
12 d

Chapter 32: Confusion and Dementia

1 a
2 b
3 d
4 d
5 b
6 b
7 a
8 d
9 c
10 a

Chapter 33: Rehabilitation and Restorative Care

1 c
2 b
3 a
4 d
5 a
6 a
7 a
8 c
9 a
10 c

Chapter 34: Caring for Mothers and Newborns

1 c
2 d
3 b
4 d
5 d
6 b
7 c
8 c
9 c
10 a
11 c
12 d
13 d
14 a
15 d
16 d
17 b
18 a
19 c
20 c

Chapter 35: Basic Emergency Care

1 b
2 a
3 b
4 c
5 d
6 c
7 b
8 c
9 b
10 c
11 a
12 d
13 b
14 a
15 d
16 b
17 b
18 c
19 c
20 b
21 b
22 c
23 a
24 a
25 b

Chapter 36: The Dying Person

1 c
2 a
3 c
4 b
5 b
6 a
7 d
8 b
9 a
10 d
11 c
12 c
13 a
14 c
15 b
16 b

GLOSSARY

abbreviation A shortened form of a word or phrase

abduction Moving a body part away from the body

abrasion A partial-thickness wound caused by the scraping away or rubbing of the skin

accountable Being responsible for one's actions and the actions of others who perform delegated tasks; answering questions about and explaining one's actions and the actions of others

acetone Ketone bodies that appear in the urine because of the rapid breakdown of fat for energy

active physical restraint A restraint attached to the person's body and to a stationary (nonmovable) object; movement and access to one's body are restricted

activities of daily living (ADL) Self-care activities a person performs daily to remain independent and to function in society

acute illness A sudden illness from which a person is expected to recover

acute pain Pain that is felt suddenly from injury, disease, trauma, or surgery; it generally lasts less than 6 months

adduction Moving a body part toward the body

admission Official entry of a person into an agency or nursing unit

adolescence A time of rapid growth and psychological and social maturity

advance directive A written document stating a person's wishes about health care when that person can no longer make his or her own decisions

affect Feelings and emotions

air embolism Air that enters the cardiovascular system and travels to the lungs where it obstructs blood flow

allergy A sensitivity to a substance that causes the body to react with signs and symptoms

alopecia Hair loss

ambulation The act of walking

AM care Routine care performed before breakfast; early morning care

amputation The removal of all or part of an extremity

anal incontinence The inability to control the passage of feces and gas through the anus; fecal incontinence

anaphylaxis A life-threatening sensitivity to an antigen

anesthesia The loss of feeling or sensation produced by a drug

antibody A substance in the blood plasma that fights or attacks *(anti)* antigens

antigen A substance that the body reacts to

anxiety A vague, uneasy feeling that occurs in response to stress

aphasia The inability *(a)* to speak *(phasia)*

apical-radial pulse Taking the apical and radial pulses at the same time

apnea The lack or absence *(a)* of breathing *(pnea)*

arrhythmia Without *(a)* a rhythm

artery A blood vessel that carries blood away from the heart

arthritis Joint *(arthr)* inflammation *(itis)*

arthroplasty Surgical replacement *(plasty)* of a joint *(arthro)*

artifact Interference on the electrocardiogram

asepsis Being free of disease-producing microbes

aspiration Breathing fluid or an object into the lungs

assault Intentionally attempting or threatening to touch a person's body without the person's consent

assessment Collecting information about the person

assistive personnel Individuals who give basic nursing care under the supervision of RNs; other titles include nursing assistants, nursing attendants, patient care assistants, patient care technicians, and nurse extenders

atrophy A decrease in size or a wasting away of tissue

autoclave A pressure steam sterilizer

base of support The area on which an object rests

battery Unauthorized touching of a person's body without the person's consent

bedsore A decubitus ulcer; a pressure sore; a pressure ulcer

benign tumor A tumor that grows slowly and within a localized area

biohazardous waste Items contaminated with blood, body fluids, secretions, and excretions and that may be harmful to others; *bio* means life, and *hazardous* means dangerous or harmful

Biot's respirations Irregular breathing with periods of apnea; respirations may be slow and deep or rapid and shallow

bisexual A person attracted to both sexes

blood pressure The amount of force exerted against the walls of an artery by the blood

blood transfusion The intravenous administration of blood or its products

body alignment The way in which body parts are aligned with one another; posture

body language Facial expressions, gestures, posture, and body movements that send messages to others

body mechanics Using the body in an efficient and careful way

body temperature The amount of heat in the body that is a balance between the amount of heat produced and the amount lost by the body

bowel movement defecation

bradycardia A slow *(brady)* heart rate *(cardia)*; the rate is less than 60 beats per minute

bradypnea Slow *(brady)* breathing *(pnea)*; respirations are fewer than 10 per minute

braille A method of writing that uses raised dots; raised dots are arranged to represent each letter of the alphabet; the first ten letters represent the numbers 0 through 9

callus A thick, hardened area on the skin

calorie The amount of energy produced from the burning of food by the body

cancer Malignant tumor

capillary A tiny blood vessel; food, oxygen, and other substances pass from the capillaries to the cells

cardiac arrest The heart and breathing stop suddenly and without warning

carrier A human or animal that is a reservoir for microbes but does not have signs and symptoms of infection

case management A nursing care pattern; a case manager (an RN) coordinates a person's care from admission through discharge and into the home setting

catheter A tube used to drain or inject fluid through a body opening

catheterization The process of inserting a catheter

cell The basic unit of body structure

chart Another term for the medical record

Cheyne-Stokes Respirations gradually increase in rate and depth and then become shallow and slow; breathing may stop (apnea) for 10 to 20 seconds

chronic illness An illness, slow or gradual in onset, for which there is no known cure; the illness can be controlled and complications prevented

chronic pain Pain lasting longer than 6 months; it may be constant or occur off and on

chronic wound A wound that does not heal easily

circadian rhythm Daily rhythm based on a 24-hour cycle

circumcision The surgical removal of foreskin

civil law Laws concerned with relationships between people; private law

clean-contaminated wound A wound occurring from the surgical entry of the urinary, reproductive, respiratory, or gastrointestinal system

clean technique Medical asepsis

clean wound A wound that is not infected; microbes have not entered the wound

closed fracture The bone is broken, but the skin is intact; simple fracture

closed wound A wound in which tissues are injured but the skin is not broken

colostomy An artificial opening between the colon and abdominal wall

coma A state of being unaware of one's surroundings and being unable to react or respond to people, places, or things

comfort A state of well-being; the person has no physical or emotional pain and is calm and at peace

communicable disease A disease caused by pathogens that spread easily; a contagious disease

communication The exchange of information—a message sent is received and interpreted by the intended person

compound fracture The bone is broken and has come through the skin; open fracture

compulsion The uncontrolled performance of an act

confidentiality Trusting others with personal and private information

conflict A clash between opposing interests and ideas

conscious Awareness of the environment and experiences; the person knows what is happening and can control thoughts and behaviors

constipation The passage of a hard, dry stool

constrict To narrow

contagious disease Communicable disease

contaminated wound A wound with a high risk of infection

contamination The process of becoming unclean

contracture The abnormal shortening of a muscle

contusion A closed wound caused by a blow to the body

convulsion A seizure

courtesy A polite, considerate, or helpful comment or act

crime An act that violates a criminal law

criminal law Laws concerned with offenses against the public and society in general; public law

culture Values, beliefs, habits, likes, dislikes, customs, and characteristics of a group that are passed from one generation to the next

cyanosis Bluish discoloration of the skin

Daily Reference Values (DRVs) The maximum daily intake values for total fat, saturated fat, cholesterol, sodium, carbohydrate, and dietary fiber

Daily Value (DV) How a serving fits into the daily diet; it is expressed in a percentage based on a daily diet of 2000 calories

dandruff The excessive amount of dry, white flakes from the scalp

decubitus ulcer A bedsore, pressure sore, or pressure ulcer

defamation Injuring a person's name and reputation by making false statements to a third person

defecation The process of excreting feces from the rectum through the anus; a bowel movement

defense mechanism An unconscious reaction that blocks unpleasant or threatening feelings

dehiscence The separation of wound layers

dehydration The excessive loss of water from tissues

delegate To authorize another person to perform a task

delirium A state of temporary but acute mental confusion that comes on suddenly

delusion A false belief

delusion of grandeur An exaggerated belief about one's own importance, wealth, power, or talents

delusion of persecution A false belief that one is being mistreated, abused, or harassed

dementia An illness that affects memory, thinking, and behavior and is caused by changes in the brain

development Changes in a person's psychological and social functioning

developmental task That which the person must complete during a stage of development

dialysis Process of removing waste products from the blood

diarrhea The frequent passage of liquid stools

diastole The period of heart muscle relaxation

diastolic pressure The pressure in the arteries when the heart is at rest

digestion The process of physically and chemically breaking down food so that it can be absorbed for use by the cells

dilate To expand or open wider

dirty wound An infected wound

disability Any lost, absent, or impaired physical or mental function

disaster A sudden catastrophic event in which many people are injured and killed and property is destroyed

discharge Official departure of a person from an agency or nursing unit

discomfort To ache, hurt, or be sore; pain

disinfection The process of destroying pathogens

distraction To change the person's center of attention

dorsal recumbent position The back-lying or supine position; the supine or back-lying examination position; the legs are together

dorsiflexion Bending backward

drawsheet A small sheet placed over the middle of the bottom sheet; it helps keep the mattress and bottom linens clean and dry; can be used to turn and move the person in bed; the cotton drawsheet

dysphagia Difficulty or discomfort *(dys)* in swallowing *(phagia)*

dyspnea Difficult, labored, or painful *(dys)* breathing *(pnea)*

dysrhythmia An abnormal *(dys)* rhythm

dysuria Painful or difficult *(dys)* urination *(uria)*

early morning care AM care

edema The swelling of body tissues with water

ego The part of the personality dealing with reality; deals with thoughts, feelings, good sense, and problem solving

ejaculation The release of semen

elective surgery Scheduled surgery a person chooses to have at a certain time

electrocardiogram A recording *(gram)* of the electrical activity *(electro)* of the heart *(cardio)*; ECG or EKG

electrocardiograph An instrument *(graph)* that records the electrical activity *(electro)* of the heart *(cardio)*

embolus A blood clot that travels through the vascular system until it lodges in a distant blood vessel

emergency surgery Unscheduled surgery done immediately to save the person's life or limb

emotional illness Mental illness, mental disorder, psychiatric disorder

enema The introduction of fluid into the rectum and lower colon

enteral nutrition Giving nutrients through the gastro-intestinal tract *(enteral)*

enuresis Urinary incontinence in bed at night

epidermal stripping Removing the epidermis *(outer skin layer)* with tape

episiotomy Incision *(otomy)* into the perineum

erythrocyte Red *(erythro)* blood cell *(cyte)*; carries oxygen to the cells

esteem The worth, value, or opinion one has of a person

ethics Knowledge of what is right conduct and wrong conduct

evaluation To measure

evening care HS care or PM care

evisceration The separation of the wound along with the protrusion of abdominal organs

expressive aphasia Difficulty expressing or sending out thoughts

expressive-receptive aphasia Difficulty expressing or sending out thoughts and difficulty receiving information

extension Straightening of a body part

external rotation Turning the joint outward

fainting The sudden loss of consciousness from an inadequate blood supply to the brain

false imprisonment Unlawful restraint or restriction of a person's movement

fecal impaction The prolonged retention and accumulation of feces in the rectum

fecal incontinence anal incontinence

feces The semisolid mass of waste products in the colon

first aid Emergency care given to an ill or injured person before medical help arrives

flatulence The excessive formation of gas in the stomach and intestines

flatus Gas or air passed through the anus

flexion Bending a body part

flow rate The number of drops per minute (gtt/min)

footdrop Plantar flexion

Fowler's position A semisitting position; the head of the bed is elevated 45 to 60 degrees

fracture A broken bone

fraud Saying or doing something to trick, fool, or deceive another person

friction The rubbing of one surface against another

full-thickness wound The dermis, epidermis, and subcutaneous tissue are penetrated; muscle and bone may be involved

functional incontinence The involuntary, unpredicted loss of urine from the bladder

functional nursing A nursing care pattern that focuses on tasks and jobs; nursing personnel have specific tasks to do

gait belt A transfer or safety belt

gangrene A condition in which there is death of tissue; tissues become black, cold, and shriveled

gastrostomy A surgically created opening (stomy) in the stomach (gastro)

gavage Tube feeding

general anesthesia Unconsciousness and the loss of feeling or sensation produced by a drug

geriatrics The branch of medicine concerned with the problems and diseases of old age and elderly persons

germicide A disinfectant applied to skin, tissues, or nonliving objects

gerontology The study of the aging process

glucosuria Sugar (glucos) in the urine (uria); glycosuria

glycosuria Sugar (glycos) in the urine (uria); glucosuria

goal That which is desired in or by the person as a result of nursing care

gossip Spreading rumors or talking about the private matters of others

graduate A calibrated container used to measure fluid

ground That which carries leaking electricity to the earth and away from an electrical appliance

growth The physical changes that can be measured and that occur in a steady, orderly manner

guided imagery Creating and focusing on an image

hallucination Seeing, hearing, or feeling something that is not real

harassment Troubling, tormenting, offending, or worrying a person by one's behavior or comments

hazardous substance Any chemical that presents a physical hazard or a health hazard in the workplace

health team Staff members who work together to provide health care

hematology The study (ology) of blood (hemat)

hematoma The collection of blood under the skin and tissues; a swelling (oma) that contains blood (hemat)

hematuria Blood (hemat) in the urine (uria)

hemiplegia Paralysis on one side of the body

hemoglobin The substance in red blood cells that carries oxygen and gives blood its color

hemolysis The destruction (lysis) of blood (hemo)

hemoptysis Bloody (hemo) sputum (ptysis meaning "to spit")

hemorrhage The excessive loss of blood in a short period of time

hemothorax The collection of blood (hemo) in the pleural space (thorax)

heterosexual A person who is attracted to people of the other sex

hirsutism Excessive body hair in women and children

holism A concept that considers the whole person; the whole person has physical, social, psychological, and spiritual parts that are woven together and cannot be separated

homosexual A person who is attracted to members of the same sex

horizontal recumbent position The dorsal recumbent position

hormone A chemical substance secreted by the glands into the bloodstream

hospice A health care agency or program for persons who are dying

HS care Care given in the evening at bedtime; evening care or PM care

hyperextension Excessive straightening of a body part

hyperglycemia High *(hyper)* sugar *(glyc)* in the blood *(emia)*

hypertension Persistent blood pressure measurements above the normal systolic (140 mm Hg) or diastolic (90 mm Hg) pressures

hyperthermia A body temperature *(thermia)* that is much higher *(hyper)* than normal

hyperventilation Respirations that are rapid *(hyper)* and deeper than normal

hypoglycemia Low *(hypo)* sugar *(glyc)* in the blood *(emia)*

hypotension A condition in which the systolic blood pressure is below 90 mm Hg and the diastolic blood pressure is below 60 mm Hg

hypothermia A very low *(hypo)* body temperature *(thermia)*

hypoventilation Respirations that are slow *(hypo)*, shallow, and sometimes irregular

hypoxemia A reduced amount *(hypo)* of oxygen *(ox)* in the blood *(emia)*

hypoxia A deficiency *(hypo)* of oxygen *(oxia)* in the cells

id The part of the personality at the unconscious level; concerned with pleasure

ileostomy An artificial opening between the ileum (small intestine) and abdominal wall

immunity Protection against a disease or condition; the person will not get or be affected by the disease

implementation To perform or carry out

impotence The inability of the male to have an erection

incision An open wound with clean, straight edges; usually intentionally produced with a sharp instrument

infected wound A wound that contains large amounts of bacteria and that shows signs of infection; a dirty wound

infection A disease state resulting from the invasion and growth of microorganisms in the body

insomnia A chronic condition in which the person cannot sleep or stay asleep throughout the night

intake The amount of fluid taken in by the body

intentional wound A wound created for therapy

internal rotation Turning the joint inward

intravenous (IV) therapy The administration of fluids into a vein; IV, IV therapy, and IV infusion

intubation The process of inserting an artificial airway

invasion of privacy Violating a person's right not to have his or her name, photograph, or private affairs exposed or made public without giving consent

involuntary seclusion Separating a person from others against his or her will; keeping the person confined to a certain area or away from his or her room without consent

irrigation The process of washing out, flushing out, clearing, or cleaning a tube or body cavity

jejunostomy A surgically created opening *(stomy)* into the middle part of the small intestine *(jejunum)*

Kardex A type of file that summarizes information found in the medical record—medications, treatments, diagnosis, routine care measures, and special equipment used by the patient

ketone body Acetone

knee-chest position The person kneels and rests the body on the knees and chest; the head is turned to one side, the arms are above the head or flexed at the elbows, the back is straight, and the body is flexed about 90 degrees at the hips

Kussmaul's respirations Very deep and rapid respirations; a sign of diabetic coma

laceration An open wound with torn tissues and jagged edges

lancet A short, pointed, disposable blade

laryngeal mirror An instrument used to examine the mouth, teeth, and throat

lateral position The side-lying position

law A rule of conduct made by a government body

lead A pair of electrodes; electrical activity is recorded between the electrodes

leukocyte White *(leuko)* blood cell *(cyte);* protects the body against infection

libel Defamation through written statements

licensed practical nurse (LPN) An individual who completed a 1-year nursing program and passed a licensing examination; called licensed vocational nurse (LVN) in some states

lithotomy position The person is in a back-lying position, the hips are brought down to the edge of the examination table, the knees are flexed, the hips are externally rotated, and the feet are supported in stirrups

local anesthesia The loss of sensation in a small area

lochia The vaginal discharge that occurs during the postpartum period

logrolling Turning the person as a unit in alignment with one motion

malignant tumor A tumor that grows rapidly and invades other tissues; cancer

malpractice Negligence by a professional person

mechanical ventilation Using a machine to move air into and out of the lungs

medical asepsis The practices used to remove or destroy pathogens and to prevent their spread from one person or place to another person or place; clean technique

medical diagnosis The identification of a disease or condition by a doctor

medical record A written account of a person's illness and response to the treatment and care given by the health team; chart

melena A black, tarry stool

menarche The time when menstruation first begins

meniscus The curved surface of a column of liquid

menopause The time when menstruation stops; it marks the end of the woman's reproductive years

menstruation The process in which the lining of the uterus breaks up and is discharged from the body through the vagina

mental Relating to the mind; something that exists in the mind or is performed by the mind

mental disorder Mental illness; emotional illness, psychiatric disorder

mental health A state of mind in which the person copes with and adjusts to the stresses of everyday living in ways acceptable to society

mental illness A disturbance in the person's ability to cope or adjust to stress; behavior and functioning are impaired; mental disorder, emotional illness, psychiatric disorder

metabolism The burning of food for heat and energy by the cells

metastasis The spread of cancer to other parts of the body

microbe A microorganism

microorganism A small *(micro)* living plant or animal *(organism)* seen only with a microscope; a microbe

micturition The process of emptying urine from the bladder; urination or voiding

mixed incontinence A combination of urge and stress incontinence

morning care Care given after breakfast; cleanliness and skin care measures are more thorough at this time

nasal speculum An instrument used to examine the inside of the nose

nasogastric (NG) tube A tube inserted through the nose *(naso)* into the stomach *(gastro)*

nasointestinal tube A tube inserted through the nose into the duodenum or jejunum of the small intestine

need That which is necessary or desirable for maintaining life and mental well-being

negligence An unintentional wrong in which a person fails to act in a reasonable and careful manner and causes harm to a person or to the person's property

nocturia Frequent urination *(uria)* at night *(noct)*

nonpathogen A microbe that usually does not cause an infection

nonREM sleep NREM sleep

nonverbal communication Communication that does not involve words

normal flora Microbes that usually live and grow in a certain location

nosocomial infection An infection acquired after admission to a health care agency

NREM sleep The stage of sleep when there is no rapid eye movement; nonREM sleep

nursing care plan A written guide giving direction about the nursing care a patient should receive

nursing diagnosis A statement describing a health problem that can be treated by nursing measures

nursing intervention An action or measure taken by the nursing team to help the person reach a goal

nursing process The method used by RNs to plan and deliver nursing care; its five steps are assessment, nursing diagnosis, planning, implementation, and evaluation

nursing team Individuals who provide nursing care—RNs, LPNs/LVNs, and assistive personnel

nutrient A substance that is ingested, digested, absorbed, and used by the body

nutrition The many processes involved in the ingestion, digestion, absorption, and use of foods and fluids by the body

objective data Information that can be seen, heard, felt, or smelled by another person; signs

observation Using the senses of sight, hearing, touch, and smell to collect information about a person

obsession A persistent thought or idea

obstetrics The branch of medicine concerned with the care of women during pregnancy, labor, and childbirth and during the 6 to 8 weeks after birth

oliguria Scant amount *(olig)* of urine *(uria);* usually less than 500 ml in 24 hours

open wound The skin or mucous membrane is broken

open fracture Compound fracture

ophthalmoscope A lighted instrument used to examine the internal structures of the eye

oral hygiene Measures performed to keep the mouth and teeth clean; mouth care

organ Groups of tissues with the same function

orthopnea Being able to breathe *(pnea)* deeply and comfortably only while sitting or standing *(ortho)*

orthopneic position Sitting up in bed *(ortho)* and leaning forward over the bedside table

orthostatic hypotension A drop in *(hypo)* blood pressure when the person stands *(ortho* and *static);* postural hypotension

ostomy The surgical creation of an artificial opening

otoscope A lighted instrument used to examine the external ear and the eardrum (tympanic membrane)

output The amount of fluid lost by the body

overflow incontinence The loss of urine when the bladder is too full

oxygen concentration The amount of hemoglobin that contains oxygen (O_2)

pain Discomfort

palpate To feel or touch using your hands or fingers

panic An intense and sudden feeling of fear, anxiety, terror, or dread

paranoia A disorder *(para)* of the mind *(noia);* false beliefs (delusions) and suspicion about a person or situation

paraphrasing Restating the person's message in your own words

paraplegia Paralysis from the waist down

partial-thickness wound A wound in which the dermis and epidermis of the skin are broken

passive physical restraint A restraint near but not directly attached to the person's body; it does not totally restrict freedom of movement and allows access to certain body parts

pathogen A microbe that is harmful and can cause an infection

pediatrics The branch of medicine concerned with the growth, development, and care of children ranging in age from the newborn to the adolescent

pediculosis capitis The infestation of the scalp *(capitis)* with lice

pediculosis corporis The infestation of the body *(corporis)* with lice

pediculosis (lice) The infestation with lice

pediculosis pubis The infestation of the pubic *(pubis)* hair with lice

penetrating wound An open wound in which the skin and underlying tissues are pierced

percussion hammer An instrument used to tap body parts to test reflexes; reflex hammer

percutaneous endoscopic gastrostomy (PEG) tube A tube inserted into the stomach *(gastro)* through a stab or puncture wound *(stomy)* made through *(per)* the skin *(cutaneous);* a lighted instrument *(scope)* allows the doctor to see inside a body cavity or organ *(endo)*

pericare Perineal care

perineal care Cleansing the genital and anal areas

peristalsis Involuntary muscle contractions in the digestive system that move food through the alimen-tary canal; the alternating contraction and relaxation of intestinal muscles

personality The set of attitudes, values, behaviors, and traits of a particular person

phantom pain Pain felt in a body part that is no longer there

phlebitis Inflammation *(itis)* of a vein *(phleb)*

phobia Fear, panic, or dread

plantar flexion The foot *(plantar)* is bent *(flexion);* footdrop

plaque A thin film that sticks to the teeth; it contains saliva, microorganisms, and other substances

plasma The liquid portion of the blood; it carries blood cells to other body cells

plastic drawsheet A drawsheet placed between the bottom sheet and the cotton drawsheet to keep the mattress and bottom linens clean and dry

platelet Thrombocyte

pleural effusion The escape and collection of fluid *(effusion)* in the pleural space

PM care HS care or evening care

pneumothorax The collection of air *(pneumo)* in the pleural space *(thorax)*

pollutant A harmful chemical or substance in the air or water

polyuria The production of abnormally large amounts *(poly)* of urine *(uria)*

postmortem After *(post)* death *(mortem)*

postoperative After surgery

postpartum After *(post)* childbirth *(partum)*

postural hypotension Orthostatic hypotension

posture The way in which body parts are aligned with one another; body alignment

preceptor A staff member who guides and teaches

prefix A word element placed at the beginning of a word to change the meaning of the word

preoperative Before surgery

pressure sore A bed sore, decubitus ulcer, or pressure ulcer

pressure ulcer Any injury caused by unrelieved pressure; a decubitus ulcer, bedsore, or pressure sore

primary care giver The person in the child's environment who is mainly responsible for providing or assisting with the child's basic needs

primary nursing A nursing care pattern; an RN is responsible for patients' total care

pronation Turning downward

prone position Lying on the abdomen with the head turned to one side

prosthesis An artificial replacement for a missing body part

pseudodementia False *(pseudo)* disorder of the mind *(dementia)*

psychiatric disorder Mental illness, mental disorder, emotional illness

psychiatry The branch of medicine concerned with the diagnosis and treatment of people with mental health problems

psychosis A serious mental disorder; the person does not view or interpret reality correctly

puberty The period when the reproductive organs begin to function and secondary sex characteristics appear

pulse The beat of the heart felt at an artery as a wave of blood passes through the artery

pulse deficit The difference between the apical and radial pulse rates

pulse rate The number of heartbeats or pulses felt in 1 minute

puncture wound An open wound made by a sharp object; entry of the skin and underlying tissues may be intentional or unintentional

purulent drainage Thick green, yellow, or brown drainage

quadriplegia Paralysis from the neck down; paralysis of the arms, legs, and trunk

radiating pain Pain felt at the site of tissue damage and in nearby areas

range of motion (ROM) The movement of a joint to the extent possible without causing pain

receptive aphasia Difficulty receiving information

recording Writing or charting patient care and observations

red blood cells (RBCs) Erythrocytes

reflex An involuntary movement

reflex incontinence The loss of urine at predictable intervals; unconscious incontinence

regional anesthesia The loss of sensation or feeling in a part of the body, produced by the injection of a drug; the person does not lose consciousness

registered nurse (RN) An individual who studied nursing for 2, 3, or 4 years and passed a licensing examination

regurgitation The backward flow of food from the stomach into the mouth

rehabilitation The process of restoring the person to the highest level of physical, psychological, social, and economic functioning possible; restorative care

reincarnation The belief that the spirit or soul is reborn in another human body or in another form of life

relaxation To be free from mental or physical stress

religion Spiritual beliefs, needs, and practices

REM sleep The stage of sleep when there is rapid eye movement

reporting A verbal account of patient care and observations

residual urine The amount of urine left in the bladder after voiding

respiration The process of supplying the cells with oxygen and removing carbon dioxide from them; the act of breathing air into (inhalation) and out of (exhalation) the lungs

respiratory arrest Breathing stops but the heart still pumps blood for several minutes

respiratory depression Slow, weak respirations that occur at a rate of fewer than 12 per minute; respirations are not deep enough to bring enough air into the lungs

responsibility The duty or obligation to perform some act or function

rest To be calm, at ease, and relaxed; to be free of anxiety and stress

restorative care Rehabilitation

restraint Any item, object, device, garment, material, or chemical that restricts a person's freedom of movement or access to one's body

reverse Trendelenburg's position The head of the bed is raised, and the foot of the bed is lowered

rigor mortis The stiffness or rigidity *(rigor)* of skeletal muscles that occurs after death *(mortis)*

root A word element containing the basic meaning of the word

rooting reflex The baby turns his or her head when the cheek or mouth is stroked; the head is turned toward the direction of the stimulus, and the baby starts to suck

safety belt A transfer belt

sanguineous drainage Bloody drainage *(sanguis)*

schizophrenia Split *(schizo)* mind *(phrenia)*

seizure Violent and sudden contractions or tremors of muscles; convulsion

self-actualization Experiencing one's potential

self-esteem Thinking well of yourself and being thought well of by others

semi-Fowler's position The head of the bed is raised 45 degrees, and the knee portion is raised 15 degrees; or the head of the bed is raised 30 degrees

serosanguineous drainage Thin, watery drainage *(sero)* that is blood-tinged *(sanguineous)*

serous drainage Clear, watery fluid *(serum)*

sex The physical activities involving the organs of reproduction; the activities are done for pleasure or to produce children

sexuality The physical, psychological, social, cultural, and spiritual factors that affect a person's feelings and attitudes about his or her sex

shearing When skin sticks to a surface and muscles slide in the direction the body is moving

shock The condition that results when there is not enough blood supply to organs and tissues

side-lying position The lateral position

signs Objective data

simple fracture closed fracture

Sims' position A side-lying position in which the upper leg is sharply flexed so that it is not on the lower leg and the lower arm is behind the person

slander Defamation through oral statements

sleep A state of unconsciousness, reduced voluntary muscle activity, and lowered metabolism

sphygmomanometer The instrument used to measure blood pressure

spore A bacterium protected by a hard shell that forms around the microbe

sputum Expectorated mucus

sterile The absence of all microbes

sterile field A work area free of all pathogens and nonpathogens (including spores)

sterile technique Surgical asepsis

sterilization The process of destroying all microbes

stethoscope An instrument used to listen to the sounds produced by the heart, lungs, and other body organs

stoma An opening; see colostomy and ileostomy

stomatitis Inflammation *(itis)* of the mouth *(stomat)*

stool Excreted feces

stress The response or change in the body caused by any emotional, physical, social, or economic factor

stress incontinence The loss of small amounts of urine with exercise and certain movements

stressor Any emotional, physical, social, or economic factor that causes stress

subconscious Memory, past experiences, and thoughts of which the person is not aware; they can be easily recalled

subjective data That which is reported by a person that you cannot observe through your senses; symptoms

suction The process of withdrawing or sucking up fluid (secretions)

suffix A word element placed at the end of a root to change the meaning of the word

suffocation When breathing stops from the lack of oxygen

sundowning Increased signs, symptoms, and behaviors of Alzheimer's disease during hours of darkness

superego The part of the personality concerned with what is right and wrong

supination Turning upward

supine position The back-lying or dorsal recumbent position

suppository A cone-shaped solid medication that is inserted into a body opening; it melts at body temperature

surgical asepsis The practices that keep equipment and supplies free of all microbes; sterile technique

symptoms Subjective data

syncope A brief loss of consciousness; fainting

system Organs that work together to perform special functions

systole The period of heart muscle contraction

systolic pressure The amount of force it takes to pump blood out of the heart into the arterial circulation

tachycardia A rapid *(tachy)* heart rate *(cardia);* the rate is more than 100 beats per minute

tachypnea Rapid *(tachy)* breathing *(pnea);* respirations are usually more than 24 per minute

tartar Hardened plaque on teeth

task A function, procedure, activity, or work that does not require an RN's professional knowledge or judgment

team nursing A nursing care pattern; the team leader (an RN) delegates the care of specific persons to RNs and LPNs/LVNs and delegates nursing tasks to assistive personnel

terminal illness An illness or injury for which there is no reasonable expectation of recovery

thrombocyte A cell *(cyte)* necessary for the clotting *(thrombo)* of blood

thrombus A blood clot

tinnitus Ringing in the ears

tissue A group of cells with the same function

tort A wrong committed against a person or the person's property

tourniquet A constricting device applied to a limb to control bleeding

transfer Moving a person from one room, nursing unit, or agency to another

transfer belt A belt used to hold onto a person during a transfer or when walking with the person; a gait belt or safety belt

transsexual A person who believes that he or she is really a member of the other sex

transvestite A person who becomes sexually excited by dressing in the clothes of the other sex

trauma An accident or violent act that injures the skin, mucous membranes, bones, and internal organs

Trendelenburg's position The head of the bed is lowered, and the foot of the bed is raised

tumor A new growth of cells; tumors are benign or malignant

tuning fork An instrument used to test hearing

umbilical cord The structure that carries blood, oxygen, and nutrients from the mother to the fetus

unconscious Experiences and feelings that cannot be remembered

unconscious incontinence Reflex incontinence

unintentional wound A wound resulting from trauma

urge incontinence The involuntary loss of urine after feeling a strong need to void

urgent surgery Surgery necessary for the person's health; it must be done soon to prevent further damage or disease

urinary frequency Voiding at frequent intervals

urinary incontinence The inablility to control the loss of urine from the bladder

urinary urgency The need to void immediately

urination The process of emptying urine from the bladder; micturition or voiding

vaginal speculum An instrument used to open the vagina so that it and the cervix can be examined

vein A blood vessel that carries blood back to the heart

venipuncture A technique in which a vein *(veni)* is punctured

verbal communication Communication that uses the written or spoken word

vertigo Dizziness

vital signs Temperature, pulse, respirations, and blood pressure

voiding Urination or micturition

word element A part of a word

work ethics Behavior in the workplace

wound A break in the skin or mucous membrane

INDEX